Overview of Sections & Units/Register der Abschnitte & Module

Part 1 — Basic Medical & Health Terms Related to Dentistry

Unit 1 Diet & Dieting, Unit 2 Food & Drink, Unit 3 Injuries, Unit 4 States of Consciousness, Unit 5 Drugs & Remedies, Unit 6 At the Dentist's, Unit 7 Ba...

Part 2 — Body Structures & Functions Relevant to Dentistry

Unit 8 Parts of the Body: The Head & Neck, Unit 9 The Teeth, Unit 10 Dentition & Mastication, Unit 11 Human Sounds & Speech, Unit 12 Nutrition

Part 3 — Medical Science

Unit 13 General Pathology, Unit 14 Medical Statistics, Unit 15 Medical Studies & Research

Part 4 — General Clinical Terms

Unit 16 Pain, Unit 17 Fractures, Unit 18 Therapeutic Intervention, Unit 19 Pharmacologic Treatment, Unit 20 Pharmacologic Agents, Unit 21 Surgical Treatment, Unit 22 Basic Operative Techniques, Unit 23 The Surgical Suite, Unit 24 Surgical Instruments, Unit 25 Perioperative Management, Unit 26 Sutures & Suture Material, Unit 27 Medical & Surgical Asepsis, Unit 28 Wound Healing, Unit 29 Fracture Management

Part 5 — Dentistry

Unit 30 Basic Dental Materials, Unit 31 Dental Lab Procedures & Equipment, Unit 32 Dental Instruments, Unit 33 Dental Imaging Techniques, Unit 34 Oral Hygiene & Prophylactic Dentistry, Unit 35 Periodontics, Unit 36 Orthodontic Dentistry, Unit 37 Orthodontic Appliances, Unit 38 TMJ Disorders, Unit 39 Cosmetic Dentistry, Unit 40 Restorative Dentistry, Unit 41 Endodontics, Unit 42 Prosthodontics, Unit 43 Dental Implantology, Unit 44 Oral Surgery, Unit 45 Maxillofacial Surgery

Part 6 — Related Medical Specialties

Unit 46 Basic Radiologic Terms, Unit 47 Basic Terms in Anesthesiology, Unit 48 Types of Anesthesia & Anesthetics, Unit 49 Basic Terms in Plastic Surgery, Unit 50 Grafts & Flaps

KWiC-Web

Fachwortschatz Zahnmedizin

Englisch

KWiC – Key Words in Context

Ingrid & Michael Friedbichler

2., korrigierte Auflage
26 Abbildungen

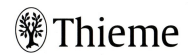

Dipl. Übers. Mag. Ingrid Friedbichler
Mag. Michael Friedbichler, M.A.
Institut für Translationswissenschaft
Universität Innsbruck
Herzog-Sigmund-Ufer 15
A – 6020 Innsbruck

Die Deutsche Bibliothek – CIP-Einheitsaufnahme

Die Deutsche Bibliothek verzeichnet diese Publikation in der Deutschen Nationalbibliografie; detaillierte bibliografische Daten sind im Internet über http://dnb.ddb.de abrufbar.

1. Auflage 2001

Wichtiger Hinweis: Wie jede Wissenschaft ist die Medizin ständigen Entwicklungen unterworfen. Forschung und klinische Erfahrung erweitern unsere Erkenntnisse, insbesondere was Behandlung und medikamentöse Therapie anbelangt. Soweit in diesem Werk eine Dosierung oder eine Applikation erwähnt wird, darf der Leser zwar darauf vertrauen, dass Autoren, Herausgeber und Verlag große Sorgfalt darauf verwandt haben, dass diese Angabe **dem Wissensstand bei Fertigstellung des Werkes** entspricht.

Für Angaben über Dosierungsanweisungen und Applikationsformen kann vom Verlag jedoch keine Gewähr übernommen werden. **Jeder Benutzer ist angehalten,** durch sorgfältige Prüfung der Beipackzettel der verwendeten Präparate und gegebenenfalls nach Konsultation eines Spezialisten festzustellen, ob die dort gegebene Empfehlung für Dosierung oder die Beachtung von Kontraindikationen gegenüber der Angabe in diesem Buch abweicht. Eine solche Prüfung ist besonders wichtig bei selten verwendeten Präparaten oder solchen, die neu auf den Markt gebracht worden sind. **Jede Dosierung oder Applikation erfolgt auf eigene Gefahr des Benutzers.** Autoren und Verlag appellieren an jeden Benutzer, ihm etwa auffallende Ungenauigkeiten dem Verlag mitzuteilen.

© 2005 Georg Thieme Verlag KG
Rüdigerstr. 14
D-70469 Stuttgart
Telefon: +49/0711/8931-0

Unsere Homepage: http://www.thieme.de
Printed in Germany

Cartoons: Dr. Stephan Schreieck, Innsbruck
Zeichnungen: Angelika Kramer, Stuttgart
Umschlaggestaltung: Martina Berge, Erbach-Ernsbach
Satz: Druckhaus Götz GmbH, D-71636 Ludwigsburg
  Satzsystem: 3B2 Version 6.05
Druck: Grafisches Centrum Cuno, D-39240 Calbe

Geschützte Warennamen werden **nicht** besonders kenntlich gemacht. Aus dem Fehlen eines solchen Hinweises kann also nicht geschlossen werden, dass es sich um einen freien Warennamen handle.

Das Werk, einschließlich aller seiner Teile, ist urheberrechtlich geschützt. Jede Verwertung außerhalb der engen Grenzen des Urheberrechtsgesetzes ist ohne Zustimmung des Verlages unzulässig und strafbar. Das gilt insbesondere für Vervielfältigungen, Übersetzungen, Mikroverfilmungen und die Einspeicherung und Verarbeitung in elektronischen Systemen.

ISBN 3-13-124942-0   1 2 3 4 5 6

Vorwort

Wir widmen dieses Buch unseren Töchtern Katrin und Dorit, die in den letzten Jahren viel Verständnis für unser „lexikographisches Kind" aufbringen mussten.

Wie in vielen anderen Fachgebieten ist mit der zunehmenden internationalen Vernetzung das Beherrschen der englischen Fachsprache in der Zahnmedizin zu einer wichtigen Zusatzqualifikation geworden. Einschlägige Hilfsmittel, mit denen sich Zahnmediziner die entsprechende sprachliche Kompetenz aneignen können, gibt es bislang aber nur ansatzweise.

Mit **KWiC-Web:** *Englischer Fachwortschatz Zahnmedizin* wurden bahnbrechende neue Materialien zur Aktivierung der produktiven Sprachkompetenz entwickelt. Auf der Grundlage von computergestützten lexikographischen Methoden und den neuesten Erkenntnissen der Spracherwerbsforschung wurde ein zukunftsweisendes Konzept entwickelt, welches Zahnmedizinern aller Fachrichtungen die Möglichkeit bietet, sich zwischendurch oder auf der Anreise zu einem Kongress mit den englischen Fachausdrücken und Wendungen eines bestimmten Fachbereichs rasch vertraut zu machen.

Neuland zu betreten bedeutet immer eine Potenzierung des Aufwandes. Wenngleich wir durch unsere Lehrtätigkeit an der Universität Innsbruck auf einen wertvollen Erfahrungsschatz in der Fachsprachenvermittlung zurückgreifen konnten, wäre dieses Buch ohne die Unterstützung eines ganzen Teams von Fachleuten und Beratern, denen wir an dieser Stelle unseren besonderen Dank aussprechen möchten, nicht realisierbar gewesen. An erster Stelle gebührt dieser Dank W. Gallagher, M.D. (FACS) und L. Cohen, D.D.S., Tucson, AZ., USA sowie N. Jones, M.D. (G.B.), die für uns die englischen Termini und Texte auf deren fachliche und sprachliche Richtigkeit überprüft haben.

Weiters bedanken wir uns bei einem Team von niedergelassenen und wissenschaftlich arbeitenden Zahnärzten, die jeweils die deutschen Entsprechungen der übersetzten Termini in ihren Fachgebieten überprüft haben und uns darüber hinaus beratend zur Seite gestanden sind. Ganz besonders hat uns Dr. P. Huemer (Zahnprophylaxe, Parodontologie, Implantologie, zahnärztliche Instrumente, Labortechnik) unterstützt. Weiters gilt unser Dank Dr. O. Barwart und Dr. G. Brodl (Kieferorthopädie), Univ.-Prof. Dr. I. Grunert (Zahnerhaltung u. -prothetik), Dr. C. Hoser (Unfallchirurgie), Dr. I. Moschen (Endodontie) und Univ.-Prof. Dr. B. Norer (MKG-Chirurgie).

Außerdem danken wir folgenden Fachleuten von der medizinischen Fakultät der Universität Innsbruck, die die nicht-zahnärztlichen Abschnitte durchgesehen haben, für Ihre Unterstützung: Dr. H. Hausdorfer (Allgemeinmedizin), Univ.-Prof. Dr. G. Helweg (Radiologie), Univ.-Prof. Dr. G. Putz (Anästhesie), Univ.-Prof. Dr. A. Stenzl (Chirurgie), Dr. H. Ulmer (Biostatistik) sowie Dr. S. Schreieck für die humorvollen Zeichnungen, die zur Auflockerung der fachlichen Materie beitragen sollen.

Last but not least verdankt dieses Buch seine Veröffentlichung dem Mut und Pioniergeist von Dr. T. Pilgrim und seinen Mitarbeitern vom Thieme Verlag, die sich nicht gescheut haben, mit **KWiC-Web** zu neuen Ufern aufzubrechen. Wir bedanken uns für das Vertrauen, das sie in uns und unsere Arbeit gesetzt haben und die weiten Wege, die sie bei der Konzeption einer benutzerfreundlichen graphischen Gestaltung und der Entwicklung einer speziellen Datenbank mit uns gegangen sind, um nur zwei der Punkte zu erwähnen, die für alle Pionierarbeit bedeutet haben.

Bleibt zu hoffen, dass dieses Buch all jenen, die sich mit der englischen Fachsprache der Zahnmedizin vertraut machen wollen, ein nützliches und effizientes Hilfsmittel sein möge, das ihnen das Tor zur internationalen Fachwelt öffnet.

Innsbruck   Ingrid & Michael Friedbichler

Table of Contents / Inhaltsübersicht

Part 1   Basic Medical & Health Terms Related to Dentistry

Unit 1	Diet & Dieting / Nahrung & Diät	1
Unit 2	Food & Drink / Essen & Trinken	4
Unit 3	Injuries / Verletzungen	8
Unit 4	States of Consciousness / Bewusstseinslagen	13
Unit 5	Drugs & Remedies / Medikamente & Heilmittel	16
Unit 6	At the Dentist's / Beim Zahnarzt	19
Unit 7	Basic Dental Equipment / Zahnärztliche Grundausrüstung	22

Part 2   Body Structures & Functions Relevant to Dentistry

Unit 8	Parts of the Body: The Head & Neck / Körperteile: Kopf & Hals	24
Unit 9	The Teeth / Die Zähne	27
Unit 10	Dentition & Mastication / Zahnen & Kauen	31
Unit 11	Human Sounds & Speech / Sprache & menschliche Laute	34
Unit 12	Nutrition / Ernährung	38

Part 3   Medical Science

Unit 13	General Pathology / Allgemeine Pathologie	42
Unit 14	Medical Statistics / Biostatistik	49
Unit 15	Medical Studies & Research / Medizinische Studien & Forschung	55

Part 4   General Clinical Terms

Unit 16	Pain / Schmerz	61
Unit 17	Fractures / Knochenbrüche	65
Unit 18	Therapeutic Intervention / Therapeutische Maßnahmen	68
Unit 19	Pharmacologic Treatment / Medikamentöse Behandlung	71
Unit 20	Pharmacologic Agents / Arzneimittel & pharmazeutische Wirkstoffe	74
Unit 21	Surgical Treatment / Der operative Eingriff	80
Unit 22	Basic Operative Techniques / Grundlegende Operationstechniken	83
Unit 23	The Surgical Suite / Der Operationstrakt	86
Unit 24	Surgical Instruments / Chirurgische Instrumente	88
Unit 25	Perioperative Management / Perioperative Maßnahmen	91
Unit 26	Sutures & Suture Material / Chirurgische Nahttechniken & -materialien	95
Unit 27	Medical & Surgical Asepsis / Medizinische & chirurgische Asepsis	98
Unit 28	Wound Healing / Wundheilung	101
Unit 29	Fracture Management / Frakturbehandlung	105

Part 5 Dentistry

Unit 30	Basic Dental Materials / Wichtige Dentalwerkstoffe	109
Unit 31	Dental Lab Procedures & Equipment / Zahntechnik	112
Unit 32	Dental Instruments / Zahnärztliche Instrumente	116
Unit 33	Dental Imaging Techniques / Bildgebende Verfahren in der Zahnheilkunde	119
Unit 34	Oral Hygiene & Prophylactic Dentistry / Mundhygiene & zahnmedizinische Prophylaxe	122
Unit 35	Periodontics / Parodontologie	126
Unit 36	Orthodontic Dentistry / Kieferorthopädie	130
Unit 37	Orthodontic Appliances / Kieferorthopädische Geräte	135
Unit 38	TMJ Disorders / Erkrankungen des Kiefergelenks	138
Unit 39	Cosmetic Dentistry / Ästhetische Zahnheilkunde	141
Unit 40	Restorative Dentistry / Konservierende Zahnheilkunde	144
Unit 41	Endodontics / Endodontie	147
Unit 42	Prosthodontics / Zahnersatz & zahnärztliche Prothetik	151
Unit 43	Dental Implantology / Zahnärztliche Implantologie	154
Unit 44	Oral Surgery / Oralchirurgie	158
Unit 45	Maxillofacial Surgery / Kiefer- u. Gesichtschirurgie	161

Part 6 Related Medical Specialties

Unit 46	Basic Radiologic Terms / Grundbegriffe der Radiologie	165
Unit 47	Basic Terms in Anesthesiology / Grundbegriffe der Anästhesiologie	169
Unit 48	Types of Anesthesia & Anesthetics / Anästhesieverfahren & Anästhetika	173
Unit 49	Basic Terms in Plastic Surgery / Grundbegriffe der plastischen Chirurgie	177
Unit 50	Grafts & Flaps / Transplantate	180

Index – English Terms · Index der englischen Fachtermini ... 184

Index – English Abbreviations · Index der englischen Abkürzungen ... 204

Index – German Terms · Index der deutschen Fachtermini ... 206

Ausführliche Benutzeranleitungen

Wozu wurde KWiC-Web Fachwortschatz Zahnmedizin entwickelt?

In den letzten Jahren sind für Mediziner, für die die englische Fachsprache im Beruf unentbehrlich geworden ist, eine Reihe von Materialen auf den Markt gekommen, darunter gleich mehrere zahnmedizinische Fachwörterbücher. Ob umfassend oder als Taschenbuch, gebunden oder auf CD-ROM, all diese herkömmlichen Wörterbücher haben für den Sprachlernenden einen entscheidenden Nachteil. Durch die alphabetische Auflistung der Wörter sind sie zwar als Nachschlagewerke ideal, für den Erwerb des Fachwortschatzes jedoch ungeeignet.

Was Sie hier in Händen halten ist eine völlig andere Art von Wörterbuch. Es ist nach dem Bausteinprinzip auf der Grundlage fachlicher Zusammenhänge aufgebaut und ermöglicht es sowohl Studenten der Zahnmedizin, die sich mit den grundlegenden Termini auseinandersetzen, niedergelassenen Zahnärzten, die sich mit den Begriffen der dentalen Implantologie vertraut machen wollen, Dentalhygienikerinnen ebenso wie Kieferchirurgen, aber auch Übersetzern von kieferorthopädischen Texten, gezielt den jeweils relevanten Wortschatz aus den entsprechenden Bausteinen (Modulen) ihren speziellen Bedürfnissen entsprechend zu aktivieren. Da sich jedes Modul auf eine überschaubare Anzahl von Fachtermini beschränkt, lassen sich diese Baustein für Baustein auf Reisen oder in schöpferischen Pausen zwischendurch leicht einprägen oder auffrischen.

Was bedeutet KWiC-Web und wie ist der Fachwortschatz strukturiert?

KWiC steht für *Key Words In Context* und **Web** für die Vernetzung in semantischen Netzwerken. **KWiC-Web** setzt in zweierlei Hinsicht neue Maßstäbe.

1. Keywords. Der zahnmedizinische Wortschatz in **KWiC-Web** ist in 50 Kapitel (Module), die in so genannte semantische Netzwerke (sinnzusammenhängende Termini, Ausdrücke oder Wendungen, die wie Nervenzellen miteinander verbunden sind) gegliedert sind, aufbereitet. Diese Module umfassen die gängigen Begriffe der verschiedenen zahnmedizinischen Fachgebiete in baumdiagrammartigen Verknüpfungen – von einfachen, die Zahnmedizin betreffenden Wörtern aus der Allgemeinsprache, wie z.B *decayed tooth (kariöser Zahn)*, bis hin zu sehr spezifischen Mehrwort-Komposita, wie z.B. *internal derangement (Diskusluxation)*, einem wichtigen Ausdruck der MKG-Chirurgie.

Zusätzlich wurden die elektronisch herausgefilterten Schlüsselwörter auf ihren didaktischen Wert hin geprüft, d.h. typische englische Bezeichnungen und Wendungen wurden gegenüber medizinischen Internationalismen und Termini, die dem Non-Native-Speaker weder in der Bedeutung noch in der Aussprache oder Verwendung Probleme bereiten, bevorzugt berücksichtigt.

Obwohl Vollständigkeit ein unerreichbares Ziel bleibt, findet man in **KWiC-Web** alle wichtigen Fachtermini und darüber hinaus viele fachspezifische Wortverbindungen, die zwar gängig sind, aber bisher noch nirgends beschrieben wurden.

2. Context. KWiC-Web geht weit über eine Liste von englisch-deutschen Wortgleichungen hinaus. Da die adäquate Einbettung der Fachtermini im Kontext für Fachleute wie auch Übersetzer und Dolmetscher meist die größte Hürde im aktiven Sprachgebrauch darstellt, ist die Kontextualisierung der Termini ein wesentliches Kriterium. Spracherwerb findet schließlich immer im Kontext statt, und Übersetzungen bieten meist nur in sehr begrenztem Maß Hilfe.

Deshalb werden in **KWiC-Web** die Schlüsselwörter nicht nur mit deutschen Entsprechungen, sondern jeweils samt ihrem typischen semantischen Umfeld in englischen Erklärungen, Beispielsätzen, und den gebräuchlichsten Wortverbindungen (Kollokationen) und Phrasen, die alle einer riesigen Fachtextsammlung entnommen sind, präsentiert. Dies gibt dem Benutzer Einblick in die authentische Verwendung der Fachausdrücke in der medizinischen Literatur.

Fachwörterbuch, Thesaurus, Kollokationswörterbuch und Wissensdatenbank in einem

KWiC-Web vereint die Vorzüge eines englischen Erklärungswörterbuches mit jenen einer einsprachigen Phraseologiesammlung und eines zweisprachigen Nachschlagewerkes.

Jedes Modul beinhaltet rund 200 morphologisch oder semantisch verwandte Ausdrücke, Phrasen, und Kollokationen die mit verwandten Modulen durch Verweise verbunden sind, sodass ein einprägsames semantisches Netzwerk (= WEB) von miteinander in enger Beziehung stehenden Termini, Erläuterungen, Wortverbindungen, lexikalischen Clustern und Fakten entsteht, das einer Wissensdatenbank gleicht. Dadurch wird nicht nur die Verwendung der Schlüsselwörter veranschaulicht, sondern auch deren Verknüpfung und Beziehung mit anderen Fachtermini aufzeigt. So wird jedes Modul zu einer Zusammenschau der wichtigsten Schlüsselwörter und Wendungen, denen man in einschlägigen Fachtexten und im Klinikalltag immer wieder begegnet. Vertraute Ausdrücke und solche, die man schon einmal gehört aber wieder vergessen hat, stehen dabei neben unbekannten, und **KWiC-Web** zeigt, wie sie untereinander vernetzt sind. Es entstehen im Unterbewusstsein Assoziationen, die das Wiedererkennen und Behalten auf lange Sicht wesentlich verbessern. Dadurch kommt das Arbeiten mit **KWiC-Web** dem Studium bzw. Querlesen Tausender Seiten von Fachtexten gleich – allerdings in kürzester Zeit, da es sich um einen stark verdichteten Auszug handelt (deshalb auch KWiC!).

Korpusgestütztes Erfassen

Ohne die Verwendung von repräsentativen elektronischen Korpora von authentischen englischen Fachtexten wäre die Selektion der Schlüsselwörter, Kontextbeispiele und Kollokationen nur mit Qualitätseinbußen und einem riesigen Zeitaufwand zu bewältigen. **KWiC-Web** basiert auf einem über 20 Millionen Wörter umfassenden medizinischen Korpus. Um die Verlässlichkeit hoch und die Fehlerhaftigkeit des Korpus gering zu halten, wurden ausschließlich authentische Quellen (Standard-Handbücher, Fachartikel, und Fachtexte englischsprachiger Autoren aus verschiedenen Fachbereichen) herangezogen.

Die moderne Computerlinguistik ermöglicht es uns, spezifische Fragen des Sprachgebrauchs, v.a. die Verwendung und Verbreitung von Fachausdrücken und Wendungen, anhand von authentischen Fachtexten per Knopfdruck zu prüfen. Da **KWiC-Web** auf der Grundlage solcher Textanalysen erstellt wurde, sind die Sprachdaten nicht nur aktuell sondern entsprechen auch jenen Termini und Wendungen, die in der Fachkommunikation tatsächlich verwendet werden.

Welches Englisch?

Die Weltsprache Englisch hat viele Ausprägungen und Varianten. In **KWiC-Web** wird grundsätzlich *Standard American* als Ausgangssprache verwendet, es wird aber auf regionale Varianten – besonders auf Unterschiede zwischen amerikanischem und britischem Englisch – verwiesen (*BE*, *espBE*) und fallweise auch erläutert (bes. bei unterschiedlicher Bedeutung oder Verwendung; siehe auch Hinweise zur Aussprache & Schreibweise, letzte Seite).

Wie sind die Module aufgebaut?

Die Aufbereitung des zahnmedizinischen Fachwortschatzes in übersichtliche Module erfolgte analog zur fachlichen Strukturierung in einzelne Fachbereiche.

Auch innerhalb der Module sind die Wortfelder nach fachlich-semantischen Kriterien angeordnet. Ähnlich wie bei einem guten Lehrbuch gelangt man den Begriffssystemen folgend von den grundlegenden Schlüsselwörtern zu immer spezifischeren Termini. Das zweite Ordnungsprinzip folgt didaktischen Kriterien. Grundlegende und häufig verwendete Ausdrücke werden jeweils vor den komplexeren und selteneren angeführt. Durch den ansteigenden Schwierigkeitsgrad kann jeder Benutzer die Eindringtiefe individuell bestimmen und einfach zum nächsten Modul/Abschnitt weitergehen, wenn er den Eindruck hat, es wird zu spezifisch. Durch die spezielle Anordnung der Schlüsselwörter innerhalb eines jeden Moduls (den Bedeutungszusammenhängen statt dem Alphabet folgend) ergeben sich zusätzliche Kopplungseffekte, wodurch die Effizienz von **KWiC-Web** weiter gesteigert wird, da die Behaltensquote vor allem für Benutzer, die mit dem betreffenden Fachgebiet in der Muttersprache bereits vertraut sind, noch höher wird. Die Einträge decken jedes Gebiet so ab, dass zwischen den Modulen keine wesentlichen Überschneidungen oder Lücken entstehen.

Die Module sind mit treffenden Überschriften versehen, die den jeweiligen Bereich klar umreißen. So findet man beispielsweise Termini wie *teeth grinding*, *exfoliated* und *gag reflex* im Modul **Dentition & Mastication**, und Einträge wie *ache*, *tender*, und *analgesic* im Modul **Pain**. Wenn sich auch in inhaltlich angrenzenden Modulen manche Ausdrücke wiederfinden, als Keywords sind sie jeweils nur einem Modul zugeordnet.

Querverweise: Am Beginn jedes Moduls wird auf Zusammenhänge mit verwandten Modulen verwiesen, in denen der Benutzer viele Kontextausdrücke samt ausführlichen Erklärungen und Übersetzungen wiederfinden kann. Auf zusätzliche Querverbindungen zwischen einzelnen Termini verschiedener Module wird jeweils beim betreffenden Wort verwiesen (z.B. →U23-14). Damit wird das Modul (Unit 23) und die Eintragsnummer (14) bezeichnet.

Wie sind die einzelnen Einträge strukturiert?

Die Einträge enthalten folgende Komponenten:

Das Hauptstichwort (Schlüsselwort): Jedes Modul wurde so angelegt, dass es 10 bis maximal 35 Einträge (Hauptstichwörter und deren Wortfelder) umfasst. Nominalformen und Nominalverbindungen machen den Großteil der Schlüsselwörter aus; die dazugehörigen Adjektive, Präpositionen und Verben findet man in den Beschreibungen, Beispielsätzen, Wortverbindungen und Phrasen (z.B. *an elective operation, to undergo an operation for a tumor, to be operated on, operative approach, operating room*). Deshalb scheint z.B. das Verb *perform* zwar nirgends als Haupteintrag auf, im Kontext taucht es allerdings immer wieder in Verbphrasen wie *to perform a study/an operation/a biopsy* bei den betreffenden Nomina auf.

Verwandte Ausdrücke: Bei jedem Schlüsselwort sind Synonyme (*syn*), Fast-Synonyme (*sim*), Antonyme (*opposite*) und verwandte Ausdrücke (*rel*) wie z.B. Unter-, Ober- und Nebenbegriffe des Haupteintrags angeführt. Bei Vorliegen mehrerer synonymer Ausdrücke werden diese nicht einfach kommentarlos aufgelistet, sondern nach Gebräuchlichkeit gewichtet. Die häufiger verwendeten werden zuerst genannt, selten gebrauchte Benennungen werden gekennzeichnet (*rare*). Zusammen mit den Angaben zur Sprachebene und den Kontextbeispielen wird dadurch für den Benutzer ersichtlich, welcher Terminus in welchem Zusammenhang bevorzugt verwendet wird.

Deutsche Übersetzungen (Marginalspalte): Für jedes Schlüsselwort sowie vorhandene verwandte Ausdrücke werden in der Marginalspalte jeweils die deutschen Entsprechungen angeführt. Zusätzlich werden Wörter oder Passagen im Kontext, die für den Benutzer schwer aus dem Zusammenhang erschließbar oder besonders wichtig oder nützlich sind, übersetzt. Die übersetzten Passagen sind im englischen Text blau markiert und über Hochzahlen den Übersetzungen in der Marginalspalte zugeordnet. Dadurch bekommt der Benutzer auch Einblick in spezielle Bedeutungen der Termini im authentischen Kontext.

Worterklärungen: Hier handelt es sich weniger um Definitionen als um beschreibende Erklärungen bzw. Paraphrasen in einfachem Englisch. Diese sind für Fachleute als Formulierungshilfe ebenso nützlich wie für Translatoren, die die Bedeutung des Fachausdrucks weder im Englischen noch in der Muttersprache kennen. Außerdem enthalten diese Umschreibungen viele weitere Über-, Neben- und Unterbegriffe zu den Haupteinträgen.

Authentische Beispielsätze (»-Symbol): Diese sind dem medizinischen Korpus entnommen und geben dem Benutzer Einblick in die authentische Verwendung der Fachtermini in der medizinischen Literatur. Bei der Auswahl der Beispiele wurde sowohl auf die sprachliche als auch die fachliche Relevanz geachtet.

Wortfamilie: Bei jedem Schlüsselwort und dessen verwandten Ausdrücken werden auch die dazugehörigen Wortfamilien (Verben, Adjektive etc.) angeführt. Man findet also beim Eintrag *diagnosis* auch *to (over)diagnose, misdiagnosis, (non)diagnostic* etc.

Hinweise zur Grammatik und Stilebene: Neben Angaben zu Wortart und grammatikalischen Besonderheiten (Plural, unregelm. Verb etc.) wird auch auf die Sprachebene, in der die Ausdrücke vorwiegend verwendet werden, verwiesen (z.B. medizinischer Fachterminus, Fachjargon, klinischer oder umgangssprachlicher Ausdruck). Bei Wörtern, die in mehr als zwei Stilebenen verwendet werden, wurde auf eine Angabe verzichtet. Aus Platzgründen konnte die Stilebene bei den verwandten Termini und den Wortfamilien nur dann angegeben werden, wenn diese von jener der Wörter davor bzw. danach abweicht. Die Stilebene von Termini ohne entsprechende Angabe entspricht daher jenen, die für die Wörter danach (verw. Termini) bzw. davor (Wortfamilie) angegeben sind. Die Kennzeichnung der Sprachebenen und deren Bedeutung ist den Erläuterungen zu den verwendeten Abkürzungen zu entnehmen (s. Umschlagklappe).

Phrasen und Kollokationen (*Use*): Diese werden ähnlich wie in Kollokationswörterbüchern jeweils in Blöcken von linken bzw. rechten Kollokationen dargestellt. Auf die Tilde wurde verzichtet; das zu ergänzende Tildewort ist kursiv/halbfett hervorgehoben. Der Eintrag **drilling** technique / device / site • twist / spiral / countersink **drill** ist also wie folgt zu lesen: drilling technique, drilling device, drilling site <neuer Block> twist drill, spiral drill, countersink drill. Bei Aneinanderreihungen von Verbphrasen, z. B. to relieve/blunt/alleviate pain (to ist jeweils zu ergänzen) und bei zusammengesetzten Wörtern, wie z. B. hypo / hyper**esthesia** oder **patho**genesis / physiology steht der Schrägstrich direkt beim betreffenden Wort(teil).

Klinische Phrasen: In vielen Fachbereichen gibt es wiederkehrende klinische Situationen, in denen bestimmte Wendungen und Aussagen ständig vorkommen. Solche Standardphrasen sind jeweils am Ende des Moduls unter Clinical Phrases in ganzen Sätzen mit der deutschen Entsprechung angeführt (in 9 Modulen).

Aussprache: Bei englischen Wörtern, deren Aussprache bzw. Betonung Probleme bereiten kann, ist die internationale Lautschrift bzw. die Betonung angegeben. Eine Erklärung der Lautschriftsymbole anhand von Beispielen findet sich in der Umschlagklappe.

Tipps und Hinweise auf Besonderheiten (Note): Bei Stichwörtern, die in Bezug auf Verwendung, Bedeutung oder Grammatik besondere Schwierigkeiten bereiten, werden diese in leicht verständlichem Englisch erläutert (Hinweis auf falsche Freunde, Verwechslungsgefahr, Nebenbedeutungen, vom Deutschen abweichende Verwendung etc.).

Kann ich KWiC-Web auch zum Nachschlagen bestimmter Suchwörter verwenden?

Alle englischen Schlüsselwörter und Übersetzungsäquivalente sind auch über einen deutschen und englischen Index auffindbar, wodurch **KWiC-Web** auch wie ein zweisprachiges Fachwörterbuch zum Nachschlagen geeignet ist. Ein Index der englischen Abkürzungen ermöglicht das Auffinden jener Akronyme im Text, die im klinischen Bereich häufig verwendet und oft zu sprachlichen Stolpersteinen werden.

Wie kann ich mit KWiC-Web arbeiten?

Es gibt grundsätzlich drei Zugangswege zu den in **KWiC-Web** aufbereiteten Materialien.

1. Über das Inhaltsverzeichnis und das Modulregister. Im Inhaltsverzeichnis finden Sie eine Übersicht der einzelnen Module (Units), Abschnitte und Fachbereiche in englischer und deutscher Sprache. Hier können Sie die relevanten Bereiche auswählen und dann die betreffenden Module nacheinander in der gewünschten Tiefe durcharbeiten. Mit Hilfe des Griffregisters finden Sie schnell zu den gesuchten Modulen.

2. Über die Querverweise. Jedes Modul sowie viele Schlüsselwörter stehen mit anderen Modulen bzw. Einträgen in Verbindung. Auf Querverbindungen zwischen den Modulen wird jeweils am Beginn jeder Einheit verwiesen (**Related Units**). Wollen Sie also ein spezielles Fachgebiet umfassend erarbeiten, folgen Sie einfach diesen Verweisen, um zu jenen Fachbereichen zu gelangen, die damit in Verbindung stehen. Auch die Querverweise zwischen einzelnen Termini sind nützliche Wegweiser zu weiteren fachlichen Zusammenhängen.

3. Über die Indices. Suchen Sie spezielle Termini oder wollen deren Bedeutung, Übersetzung oder Verwendung nachschlagen, können Sie dies mit Hilfe des deutschen bzw. englischen Index tun. Mit dem Index können Sie auch schnell zu anderen Schlüsselwörtern und ihrem sprachlichen Umfeld gelangen, selbst wenn kein direkter Zusammenhang besteht.

Wer kann mit KWiC-Web arbeiten?

Grundsätzlich jeder, der über grundlegende Englischkenntnisse aus der Schulzeit verfügt (upper intermediate). Durch die differenzierte Aufbereitung des reichhaltigen Sprachmaterials ist **KWiC-Web** für mehrere Benutzergruppen optimal verwendbar.

Studenten und Ärzte in Ausbildung, die mit englischen Lehrbüchern und internationalen Fachzeitschriften arbeiten, ihre Dissertation in englischer Sprache verfassen oder ein Auslandsjahr in Boston, Edinburg, Kapstadt oder Sydney anstreben.

Zahnärzte in Klinik und Forschung, die sich mit Hilfe von englischen Fachartikeln weiterbilden, internationale Kongresse besuchen oder einen Artikel in einer renommierten amerikanischen Fachzeitschrift veröffentlichen wollen.

Übersetzer und Dolmetscher, die im zahnmedizinischen Bereich arbeiten. Ob Sie sich in ein neues Fachgebiet einarbeiten oder spezielle Kollokationen oder Phrasen suchen, in *KWiC-Web* finden Sie auf kleinstem Raum eine Fülle von sprachlichen und fachlichen Informationen, die Sie sonst aus verschiedenen Nachschlagewerken erst mühsam zusammensuchen müssen oder überhaupt in keinem anderen Behelf finden können.

Zahnmedizinisches Personal (DentalassistentInnen, MundhygienikerInnen, Dentaltechniker etc.), die mit den wichtigsten englischen Begriffen und Wendungen in ihrem Fachbereich vertraut sein müssen. Durch die didaktische Gliederung der Schlüsselwörter (Grundlegendes zuerst) müssen Sie die relevanten Termini nicht erst mühsam aus einer Fülle von Informationen herausfiltern.

Diet & Dieting **BASIC MEDICAL & HEALTH TERMS 1**

Unit 1 Diet & Dieting
Related Units: 2 Food & Drink, 12 Nutrition, 10 Dentition & Mastication

ingest [ɪndʒest] v term   syn **take in** v phr, sim **eat**[1] [iːt]-**ate** [eɪt‖et]-**eaten** v irr
to take in food, drink or medication via the mouth for digestion[2] [daɪdʒestʃən‖dɪ-]
ingestion[3] n term • ingestants[4] n • intake[5] n • overeat[6] v clin • eater n • eating n
» Ingested food is mixed with salivary amylase [eɪ] before it reaches the stomach [k]. Hospitalize patients who have ingested mushrooms[7] [ʌ] known to cause serious [ɪə] poisoning[8]. Adequate intake of fluids should be encouraged [ɜː] in immobilized patients. Many depressed patients eat little and are frequently constipated[9]. Eat up[10] before it gets cold. You should not eat a late meal before bedtime.
Use **to ingest** food / foreign [fɒrɪn] bodies[11] • **ingested** eggs / fluid / drugs / poison • milk / accidental[12] / toxin / caustic[13] [ɒː] co**ingestion** • **to eat** less / enough / well / like a horse[14] / without help / cooked foods / a regular diet[15] / out[16] • to have sth./be unable/to refuse **to eat** • ready[17]-**to-eat** • to be a big / small / fussy [ʌ] or picky[18] / compulsive [ʌ] **eater** • **eating** habits[19] / disorder[20] • binge[21] [bɪndʒ] **eating** • obsessive, compulsive[22] **overeating**

einnehmen, zu sich nehmen
essen[1] Verdauung[2] (Nahrungs)aufnahme, Einnahme (Medikament)[3] aufgenommene Nahrung, Ingesta[4] Ein-, Aufnahme, Zufuhr[5] s. überessen[6] Pilze[7] Vergiftung[8] verstopft, obstipiert[9] iss auf[10] Fremdkörper verschlucken[11] akzidentelle / versehentliche Einnahme[12] E. von Ätzmitteln[13] essen für vier[14] normale Kost zu s. nehmen[15] (ins Restaurant) essen gehen[16] fertig zubereitet[17] heikel b. Essen[18] Essgewohnheiten[19] Essstörung[20] Fressgelage[21] Fresssucht[22]   1

consume [uː] v term   sim **have**[1], **dine**[2] [aɪ] v, **lunch**[3] [lʌntʃ] v & n
consumption[4] [ʌ] n • dining n • dinner[5] [ɪ] n • diner[6] [aɪ] n
» Nutritional [ɪʃ] needs can be met quite easily by adults who consume dairy [eə] products[7]. Alcohol when consumed in excess for prolonged periods typically causes these symptoms. Why don't you have another toast? They lunched on fast food every day.
Use **to consume** a varied diet [daɪət]/ little dietary fiber[8] / large quantities of beer • **consumption of** contaminated food[9] / heavy [e] meals[10] • coffee / alcohol / seafood[11] / excessive **consumption** / safe for **consumption**[12] • **to dine** out with sb. • dining hall[13] / room / table / car[14] • to have/go out for **lunch** • buffet [eɪ]/ business **lunch** • **lunch**time / break or hour[15] • candlelight **dinner**

konsumieren, verzehren, zu sich nehmen
essen, trinken, zu sich nehmen[1] speisen, dinieren[2] (zu) Mittag essen, Mittagessen[3] Konsum, Verzehr[4] Hauptmahlzeit, Abendessen[5] Esslokal[6] Milchprodukte[7] wenig Ballaststoffe zu s. nehmen[8] Konsum verdorbener Lebensmittel[9] K. schwerverdaulicher Gerichte[10] Konsum v. Meeresfrüchten[11] für den Verzehr geeignet / mindestens haltbar bis[12] Speisesaal[13] Speisewagen[14] Mittagspause[15]   2

feed [fiːd] -**fed**-**fed** [e] v irr   sim **nourish**[1] [nɜːrɪʃ] v → U12-1
(i) to give food to a baby, animals or persons who cannot eat without help (ii) to supply with nutriment[2] [uː]
feed(ing)[3] n • underfeeding[4] n • underfed adj
» Generally, infants[5] weighing [eɪ] less than 1200 g require 2-hour feedings, whereas larger infants are fed at 3-hour intervals. How often does your baby feed[6]?
Use **to feed** sb. honey [ʌ]/ sb. with a spoon / poorly[7] • **feeding** bottle[8] / cup[9] / method / pattern[10] / problem / tube [uː]/ regimen[11] [dʒ] • breast[12]- [e]/ bottle-/ adequately[13] / well / tube-**fed** • tube[14] / intravenous [iː]/ forced[15] / breast **feeding** • to be a heavy[16] [e]/ poor **feeder**

(i) füttern, Nahrung zuführen
(ii) (er)nähren, mit Nahrung versorgen
(er)nähren[1] Nahrung[2] Stillen, Füttern, Ernährung[3] Unterernährung[4] Säuglinge[5] trinken, nach d. Brust / Flasche verlangen[6] wenig zu sich nehmen / trinken (Baby)[7] Saugflasche[8] Schnabeltasse[9] Stillzeiten[10] Ernährungsplan[11] gestillt[12] ausreichend ernährt[13] Sondenernährg.[14] Zwangsernährg.[15] e. starker Esser sein[16]   3

wolf [ʊ] **down** v phr inf   sim **gulp** [ʌ] **down**[1], **bolt down**[2], **gobble (up)**[2] v phr inf
to take big bites[3] and swallow[4] hurriedly or greedily[5] [iː] without chewing [tʃuːɪŋ] or drink in one swallow[6] [swɒːloʊ]

(Speisen) hinunterschlingen
hinunterstürzen (Getränk), -schlingen (Essen)[1] gierig essen, verschlingen[2] Bissen[3] schlucken[4] gierig[5] Zug[6]   4

nonedible or **inedible** [e] adj   opposite **edible**[1] adj, rel **palatable**[2] adj
unfit for human consumption, e.g. past its sell-by date[3]
unpalatable[4] adj • palatability[5] n
» Vitamin K1 is present in most edible vegetables, especially in green leaves. A diet with normal fat content is more palatable and just as effective as a low-fat diet.
Use **nonedible** plants

nicht essbar, ungenießbar
ess-, genießbar[1] wohlschmeckend, schmackhaft[2] nach dem Ablaufdatum[3] nicht schmackhaft; ungenießbar[4] Schmackhaftigkeit[5]   5

2 BASIC MEDICAL & HEALTH TERMS — Diet & Dieting

food [fuːd] n   sim **foodstuffs**[1], **groceries**[2] [oʊs], **victuals**[3] n BE, *****grub**[4] [ʌ] n inf

any substance [ʌ] that can be metabolized[5] by an organism to give energy and build up tissue
» Enjoy your food. Asking the patient to keep a diary[6] [daɪəri] of foods eaten may prove helpful. Fortification[7] of foodstuffs with vitamins etc. has nearly eliminated once-common deficiency states[8] [ɪʃ].
Use to refuse/prepare[9]/(BE) be off one's[10] **food** • **food** intake[11] / additives[12] / preservatives[13] / supplement • bolus[14] of / fatty / ingested / junk[15] [dʒʌŋk]/ fast / health[16] [e] **food** • (un)cooked / solid[17] / spicy [spaɪsi]/ spoiled[18] **food** • **food** craving[19] [eɪ] / intolerance[20] / particles / poisoning[21] • **food** aversion[22] / debris[23] [iː]/ choices / sources / chain[24] [tʃeɪn] • undigested / baby[25] / regurgitated[26] [ɡɜːrdʒ] **food** • **food**-borne infection[27] • fortified / contaminated[28] / aspiration of **foodstuffs**

> **Note:** *Food* is normally used in the singular. In the *plural* it is used synonymously with *foodstuffs* to refer to different types of food.

Nahrung, Essen
Nahrungsmittel[1] Lebensmittel[2] Lebensmittel, Proviant[3] Fressalien[4] abbauen, umwandeln[5] Tagebuch[6] Anreicherung[7] Mangelzustände[8] E. zubereiten[9] keinen Appetit haben[10] Nahrungsaufnahme[11] Lebensmittelzusatzstoffe[12] Konservierungsmittel[13] Bolus, Bissen[14] N. mit geringem Nährwert[15] Reformkost[16] feste N.[17] verdorbene N.[18] Essensgelüste[19] Nahrungsmittelunverträglichkeit[20] Nahrungsmittelvergiftung[21] Abneigung gegen Speisen[22] Speisereste[23] Nahrungskette[24] Säuglingsnahrung[25] erbrochenes Essen[26] Lebensmittelinfektion[27] kontaminierte Lebensmittel[28]   6

---

meal [miːl] n

food served and eaten at one time (e.g. breakfast, brunch[1] [ʌ], lunch, barbeque[2], afternoon tea, supper[3], dinner[4])
» Cafeterias [ɪə] and buffet [eɪ] meals should be avoided by anyone on a weight-reducing [weɪt] diet. Certain foods or meal patterns can change drug effectiveness.
Use to eat/ingest[5]/miss[6] a **meal** • the major[7] **meal** • before / after / in-between **meals** • at **meal**time • **meals** on wheels[8] [iː] • large / light / heavy[9] / fatty / solid[10] / test / evening / bedtime **meal** • **meal** planning / patterns[11]

Mahlzeit; Essen, Kost
Brunch, Frühstück u. Mittagessen in einem[1] Grillen (im Freien)[2] Abendessen[3] Hauptmahlzeit, (Fest)essen[4] Mahlzeit einnehmen[5] M. auslassen[6] Hauptmahlzeit[7] Essen auf Rädern[8] schwerverdauliches Gericht[9] feste Kost[10] Essgewohnheiten[11]   7

---

dish [dɪʃ] n

(i) food prepared in a particular way (ii) dishware for serving food (pl) (iii) a shallow[1] container, e.g. a Petri dish
dish out[2] / up[3] v • dish towel [aʊ]/ cloth[4] [ɒː] n or tea towel[4] BE
» These infections are mostly due to raw [rɒː] fish dishes. This dish is best when served cold. They dished up the finest of meals.
Use to do or wash[5] the dishes • favorite[6] [eɪ] dish • dish washer[7] / water[8] / rack[9]

(i) Gericht, Speise (ii) Geschirr (iii) Schale, Schüssel
flach[1] austeilen[2] anrichten, auftragen[3] Geschirrtuch[4] Geschirr spülen / abwaschen[5] Lieblingsspeise[6] Spülmaschine, Geschirrspüler[7] Abwasch-, Spülwasser[8] Geschirrkorb, -ständer[9]   8

---

serving [ɜː] n   syn **helping** n , sim **course**[1] [kɔːrs] n

a portion of food or drink
serve[2] v • service[3] n • server[4] n
» Do you want a second helping? Frying[5] [aɪ] the food before serving may not destroy the toxins.
Use standardized **serving** size[aɪ] • **serving** spoon [uː] • salad server[6] • a four-**course** meal[7]

Portion
Gang[1] servieren[2] Bedienung[3] Vorlegebesteck[4] (ab)braten[5] Salatbesteck[6] 4-gängiges Menü[7]

  9

---

snack n & v

(n) a light informal meal, e.g. tea or coffee break[1] [eɪ] where you have some refreshments[2]
» Dietary strategies to increase appetite or intake include providing salty foods, nutrient-dense beverages[3] [rɪdʒɪz] such as fruit juice, and easy-to-eat snacks. What are you snacking on?
Use to have a[4] **snack** • **snack** food / bar[5]

Imbiss, Zwischenmahlzeit; Imbiss zu sich nehmen
Kaffeepause[1] Erfrischungen[2] nährstoffreiche Getränke[3] eine Kleinigkeit essen[4] Imbissstube[5]
  10

Diet & Dieting BASIC MEDICAL & HEALTH TERMS 3

appetite [æpətaɪt] *n*   *rel* **hungry**[1] [ʌ], **thirsty**[2] [ɜː] *adj*, **hunger**[3], **thirst**[4] *n & v*
(i) normal desire to eat (ii) to have a craving[5] [eɪ] for special foods
appetizer[6] *n* -iser *espBE* • appetizing[7] *adj* -ising *BE*
» The patient's appetite is poor. Are you hungry for[8] some meat? Some medications enhance the sensation of thirst[9] by causing a dry mouth.
Use to work up[10] / it gives me[11] **an appetite** • loss of[12] / healthy[13] / inability to control one's **appetite** • to spoil *or* ruin[14] / lose **your appetite** • to be/feel **hungry** • wolfish[15] [ʊ]/ salt / air **hunger** • **hunger** pain[16] / strike / cry / behavior [eɪ] • **appetite** suppressant[17] • to experience **thirst** • **thirst** mechanism [k]/ center / sensation[9]

Appetit
hungrig[1] durstig[2] Hunger; hungern[3] Durst; dürsten[4] Verlangen, Lust[5] Appetitanreger, -happen, Vorspeise[6] appetitanregend, lecker[7] A./ Lust haben auf[8] Durstgefühl[9] s. einen Appetit holen[10] A. anregen[11] Appetitlosigkeit[12] guter/gesunder A.[13] A. verderben[14] Wolfshunger[15] Nüchtern-, Hungerschmerz[16] Appetitzügler[17]   11

wholesome [hoʊlsəm] *adj*   *syn* **healthy** [helθi], **healthful** *adj*
food supposed to be good for your health because it is rich in nutrients[1] or low in artificial ingredients [iː]
wholefood(s)[2] *n espBE* • whole wheat[3] [wiːt] *n* • whole bread[4] [e] *n*
» The wholesome ingredients[5] of their breads are well documented.

gesund, bekömmlich
reich an Nährstoffen[1] Vollwertprodukte[2] Voll(korn)weizen[3] Vollkornbrot[4] Zutaten[5]   12

diet [daɪət] *v & n*
v to eat sparingly[1] [eə] *n* (i) prescribed selection of foods (ii) usual food and drink consumed by a person
dietary[2] *adj & n* • dietician *or* -tian[3] *n* • dietetics[4] *n* • dietetic[2] *adj*
» A healthy person consuming a variety [aɪə] of foods is unlikely to have a dietary deficiency[5] [ɪʃ]. I have been on this diet for weeks but to no effect. Regaining body weight after dieting is referrred to as weight cycling.
Use to be on[6]/go on/observe[6]/follow[6]/adhere [ɪə] to[6] **a diet** • to put sb. on[7]/prescribe/tolerate[8] **a diet** • strict[9] / well-balanced[10] / a 1000-calorie / high-fiber[11] [aɪ] **diet** • low-fat / diabetic [e]/ bland [æ] *or* ulcer[12] [ʌlsɚ] **diet** • full- *or* clear-liquid[13] / modified / (weight [weɪt]) reducing *or* slimming down[14] / soft[15] **diet** • changes in / staple[16] [eɪ] **diet** / dietary assessment / history / allowance[17] [aʊ]/ risk factors / service / counselor[18] [aʊ] • **dieting** with exercise / patient • **diet** free of / high in proteins / of fruits[19]

Diät halten; (i) Diät, Schon-, Krankenkost (ii) Nahrung, Kost
in Maßen, wenig[1] diätetisch; Diätvorschrift[2] Diätetiker(in)[3] Diätetik, Ernährungslehre[4] Mangelernährung[5] D. halten[6] auf D. setzen[7] Kost vertragen[8] strenge D.[9] ausgewogene K.[10] ballaststoffreiche K.[11] reizarme / blande Diät[12] flüssige Nahrung[13] Schlankheitsdiät, Reduktionskost[14] leichte K., Breikost[15] Hauptnahrung[16] Diätempfehlung, empfohlene Nahrungszufuhr[17] Ernährungsberater[18] Obstdiät[19]   13

starve [stɑːrv] *v*
(i) to die *or*–informally–suffer (extremely) from lack of food (ii) not to give someone any food
(semi-)starvation[1] [eɪ] *n* • starving[2] *adj & n*
» She has been starving herself. They died of starvation. Total starvation causes a loss of approximately 0.4 kg of body weight per day.
Use to be **starving**[3] • **to starve** to death[4] • **starvation** diet[5] • to die of / total / prolonged / oxygen[6] [ɒːksɪdʒən] **starvation**

(ver)hungern (lassen), fasten
(Ver)hungern, Hungertod[1] (ver)hungernd; (Aus)hungern[2] halb verhungert sein, vor Hunger umkommen[3] verhungern[4] Hungerkur[5] Sauerstoffhunger[6]   14

fast [fæst] *v & n*   *sim* **fasting**[1] [fæstɪŋ] *adj & n*
to abstain [eɪ] from[2] (certain) food over a specific period of time for therapeutic [uː] or religious [dʒ] reasons
» Patients are fasted under close supervision [ɪʒ] for up to 72 h. Diarrhea [daɪəriːə] of any cause often improves or resolves with fasting[3]. They also recommend obtaining a fasting lipid profile.
Use prolonged periods of / avoidance of / after **fasting** • **fasting** blood sugar *or* glucose levels[4] • in the fed and **fasted** states[5] • under **fasting** conditions

fasten, hungern; Fasten(zeit)
nüchtern, hungernd; Fasten[1] sich enthalten[2] sistiert bei Nahrungskarenz[3] Nüchternblutzucker[4] nüchtern und mit vollem Magen[5]   15

vegetarian [vedʒɪteəˑrɪən] *n & adj*   *sim* **vegan**[1] [viːɡən] *adj & n*,
    rel **vegetarianism**[2] *n*
(n) person who does not eat meat or fish or (often) any animal products (adj) excluding meat
» A vegan diet can be nutritionally adequate, although more thoughtful [3] [θɒːtfˀl] food choices and supplementation[4] with fortified foods[5] may be necessary.
Use **vegetarian** food • ovo-/ ovo-lacto/ strictly **vegetarian** diet[6]

Vegetarier(in); vegetarisch
streng vegetarisch; strenge(r) V.[1] Vegetarismus, veget. Lebensweise[2] wohlüberlegt[3] Ergänzung[4] angereicherte Nahrungsmittel[5] streng vegetarische Kost[6]   16

4 BASIC MEDICAL & HEALTH TERMS — Food & Drink

health freak [i:] n inf
person very enthusiastic [u:] about a healthy life-style, esp. health food, often to the point of being obsessed[1] with it
» Oat bran[2] [oʊt bræn] has become the favorite [eɪ] of health freaks.

Gesundheitsapostel
besessen sein[1] Haferkleie[2]
17

Clinical Phrases

Try to keep off salty food. Salzhaltige Speisen sollten Sie nach Möglichkeit meiden • She has a sweet tooth. Sie isst gern Süßigkeiten. • I don't have a stomach for milk any more. Mir schmeckt die Milch nicht mehr. • I couldn't stomach it. Ich habe es nicht vertragen. • Thanks, I'm full. Danke, ich bin satt. • I made a real pig of myself stuffing myself with sweets. Ich habe mir den Bauch mit Süßigkeiten vollgeschlagen. • He just couldn't stay off the booze. Er griff immer wieder zur Flasche. • I've hardly touched any food for a week. Ich habe schon eine Woche kaum etwas gegessen. • Most infants will want to feed every two or three hours. Die meisten Säuglinge wollen alle 2-3 Stunden gefüttert werden. • The baby's refused the bottle ever since. Seither hat das Baby die Flasche verweigert. • It seems the boy's practically living on chips and sweets. Der Bub ernährt sich anscheinend nur von Chips und Süßigkeiten. • It makes my mouth water. Mir läuft das Wasser im Mund zusammen. • I've been off my food for the past few weeks. (BE) Ich hatte in den letzten paar Wochen keinen Appetit. • I am starved / starving. Ich komme fast um vor Hunger. • For them lunch is just a snack. Sie essen mittags nicht viel.

Unit 2   Food & Drink
Related Units: 2 Food & Drink, 12 Nutrition, 10 Dentition & Mastication

meat [i:] n
flesh of animals that is cooked and eaten; types include pork (from pigs), beef[1] (cows), veal[2] [i:] (calf [kæf]), mutton[3] [ʌ] (sheep), lamb, poultry[4] [oʊ] (chicken, turkey[5], etc.), and venison or game[6] (from wild animals, e.g. deer[7] [ɪ]). Meat can be eaten as bacon[8], ham[9], steak, cutlet[10] [ʌ], chop[11], hamburger, sausage[12] [sɒ:sɪdʒ], hot dog[13], etc.
meaty adj • meatloaf[14] [oʊ] n • meatballs[15] n
» Do you like your steak medium-rare[16] or well-done? Excessive intake of purine from meat, fish and poultry may favor stone formation. You should not pour any gravy[17] [eɪ] on your meat. Tofu is used as a meat substitute.
Use raw / (under)cooked[18] / fried / roast / lean[19] [i:] **meat** • fatty / red / white / ground[20] [aʊ] / tough[21] [tʌf] / tender[22] **meat** • **meat** tenderizer / substitute[23] • corned[24] **beef** • **chicken** soup

Fleisch
Rindfl.[1] Kalbfl.[2] Schaffl.[3] Geflügel[4] Truthahn[5] Wild[6] Rotwild[7] Speck[8] Schinken[9] Schnitzel[10] Kotelett[11] Wurst[12] Würstchen[13] Fleischkäse[14] Fleischklöße[15] halb durch[16] Soße[17] (nicht) durchgegartes Fl.[18] mageres Fl.[19] Hackfleisch[20] zähes Fl.[21] zartes Fl.[22] Fleischersatz[23] Dosenfleisch[24]
1

fish v & n usu sing
types of fish commonly eaten include trout[1] [aʊ], cod[2], herring, sardine, salmon[3] [sæmən], mackerel, and tuna[4].
» Shall we have fish for lunch? I'd like the cod fillets. Do you like tuna canned in oil?
Use freshwater[5] / marine[6] / fatty / smoked[7] / baked / broiled[8] / canned[9] / breaded[10] [e] **fish** • **fish** stick or finger[11] • filleted sole[12] [soʊl]

fischen; Fisch
Forelle[1] Dorsch[2] Lachs[3] Thunfisch[4] Süßwasserfisch[5] Meeres-, Seefisch[6] Räucherfisch[7] gegrillter F.[8] Dosenfisch[9] panierter F.[10] Fischstäbchen[11] Seezungenfilet[12]
2

seafood n
edible marine fish and shellfish[1], e.g. octopus or squid[2], shrimps[3], roe[4] [roʊ], lobster[5] [ɒ:], crab, mussel[6] [ʌ], oyster[7].
» Most cases of food poisoning[8] were linked to ingestion[9] [dʒ] of undercooked seafood.
Use **seafood** restaurant / consumption[9] / ingestion • raw [ɒ:] **seafood**

Meeresfrüchte
Schalentiere[1] Tintenfisch[2] Garnelen[3] Rogen[4] Hummer[5] Miesmuscheln[6] Austern[7] Lebensmittelvergiftung[8] Konsum v. Meeresf.[9]
3

milk n & v
» The patient should not drink any cold milk. This milk has turned / gone sour[1] [saʊɚ]. A glass of milk usually relieves[2] the pain.
Use whole[3] [hoʊl]/ skim(med)[4] / raw / cow / goat's[5] / breast[6] [e] **milk** • (un)pasteurized [tʃə]/ certified[7] / fortified vitamin D[8] / butter **milk** / scalded[9] [ɒ:] / low-fat[4] / condensed[10] / acidophilus[11] / coconut / dry or instant[12] **milk** • **milk**shake / sugar / powder [aʊ]

Milch; melken
sauer werden[1] lindert[2] Vollmilch[3] Magermilch[4] Ziegenmilch[5] Muttermilch[6] Vorzugsmilch[7] mit Vitamin D angereicherte M.[8] abgekochte M.[9] Kondens-, Dosenmilch[10] Sauermilch[11] Trockenmilch[12]
4

Food & Drink　　　　　　　　　　　　　　　　　　　　　　　　　　　　　　　　　　　　　　**BASIC MEDICAL & HEALTH TERMS** 5

dairy [deəɪ] **products** *or espBE* **produce** *n*

foods made from milk such as cheese, cr<u>ea</u>m[1] [iː], butter, c<u>ur</u>d[2] [ɜː], yog(ho)urt [jougət], and whey[3] [ʰweɪ]

» The fruit c<u>u</u>stard[4] [ʌ] may have been mouldy[5] and the mild<u>ew</u>[6] [duː] has probably pr<u>e</u>cipitated[7] his symptoms.

Use peanut[8] / melted[9] **butter** • (un)grated[10] [eɪ] / cream[11] / soft[12] / Swiss / cottage **cheese** • (un)whipped / whipping[13] **cream** • **dairy** farm / cow

Milch-, Molkereiprodukte

Obers, Sahne[1] Quark, Topfen[2] Molke[3] Fruchtcreme[4] schimmelig[5] Schimmel[6] auslösen[7] Erdnussbutter[8] zerlassene B.[9] geriebener Käse[10] (Doppelrahm-)frischkäse[11] Weichkäse[12] Schlagsahne, -rahm[13]　　　　　　　　5

vegetable [vedʒətəbl] *n usu sing*　　*sim* **legumes**[1] [legjuːmz] *n*

edible seeds[2], roots[3], stems[4] or leaves or nonsweet fruits of many plants such as potatoes, beets[5], asparagus[6], cabbage[7], cauliflower[8] [ɒː], lettuce[9] [letɪs], cucumbers[10], rhubarb, horseradish[11], carrots, beans[12], peppers[13], sweet corn[14], <u>o</u>nions[15] [ʌ], green peas[16], turnips[17], egg plants[18], pumpkins[19], spin<u>ach</u> [ɪtʃ], br<u>o</u>ccoli, lentils[20], etc.

» Travelers can reduce their risk of diarrhea [daɪəriːə] by avoiding uncooked vegetables, salads, and unpeeled[21] fruit. Vitamin K1 is present in most edible vegetables, particularly in green leaves.

Use fresh / (green) leafy / root / starchy[22] [tʃ] / raw / grated[23] **vegetables** • **vegetable** proteins / oils / soup • **salad** dressing[24] • dried **beans** • meshed **potatoes**[25]

Gemüse

Hülsenfrüchte[1] Samen[2] Wurzeln[3] Stiele[4] Rüben, Bete[5] Spargel[6] Kohl[7] Blumenkohl[8] Kopfsalat[9] Gurken[10] Meerrettich[11] Bohnen[12] Paprika[13] Zuckermais[14] Zwiebel[15] grüne Erbsen[16] weiße Rüben[17] Auberginen[18] Kürbisse[19] Linsen[20] ungeschält[21] stärkehaltiges Gemüse[22] geraspeltes G.[23] Salatsoße[24] Kartoffelpüree[25]　　　　　　　　6

fruit [fruːt] *n usu sing*

ripened[1] [aɪ], mostly edible reproductive parts of a plant containing the seeds, e.g. apples, pears[2] [eə], peaches[3] [iːtʃ], tangerines[4] [dʒ], cherries[5], pineapples[6] [aɪ], apricots, grapes[7] [eɪ], plums[8] [ʌ], prunes[9] [uː], dates[10] [eɪ], figs[11], melons, etc.

» Fructose is a natural or added sweetener in fruit. Many fruits are a good source of vitamin C and di<u>e</u>tary [aɪə] fiber[12] [aɪ]. Consume at least 5-9 servings of fruits and vegetables per day.

Use fresh / dried[13] / canned[14] / (un)peeled[15] **fruit** • c<u>i</u>trus [saɪ]/ kiwi / tropical / raw / unripened / fallen[16] **fruit** • **fruit** sugar / juice / pulp[17] / s<u>a</u>lad / in heavy/light syrup • **fruit**cake • **apple** pie[18] [paɪ]/ sauce[19] • sl<u>i</u>ced [aɪ] **peaches**[20]

Obst, Früchte; Frucht

gereift[1] Birnen[2] Pfirsiche[3] Mandarinen[4] Kirschen[5] Ananas[6] Weintrauben[7] Zwetschgen, Pflaumen[8] gedörrte Zwetschgen, Dörrpflaumen[9] Datteln[10] Feigen[11] Ballaststoffe[12] Trockenfrüchte[13] Dosenfrüchte[14] (un)geschältes Obst[15] Fallobst[16] Fruchtfleisch[17] Apfelkuchen[18] Apfelmus[19] Pfirsichspalten[20]　　　　　　　　7

berries *n pl*

pulpy[1] [ʌ] and mostly edible small fruit from low bushes [ʊ], e.g. strawberry[2] [ɔː], blueberry[3], blackberry[4], black and red currant[5] [ɜː], cranberry[6], raspberry[7] [ræzberi]

Use **raspberry** tart[8] / pie[9] / jam[10] / jello[11] [dʒeloʊ] • p<u>oi</u>sonous[12] **berry**

Beeren

fleischig[1] Erdbeere[2] Heidel-, Blaubeere[3] Bromb.[4] Johannisb.[5] Preiselb.[6] Himb.[7] Himbeertörtchen[8] Himbeertorte[9] Himbeermarmelade[10] Himbeergelee[11] giftige B.[12]　　8

bread [bred] *n*　　*sim* **breadstuff**[1] *n*

food made from flour[2] [flaʊə], water and yeast[3] [jiːst] mixed into a dough[4] [doʊ] and baked in the <u>o</u>ven[5] [ʌ]; bread products include rolls[6], buns[7] [ʌ], doughnuts[8], wafers[9] [eɪ] / waffles[9] [ɒː], toasts, etc.

breading[10] *n* • breaded[11] *adj*

» In patients with heart failure specially pr<u>o</u>cessed breads[12] and salt s<u>u</u>bstitutes are advisable.

Use white / dark / rye[13] [raɪ]/ barley / wh<u>ea</u>t[14] [iː]/ (un)enriched / whole grain[15] / crisp**bread**[16] / garlic[17] / French / r<u>ai</u>sin[18] [eɪ]/ sourdough[19] / gluten(-free) / ginger**bread**[20] [dʒ] / a slice[21] of / l<u>oa</u>f[22] [oʊ] of **bread** • **bread** products / crumbs[23] [krʌmz]

Brot

Brot(getreide)[1] Mehl[2] Hefe, Germ[3] Teig[4] Backofen, -rohr[5] Brötchen, Semmeln[6] süße Brötchen[7] Krapfen, Berliner[8] Waffeln[9] Paniermehl[10] paniert[11] speziell hergestellte Brotsorten[12] Roggenbrot[13] Weizenb.[14] Vollkornb.[15] Knäckeb.[16] Knoblauchb.[17] Rosinenb.[18] Sauerteigbrot[19] Lebkuchen[20] eine Scheibe Brot[21] Brotlaib[22] Brotkrümel, Brösel[23]　　　　　　　9

pastry [peɪstri] *n*　　*rel* **frosting**[1] *n, BE* **icing** [aɪsɪŋ] *n*

dough of flour, water, baking powder[2], and shortening[3] to make pies[4], cakes, strudel, pancakes[5], soufflés [sufleɪz], etc.

» Apple pie and c<u>u</u>stard[6] [ʌ] was his st<u>a</u>ple food[7] [eɪ]. You should avoid cookies[8] and pastries.

Use French **pastry** • **pastry** cook[9] • apple / pumpkin[10] / meat / rhubarb / deep-dish **pie** • chocolate [tʃɒːklət] **frosting**[11]

(Fein)gebäck

Zuckerguss, Glasur[1] Backpulver[2] Backfett[3] Törtchen, Obstkuchen, Pasteten[4] Pfannkuchen, Omelette[5] Vanillesoße, -pudding[6] Hauptnahrung[7] Kekse, Plätzchen[8] Konditor(in)[9] Kürbiskuchen[10] Schokoladeglasur[11]　　　　　　10

6 BASIC MEDICAL & HEALTH TERMS — Food & Drink

pasta n

types of pasta include spaghetti, noodles [uː], macaroni, tortellini, etc.

» *The Food Guide Pyramid recommends 6-11 daily servings of bread, pasta, rice, and cereals.*

Use **spaghetti** with meatballs[1] / in tomato sauce[2] • egg[3] / tender-stage[4] **noodles**

Teigwaren

Spaghetti bolognese[1] Pasta asciuta[2] Eiernudeln[3] Nudeln al dente[4]

11

cereals [sɪəˑɪəlz] n pl   syn **cornflakes** n espBE

(i) starchy [tʃ] grains[1] used as food, e.g. rice[2], wheat, rye, barley[3], oats[4] [oʊ], corn[5], buckwheat[6] [ʌ], millet[7], etc. (ii) breakfast food prepared from grain

» *Oatmeal[8] is among the most nourishing [ɜː] ingredients[9] in cereals. How about Graham crackers[10]?*

Use whole-grain[11] **cereals** • **cereal**-based formulation / grains

(i) Getreideflocken (ii) Muesli

stärkehaltige Getreidesorten[1] Reis[2] Gerste[3] Hafer[4] Mais[5] Buchweizen[6] Hirse[7] Haferflocken[8] nahrhafte Bestandteile[9] Graham-, Weizenschrotcrackers[10] Vollkornflocken[11]

12

egg n

thin-shelled female reproductive body laid by e.g. hens containing the ovum or embryo together with nutritive[1] (yolk[2] [joʊk]) and protective envelopes (egg white[3] and shell[4])

» *Some gastric infections are associated with ingestion of cracked[5] eggs.*

Use hard-boiled[6] / soft-boiled / raw / whole [hoʊl] / scrambled[7] / fried[8] [aɪ] **egg** • hen's / half a dozen [ʌ] / ham and / free-range[9] / commercial henhouse[10] **eggs** • **egg** protein / products / nog[11] / cup /-timer[12] / allergy

Ei

nahrhaft[1] Eigelb, Dotter[2] Eiweiß[3] Schale[4] gesprungen[5] hart gekochtes E.[6] Rührei, Eierspeise[7] Spiegelei[8] Freilandeier[9] Batterieeier[10] Eierlikör[11] Eieruhr[12]

13

nuts [nʌts] n usu pl

large, hard-shelled seeds, e.g. peanuts[1], walnuts[2] [ɔː], almonds[3] [ɑːl], pignolia[4], cashew nuts or coconuts

nutcracker[5] n • nutshell[6] n

» *Seeds and nuts are good sources of vitamin E.*

Nüsse

Erdnüsse[1] Walnüsse[2] Mandeln[3] Pinienkerne[4] Nussknacker[5] Nussschale[6]

14

oil n & v   sim **(cooking) fats**[1] n

(n) greasy[2] [iː], viscous [vɪskəs] liquid used for cooking, in ointments[3], lubricants[4] [uː], etc.

oily adj • oilcloth[5] n • fatty[6] adj

» *Take margarine [dʒ] instead of lard[7] or butter as a cooking fat, but use it sparingly.*

Use animal / vegetable[8] / dietary[1] **fats** • soybean / olive / corn[9] / wheat germ[10] [dʒ]/ rapeseed[11] **oil** • fish[12] / cod [ɔː] liver[13] / greasy **oil**

Öl; (ein)ölen

Speisefette[1] fett(ig), schmierig[2] Salben[3] Schmier-, Gleitmittel[4] Wachstuch[5] fett(haltig)[6] Schweineschmalz[7] pflanzliche Fette[8] Maiskeimöl[9] Weizenkeimöl[10] Rapsöl[11] Tran[12] Lebertran[13]

15

sugar n & v   sim **(mono-/di-** [aɪ]**)saccharide**[1] [k], rel **molasses**[2] n term

sweet crystalline [ɪ] carbohydrate [aɪ] (fructose [uː], lactose, sucrose [uː], dextrose, and glucose) which works as a sweetener and a source of energy for the body

sugared[3] adj • sugary[4] adj • sugar-coated[5] adj

» *High-fiber, sugar-free cereals should be encouraged. Aspartame (NutraSweet) is an artificial sweetener very popular with diabetics [aɪə].*

Use a lump [ʌ] of[6] **sugar** • table / brown[7] / refined[8] / granulated / powdered[9] / cane[10] [eɪ]/ maple[11] [eɪ]/ invert[12] **sugar** • **sugar** beet[13] [iː] / cube[6] / substitute[14] / uptake /-containing foods • sugared almonds[15]

Zucker, Saccharose; süßen, zuckern

Saccharid[1] Melasse[2] gezuckert[3] zuckerhaltig, süß[4] m. Z. überzogen, dragiert[5] e. Stück Zucker[6] brauner Zucker[7] raffinierter Z.[8] Staubzucker[9] Rohrzucker[10] Ahornsirup[11] Invertzucker[12] Zuckerrübe[13] Zuckerersatz[14] kandierte Mandeln[15]

16

candy n sing   syn **sweet(ie)** n BE

rich sweet made of flavored[1] [eɪ] sugar often with chocolate, caramel, honey, liquorice[2] [lɪkəɪs], nougat [uː], fruit or nuts; merchandized [tʃ] as candy bars, lollipops[3] or suckers[3], pralines, crisps[4], marshmellows, chewing gum, etc.

sweetener[5] n • sweet adj • sweeten[6] v

» *Younger children may suck on hard candy[7]. A high intake of sucrose (table sugar) in such items [aɪ] as soft drinks, candy, syrup[8], and sweetened cereals is a major risk factor for caries.*

Use artificial / nonnutritive[9] **sweetener** • **candy** bar[10] / store / floss[11] (BE) • hard / cotton[11] **candy** • **sweet** smelling[12] / potatoes[13] • to have a **sweet** tooth[14]

Note: In BE a **sweet**[15] can also be the last course of a meal (dessert[15] in AE).

Süßigkeiten, Bonbons

aromatisiert[1] Lakritze, Süßholz[2] Lutscher[3] Knabbergebäck[4] Süßstoff[5] (ver)süßen[6] Bonbon[7] Sirup[8] kalorienarmer Süßstoff[9] Riegel[10] Zuckerwatte[11] wohlriechend[12] Süßkartoffeln[13] e. Schwäche für Süßkeiten haben[14] Nachspeise, Dessert[15]

17

seasoning [i:] *n* *syn* **seasoner** *n, rel* **salt** *n*

substances added to food to give it more flavor[1], including salt, pepper, herbs[2] [ɜːrbz] and spices

season[3] *v* • (un)salted[4] *adj* • salt-rich[5] *adj* • salt-restricted[6] *adj*

» Counseling should be offered about seasoning the food with spices (e.g. pepper).

Use well **seasoned**[7] • table / rock[8] /a pinch [tʃ] of[9] **salt** • **salt** intake[10] • **salted** butter / water • **salt**-restricted diet[11] / depletion[12] [iː]

Würze, Würzen
Geschmack[1] Kräuter[2] würzen[3] (un)gesalzen[4] stark gesalzen[5] salzarm[6] gut gewürzt[7] Steinsalz[8] eine Prise Salz[9] Salzkonsum[10] salzarme Diät[11] Salzmangel, -verlust[12]   18

spices [spaɪsiːz] *n usu pl*

intensely aromatic vegetable substances used for seasoning food, e.g. mustard[1] [ʌ], garlic[2], cinnamon[3], ginger[4] [dʒ], cloves[5] [oʊ], nutmeg[6], cayenne pepper, chili powder[7], curry, etc.

spicy[8] *adj* • spice (up)[9] *v*

» The veal was spiced with black pepper. Rely on a mild and bland diet[10] and avoid spicy food.

Use hot and **spicy**[11] • to cut down on **spicy** dishes[12]

Gewürze
Senf[1] Knoblauch[2] Zimt[3] Ingwer[4] Gewürznelken[5] Muskat[6] Chilipulver[7] würzig[8] (pikant) würzen[9] blande / reizarme Diät[10] scharf gewürzt[11] Konsum stark gewürzter Speisen reduzieren[12]   19

herbs [ɜːrbz] *n pl* *syn* **potherbs** *n*

(i) dried aromatic plants used in cookery[1] for its savory[2] [eɪ] qualities (chives[3] [tʃaɪvz], parsely[4], basil[5], dill, fennel[6], thyme[7] [θaɪm], sage[8] [seɪdʒ], rosemary[9], mint[10] etc. (ii) plants used for medicinal purposes, e.g. camomile[11], arnica, etc.

herbal[12] *adj & n* • herbaceous[12] [hɚˈbeɪʃəs] *adj* • herbarium[13] *n* • herbalist[14] *n*

» Clinical research showed that Chinese herbal medicine is effective in controlling eczema [eks]. Many herbal folk remedies[15] are prepared by immersing[16] dried leaves or flowers in hot water.

Use **herbal** tea[17] / extract / remedies / medicines • garden / officinal[18] [fɪʃ] **herbs**

(Küchen)kräuter
Kochen[1] schmackhaft[2] Schnittlauch[3] Petersilie[4] Basilikum[5] Fenchel[6] Thymian[7] Salbei[8] Rosmarin[9] Minze[10] Kamille[11] krautartig, Kräuter-; Kräuterbuch[12] Herbarium, Kräutersammlung[13] Kräutersammler, -doktor[14] pflanzliche Hausmittel[15] ansetzen[16] Kräutertee[17] pflanzliche Drogen, Heilkräuter[18]   20

food substitute *or* **replacer** *n*   *rel* **food exchange list**[1] *n*

foods similar in nutritive value and/or taste that are used to replace foodstuffs a person must strictly avoid[2]

substitute[3] *v* • substitution[4] *n* • replace[3] *v* • replacement[4] *n*

» Substitution with any food low in saturated fat such as bran[5] or nuts will have positive effects.

Use fat / meat / coffee / milk[6] **substitute** • **substitution** of margarine for butter

Nahrungsmittelersatz(stoff)
Nährwert-, Lebensmitteltabelle[1] meiden[2] ersetzen[3] Ersatz, Substitution[4] Kleie[5] Milchersatz[6]

21

nutritional supplement *n term*   *rel* **food additives**[1] *n term*

enrichment of foods with nutrients[2] such as vitamins to improve dietary intake according to specific needs

supplement[3] *v* • supplementary, -al[4] *adj* • additional[5] *adj*

» The first dietary measure [eʒ] is a low-fat diet supplemented with medium-chain triglycerides [aɪ]. Claims that dyes[6] [daɪz], emulsifiers[7], stabilizers[8], and other food additives may contribute to hyperactivity in children are controversial.

Use diet(ary) / (multi)vitamin / mineral / calcium / iron[9] / daily high fiber[10] / weight-loss **supplement** • iron-**supplemented** • dietary bulk[10] **additive** • **additive**-free baby food[11]

Nährstoffanreicherung
Lebensmittelzusatzstoffe, Additive[1] Nährstoffe[2] ergänzen[3] ergänzend[4] zusätzlich[5] Lebensmittelfarbstoffe[6] Emulgatoren[7] Stabilisatoren[8] Eisenanreicherung[9] Ballaststoffanreicherung[10] zusatzstofffreie Kindernahrung[11]

22

cooked *adj*   *opposite* **raw**[1] [rɒː], **uncooked**[1] *adj*

food prepared for consumption by heating; it can be baked[2] (dry oven heat), boiled[3] (in hot water) fried[4] (in hot oil), steamed[5] [iː] (in water vapor [eɪ]), stewed[6] [stuːd], roasted[7], broiled[8] or barbequed (abbr BBQ)

(pre/over/pressure-)cook[9] *v* • cooking *n* • cookery *n* • cookbook *n*

» Do you want your chicken roasted, fried or with stuffing[10]?

gekocht
roh, ungekocht[1] gebacken[2] gekocht, -sotten[3] gebraten[4] gedünstet[5] gedünstet, -schmort[6] geröstet[7] gegrillt[8] (vor-/ver-/m. Dampf) kochen[9] Füllung[10]   23

8 BASIC MEDICAL & HEALTH TERMS — Injuries

beverage [bevərɪdʒ] n   syn **drinks** n usu pl

any liquid suitable for drinking including mineral water, fruit juice[1], tea, carbonated[2] and alcoholic drinks

drink-drank-drunk v irr • drinkable[3] adj • drinking[4] adj & n • drinker[5] n

» How much do you ordinarily drink? Did you have any artificially sweetened beverages? He is a heavy drinker[6].
Use carbonated / alcoholic **beverages** • to have a **drink**[7] • hard / long / soft[8] **drinks** • **drinking** water[9] / soda / age / bout[10] [aʊ] • beer / wine / tea / social[11] **drinker**

> Note: Both in colloquial and clinical situations drink, drinking and drinker are frequently used to refer to alcohol intake (esp when not further specified).

Getränk
Fruchtsaft[1] kohlensäurehaltig[2] trinkbar[3] Trink-; (Be)trinken[4] Trinker(in)[5] Alkoholiker(in), Säufer(in)[6] etwas trinken[7] alkoholfreie G.[8] Trinkwasser[9] Trinkgelage, Zecherei[10] Gesellschaftstrinker(in)[11]

24

---

juice [dʒuːs] n

(i) liquid that can be extracted from fruit and vegetables (ii) body fluid, e.g gastric juice[1]
juicy[2] adj

» Pour [ɔː] some lemon juice[3] over the cutlet[4] [ʌ]. Is your steak juicy?
Use orange / grapefruit / apple / tomato [eɪ] **juice** • **juice** bar

Saft
Magensaft[1] saftig[2] Zitronensaft[3] Schnitzel[4]

25

---

caffein(e) [kæfiːn] n

bitter alkaloid contained in coffee, cocoa[1] [koʊkoʊ], and tea that is responsible for their stimulating effects

caffeinism[2] n • caffea[3] n • café[4] [kæfeɪ] n • (de)caffeinated[5] adj

» A few cups of coffee can significantly disturb sleep in some patients.
Use **caffeine** withdrawal[6] [ɒːəl] • ground[7] [aʊ] **coffee** • **coffee** bean[8] • black / green / iced **tea**

Koffein
Kakao[1] Koffeinvergiftung[2] Kaffeestrauch[3] Kaffeehaus[4] koffeinhaltig; -frei[5] Koffeinentzug[6] gemahlener Kaffee[7] Kaffeebohne[8]

26

---

alcoholic drinks n   sim **brew(age)**[1] [bruːɪdʒ] n , **booze**[2] [buːz] n inf

fermented brew or distilled alcohol-containing drinks, e.g. beer, wine, cider[3] [saɪdər], etc.
alcohol n • alcoholic[4] adj & n • alcoholism[5] n

» Alcohol consumption also raises [eɪ] the blood pressure. He's been an alcoholic for years.
Use **alcoholic** excess[6] / patient • **alcohol** ingestion or consumption[7] / abuse[8] /-dependent[9] • **Alcoholics** Anonymous[10]

alkoholische Getränke
Gebräu[1] Alkohol, Schnaps[2] Apfelwein, Most[3] alkoholisch, -haltig; Alkoholiker(in)[4] Alkoholabhängigkeit, Alkoholismus[5] Alkoholexzess[6] Alkoholkonsum[7] Alkoholmissbrauch[8] alkoholabhängig[9] Anonyme Alkoholiker[10]

27

---

liquor [lɪkər] n   syn **spirits** n pl BE

hard (alcoholic) drinks[1] which are distilled[2] rather than fermented[3], e.g. whiskey, vodka, brandy, gin, tequila

» Heavy users of hard liquor and wine account for[4] 40% of cases of pancreatitis [aɪtɪs].
Use **liquor** store[5] • to drown in[6] [aʊ]/ intoxicating[7] / bottles of **liquor**

> Note: In medical English liquor is practically never used to refer to body fluids, e.g. the amniotic or the cerebrospinal [aɪ] fluid[8].

Spirituosen
harte Getränke[1] gebrannt[2] vergoren[3] ausmachen[4] Spirituosengeschäft[5] (Sorgen) im A. ertränken[6] berauschendes Getränk[7] Zerebrospinalflüssigkeit, Liquor (cerebrospinalis)[8]

28

Unit 3   Injuries
Related Units: **17** Fractures, **16** Pain, **13** General Pathology, **28** Wound Healing, **29** Fracture Management

---

injure [ɪndʒər] v usu pass   syn **hurt, wound** [uː] v → U16-3

to hurt oneself or harm somebody else
injury[1] n • (un)injured / (un)hurt adj • the injured[2] n

» Do not rub or massage [-ɑː(d)ʒ] injured tissues or apply ice or heat. The injured area should be cleansed [e] with soap or antiseptic and sterile dressings[3] applied.
Use badly / seriously [ɪə]/ critically / fatally[4] **injured** • **injured** extremity / area / head / party[5] / tissue / epithelium [iː] • **to hurt** oneself / one's back

> Note: Do not confuse to injure and injury with insure[6] [ɪnʃʊər] and insurance[7].

(sich) verletzen, verwunden
Verletzung[1] Verletzte(r)[2] Verband[3] tödlich verletzt[4] verletzte Person / Partei[5] versichern (lassen)[6] Versicherung[7]

1

Injuries BASIC MEDICAL & HEALTH TERMS

injury [ˈɪndʒəi] n   syn **trauma** [ˈtrɔːmə] n term

damage or wound inflicted[1] on the body by external forces

injurious[2] [ɪndʒʊəˈɪəs] adj • injury-free adj

» Many patients find even minor injuries (such as venipuncture) unbearable[3] [eə]. Tell me about the circumstances of your injury. Where is your injury? Excess carotene is not injurious.

Use to sustain[4]/receive **an injury** • **injury** to the breast[5] [e]/ from exposure to cold[6] • site / type / degree / mechanism [k]/ pattern **of injury** • head / brain / spinal [aɪ] cord[7] / blast[8] / whiplash[9] / facial [ˈfeɪʃəl] **injury** • work(-related) / sports / thermal / cold[6] / radiation / renal [iː]/ self-inflicted[10] / bodily[11] **injury** • superficial / blunt[12] [ʌ]/ closed / penetrating / needle stick[13] / crush(ing)[14] [ʌ]/ soft tissue[15] / impalement[16] [eɪ] **injury** • **injured** extremity / area / head • **injurious** effect / agent[17]

Verletzung, Trauma
zugefügt[1] schädlich[2] unerträglich[3] V. erleiden[4] Brustverletzung[5] Erfrierung[6] Rückenmarkverletzung[7] Explosionstrauma[8] Schleudertrauma[9] Selbstverstümmelung[10] Körperverletzung[11] stumpfe V.[12] Nadelstichverletzung[13] Quetschung[14] Weichteilverletzung[15] Pfählungsverletzung[16] schädliche Substanz[17]

2

wound [wuːnd] v & n   syn **traumatize** v term, **injure** v, sim **harm**[1] v

(v) to cause an injury, esp one that breaks the skin (n) injury to the skin or an internal organ caused by violence [aɪ] or a surgical incision

wounded[2] n & adj • harm n • unharmed[3] adj

» The wound was dressed with a plain pad[4] and bandage. It was a simple through-and-through bullet [ʊ] wound[5]. The wound exudate[6] was quite frothy[7]. Explore and debride [iː] the wound carefully.

Use to inflict/cause/approximate[8]/clean/cover/dress[9]/swab[10] [ɒː]/close **a wound** • **wound** healing / care[11] / cleanser[12] [e]/ closure • deep / burn / bite / flesh / open / penetrating **wound** • gunshot / puncture or stab[13] / clean / contaminated / gaping[14] [eɪ]/ surgical **wound** • **wound** cavity / abscess / discharge[6] / margins[15] [dʒ]/ edges[15] / surface • to do sb[16] / to come to / bodily[17] **harm**

verletzen, verwunden; Wunde, Verwundung
verletzen, Schaden zufügen[1] Verletzte(r); verwundet[2] unverletzt, -versehrt[3] Wundauflage[4] Durchschuss[5] Wundsekret[6] trüb[7] Wundränder adaptieren[8] W. verbinden[9] W. abtupfen[10] Wundversorgung[11] Wundreinigungsmittel[12] Stichwunde[13] klaffende W.[14] Wundränder[15] jem. Schaden / e. Verletzung zufügen[16] Körperverletzung[17]

3

trauma [ˈtrɔːmə] n term, pl **-s** or **-ata**   syn **injury, wound** n

physical or psychic [ˈsaɪkɪk] injury caused by accidents, violent action, toxic substances, emotional shock, etc.

traumatic adj term • traumatize v • -trauma, trauma(to)- comb

» There was eyelid swelling from blunt trauma to the orbit. The CNS bleeding occurred without evidence of antecedent [siː] trauma or of a specific lesion.

Use **trauma** center / care / index • high risk for **trauma** • acoustic[1] [kuː]/ birth / facial / arterial **trauma** • emotional / major[2][eɪdʒ]/ multiple[3] **trauma** • a/ non/ post-**traumatic** • **traumatic** death[4] [e]/ in origin / pain / shock / event[5] / (brain) injury / sexual experience • **traumatized** zone [zoʊn]/ patient[6] • **traumatology** /genic • baro/ microtrauma

Trauma, Wunde, seelische Erschütterung
Schalltrauma[1] schweres T.[2] Polytrauma[3] Unfalltod[4] traumatisches Ereignis[5] Traumapatient(in)[6]

4

lesion [ˈliːʒən] n term → U13-3   sim **sore**[1] [sɔːr] n clin → U16-11

(i) wound or injury (ii) broad term for all kinds of tissue damage (skin sores[2], ulcers [ʌls], tumors, etc.)

» If the carious lesion progresses, infection of the dental pulp may occur, causing acute pulpitis [-aɪtɪs].

Use gross[3] [oʊ]/ deep seated / occult / palpable / nodular / localized / focal[4] / irritative / polypoid / premalignant[5] / necrotic **lesion** • skin[2] / scalp[6] / vaginal [dʒ] wall / rib / solitary[7] / recurrent[8] [ɜː|ʌ] **lesions** • bed or pressure[9] / running[10] / oriental / cold[11] **sore**

(i) Verletzung (ii) Läsion, Schädigung, Tumor
wunde Stelle, Geschwür[1] Hautläsionen[2] makroskopische Läsion[3] Herdläsion[4] Präkanzerose[5] Kopfhautverletzungen[6] Solitärläsionen[7] Rezidive[8] Dekubital-, Druckgeschwür[9] eiternde Wunde[10] Herpes simplex, Fieberbläschen[11]

5

cut n & v   sim **slash**[1], **slice**[2] [aɪ] n & v clin, **incision**[3] n term → U21-9

(n) wound made by cutting (v) incise the skin or tissue by accident[4] or intention with a knife [naɪf], scalpel, scissors [ˈsɪzɚz], etc.

cutdown[5] n term → U22-18 • cut through/away/off[6]/in v jar

» He had a bad cut on his shin[7]. She cut her soles[8] on the broken glass. Cut the umbilical cord[9].

Use slight / superficial / deep **cut** • venous[5] [iː] • **cutdown** • **cut** edge[10] / surface[11] / section / ends / into slices [aɪ] • vein [eɪ] was **cut** and ligated[12] [aɪ] • **to slash** one's wrists[13] [rɪsts]

Schnittwunde, -verletzung; (ein/ab/durch/zer)schneiden
(langer / tiefer) Schnitt; aufschlitzen[1] Scheibe; (Scheiben) schneiden[2] (Ein)schnitt, Inzision[3] versehentlich[4] Venae Sectio, Venenschnitt[5] ab-, wegschneiden[6] Schienbein[7] Fußsohlen[8] Nabelschnur[9] Schnittrand[10] Schnittfläche[11] V. wurde ligiert u. durchtrennt[12] s. die Pulsadern aufschneiden[13]

6

BASIC MEDICAL & HEALTH TERMS — Injuries

laceration [læsəreɪʃ°n] n term · sim tear¹ [teə·] n clin

(i) a torn external or internal wound with rough [rʌf] margins²; not a cut or incision
(ii) the act of lacerating

lacerated³ adj term • lacerate v usu pass • lacerable adj • torn adj

» Bleeding from the external ear is most commonly due to⁴ local laceration or abrasion. A tear had developed in the intima of the aorta [eɪ].

Use **lacerated** wound / tendon⁵ • scar from / skin / pelvic floor⁶ / puncture⁷ / flap-type **laceration** • **laceration of the** liver / pleura [ʊ]/ cervix / perineum⁸ • **torn** dura / vessel⁹ • retinal / esophageal [dʒɪəl] **tear**

Riss-, Platzwunde; Zerreißung
(Ein)riss, Ruptur¹ ausgefranste Ränder² ein-, aufgerissen, zerfetzt³ zurückzuführen auf⁴ Sehnenriss, -ruptur⁵ Beckenbodenriss⁶ Stichwunde⁷ Dammriss⁸ Gefäßruptur⁹

7

abrasion [əbreɪʒ°n] n term · syn graze [eɪ] n & v clin, sim chafe¹ [tʃeɪf] v & n, excoriation² n term

(i) wound caused by scraping [eɪ] the skin against a rough object
(ii) pathologic or therapeutic grinding or wearing [eə·] away³ of superficial tissue layers, e.g. of tooth substance, skin layers, uterine mucosa, etc.

abrasive⁴ adj & n term • abrade⁵ v • excoriated adj

» Abrasions such as a skinned knee⁶ [niː] or a floor burn⁷ should be washed, a mild antiseptic ointment⁸ applied, and covered with sterile gauze⁹ [ɔː].

Use superficial [ɪʃ]/ facial / scalp / corneal¹⁰ / multiple **abrasion** • **abrasions and/or** contusions [juː]/ lacerations • derm**abrasion**

(i) Schürfwunde, Abschürfung, Schramme (ii) Abrieb, Abrasion, Abschabung
aufscheuern, wundreiben; wundgeriebene Stelle¹ Exkoriation² Abtragung³ abreibend; Schleifmittel⁴ abschürfen, -reiben⁵ aufgeschürftes Knie⁶ Abschürfung durch mechan. Reibung⁷ Salbe⁸ (Verbands)mull⁹ Hornhautabschabung, Abrasio corneae¹⁰

8

scratch [skrætʃ] v & n clin · syn scrape [eɪ] v & n clin

(v) (i) to inflict small shallow cuts¹ with a sharp object (ii) scrape or rub oneself with one's fingernails to relieve itching [ɪtʃɪŋ] (n) a small abraded area where the skin is torn or worn off

» The lesions were found along linear scratch marks². The itch³ provokes a desire to scratch.

Use **scratch**-type incision / test⁴ • vigorously [ɪg] **scraped** area • skin / tissue / corneal / uterine⁵ **scrapings** • iris [aɪ] **scraped** free • cat-**scratch** fever⁶ [iː]

(sich) kratzen, schaben; Kratzer, Schramme
oberflächliche Schnittverletzungen¹ Kratzspuren² Juckreiz³ Skarifikations-, Kratztest⁴ Kürettagematerial a.d. Uterus⁵ Katzenkratzkrankheit⁶

9

sting [stɪŋ]-stung-stung v irr & n · sim bite¹-bit-bitten v irr & n, prick² v & n, puncture³ [ʌ] v & n term

(n) wound caused by certain insects (e.g. hornets⁴, wasps [ɒː], fire ants⁵), plants (e.g. nettles⁶, poison ivy⁷ [aɪvi]) and animals (esp marine animals like jellyfish⁸ [dʒ], stingrays⁹, etc.) typically associated with exposure to irritating chemicals or venoms¹⁰

stinging¹¹ adj • biting adj • stinger¹² n • punctured adj term

» Usually the barbed venomous stinger¹³ can be found in place after a bee sting. The girl was stung by several honeybees. Hospitalize all patients who have been bitten by poisonous snakes.

Use insect / scorpion **stings** • animal / dog / cat / mosquito / snake / tick¹⁴ / human / stork¹⁵ **bite** • **bite** wound¹⁶ / injury • flea¹⁷-[iː]/ frost¹⁸-**bitten** • **biting** sensation / louse [aʊ] • **puncture** wound / site¹⁹ • needle / lumbar²⁰ [ʌ]/ acu**puncture** • **to prick** one's finger • **prick** (skin) test²¹

stechen, brennen; (Insekten)stich, Biss, Stachel (BE)
beißen; Biss¹ (ein-, auf-, durch)stechen; (Ein)stich² punktieren, (durch)stechen; Punktion, Einstich³ Hornissen⁴ Feuerameisen⁵ (Brenn)nessel⁶ Gifteffeu⁷ Quallen⁸ Stachelrochen⁹ tierische Gifte¹⁰ stechend, brennend¹¹ Stachel¹² Giftstachel m. Widerhaken¹³ Zeckenbiss¹⁴ Storchenbiss¹⁵ Bisswunde¹⁶ voller Flohbisse¹⁷ erfroren¹⁸ Punktionsstelle¹⁹ Lumbalpunktion²⁰ Pricktest²¹

10

burn [bɜːrn] n & v clin · sim scald¹ [skɔːld] v & n clin

(n) injury to tissues resulting from fire, hot liquids, steam² [iː], acid chemicals, lightning³, electricity or radiation (v) to cause a lesion by heat exposure or suffer pain from heat

scalding⁴ adj clin • sunburn⁵ n • postburn adj term

» Burn scars are often unsightly⁶ [saɪt] and total resolution⁷ is not possible in many cases. The mainstay of treatment of any chemical burn is copious⁸ irrigation with large amounts of tap water⁹. Be careful not to scald the anesthetized tissues.

Use minor / major / deep thermal / 1st degree¹⁰ / contact / friction¹¹ [kʃ] **burns** • chemical or acid¹² / electrical / depth of **burn** • **burn** victim / trauma / coma / care • **burned** body surface • **burning** pain / sensation¹³ / feet / tongue [tʌŋ]/ on urination¹⁴ • **scald(ing)** burn¹ • **scalded** skin¹⁵

Verbrennung, Brandwunde; (sich) verbrennen
(sich) verbrühen; Verbrühung¹ Dampf² Blitzschlag³ siedend (heiß)⁴ Sonnenbrand⁵ hässlich, unansehnlich⁶ Rückbildung⁷ gründlich⁸ Leitungswasser⁹ V. 1. Grades¹⁰ Verbrennungen durch mech. Reibung¹¹ Verätzung¹² Brennen, brennendes Gefühl¹³ Brennen beim Urinieren¹⁴ verbrühte Haut¹⁵

11

Injuries   BASIC MEDICAL & HEALTH TERMS **11**

frostbite [frɒːstbaɪt] n clin   sim **chilblain** [tʃɪlbleɪn] or
                                        (erythema) [iː] pernio[1] n term
  blanching[2], paresthesias[3] [iː], edema [ɪdiːmə] and local tissue destruction as a result of exposure
  to extreme cold
  frostbitten[4] adj clin • frostnip[5] n
» After rewarming the frostbitten area becomes purple [ɜː], painful and tender. Chil-
  blains are red, itching, blistering[6] skin lesions without actual freezing of the tissues.
Use deep / superficial / severe[7] *frostbite* • *frostbitten* toes / digits [dʒ]

bruise [bruːz] n & v clin   syn **contusion** [uː] n,
                                   sim **hematoma**[1] [hiːmətoʊmə] n term → U13-26
  (n) injury to soft tissues produced by blunt trauma (e.g. a blow[2], kick, or fall) producing a
  subcutaneous hematoma from ruptured blood vessels
  (v) to cause a contusion, e.g. by bumping into[3] [ʌ] sth.
  bruising[4] n • contuse v • black eye or shiner[5] [aɪ] n clin
» How did you bruise your forearm? She was treated for cuts and bruises. The left
  kidney is mildly contused. How do you differentiate subdural hematomas from
  cerebral contusion without hematoma?
Use skin **bruises** • to be easily[6] **bruised** • ecchymosis [kɪ] and **bruising** • cerebral[7]
  contusion • **contusion** of the spinal [aɪ] cord • *contused* wound[8]

concussion [kənkʌʃən] n clin & term   syn **commotio** [kəmoʊʃioʊ] n term rare
  (i) generally, a collision [ɪʒ] or violent shaking (ii) the resulting injury to soft tissues, esp. the
  brain or retina
  be concussed[1] phr • concussive[2] adj • postconcussion adj
» Concussion affects only mentation[3], with return of consciousness moments or minutes after impact[4]. Amnesia[5] [iːʒ] after concussion typically follows a few moments
  of unresponsiveness[6].
Use **concussion of the** brain[7] / spinal cord[8] • to suffer a[9] / cerebral / cochlear [k]/
  grade 3 **concussion** • **concussive** effect / blow / (head) injury / state • **postconcussion** headache / syndrome[10]

swelling n clin   sim **puffiness**[1] [ʌ] n clin,
                        tumescence[2], **edema**[3] [ɪdiːmə] n term
  abnormal localized enlargement due to accumulation of fluid[4] in the tissue
  swell[5]-swelled-swollen v irr • puffy[6] adj • edematous[7] [e] adj
» Is the painful swelling in her breast [e] due to bruising? Venous stasis [eɪ] may
  sometimes affect lymphatic vessels, producing a permanent swelling called solid
  edema[8].
Use **swelling** subsides[9] • **swollen** lymph nodes / joints / ankle / nasal mucosa • acute
  / local(ized) / diffuse / inflammatory[10] / marked[11] / painful or tender **swelling** •
  facial / soft tissue / ankle / eyelid[12] / cloudy[13] [aʊ] **swelling** • **puffiness** about the
  eyes

sprain [eɪ] n & v clin   sim **torsion**[1] [ʃ] n term
  (n) injury to the tendons[2], ligaments[3] and/or capsule around a joint (v) to twist[4] a joint
  torsional[5] adj • distort[6] v • distortion[7] n
» It was just a sprain, the ligament was not torn and there was no avulsion fracture[8].
  How did you sprain your ankle?
Use ankle / foot / knee / collateral ligament[9] / (un)stable **sprain** • **sprain** fracture[8] •
  sprained ankle[10] / wrist [rɪst] • (internal/external) tibial / testicular[11] **torsion** •
  torsional movement / displacement[12] / stress • outward / medial / radiographic
  / mandibular[13] **distortion** • **distorted** face[14] / anatomy / body image

  ▪ Note: In English medical usage *distortion* and *sprain* are not synonymous.

Erfrierung, Congelatio
Frostbeule, Pernio[1] Blässe, Blass-
werden[2] Parästhesien, Sensibili-
tätsstörungen[3] erfroren[4] leichte Erfrierung[5] mit Blasenbildung[6]
schwere / hochgradige Erfrierung[7]
                                    12

**Quetschung, Prellung, Kon-
tusion, Bluterguss; quetschen,
s. einen blauen Fleck holen**
Hämatom, Bluterguss[1] Schlag,
Stoß[2] stoßen gegen[3] Prellungen,
blaue Flecke(n)[4] blaues Auge, Veil-
chen[5] leicht blaue Flecke(n) bekommen[6] Hirnprellung, Contusio
cerebri[7] Quetschwunde[8]
                                    13

**(Gehirn)erschütterung,
Commotio**
(Gehirn)erschütterung haben[1] er-
schütternd[2] mentale Funktionen[3]
Aufprall, Stoß[4] Amnesie, Erinnerungslücke[5] Nichtansprechbarkeit[6]
Commotio cerebri[7] Commotio spi-
nalis, Rückenmarkerschütterung[8]
eine Gehirnerschütterung erleiden[9]
postkommotionelles Syndrom[10] 14

(An)schwellung
Aufgedunsenheit[1] Tumeszenz, (diffuse) Anschwellung[2] Ödem[3] Flüssigkeitsansammlung[4] (an)schwel-
len[5] verschwollen[6] ödematös[7]
Myxödem[8] Schwellung klingt ab[9]
entzündliche Schwellung[10] starke
Schwellung[11] Lidschwellung[12]
trübe Schwellung[13]
                                    15

**Verstauchung, Zerrung, Dis-
torsion; zerren, verstauchen,
überdehnen**
Torsion, (Ver)drehung[1] Sehnen[2]
Bänder[3] verdrehen, -stauchen, um-
knicken[4] Dreh-, Torsions-[5] verdrehen, -zerren[6] Verzerrung[7] Abrissfraktur[8] Seitenbandzerrung[9] ver-
stauchter Knöchel[10] Hodentorsion[11]
Drehfehlstellung[12] Unterkieferasymmetrie[13] verzerrtes Gesicht[14] 16

12 BASIC MEDICAL & HEALTH TERMS — Injuries

strain [eɪ] *v & n clin*   *sim* **pull**[1] *v* , **sprain** *v & n clin*

(v) to overstretch[2] or overexercise a muscle [mʌsl] or ligament (n) damage (usually muscular [kjʊ]) resulting from excessive physical effort[3]

straining[4] *n* • strenuous[5] [e] *adj*

» You must avoid flexing[6], lifting and straining. Causes of chronic low back pain may also include back strain due to poor posture[7] [pɒːstʃɚ] or poor conditioning[8] that is aggravated[9] by mechanical factors (e.g. overuse[10] or obesity [iː]).

Use to strain *or* pull[1] **a muscle** • (low) back[11] / muscle[12] / abduction / right heart[13] / emotional[14] **strain** • abdominal[15] **straining**

überdehnen, -lasten, zerren; Überdehnung, -belastung, Zerrung
(Muskel) zerren[1] überdehnen[2] körperliche Überanstrengung[3] Anstrengung, Belastung[4] anstrengend[5] Beugen, Bücken[6] schlechte Haltung[7] schlechter Trainingszustand[8] verschlechtert[9] Überbelastung, -training[10] überanstrengter/s Rücken / Kreuz[11] Muskelzerrung[12] Rechtsherzbelastung[13] seelische Belastung[14] Bauchpresse[15]   17

---

rupture [rʌptʃɚ] *n & v term*   *syn* **tear** [teɚ] -tore-torn *n & v irr clin*,   *sim* **disruption**[1] [ʌ] *n term*

(n) a break [eɪ] or tear in continuity[2] of soft tissues (tendons, vessels)

(un)ruptured *adj* • tearing *n* • disrupt[3] *v* • disruptive[4] *adj*

» On laparoscopy blunt diaphragmatic rupture was diagnosed. There was a tear of the middle meningeal artery.

Use traumatic / spontaneous[5] [eɪ] **rupture** • tendon[6] / partial[7] / delayed [eɪ]/ free / contained[8] [eɪ] **rupture** • splenic[9] [e]/ bladder[10] / aortic [eɪ] **rupture** • **rupture of** the diaphragm [æm]/ an aneurysm [ænjərɪzᵊm]/ membranes[11] / longitudinal ligaments • **ruptured** eardrum[12] / vessels / scar[13] / ligamentous[14] / partial[15] / neural / family[16] **disruption** • **disrupted** muscle / sleep[17] / speech • **disruptive** behavior[18] / child / patient • **tear** injury • wear-and-[19] [eɚ]/ hamstring[20] / meniscal **tear**

Note: Mark the difference in pronunciation and meaning in tear[21] [ɪɚ] and tearing[22] [ɪɚ].

Ruptur, Riss, (Durch)bruch, Hernie; reißen, platzen, rupturieren
Zerreißung, Spaltung[1] Kontinuität[2] (zer)stören, zerreißen, spalten[3] zerreißend, -störend[4] Spontanruptur[5] Sehnenriss, -ruptur[6] Einriss[7] gedeckte Ruptur[8] Milzruptur[9] Blasenruptur[10] Blasensprung[11] Trommelfellruptur[12] Narbenbruch[13] Bänderriss[14] Zerrung[15] zerrüttete Familienverhältnisse[16] gestörter Schlaf[17] störendes / destruktives Verhalten[18] Abnutzung, Verschleiß[19] Zerrung / Riss der Oberschenkelbeuger[20] Träne[21] Tränen(träufeln); tränend[22]   18

---

hemorrhage [hemərɪdʒ] *n term*   *syn* **bleeding** *n clin*, **bleed** *n jar* → U13-26

internal or external bleeding usually from a ruptured vessel, e.g. prolonged minor oozing [uːzɪŋ] of blood[1] from minute[2] [maɪnuːt] vessels or acute and massive extravasation[3]

hemorrhagic *adj* • nosebleed[4] *n* • bleeder[5] *n* • bleed-bled-bled *v irr*

» In an arterial [ɪɚ] hemorrhage the blood is bright red in color and comes in spurts[6] [ɜː].

Use to arrest *or* stop a[7] **hemorrhage** • acute / major[8] / brisk[8] / profuse[8] / intracranial / internal[9] **hemorrhage** • petechial [k]/ capillary / postextraction / postpartum[10] / essential / concealed[11] [siː]/ secondary[12] **hemorrhage** • **hemorrhagic** disease of the newborn[13] / fever

Blutung, Hämorrhagie
Sickerblutung[1] kleinste[2] Blutaustritt, Blutung[3] Nasenbluten[4] Bluter(in), Hämophile(r)[5] pulssynchron spritzen[6] Blutung stillen[7] starke B.[8] innere B.[9] Nachgeburtsblutung[10] okkulte B.[11] Nachblutung[12] hämorrhagische Diathese d. Neugeborenen[13]   19

---

dislocation *n term*   *rel* **displacement**[1] *n*, **fracture**[2] *n & v term* → U17-1ff

displacement of the articular surface of a bone from its joint; in displaced fractures the main bony fragments are widely separated

dislocate[3] *v term* • displace[4] *v* • (un)displaced *adj*

» Proper positioning of the x-ray tube[5] will improve identification of the radial head dislocation. Swelling may mask the bone displacement.

Use hip / elbow (joint) / carpal / traumatic / fracture-[6]/ (un)complicated / recurrent[7] [ɜː:‖ʌ] **dislocation** • **dislocation of the** shoulder / jaw [dʒɔː]/ thumb[8] [θʌm] • downward / anterior / medial / lateral **displacement** • degree[9] / direction **of displacement** • double / (non)displaced[10] / old (healed) / (un)stable[11] **fracture** • **fracture** site[12] [aɪ]/ fragments / reduction[13] / nail / healing • **fractured** rib / limb [lɪm]/ jaw[14]

Verrenkung, Luxation
Verschiebung, Fehlstellung, Dislokation[1] (Knochen)fraktur, -bruch; (Knochen) brechen / frakturieren[2] verrenken, luxieren[3] verschieben, dislozieren[4] Röntgenröhre[5] Luxationsfraktur[6] habituelle L.[7] Daumenluxation[8] Grad der Fehlstellung[9] dislozierte Fraktur[10] (in)stabile F.[11] Bruchstelle[12] Reposition d. Fraktur[13] Kieferbruch[14]   20

Unit 4   States of Consciousness

Related Units: 3 Injuries, 47 Anesthesiology, 21 Surgical Treatment, 25 Perioperative Care

conscious [kɒnʃəs] *adj*, **-ly** *adv*   opposite **unconscious**[1] *adj*

(i) associated with thought, will, or perception[2] (ii) related to consciousness (iii) awareness undulled[3] [ʌ] by sleep, faintness, or stupor

(un/sub)**consciousness**[4] *n* • semi**consciousness**[5] *n* • self/subconscious *adj*

» Some patients may consciously or unconsciously engage in forceful air swallowing. She became conscious[6] after the anesthesia wore off[7]. The clinical definition of consciousness ranges from alert wakefulness[8], to mild lethargy, stupor, and deep coma.

Use loss of / to lose / to regain or return to[9] / clouding of[11] [aʊ] **consciousness** • alteration of[10] [ɔː]/ altered state of[10] / to assess the level of **consciousness** • full / impaired[11] [eə]/ compromised[11] / dull[11] / waxing-waning[12] [eɪ] **consciousness** • to lapse or fall into[13]/verify **unconsciousness** • to become[13]/be **unconscious** • **unconscious** patient / guilt[14] [gɪlt]/ motivation [eɪ] • **(un)conscious** process / control • weight [weɪt]/ health[15] [helθ] **conscious**

> Note: Do not confuse self-conscious (inhibited)[16] and self-confident (=self-reliant)[17] [aɪ] as well as conscious and conscience[18] [kɒnʃəns] and conscientious[19] [-ʃɪenʃəs].

bewusst
bewusstlos; unbewusst[1] Wahrnehmung[2] ungetrübt[3] (Unter)bewusstsein[4] Dämmerzustand[5] B. erlangen[6] nachlassen[7] Vigilanz, Wachheit[8] B. wiedererlangen[9] Bewusstseinsstörung, -veränderung[10] Bewusstseinstrübung[11] schwankende Bewusstseinslage[12] Bewusstsein verlieren, bewusstlos werden[13] nicht bewusste Schuld[14] gesundheitsbewusst[15] befangen, gehemmt[16] selbstbewusst[17] Gewissen[18] gewissenhaft[19]

1

alert [əlɜːrt] *adj & v & n term & clin*   sim **arousal**[1][aʊ], **vigilance**[2] [dʒ] *n term*

(adj) be wide awake[3] [eɪ], watchful or mentally responsive, fully aware, (v) to alarm (n) warning signal

alertness[2] *n clin* • **arouse**[4] [aʊ] *v* • **vigilant**[5] *adj*

» An alert, wakeful patient responds immediately and appropriately to all stimuli [aɪ]. A stuporous patient responds only when aroused by vigorous[6] [vɪgərəs] stimulation.

Use quiet/active **alert** state • patient is awake, **alert** and oriented/cooperative • medic-**alert** tag[7] • be **alert** to • be on the[8] **alert** • mental **alertness** and arousal

wach, rege; warnen, alarmieren; Alarm
Erwachen, Erhöhung d. Wachheitsgrades, Arousal[1] Wachheit, Vigilanz[2] hellwach[3] (auf)wecken, erregen[4] wach, rege[5] stark[6] mediz. Informationsplakette[7] einsatzbereit / auf der Hut sein[8]

2

lucid [luːsɪd] *adj term*

mentally clear, not confused, and able to be understood, esp between periods of clouded consciousness

lucidity[1] *n clin* • **lucidness**[1] *n*

» The level of alertness fluctuated considerably[2] with the occurrence of episodic confusion and lucid intervals[3] suggesting delirium.

Use **lucid** periods[3] [ɪə] / intervals[3] / lethargy • periods of[3] **lucidity**

bei Bewusstsein, hell, klar (denkend)
Klarheit, bei klarem Verstand[1] stark schwanken[2] helle Augenblicke / Phasen[3]

3

faint [feɪnt] *v & n & adj term & clin*   sim **blackout**[1], **breakdown**[2] *n clin*, **syncope**[3] [sɪŋkəpi] *n term*

(v) to collapse[6] or pass out[4] (n) temporary loss of consciousness usually due to cerebral hypoxia

faintness[5] *n clin* • break down[6] *v* • syncopal *adj term*

» Shouting and gentle shaking are usually enough to revive[7] [rɪvaɪv] a person who may have fainted or may be just sleeping. The pain may be so severe that the patient faints.

Use to precipitate/produce[8] a **faint** • **syncopal** attack[1] • **fainting** fit or spell[1] • cardiac / vasovagal [eɪ]/ sudden **faint**

> Note: As an adjective faint is also used in medicine to mean weak or hard to hear, see etc. (faint pulse[9]/heart sound/macules)

ohnmächtig werden; Ohnmacht; schwach
(kurze) Ohnmacht, Blackout[1] Kollaps[2] Synkope[3] ohnmächtig werden[4] Schwäche(gefühl)[5] kollabieren[6] ins Bewusstsein zurückholen[7] Ohnmacht verursachen / auslösen[8] schwacher Puls[9]

4

light-headed *adj clin*   sim **(to feel) faint**[1]*phr*, **drowsy**[2] [draʊzi], **dizzy**[3] [dɪzi] *adj clin*

to feel weak or dizzy and likely to lose consciousness

light-headedness[4] *n clin* • **drowsiness**[5] *n*

» Both drowsiness and stupor are usually attended by[6] some degree of mental confusion. Faintness, dizziness, or light-headedness may indicate an impending[7] loss of consciousness.

benommen
einer Ohnmacht nahe sein[1] schläfrig, benommen[2] schwindlig[3] Benommenheit[4] Schläfrigkeit[5] einhergehen mit[6] bevorstehend, drohend[7]

5

14 BASIC MEDICAL & HEALTH TERMS — States of Consciousness

pass out v inf　　sim **be out**[1] v jar, opposite **come to**[2] v clin, BE **come round**[2] phr

to lose consciousness

» When she heard [hɜːrd] about her father's death she passed out.

in Ohnmacht fallen, ohnmächtig werden
bewusstlos / weg sein[1] wieder zu sich kommen[2]　　6

---

unresponsive adj term & jar　　opposite **responsive**[1] adj term & jar

(i) failing to respond to sensations or verbal stimuli (ii) failing to respond to treatment

(un)responsiveness[2] n term • respond (to)[3] v • response[4] n

» Certain psychiatric [saɪkɪætrɪk] states can mimic[5] coma by producing an apparent [e] unresponsiveness.

Use **unresponsive** pupils[6] [pjuːpᵊlz]/ to stimuli / to light • not **responsive** to therapy

(i) nicht ansprechbar (ii) nicht reagierend / ansprechend
ansprechbar[1] Ansprechbarkeit, Reaktionsfähigkeit, Reagibilität[2] reagieren, ansprechen (auf)[3] Reaktion[4] vortäuschen[5] lichtstarre Pupillen[6]　　7

---

disorientation n　　sim **confusion**[1] [-fjuːʒᵊn] n,
　　　　　　　　lose one's bearings[2] [eə·] phr inf

be bewildered[3] [ɪ] or perplexed[4]; reactions to one's surroundings[5] (esp. time, place, person) are inappropriate

(dis)oriented adj • confused[3] adj • orientation n

» Patients with psychotic disorders may be fully oriented or exhibit a disorientation as to person that is at least as great as their disorientation as to time and place.

Use patient is **disoriented** and confused • well-**oriented** to time, place, and person[6] • **disoriented** behavior • acute **disorientation** • confusional state[7]

Desorientiertheit, fehlende Orientierung
Verwirrtheit, Verwirrung[1] Orientierung verlieren[2] verwirrt[3] verblüfft, perplex[4] Umgebung[5] orientiert zu Zeit, Raum, Person[6] Verwirrtheitszustand[7]
　　8

---

stunned [stʌnd] adj inf　　sim **dazed**[1] [deɪzd] adj inf, *****spaced out**[2] [eɪ] adj

(i) knocked out by a heavy blow (ii) mental numbness[3] [nʌmnəs] esp. due to a shock, great surprise or intense light

» Suspect lightning injury[4] in persons found dazed or unconscious after a thunderstorm[5].

(i) betäubt (durch einen Schlag) (ii) benommen, (wie) gelähmt, fassungslos
benommen, verwirrt[1] (wie) unter Drogen, weg, high[2] Benommenheit[3] Verletzung durch Blitzschlag[4] Gewitter[5]　　9

---

obtunded [ʌ] adj term　　sim **blunt**[1] [ʌ], **dull**[2] [ʌ] adj & v clin

reduced level of consciousness; insensitive to pain as a result of an analgesic[3] [-dʒiːsɪk] or anesthetic[4]

obtundent[5] adj & n • obtundation n

» If lavage [ləvɑːʒ] is done in an obtunded or comatose patient, prophylactic insertion of a cuffed [ʌ] endotracheal [eɪk] tube[6] is recommended to prevent aspiration. Brain function may range from alertness to obtundation.

Use be/become **obtunded** • deeply[7] **obtunded** • state of mental / prolonged **obtundation**

teilnahmslos, abgestumpft, gedämpft
abgestumpft; abstumpfen[1] teilnahmslos; abstumpfen, dämpfen[2] Schmerzmittel[3] Narkotikum[4] dämpfend; dämpfendes Mittel[5] Endotrachealtubus m. Cuff[6] stark gedämpft[7]
　　10

---

stupor [st(j)uːpɚ] n term

impaired[1] [eə] or reduced consciousness with marked decrease in responsiveness to stimulation

(semi-)stuporous[2] adj term • stupefaction[3] n • stupefacient[4] [-feɪʃᵊnt] adj & n

» In stuporous catatonia the patient is subdued[5], mute[6] [mjuːt], and negativistic, accompanied by varying combinations of staring [eə], rigidity [dʒɪ], and cataplexy.

Use alcoholic / anergic [ənɜːrdʒɪk]/ benign [aɪn] / catatonic[7] / depressive / delusion[8] / epileptic / postseizure[9] [iː3] **stupor** • **stuporous** patient

Stupor, Reaktionsunfähigkeit
eingeschränkt[1] stuporös[2] Betäubung, Benommensein[3] betäubend; Betäubungsmittel[4] gedämpft[5] stumm[6] katatoner Stupor[7] schizophrener S.[8] Stupor nach epileptischem Anfall[9]
　　11

---

lethargy [leθɚdʒɪ] n term　　sim **apathy**[1] [æ] n, opposite **hyperactivity**[2],
　　　　　　　　agitation[3] [dʒ] n term

a state of abnormal indifference[4], listlessness[5], sluggishness[6] [ʌ], lassitude[6], languor[6] [gɚ] or stupor

lethargic adj term • apathetic adj • hyperactive adj • agitated[7] adj

» Apathy, drowsiness, and confusion improve more gradually. Hepatic encephalopathy may begin with irritability[8] and mild confusion and slowly progress to agitation, lethargy, change in personality and difficulties in judgment[9] and orientation.

Use fatigue [fətiːg] and[10] **lethargy** • depression, withdrawal[11] [-drɒːᵊl] and **apathy** • **apathetic** state / hyperthyroidism [aɪ]

Lethargie
Apathie[1] Hyperaktivität[2] psychomotor. Unruhe, Agitiertheit[3] Gleichgültigkeit[4] Antriebs-, Teilnahmslosigkeit[5] Trägheit, Mattigkeit[6] agitiert[7] Gereiztheit[8] Urteilsvermögen[9] Müdigkeit u. Lethargie[10] Zurückziehen[11]
　　12

States of Consciousness | BASIC MEDICAL & HEALTH TERMS 15

somnolence n term & clin sim **sopor**[1] [soʊpɚ] n term

(i) semicomatose state (ii) state of unnatural drowsiness

somnolent adj term • **soporific**[2] adj & n • **soporiferous**[2] adj

» The patient complained of excessive daytime somnolence, morning sluggishness and fatigue. Her lethargy deepened into somnolence.

Use episodes of **somnolence** • **somnolent** and lethargic / metabolic rate

(i) schläfrige Teilnahmslosigkeit (ii) Somnolenz

Sopor, schlafähnl. Zustand[1] einschläfernd; Schlafmittel[2]

13

coma [koʊmə] n term & clin

profound [aʊ] unconsciousness[1] from which a patient cannot be aroused even by powerful stimuli [aɪ]

comatose[2] [-toʊs] adj term • semi-comatose adj • coma-like[3] adj

» CNS symptoms include lethargy, coma, and convulsions [ʌ]. Pinpoint pupils[4], coma, and hypertension are suggestive [dʒe] of[5] cerebellar hemorrhage [e].

Use to lapse into[6]/be in/lie in / induced[7] **coma** • alcoholic / deep hepatic / diabetic [e] or hypoglycemic [-glaɪsi:]/ thyrotoxic[8] [aɪ]/ uremic [i:] **coma** • Glasgow **coma** scale[9] [eɪ] • to be/become **comatose** • deeply[10] **comatose**

Koma

tiefe Bewusstlosigkeit[1] komatös[2] komaartig[3] stecknadelkopfgroße Pupillen[4] sind ein Anzeichen für[5] ins Koma fallen[6] künstl. Tiefschlaf[7] thyreotoxisches Koma[8] Glasgow-Komaskala[9] tief komatös[10]

14

trance [træns‖trɑːns] n term

(i) altered state of consciousness as in hypnosis [ɪ], hysteria [ɪ], or ecstasy (ii) dazed or stuporous state (iii) detachment[1] [ætʃ] from one's surroundings (e.g. in deep concentration or daydreaming[2])

» A history of trancelike states[3] during which simple motor behaviors persist corroborates[4] the presence of daytime somnolence.

Use alcoholic / hypnotic[5] / induced[5] / death[6] **trance** • **trance**-like state / attack

Trance(zustand)

Losgelöstsein[1] Tag-, Wachträumen[2] tranceähnliche Zustände[3] bestätigt, erhärtet[4] hypnotischer Schlaf[5] Scheintod[6]

15

delirium n term

clouded state of consciousness and confusion, marked by difficulty in sustaining attention to stimuli, anxiety[1] [æŋzaɪəti], illusions and hallucinations, disordered sleep-wakefulness cycles[2] [saɪklz], motor disturbances; etc.

delirious[3] adj term

» Delirium is an acute confusional state associated with a change in level of consciousness ranging from lethargy and withdrawal to agitation. Symptoms and signs of delirium tremens include profoundly delirious states associated with tremulousness[4] and agitation.

Use delirious patient • **delirium** tremens[5] (abbr DT) / of persecution[6] • acute / exhaustion[7] [ɪgzɔːstʃ°n]/ traumatic / febrile[8] [e‖iː] **delirium**

Delir, Delirium

ängstl. Erregung, Angst(zustände)[1] gestörter Schlaf-Wach-Rhythmus[2] delirant[3] Zittern[4] Delirium tremens, Alkohol-, Entzugsdelir[5] Verfolgungswahn[6] Erschöpfungsdelirium[7] Fieberdelir[8]

16

persistent vegetative [vedʒ-] **state** n term, abbr **PVS** syn **vigil** [dʒ] **coma** n, rel **akinetic** [eɪkaɪnetɪk] **mutism**[1] [juː] n term

state of unresponsiveness due to diffuse cortical or brain stem damage[2]

» PVS patients may show some improvement from an initially comatose state and appear to be awake but lie motionless and without evidence of awareness or higher mental activity.

apallisches Syndrom, Coma vigile, Wachkoma

akinetischer Mutismus[1] Hirnstammschädigung[2]

17

brain death [deθ] n term syn **irreversible coma**

cessation [s] and irreversibility[1] of brain function; legal definitions vary from state to state

brain-dead[2] adj term

» The criteria [aɪ] for brain death must persist[3] for 6 hours with a confirmatory isoelectric [aɪ] (flat) EEG[4].

Use to confirm/declare/establish[5]/mimic **brain death** • diagnosis of / diagnostic criterion [kraɪtɪɔːrɪ°n] for **brain death** • **brain death** legislation [dʒ]

Hirntod

irreversibler Ausfall[1] hirntot[2] bestehen, andauern[3] isoelektr. / Nulllinien-EEG[4] Hirntoddiagnose sicherstellen[5]

18

Unit 5 Drugs and Remedies

Related Units: 19 Pharmacologic Treatment, 20 Pharmacologic Agents, 48 Types of Anesthesia & Anesthetics

medication n term　　syn **medicine** n clin & inf, **medicament** n rare

(i) medicinal preparations[1] (ii) administration[2] of remedies
medicinal[3] adj term • medical[4] adj • medicate[5] v • self-medication n

» Relapses[6] can be treated with a second course[7] of these medications. Don't forget to take your medicine! Are you on any medication?

Use to take/start/receive [iː]/continue/discontinue[8]/review[9] [vjuː] **medication** • oral / pre[10]/ transdermal / sodium-containing[11] / pain **medication** • preoperative / daily schedule [skǁʃ] of / life-long[12] **medication** • **medicinal** drug[13] / herbs[14] [ɜːrbz]/ iron supplementation [ʌ] • **medical** therapy[15] • **medicated** bath / shampoo[16] / soap [oʊ]/ area

(i) Medikament(e) (ii) Arznei-(mittel)verordnung, -anwendung, Medikation
Präparate[1] Verabreichung[2] medizinisch, Heil-[3] medizinisch, ärztlich[4] medikamentös behandeln[5] Rückfälle, Rezidive[6] Zyklus, Kur[7] Medikament absetzen[8] Med. überprüfen[9] Prämedikation[10] natriumhaltiges Med.[11] Dauermedikation[12] Arzneidroge[13] Heilkräuter[14] medikamentöse Beh.[15] medizinisches Shampoo[16]　　1

remedy [remədi] n & v clin　　rel **remediation**[1] [iː] n term

(n) substance or treatment that can cure[2] [kjʊɚ] a disease or relieve[3] pain or other symptoms
(v) to cure
remediable[4] [iː] adj clin • remedial[5] adj

» The cause of his hearing loss (impaction of ear wax[6]) was easily remediable. Hot showers are an age-old remedy for itching disorders[7]. Obstructive [ʌ] causes must be excluded or remedied.

Use pain-relieving / herbal[8] (folk) / home[9] / over-the-counter[10] / cold[11] **remedy** • **remedy for** internal/external use[12] / burns • **remediable** condition

(Heil- / Arznei)mittel; bessern, heilen
Behandlung, Besserung[1] kurieren, heilen[2] lindern[3] heil-, behebbar[4] heilend, Heil-[5] Zeruminalpfropf[6] bewährtes Mittel gegen Juckreiz[7] pflanzliche Droge[8] Hausmittel[9] rezeptfreies Arzneimittel[10] Mittel gegen Erkältungen[11] M. zur äußeren Anwendung[12]　　2

drug [ʌ] n term & clin & inf　　sim **agent**[1] [eɪdʒənt] n term

n (i) any substance other than food used for preventing, diagnosing, treating, and curing disease
(ii) in genE it also refers to stimulating or depressing substances that can be addictive[2], esp. narcotics[3]
drug-induced [uːs] adj • drug-related adj • drug[4] v usu pass

» This is the drug of choice[5] for the treatment of uncomplicated urinary tract infections.

Use to administer[6]/be on or take[7] **drugs** • street or illicit[8] / recreational[9] / designer / potent[10] / powerful **drug** • crude[11] / scheduled / (non)prescription[12] / over-the-counter[13] (abbr OTC) **drug** • oral / experimental or investigational new[14] (abbr IND) **drug** • **drugs** for hay [heɪ] fever[15] [iː] • **drug** administration / dependence[16] / dispensing[17] / incompatibility[18] / interaction /-related deaths[19] • sustained/prolonged release[20] **drug** • **adverse** drug event (abbr ADE) or drug reaction[21] (abbr ADR) • therapeutic / blocking / antiallergic **agent** • **drug-induced** jaundice[22] [dʒɒːndɪs] / parkinsonism

> **Note:** In view of its double meaning the expression *drug* is best avoided when talking to patients about *medication* as it may give rise to misunderstandings. Among physicians and in the literature, however, the term is widely used. While patients are likely to interpret *Is he on drugs?* as a reference to cocaine or LSD, doctors commonly use terms like *drug-related disease* or *drug therapy*[23].

(i) Medikament, (Arznei)mittel (ii) (Rausch)droge, Suchtgift
Wirkstoff[1] abhängig / süchtig machend[2] Narkotika, Rausch-, Betäubungsmittel[3] (starke) Medikamente geben, D. nehmen, betäuben[4] M. der Wahl[5] M. verabreichen[6] D. nehmen, drogenabhängig sein[7] illegale Droge[8] Psychopharmakon[9] hochwirksames M.[10] Ausgangsdroge[11] rezeptpflichtiges Medikament[12] rezeptfreies M.[13] Testmed.[14] M. gegen Heuschnupfen[15] Drogenabhängigkeit[16] Arzneimittelhandel[17] Arzneistoffinkompatibilität[18] Drogentote[19] Depot-, Retardpräparat[20] Nebenwirkung, unerwünschte Arzneimittelwirkung[21] Drogenikterus[22] medikamentöse Behandlung[23]　　3

pharmacy [fɑːrməsi] n clin & term　　sim BE **chemist('s)**[1] [kemɪst] n

(i) retail[2] store where medicinal preparations and supplies[3] are sold
(ii) a branch of pharmacology
pharmacist[4] n term • druggist[5] n inf • pharma(co)- comb

» In general, the prescribing physician[6] provides or asks the dispensing pharmacist to provide written drug use information for the patient.

Use hospital[7] **pharmacy** • **pharmacist**-on-call[8] • **pharmaco**chemistry /therapy[9] /logy

> **Note:** In America *drugstores* are retail shops which sell drinks, snack, cosmetics, household goods, etc.; they may, however, include a *pharmacy* where prescription drugs are dispensed.

(i) Apotheke (ii) Pharmazie, Pharmazeutik
Apotheke u. Drogerie[1] Einzelhandels-[2] Arzneimittel u. Ärztebedarf[3] Apotheker(in), Pharmazeut(in)[4] Apotheker(in), Drogist(in)[5] verschreibende(r) Arzt / Ärztin[6] Anstalts-, Klinikapotheke[7] diensthabende(r) Apoth.[8] medikamentöse Behandlung[9]　　4

Drugs and Remedies BASIC MEDICAL & HEALTH TERMS **17**

dispense *v term*

to prepare, compound[1] [aʊ], label[2] [eɪ], sell and give out medications to patients

dispensatory[3] *n term* • dispensary[4] *n clin* • dispenser[5] *n*

» Today these drugs are increasingly dispensed without prescription[6]. It may not be sold or dispensed directly to the patient. Dispense in dropper bottle[7] or amber[8] [æ] glass container.

Use **dispensing** chemist[9] *(BE)* • soap **dispenser**

(Arznei) (zu)bereiten u. abgeben

(ab)mischen[1] etikettieren[2] Arzneimittel-Codex, Ergänzung z. amtl. Arzneibuch[3] Anstalts-, Klinikapotheke[4] Spender, Dispenser[5] rezeptfrei[6] Tropfflasche[7] bernsteinfarben[8] Apotheker(in), Drogist(in)[9] 5

dosage [doʊsɪdʒ] **form** *n term*   *sim* **dosage formulation**[1] *n term*

describes how a drug is supplied[2] (as a tablet or cream [iː], powdered [aʊ], in liquid form, etc.)

formulate[3] *v term*

» Special coatings[4] [oʊ] are used to retard[5] the disintegration[6] of solid dosage forms in the gut[7] [ʌ]. This solution is specifically formulated for exclusive application to the oral mucosa.

Use oral[8] / topical / solid[9] / liquid / oral suspension[10] **dosage form** • parenteral / pediatric [iæ]/ controlled- or slow-release[11] **dosage form** • commercial [ɜː]/ metered [iː] spray[12] / water-in-oil / delayed-[11] [eɪ]/ extended-[11] / prompt-release[13] / capsule **formulation**

Arznei-, Darreichungsform

Zubereitungsform[1] hergestellt, vertrieben[2] zubereiten[3] Überzug[4] verzögern[5] Zerfall[6] Darm[7] perorale Arzneiform[8] feste A.[9] Mixtur[10] Retardpräparat[11] Dosieraerosol[12] schnell zerfallende Arzneizubereitung[13]

6

tablet *n & v, abbr* **tabs**   *sim* **capsule**[1] [kæpsəl‖sjuːl] *n term & clin*, **pill**[2] *n clin & inf*

solid dosage form varying in shape (disk-like) and size, and method of manufacture (molded[3] [oʊ], compressed[4]); a caplet is a mixture between a tablet and a capsule-shaped dosage form

» Dissolve[5] the tablet under the tongue. Swallow [ɒː] the capsule whole[6]. Take the tablet with a glass of water.

Use enteric-coated[7] / chewable[8] [uː]/ scored[9] / sublingual **tablet** • buffered [ʌ]/ half-, regular-, double-strength[10] / rapidly dissolving **tablet** • dispersable[11] [ɜː]/ slow-release[12] [iː]/ coated[13] / dry-coated[14] / film-coated[15] **tablet** • (hard/soft) gelatin [dʒe]/ translucent [uːs] **capsule** • sleeping / contraceptive[16] [se]/ multiphasic[17] [eɪ] **pill**

Tablette; tablettieren

Kapsel[1] Pille[2] geformt[3] gepresst[4] zergehen lassen[5] unzerkaut schlucken[6] magensaftresistente T.[7] Kautablette[8] T. m. Teilungs-, Bruchkerbe[9] forte Tabl.[10] Brause-, Lösungstablette[11] Retardpräparat[12] überzogene Tabl., Dragée[13] Manteltablette[14] Filmtablette[15] Antibabypille[16] Mehrphasenpille[17] 7

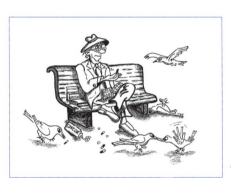

...strictly for the birds!

ointment [ɔɪ] *n term or* **salve** [sæv] *n clin, abbr* **oint.** *or* **UNG**   *sim* **gel**[1] [dʒel], **paste**[2] [eɪ], **cream**[3], **balm** [bæːm‖bɑːm] *or* **balsam**[4] [ɒː] *n clin*

semisolid medicinal preparations for application to the skin which are suspended[5] in fatty or greasy[6] [iː] material

creamy *adj*

» Oils, powders[7], and ointments should not be routinely used. Lindane 1% cream is also effective but may irritate the skin. Apply[8] the ointment topically and spread[9] [e] it with gauze[10] [gɒːz].

Use to use/rub in **an ointment** • ophthalmic [fθæl] *or* eye[11] / rectal / emulsifying[12] [ʌ]/ 5% / water-soluble **ointment** • emollient or soothing[13] [uːð] / steroid [iɚ]/ iodine[14] [aɪ] **ointment** • **ointment** dosage form / tube / application • coal tar / lidocaine / film-forming / regular-strength **gel** • (emollient) dental / zinc[15] (oxide) / gelatin [dʒe] **paste** • corticosteroid / (sun block) lip **balm** • vaginal [dʒ]/ moisturizing[16] [tʃ]/ cold[17] **cream**

Salbe, Unguentum

Gel[1] Paste[2] Creme[3] Balsam[4] suspendiert[5] fettig, schmierig[6] Puder[7] auftragen[8] verteilen[9] Gaze, Verbandsmull[10] Augensalbe[11] emulgierende S.[12] weiche Salbe, Ung. molle[13] Iodsalbe[14] Zinkpaste[15] Feuchtigkeitscreme[16] Kühlsalbe[17]

8

BASIC MEDICAL & HEALTH TERMS — Drugs and Remedies

powder [paʊdɚ] n & v term & clin   sim **pellet**[1] n term & clin

solid preparation dispensed in the form of small particles; pellets are small cylindrical or ovoid pills of compressed agents, e.g. steroid hormones for subcutaneous implantation and slow release

powdery[2] adj • powdered[3] adj

» Dissolve one 2-gram package [pækɪdʒ] of powder in a full glass (8 ounces [aʊ]) and stir [stɜːr] well[4]. The diluent[5] [ɪ] is slowly injected into the vial [vaɪəl] which is then gently [dʒ] swirled[6] [ɜː] until the pellet is dissolved.

Use absorbent / oral / topical / antifungal[7] / activated charcoal[8] [tʃ]/ sprinkle[9] / aerosol [eɚ] **powder** • freeze-dried[10] [aɪ] **pellets**

Puder, Pulver; (ein)pudern, pulverisieren

Granulat, Pellet[1] pulverförmig[2] pulverisiert[3] gut umrühren[4] Verdünnungsmittel[5] vorsichtig schwenken[6] fungizider Puder[7] Aktivkohle, Carbo medicinalis[8] Streupuder[9] gefriergetrocknete Granula[10]

9

---

tincture [tɪŋktʃɚ] n term   sim **lotion**[1] [oʊʃ] n term & clin

medicinal agents suspended in an alcohol-containing solution

» Preparations containing tincture of benzoin can be removed by swabbing[2] them with rubbing alcohol. The gel is spread onto the ulcer as a thin continuous film. Apply enough gel and rub in[3] gently.

Use iodine[4] [aɪə]/ hydroalcoholic[5] / benzoin [z] opium[6] **tincture** • shake[7] / drying / (back) rub[8] / antifungal [ʌŋg]/ cleansing[9] [e]/ aftershave **lotion**

Tinktur

Lotion[1] Wegwischen[2] einreiben[3] Iodtinktur[4] Äthanol-Wassergemisch[5] benzoesäurehalt. Opiumtinktur[6] Schüttelmixtur[7] Einreibemittel[8] Reinigungslotion[9]

10

---

drops n term & inf usu pl, abbr **gtt.**   sim **solution**[1] [uːʃ], **syrup**[2] [sɪrəp] n term & clin abbr **Liq**

(i) dosage for medications (ii) popular term for tinctures, eyewashes[3], etc.

solvent[4] n term • solute[5] n • soluble[6] adj • solubility[7] n

» Some recommend a dose of 2 drops of ophthalmic solution. 5mL of a 20% solution should be instilled[8] with a syringe[9] [dʒ] connected to the catheter. Ipecac [ɪ] syrup[10] is now used as a centrally acting emetic[11] in acute oral drug overdose.

Use eye / nose / stomach[12] [k] **drops** • maple[13] [eɪ]/ flavored [eɪ]/ demulcent [ʌls]/ glucose / cough[14] [kɒːf] **syrup** • clear / cloudy[15] [aʊ]/ discolored / diluted[16] [uː]/ aqueous[17] [eɪkwɪəs] **solution** • concentrated / IV / nasal / oral / saline[18] [eɪ] **solution**

Tropfen, Guttae

Lösung[1] Sirup[2] Augenwässer, Collyria[3] Lösungsmittel[4] gelöster Stoff[5] löslich[6] Löslichkeit[7] eingeträufelt, instilliert[8] Spritze[9] Ipecacuanha-, Brechwurzelsirup[10] Emetikum[11] Magentropfen[12] Ahornsirup[13] Hustensaft, -sirup[14] trübe Lösung[15] verdünnte L.[16] wässrige L[17] Kochsalzlösung[18]

11

---

suppository [səpɒːzətɔːri] n term

solid cone-shaped[1] [oʊ] dosage form for introduction into the rectum or vagina [dʒ] that readily [e] melts[2] at body temperature

» Moisten[3] the suppository by placing it in a cup of water for 10 sec before rectal insertion. For best results the suppository should be retained[4] for at least 3 hours.

Use to place/insert[5] **a suppository** • vaginal[6] / intraurethral / pile[7] [aɪ] / laxative[8] **suppository**

Zäpfchen, Suppositorium

kegelförmig[1] schmilzt[2] befeuchten[3] im Körper verbleiben[4] Z. einführen[5] Vaginalzäpfchen[6] Hämorrhoidenzäpfchen[7] Stuhlzäpfchen[8]

12

---

vial [vaɪəl] or **phial** [faɪəl] n term   sim **ampul(e)** or **ampoule**[1] [æmpʲuːl] n term

small receptacle[2] [se] (usually of glass) for holding liquids, and esp. medicines which are typically withdrawn[3] [ɔːn] with syringes for IV or IM injection; ampuls are hermetically sealed[4] [iː] vials which need to be broken for use

» Discard[5] opened vials after 96 hours. Remove the vial from packaging[6] just before use and shake well. The vial should be rolled not shaken to dissolve the drug. 0.05 mg/mL is packaged as single-use ampuls[7], all other strengths[8] as multiple-dose vials.

Use plastic / reaction / diluent [ɪ] / multiple dose[9] **vial** • opened / 4-mL size **ampul**

Stechampulle, Vial, Ampullenflasche

Ampulle[1] Behälter[2] entnommen[3] verschlossen[4] entsorgen[5] Verpackung[6] Einzeldosisampullen[7] Konzentrationen[8] Mehrfachentnahmeflasche[9]

13

---

lozenge [lɒːzəndʒ] n clin   syn **pastil(le)** [pæstᵊl‖pæstiːəl] n clin

(i) a dose of medicine in the form of a small pellet (ii) a small aromatic or medicated candy

» Dissolve slowly in the mouth, do not bite or chew [tʃuː] lozenges or swallow [ɒː] them whole[1] [hoʊl]. He was sucking[2] [ʌ] a lozenge.

Use menthol / iron / cough[3] [kɒːf] / sore throat[4] / benzocaine [keɪ]/ chloraseptic **lozenge** • fruit / throat[4] **pastille**

Pastille, Lutschtablette

ganz schlucken[1] lutschen[2] Hustenpastille, -bonbon[3] Lutschtablette gegen Halsschmerzen[4]

14

---

antidote [æntɪdoʊt] n & v

drugs that can neutralize [uː] toxic substances[1] or counteract[2][aʊ] their effects

» This medication is to be used as an antidote for emergency use in poisoning[3].

Use universal / physiologic [fɪz]/ chemical[4] [ke] **antidote** • **antidote** to / against

Gegenmittel, -gift, Antidot; G. verabreichen

Gift(stoff)e[1] entgegenwirken[2] bei Vergiftungsnotfällen[3] chemisches Gegenmittel[4]

15

At the Dentist's | BASIC MEDICAL & HEALTH TERMS **19**

pack(age) [pækɪdʒ] *n & v*   *sim* **packet**[1][pækɪt]**, carton**[2] [ɑː] *n*

(n) container (glass bottle, carton, packets for powders etc.) for dispensing drugs in adequate doses

packaging[3] *n* • repackaging *n*

» Keep in the protective packaging until used. Each blister card[4] contains one day's dosage (14 cards per package). Dispense in the original carton to protect the solution from light.

Use dose / triple [ɪ] card / hospital[5] **pack** • double-barrier / child-resistant[6] / unit-dose[7] **packaging**

Packung; verpacken
Schachtel, Packung[1] (Papp)karton[2] Verpackung[3] Blisterpackung[4] Klinik-, Anstaltspackung[5] kindersichere Verpackung[6] Einzeldosispackung[7]

16

package insert *n term*   *syn* **patient instruction** [ʌ] **leaflet** [iː] *n clin & inf*

important product information for the patient (composition[1], mode of action[2], dosage[3], administration[4], indications, contra-indications[5], side effects[6], precautions [ɔː] etc.)

» Carefully read the package insert for specific dosing guidelines[7] [aɪ].

Packungsbeilage, Beipackzettel
Zusammensetzung[1] Wirkungsweise[2] Dosierung[3] Anwendungsweise[4] Gegenanzeigen, Kontraindikationen[5] Nebenwirkungen[6] Dosierungsrichtlinien[7]

17

precautions [prɪkɔːʃənz] *n*

these are warnings to take preventive[1] or security measures[2] [eɪ], e.g. not to exceed [iː] the recommended dosage[3], do not take with alcohol, avoid excessive heat, keep drugs out of the reach of children, etc.

precautionary[1] *adj* • caution[4] [kɔːʃən] *n & v*

» Caution in increasing dosage is recommended. These precautions do not apply to short-term IV use unless otherwise specified. Use caution when driving or operating machinery because of possible drowsiness[5] [aʊz], impairment [eə] of motor skills[6] and/or judgement [dʒʌdʒ-] of distance[7], etc.

Use **precautions** to consider[8] / while using this medication • to **caution** against[9]

Vorsichtsmaßnahmen
vorbeugende Maßnahmen[1] Sicherheitsmaßn.[2] empfohlene Dosis nicht überschreiten[3] Vorsicht; warnen[4] Schläfrigkeit, Benommenheit[5] Beeinträchtigung d. Fahrtüchtigkeit[6] Distanzeinschätzung[7] zu berücksichtigende V.[8] warnen vor[9]

18

storage [stɔːrɪdʒ] *n*

the conditions under which drugs are kept[1] are decisive [aɪ] for their shelf life[2] and stability[3]

» Store below 40°C (104°F) in a tight [taɪt], light-resistant[4] container and protect from freezing. Fomepizole is stable [eɪ] for at least 48 hs when refrigerated [dʒ] or if stored[1] at room temperature. The tablet will maintain potency[5] through the expiration date[6] provided the bottle cap is replaced tightly after each use.

Lagerung
gelagert / aufbewahrt werden[1] Haltbarkeit[2] Stabilität[3] lichtundurchlässig[4] Wirkung behalten[5] über das Verfalldatum hinaus[6]

19

Clinical Phrases

These tablets should be taken on an empty stomach. Diese Tabletten sollten auf nüchternen Magen eingenommen werden. • Take these capsules with meals. Nehmen Sie diese Kapseln zu den Mahlzeiten ein. • The drug is well tolerated. Das Medikament ist gut verträglich. • Protect from light! Lichtschutz erforderlich. • This drug has a particularly swift onset of action. Dieses Medikament wirkt besonders rasch. • Consult your family doctor if symptoms persist. Bei anhaltenden Beschwerden sollten Sie Ihren Hausarzt aufsuchen. • Store in a cool, dry place. Protect from heat and moisture. Kühl und trocken aufbewahren! • For expiration date see bottom of container. Verfalldatum auf der Unterseite des Behälters beachten!

Unit 6   At the Dentist's
Related Units: 7 Basic Dental Equipment, Dentistry

dentist *n*   *syn* **dental practitioner** [tɪʃ] *or* **surgeon** [sɜːrdʒən] *n term*

a doctor licenced [aɪs] to treat the teeth and the associated structures in the oral cavity; dentists may be specialized in various fields of dentistry, e.g. orthodontists[1], endodontists, or pedodontists[2] [iː]

» More than 90% of patients who see a dentist less than once a year suffer tooth loss.

Use to see/visit/consult **the dentist** • general **dentist** • preventive / restorative[3] / four-handed[4] **dentistry** • oral[5]/ maxillofacial[6] [-feɪʃəl] **surgeon** • **dentist**-patient relationship

Zahnarzt
Kieferorthopäden[1] Kinderzahnärzte[2] konservierende Zahnheilkunde, Zahnerhaltung[3] assistierte Zahnheilkunde[4] Oralchirurg(in)[5] Gesichts- u. Kieferchirurg(in)[6]

1

dental practice n   sim **dental office** or BE **dental surgery**[1] n

(i) rooms where dentists see and treat patients (ii) daily routine of a practitioner

» This is essential for all dentists in private practice. This can be seen daily in the practice office. Time with the patient in the office is limited.

Use to run a[2] **practice** • private / clinical **practice** • practice[1] **office** • **office** hours[3] [aʊɚz]/ setting or envir**o**nment [aɪ]/ **schedule**[4] [skǁʃ]/ visit • **surgery** hours[3] (BE) • **in-office** contr**o**l

(i) **Zahnarztpraxis** (ii) **Praxisalltag, -management**
Zahnarztpraxis, Ordination[1] eine Praxis führen[2] Ordinationszeiten[3] Praxisablauf[4]

2

staff [stæf] n   syn **personnel** n espBE

Use to h**i**re[1] [aɪ]/train/fire **staff** • new / nursing / anc**i**llary[2] [sɪ] **staff** • **staff** recr**u**itment[3] [uː]/ member / meeting

Personal, Belegschaft
Personal einstellen[1] Hilfspersonal[2] Personaleinstellung[3]

3

dentist's or **dental assistant** n

a key member of the support personnel who directly assists the dentist at ch**ai**rside[1] and may also be del**e**gated[2] to provide intraoral dental services that do not require the skill and judgement of a dentist

chairside assistance n

» Today's assistants are no longer just responsible for passing instruments[3] and materials but also provide hands-on care[4].

Zahnarztassistent(in), -helfer(in)
am Behandlungsstuhl[1] angewiesen, abgestellt[2] Instrumentieren[3] selbständig eine Behandlung durchführen[4]

4

dental (laboratory) technician [teknɪʃən] n

profess**i**onal trained in making d**e**ntal prostheses [prɒːsθiːsɪz], orthod**o**ntic appl**i**ances [aɪ], etc. on a dentist's orders within a dental office or in his own lab

» Then the laboratory technician can apply porcelain [pɔːrsəlɪn] and form the profile of the restoration.

Use x-ray [eks] or radi**o**logy[1] **technician**

Zahntechniker(in)
Röntgenassistent(in)[1]

5

receptionist [rɪsepʃənɪst] n

assistant at the reception desk[1] who manages the appointments, telephone calls, office schedule, etc.

» The receptionist is not only the up-front contact for the patient but is also involved in book-keeping or backing up[2] in the lab, all of which require a considerable amount of insight. All right, I'll try to squeeze[3] [iː] you in today.

Sprechstundenhilfe, Rezeptionsassistent(in)
Anmeldung[1] aushelfen[2] einschieben[3]

6

waiting room n   syn **reception room** n

Use **waiting** list / p**e**riod [ɪɚ]/ time

Warteraum, -zimmer

7

practice leaflet [liːflət] n

contains information on office hours, fac**i**lities[1] [sɪl], dental care (e.g. dental hyg**i**enist[2] [aɪdʒ]), appointment system, treatment available (domic**i**liary visits[3], etc.), fees[4] [iː] and charges[5] [tʃɑːrdʒɪːz], practice phil**o**sophy, etc. for **a**ctual and pot**e**ntial p**a**tients

Patienteninformation
Einrichtungen[1] Dentalhygieneassistent(in)[2] Hausbesuche[3] Honorare[4] Gebühren[5]

8

appointment n   sim **visit**[1] n

visit to the dentist arranged in adv**a**nce[2]

(re)app**o**int[3] v • interappointment adj

» My receptionist will give you a new appointment. We'll have to reappoint Mr Hill.

Use to fix/arrange/give/make/have **an appointment** • broken[4] / examination / impress**i**on[5] [eʃ]/ try-in[6] / del**i**very **appointment** • review or checkup[7] / followup / maintenance[8] / rec**a**ll / scheduled[9] **appointment** • **appointment** card / book • by appointment only[10] • return **visit** • a five-**appointment** prot**o**col[11] • inter**appointment** fl**a**reup[12] [eɚ]

Behandlungstermin
Arztbesuch, Hausbesuch[1] im Voraus[2] (neuen) Termin geben[3] nicht eingehaltener T.[4] T. für Abdrucknahme[5] Ein-, Anprobetermin[6] Kontrolltermin[7] Nachsorgetermin[8] festgelegter / geplanter Termin[9] nur nach Vereinbarung[10] Behandlungsplan m. 5 Sitzungen[11] akute Verschlechterung vor dem nächsten Termin[12]

9

cancellation n clin

» A backup list of patients who will come in at short notice[1] is necessary for last-minute[2] cancellations.

Terminabsage
auf Abruf[1] kurzfristig[2]

10

At the Dentist's

BASIC MEDICAL & HEALTH TERMS

consultation [kɒːnsʌlteɪʃən] *n*

meeting with your dentist where (s)he discusses your treatment plan

con**sult**[1] *v* • con**sul**ting *adj* • con**sul**tant[2] *n*

» You should *seek* [iː] *the consultation*[3] *of an endodontist. Casts*[4] *on a semiadjustable* [dʒʌ] *articulator*[5] *were used for surgical consultation and patient education.*

Use dental / presurgical / prosthodontic[6] / implant / comprehensive[7] **consultation** • **consultation** room / hours[8]

ärztliche Beratung, Konsultation

zu Rate ziehen, konsultieren[1] Konsiliarius; leitender Facharzt (i. brit. Krankenhaus)[2] hinzuziehen[3] Modelle[4] teiljustierbarer Artikulator[5] (zahn)prothetische Beratung[6] eingehende Beratung[7] Sprechstunde[8]

11

referral *n term & clin*

directing or redirecting patients to a specialist or a specialized medical center for definitive treatment

refer to *v term* •referring *adj*

» *The patient was referred back to his dentist for the final restoration. She was referred for a medical evaluation*[1] *which resulted in a diagnosis of osteoporosis.*

Use the **referring** dentist • self-**referral**[2] • **referral** form[3] / assistance

Überweisung

zur medizinischen Abklärung[1] erwünschte Überweisung[2] Überweisungsschein[3]

12

treatment or **management plan** *n*

sheet of paper or special index card[1] used to record treatment progress

» *A combined consultation involving a restorative dentist and maxillofacial surgeon is critical for optimal treatment planning and coordination of implant-retained* [eɪ] *prostheses*[2] [prɒsθiːsɪz].

Use **treatment** approach / options[3] [ɒpʃənz]/ alternative / considerations / decisions

Therapie-, Behandlungsplan

Karteikarte[1] implantatgestützter Zahnersatz[2] Behandlungsmöglichkeiten[3]

13

dental chart [tʃɑːrt] *n clin*   *syn* **treatment** or **medical card** *n term* BE

file or index card used to record the patient's history (carious teeth, etc.) and treatment progress

» *The number of x-rays*[1] *taken should be recorded on the patient's chart.*

Use periodontal[2] **charting** • followup appointment **card**

Patientenbogen, Karteikarte

Röntgenbilder[1] Periodontalbefundung[2]

14

checkup *n clin*   *sim* **followup**[1], **recall**[2] *n term*

dental visit where the condition of the teeth is inspected for asymptomatic lesions [iːʒ]

» *This patient did not come for a regular checkup–this was an out-of-hours emergency* [ɜːrdʒ] *visit*[3]*. At each checkup the restorations are inspected for mobility.*

Use to have/go for **a checkup** • annual[4] / routine **checkup** • regular **checkups** • **followup** exam(ination)[1] • **recall** system[5] / interval

Note: Many dental offices have a recall system administered by the receptionist who invites the patients at regular intervals (telephone calls or appointment cards).

Vorsorge-, Kontrolluntersuchung

Nachuntersuchung, Nachsorge[1] Wiederbestellung[2] Notfallbehandlung außerhalb der Ordinationszeit[3] jährliche Kontrolle[4] Recall-, Vormerksystem[5]

15

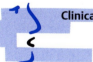

Clinical Phrases

When was the last time you saw a dentist? Wann waren Sie das letzte Mal beim Zahnarzt? • What kind of dental treatments have you had previously? Welche Behandlungen wurden schon durchgeführt? • Do you occasionally grind your teeth or bite your nails? Knirschen Sie manchmal mit den Zähnen oder kauen Sie an den Nägeln? • Which tooth is causing the problem? Welcher Zahn tut Ihnen weh? • Do you get pain with hot or cold liquids? Haben Sie Schmerzen, wenn Sie heiße oder kalte Flüssigkeiten trinken? • Have your gums been bleeding? Hatten Sie Zahnfleischbluten? • I will now tap your teeth with my mirror to find out where they are sore. Ich werde jetzt mit dem Zahnspiegel leicht auf die Zähne klopfen, um festzustellen, wo es weh tut. • How do you feel about the appearance of your teeth? Sind Sie kosmetisch mit Ihren Zähnen zufrieden? • Have you ever noticed any popping sounds in your jaw joints? Haben Sie jemals ein Knacken im Kiefergelenk bemerkt? • Which tooth is loose? Welcher Zahn wackelt? • Do you bleed a lot after extraction? Bluten Sie stark bei Extraktionen? • Are you currently attending your doctor for any medical condition? Sind Sie derzeit in ärztlicher Behandlung? • Are you on any medication? Nehmen Sie derzeit irgendwelche Medikamente? • Have you ever been hospitalized? Waren Sie jemals in stationärer Behandlung? • Come back in six months for a check-up. Kommen Sie in 6 Monaten zur Kontrolle.

Unit 7 Basic Dental Equipment

Related Units: 6 At the Dentist's, 30 Basic Dental Materials, 24 Surgical Instruments, 31 Dental Lab Procedures & Equipment 32 Dental Instruments

dental chair n

seat with a foot and head rest[1] in which the patient can be positioned for treatment as required
chairside adj term
» *All patients were seated comfortably in a dental chair in an upright position. Now we'll whisk you backwards[2] a little. This test can be performed at chairside and takes only a few minutes to complete.*
Use to be recumbent [ʌ] in the **dental chair**[3] • to make a consultation **at chairside** • **chairside** monitoring / assistance[4] / procedure / techniques / sterilization • **chair time**[5]

Behandlungs-, Patientenstuhl
Kopfstütze[1] Rückenlehne absenken[2] auf dem Behandlungsstuhl liegen[3] Stuhlassistenz[4] Behandlungszeit, -dauer[5]

1

dental unit n

central apparatus [eɪ] in the treatment room that is supplied with all the main tools and equipment required for standard dental therapy
Use portable **dental units**

(Zahn)arztelement, (Behandlungs)einheit

2

dental engine [endʒɪn] n

motor that drives a handpiece with drills with the help of electricity or pressed air
» *Most dental engines can be operated[1] via a foot control[2].*

Elektro-, Luftmotor
bedient[1] Fußschalter[2]

3

chip-blower [tʃɪp bloʊɚ] n clin   syn **chip** or **air syringe** [sɪrɪndʒ] n term

instrument with a pressure tank and a metal nozzle[1] [nɒːzl] for drying or blowing the debris[2] [iː] out of a tooth cavity that is being excavated for a filling

Luft-, Spanbläser
Ansatzstück[1] Bohrstaub[2]

4

water syringe n   rel **cooling**[1], **irrigation**[2] n

fluid channel [tʃ] usually integrated in the handpiece[3] for cooling and irrigating the drill site
» *An additional air-water spray from a triple [ɪ] syringe was used.*
Use internally / externally **irrigated drill** • air-water spray[4] • **cooling** • **cooling** agent [eɪdʒᵊnt] *or* coolant[5]

Wasserspritze
Kühlung[1] Spülung[2] Handstück[3] Spraywasser-Luftkühlung[4] Kühlmittel[5]

5

hypodermic [aɪ] **needle** n   rel **syringe**[1] n

thin hollow needle attached to a syringe used mainly for subcutaneous injection of fluids (e. g. anesthetics, vaccines[2] [væks-] and other medications) but also for aspiration and irrigation purposes
» *Slightly retract the skin overlying the vessel superior to the point of needle entry[3].*
Use fine / ultra-thin / 19-gauge [geɪdʒ] / butterfly / IV (intravenous [iː]) infusion / large-bore[4] [bɔːr]/ syringe **needle** • **needle** site[3] [aɪ]/ electrode / biopsy [aɪ]/ puncture [ʌ] mark[5] / stick injury

Injektionsnadel, -kanüle
Injektionsspritze[1] Impfstoffe[2] Einstichstelle[3] großlumige Hohlnadel[4] Punktionsnarbe[5]

6

saliva [aɪ] **ejector** [ɪdʒektɚ] n   syn **aspirator** n term

suction [ʌ] device[1] usually operated by the assistant to aspirate saliva or coolants from the oral cavity
aspiration n term • aspirate[2] [v æspɚeɪt‖n æspɚət] v & n → U22-16
» *Saliva pooling[3] at the corners of the mouth needs to be removed with the saliva ejector. The aspirator must be inserted farther. There was the constant slurping[4] [ɜː] sound of the aspirator tip picking up the copious[5] flow of saline [seɪlaɪn‖-liːn] coolant. Saliva was aspirated and enamel powder was washed with 0.5 ml of KCl buffer.*

Speichelsauger, Saugkanüle
(Ab)saugvorrichtung[1] (ab)saugen, aspirieren; Aspirat[2] ansammeln[3] schlürfend[4] reichlich[5]

7

cuspidor [ʌ] n clin & term   syn **bowl** [oʊ], **spitoon** [uː] BE n clin

bowl with a tumbler[1] [ʌ] of rinsing water for the patient to flush[2] [ʌ] debris, saliva, blood or fluids
» *Have a rinse[3], please! Flush the debris thoroughly [θɜːrəli] to make the bitter taste go away.*
Use timed **bowl** rinse[4]

Spülbecken, Speischale
(Mund)spülbecher[1] wegspülen[2] (aus)spülen[3] zeitlich programm. Speischalenrundspülung[4]

8

BASIC MEDICAL & HEALTH TERMS

Basic Dental Equipment

dental or **task light** n   sim **operating light**[1] n
lights that can be positioned by means of a swivel arm[2] to allow for good visualization [ʒ] of the oral cavity or operative site
Use surgical **light** source[1] [sɔːrs] • head**light**[3]

Behandlungsfeldleuchte
Operationsleuchte[1] Schwenkarm[2] Stirnlampe[3]

9

protective spectacles n   syn **safety specs** or **goggles** BE n
eyewear [eɚ] for the patient used mainly to shield the eyes as a major protective measure [eʒ]
» Dark eyeglasses were used to slightly discourage [ɜː] the patient from directly observing the passage of the instrument. The patient is provided with protective spectacles and draped[1] [eɪ] with a protective napkin[2] to preclude soiling[3] of clothes.

Schutzbrille
abgedeckt[1] Abdecktuch[2] Beschmutzen[3]

10

instrument table n
mostly a tray[1] mounted [aʊ] on a swivel arm; this is where the assistant lays out[2] [leɪz] the instruments needed
instrument cupboard[3] [kʌbɚd] n

Instrumententisch, -ablage
Auflagetablett, Tray[1] auflegen[2] Instrumentenschrank[3]

11

pager [peɪdʒɚ] n   syn **beeper** [iː], **bleep** [iː] n inf BE
device that makes a bleeping noise when the doctor is wanted on the telephone
page sb[1] v • bleep[1] v inf & jar
» You are asked to carry this pager with you so that you can quickly respond in case of an emergency [ɚːdʒ].

Piepser
auspiepsen[1]

12

intercom n
device enabling people in different rooms of a building to communicate

Gegensprechanlage

13

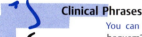

Clinical Phrases

You can lean back now. Sie können sich jetzt zurücklehnen. • Are you comfortable? Sitzen Sie bequem? • Open your mouth as wide as you can, please. Bitte den Mund ganz weit aufmachen. • Try to avoid swallowing now. Bitte jetzt nicht schlucken. • Press your tongue against the roof of your mouth. Die Zunge jetzt an den Gaumen drücken. • Unclench your teeth. Unterkiefer ganz locker, bitte. • We'll have to take the bite now. Wir müssen jetzt einen Abdruck machen. • Do not rinse out your mouth for the rest of today. Heute sollten Sie nicht mehr den Mund spülen. • You must not have any solid food for five hours. Sie dürfen erst in 5 Stunden wieder feste Nahrung zu sich nehmen. • Can you take out your dentures, please. Nehmen Sie bitte die Zahnprothese heraus.

Unit 8   Parts of the Body: The Head & Neck
Related Units: 9 The Teeth

head [hed] n

(i) top part of the body on the neck including the face, skull[1] [ʌ], and brain (ii) major end of long bones, e.g. the femoral [e] head[2] (iii) top position in a team or a department

head[3] v • bareheaded[4] [eɚ] adj • headache [hedeɪk] n • headless adj

» Tilt[5] your head backward and elevate the chin. It's important to keep his head covered.

Use to shake/turn/flex[6]/hold **one's head** • **head** and neck region [riːdʒ⁽ə⁾n] • **head** position / rotation / elevation[7] / examination / injury / film[8] • **head** rest or support[9] / mirror[10] / screw[11] [skruː]/ implant **head** • sense of **head** fullness • to be big-[12]/ bald-[13] [ɔː] **headed** • to lose one's **head** • **head** first • to **head** for[14]

(i) Kopf; (ii) Caput; (iii) Leiter
Schädel[1] Oberschenkelkopf, Caput femoris[2] an d. Spitze stehen[3] ohne Kopfbedeckung[4] neigen[5] K. nach vorne neigen[6] Hochlagerung d. K.[7] Schädelröntgen[8] Kopfstütze[9] Stirnspiegel[10] Schraubenkopf[11] eingebildet[12] glatzköpfig[13] zusteuern auf[14]

1

face [feɪs] n & v

(n) the front of the head including the forehead[1] [fɔːrhed], the chin, the temples[2], and cheeks

facial [feɪʃ⁽ə⁾l] adj • -faced adj • facies[3] [feɪʃiːiːz] n term

» The first eruptions[4] are seen on the face around the eyes and nose. Did you notice the puzzled expression on her face[5]?

Use **facial** expression or gestures[6] [dʒestʃɚz]/ muscles [mʌslz] / nerve / hair / injuries / deformity / palsy[7] [pɔːlzi] • coarse [kɔːrs] **facial** features[8] [fiːtʃɚz] • sad / angry / flushed[9] [ʌʃ]/ mask-like **face** • to lose one's / to make a[10] **face** • **face** mask / lift / pack[11] / cream [iː] • abnormal / moon / bird-like[12] / adenoid **facies** • red-/ purple-/ round-**faced** • to **face** a problem / death

Gesicht; gegenüberstehen, konfrontiert sein
Stirn[1] Schläfen[2] Gesicht(sausdruck), Facies[3] Ausschlag[4] verdutzter Gesichtsausdruck[5] Gesichtsausdruck, Mimik[6] Gesichts-, Fazialislähmung[7] grobe Gesichtszüge[8] gerötetes G.[9] d. Gesicht verziehen[10] Gesichtspackung[11] Vogelgesicht[12]

2

eye [aɪ] n & v

paired organ of sight [saɪt] located in the eye sockets [ɒː] (orbits)[1] including the pupil[2], lense and retina

(eye)lid[3] n • eyebrow [aʊ] n • eyelashes[4] [æ] n • eyeball[5] n • cross-eyed[6] adj

» Keep your eyes closed. There was infrequent blinking and fluttering[7] [ʌ] of the closed eyelids. This is not visible to the naked [neɪkɪd] eye[8].

Use to close/open the **eyes** • bags under the[9] **eyes** • watery / red / bloodshot[10] / dry **eyes** • black[11] / glass **eye** • **eye** contact / blinking[12] / charts[13] [tʃ]/ patch[14] [tʃ]/ drops /-sight[15] / piece[16] / witness[17] • to raise [eɪ] the / upper / lower **eyelids**

Auge; ansehen, mustern
Augenhöhlen, Orbitae[1] Pupille[2] (Augen)lid[3] Wimpern[4] Augapfel[5] schielend[6] Zucken[7] mit bloßem Auge[8] Tränensäcke, Ringe unter den Augen[9] blutunterlaufene A.[10] blaues Auge[11] Blinzeln, Augenwinkern[12] Sehprobentafeln[13] Augenklappe[14] Sehkraft[15] Okular[16] Augenzeuge[17]

3

nose [noʊz] n & v

covering of the nasal cavity[1] with the nostrils or nares[2] [nɚːz] (term) through which we breathe [briːð] and smell

nasal [neɪz⁽ə⁾l] adj • naso- comb • nosebleed[3] n

» A nose with a markedly depressed bridge is called saddle nose. These patients have coarse facial features, a broad, flat nose, and widely set eyes. There is blood in the nasal sinuses[4] [aɪ].

Use to blow one's[5] **nose** • to speak/breathe through **the nose** • tip / root[6] [uː]/ back or bridge[7] **of the nose** • runny / blocked-up[8] **nose** • **nasal** height [haɪt]/ concha[9] [kɒŋkə]/ septum / bone / cavity / decongestant [dʒe] spray[10] • **nose** job[11]

Nase; herumschnüffeln
Nasenhöhle[1] Nasenlöcher, Nares[2] Nasenbluten[3] Sinus paranasales, Nasennebenhöhlen[4] s. d. Nase putzen, s. schnäuzen[5] Nasenwurzel[6] Nasenrücken[7] verstopfte N.[8] Nasenmuschel, Concha nasalis[9] Nasenspray[10] Nasenoperation[11]

4

cheek [tʃiːk] n   syn bucca [bʌkə] n term

the fleshy part at either side of the face below the eyes

-cheeked adj • buccal[1] adj term • bucco- comb

» The lower lid sagged[2] [sægd] permitting tears [tɪɚz] to spill over the cheeks. Her cheeks had a rosy hue[3] [hjuː].

Use fat / upper / lateral / sunken[4] [ʌ]/ rosy[5] **cheeks** • **cheek**bone[6] / contours / biting[7] [aɪ]/ bite • red-/ chubby[8]-**cheeked** [tʃʌbi] • **buccal** mucosa[9] / surface / vestibule • **bucco**labial [eɪ]/lingual

Wange, Backe, Bucca
bukkal[1] hing herunter[2] Farbe[3] eingefallene W.[4] gerötete Wangen[5] Joch-, Wangenbein, Os zygomaticum[6] Wangenbeißen[7] pausbäckig[8] Wangenschleimhaut[9]

5

Parts of the Body: The Head & Neck — BODY STRUCTURES & FUNCTIONS

chin [tʃɪn] n   *syn* **mentum** n term

the protruding[1] front portion of the lower jaw[2] formed by the mental protuberance[3]

mental *adj* term • genial [dʒɪnaɪəl] *adj* • mento-, genio- [dʒiːnioʊ] *comb*

» Test eyebrow elevation, smiling, lip pursing[4], cheek puff[5] and chin muscle contraction. The head must be tilted and the chin lifted so that the oropharynx can be explored.

Use **chin** reflex[6] / protuberance[3] / tilt / lift / rest[7] / musculature / cap[8] • unshaven / prominent[9] / firm [ɜː] / sagging[10] / double[11] **chin** • square[12]-**chinned** • **mental** foramen [eɪ] *or* canal[13] / nerve / region • **genial** tubercle[14] • **genio**plasty[15] /hyoid [aɪ] muscle • **mento**labial /plasty[15]

Kinn, Mentum

vorspringender[1] Unterkiefer[2] Kinnvorsprung, Protuberantia mentalis[3] Mundspitzen, Vorstülpen d. Lippen[4] Aufblasen d. Wangen[5] Masseterreflex[6] Kinnstütze[7] Kinnkappe[8] vorspringendes K.[9] schlaff herabhängendes K.[10] Doppelkinn[11] m. kantigem K.[12] Foramen mentale[13] Tuberculum mentale, Kinnhöcker[14] Kinn-, Genioplastik[15]   6

jaws [dʒɔːz] n   *sim* **jawbone**[1] n term

bones of the skull (maxilla[2] and mandible[3]) and adjacent [ədʒeɪsənt] soft tissues that frame the mouth and hold the teeth

» In edentulous [-tʃələs] jaws[4] of elderly persons, atrophy of the alveolar process is common. The skin of the lateral cheeks, jawline[5], and neck is dissected free in the subcutaneous plane. The pain is localized to the jaw, base of the tongue, pharynx or larynx, tonsillar area, and ear.

Use upper[2] / lower[3] / opposing / broken / protrusive **jaw** • both / clenched[6] [tʃ]/ retrusive **jaws** • angle[7] [æŋgl]/ spasms / weakness **of the jaw** • **jaw** position / relation[8] / movement / muscle / (jerk [dʒɜːrk]) *or* reflex[9] / clenching[10] / support / exercises • **jaw** stiffness / clicking[11] / fracture / winking[12] • **jawbone** anatomy / architecture / defect / resorption / segment

Kiefer

Kieferknochen[1] Oberkiefer, Maxilla[2] Unterkiefer, Mandibula[3] zahnlose Kiefer[4] Unterkieferrand[5] zusammengepresste K.[6] (Unter)kieferwinkel, Angulus mandibulae[7] Kieferrelation[8] Masseterreflex[9] Zähnepressen[10] Kiefergelenkknacken[11] Kiefer-Lid-Phänomen[12]   7

mouth [maʊθ] n   *sim* **oral** [ɔː] **cavity**[1] n term

opening to the lungs and stomach [k] including the throat, soft and hard palate[2], teeth, tongue [tʌŋ], the upper and lower lips

mouthful[3] n • mouthwash[4] n • oral[5] *adj* term • stomat-, oro-[6] *comb*

» These patients should not be given barium [eə] by mouth[5]. The patient complained of a sore mouth[7] and difficulty swallowing.

Use to open/close **one's mouth** • wide / dry / nothing by[8] (*abbr* NPO) **mouth** • to make one's **mouth** water[9] • roof / floor / corner[10] **of the mouth** • **mouth** opening / rinse[4] / breathing[11] [iː]/-watering[12] / flora / guard[13] [ɡɑːrd] / **oral** health / mucosa / hygiene [haɪdʒiːn] / status [eɪ]/ administration[14] / contraceptive • **oro**pharynx /antral /nasal /facial • **stomat**ology /itis[7] [aɪ]/ognathic system

Mund

Mundhöhle, Cavitas oris[1] weicher / harter Gaumen[2] Bissen, Schluck[3] Mundwasser[4] oral[5] d. M. betreffend, Stomato-[6] Mundschleimhautentzündung, Stomatitis[7] nüchtern[8] d. M. wässrig machen[9] Mundwinkel[10] Mundatmung[11] lecker[12] Zahnschutz[13] orale Verabreichung[14]   8

lip n   *syn* **labium** [eɪ] n term, *pl* **labia**, *sim* **prolabium**[1] n term

(i) one of the two fleshy muscular folds with an outer mucosa surrounding the mouth
(ii) a liplike structure bounding[2] [aʊ] a cavity or groove[3] [uː]

lipstick[4] n • labial[5] [eɪ] *adj* term • labio- or cheil(o)- [kaɪl] *comb*

» The oral cavity is bounded anteriorly by the vermilion border of the lips[6]. Vesiculation[7], scabbing[8], and crusting around the lips occurred over the next few days. The infranasal groove in the midline of the upper lip is called the philtrum[9] [f].

Use to pout[10] [aʊ] /chew [tʃuː]/bite/suck [ʌ]/lick or smack[11]/burn **one's lips** • (short) upper / lower / double / cleft[12] or hare**lip** [eə] • inner / red of the / open / closed / pouted / dry **lips** • cracked or fissured[13] / thick[14] / swollen / scaling[15] [eɪ] **lips** • **lip** of a wound[16] [uː] / reading / balm[17] [bɑːlm] • **lip** mucosa / musculature / support / contour[18] / closure[19] [oʊʒ] / line[20] / (in)competence[21] / biting / retractor[22] • **labial** tooth surface / vestibule[23] / margin / frenulum[24] / consonant[25] / ulcer [ʌ] • **labio**palatal /buccal space • **cheil**osis /itis[26] [aɪ]/oplasty

Lippe, Labium

Lippenwulst, -rot, Prolabium[1] begrenzen[2] Furche, Sulcus[3] Lippenstift[4] labial, Lippen-[5] Lippensaum[6] Bläschenbildung[7] Schorfbildung[8] Oberlippengrübchen, Philtrum,[9] Lippen schürzen / vorstülpen[10] sich d. L. lecken[11] Lippenspalte, Labium fissum, Hasenscharte[12] aufgesprungene L.[13] breite / wulstige L.[14] s. schuppende L.[15] Wundrand[16] Lippenbalsam[17] Lippenprofil[18] Lippenschluss[19] Lippenschlusslinie[20] Lippen(in)kompetenz[21] Lippenhalter[22] labialer Mundvorhof[23] Lippenbändchen, Frenulum labii[24] Labial-, Lippenlaut[25] Lippenentzündung, Cheilitis[26]   9

(oral) vestibule [vɛstɪbjuːl] *n term*   *syn* **buccal** [ʌ] **cavity**,
                                  vestibulum oris *n term*

part of the mouth ouside the teeth and/or gums bounded[1] [aʊ] laterally by the lips and the cheeks, and by the reflections of the mucosa[2] from the lips and cheeks to the gums
vestibular[3] *adj term* • vestibulo- *comb*

» The patient presented with a severely resorbed mandible and a shallow vestibule[4]. The local vestibular swelling responded well to antibiotic therapy.
Use to extend into[5]/reconstruct/deepen **the vestibule** • **vestibule of the** mouth / nose[6] • labial / (labio)buccal **vestibule** • **vestibular** surface / space / depth[7] / mucosa / incision / sulcus [ʌ] • **vestibulo**plasty[8]

(Mund)vorhof, Vestibulum oris
begrenzt[1] Umschlagfalten d.Schleimhaut[2] vestibulär[3] flaches V.[4] i.d. Mundvorhof hineinreichen[5] V. nasi, Naseneingang[6] Mundvorhoftiefe[7] Vestibulum-, Mundvorhofplastik[8]

                                10

tongue [tʌŋ] *n*   *syn* **lingua** [lɪŋgwə] *n*, **glossa** [ɒ:∥ɔː] *n term*

(i) mobile muscular organ of taste[1] and speech on the floor of the oral cavity covered with mucous membrane[2] which assists in chewing, swallowing[3], and articulation[4] (ii) language
lingual[5] *adj term* • glossal[5] *adj* • gloss-, -glossia *comb*

» The anterior two-thirds of the tongue (oral tongue) is limited posteriorly by the circumvallate [-vælɛɪt] papillae[6] [iː] and includes the tip, dorsum, lateral borders, and undersurface of the mobile tongue. To increase mobility of the tongue, the lingual frenum [iː] may need cutting. Untreated tongue-tie[7] may affect speech and interfere with[8] mastication and passive cleansing [e] of the teeth.
Use to put out[9]/hold[10]/bite **one's tongue** • clean / furred [ɜː] or coated[11] / moist / parched [tʃ] or dry / fissured [ɪʃ] or scrotal or grooved[12] [uː]/ burning / bald [ɔː] or glossy or glazed[13] [eɪz] **tongue** • tip / base[14] / margin [dʒ] / anterior/posterior third / thickening **of the tongue** • mappy or geographic[15] / bitten / inflamed [eɪ]/ strawberry[16] / smoker's / black hairy[17] / cleft or bifid[18] **tongue** • **tongue** space / function / movement / pressing / depressor[19] • **lingual** nerve / tonsil[20] / artery • **linguo**labial • **glossal** surface / ulcer • **glosso**pharyngeal muscle /epiglottic folds /palatine nerve /dynia [ɪ]/ptosis • **gloss**itis[21]

(i) Zunge, Lingua, Glossa
(ii) Sprache
Geschmacksorgan[1] Schleimhaut[2] Schlucken[3] Aussprache, Artikulation[4] lingual, zungenseitig[5] Zungenpapillen, Papillae linguales[6] Ankyloglossie, Zungenverwachsung[7] behindern[8] Z. herausstecken / zeigen[9] d. Mund halten[10] belegte Z.[11] Faltenzunge, L. plicata[12] Lackzunge[13] Zungengrund, Radix linguae[14] Landkartenz., L. geographica[15] Himbeer-, Erdbeerz.[16] schwarze Haarzunge, Melanoglossie[17] Spaltzunge, L. bifida[18] Zungenspatel, -halter[19] Zungenmandel, Tonsilla lingualis[20] Zungenentzündung, Glossitis[21]   11

throat [θroʊt] *n*   *syn* **pharynx** [færɪŋks] *n*, *sim* **fauces**[1] [fɔːsiːz] *n pl term*

(i) the fauces and pharynx (ii) in genE, the front part of the neck between the chin and the clavicle[2]
throaty[3] *adj clin* • pharyngeal [-dʒɪəl] *adj term* • faucial [fɔːʃəl] *adj*

» Wrap[4] [ræp] this scarf[5] around your throat. You need warm throat irrigations[6] or gargles[7].
Use to clear one's[8] **throat** • sore[9] / scratchy[10] [tʃ]/ dry **throat** • **throat** swab[11] [ɒː]/ infection / culture • ear, nose and **throat** (abbr ENT)[12] • injected[13] [dʒe] **fauces** • pharyngeal or faucial[14] **tonsil** • **throaty** voice[15]

(i) Rachen, Schlund, Pharynx
(ii) Hals, Kehle
Schlund(enge), Fauces[1] Schlüsselbein, Clavicula[2] heiser, rauh; guttural[3] wickeln[4] Schal[5] Halsspülungen[6] Gurgelmittel[7] s. räuspern[8] Halsschmerzen[9] Halskratzen[10] Rachenabstrich[11] HNO[12] entzündeter / geschwollener Rachen[13] Rachenmandel, Tonsilla pharyngealis[14] rauhe Stimme[15]   12

neck *n*   *syn* **cervix** [sɜːrvɪks] *n term*, *sim* **nape** [neɪp]
                   or **nucha**[1] [njuːkə] *n term*

(i) narrowed connection between the trunk [ʌ] and the head (ii) neck-like narrowing in bones, teeth, etc.
cervical[2] *adj term* • nuchal[3] *adj* • neckline[4] *n clin*

» The neck was supple[5] [ʌ]. Her neck muscles [mʌslz] were tight[6] [taɪt] and she complained of a headache. Pruritic lesions are particularly common around the neckline.
Use to twist[7]/break **one's neck** • back of the[1] **neck** • **neck** pain / stiffness[8] / tie[9] /lace[10] [-ləs]/ veins / extension • bladder[11]/ femoral[12] [e] **neck** • **nuchal** rigidity[8] [rɪdʒɪdəti] • **cervical** rib[13] / spine[14] [aɪ]/ nodes [oʊ]/ collar[15]

(i) Hals, Nacken (ii) Zervix, Collum
Nacken[1] zervikal, Hals-[2] Nacken-[3] Ausschnitt, Dekolletee[4] beweglich, weich[5] verspannt[6] H. (ver)drehen[7] Nackensteifigkeit[8] Krawatte[9] Halskette[10] Blasenhals[11] Oberschenkelhals, Collum femoris[12] Halsrippe, Costa cervicalis[13] Halswirbelsäule[14] Halskrause[15]   13

Adam's apple *n clin*   *syn* **laryngeal** [-dʒ(ɪ)əl] **prominence** *n term*

cartilage[1] [kɑrtəlɪdʒ] of the voice box (larynx)[2] [lærɪŋks] moving up and down in the front of the neck, esp prominent in men

» The cricothyroid [aɪ] membrane is about 1.5 fingerwidths below the laryngeal prominence and is bounded[3] [aʊ] caudally by the cricoid cartilage[4].

Adamsapfel, Prominentia laryngea
Knorpel[1] Kehlkopf, Larynx[2] begrenzt[3] Ringknorpel, Cartilago cricoidea[4]   14

The Teeth   BODY STRUCTURES & FUNCTIONS **27**

ear [ɪɚ] *n*
  organ of hearing [ɪɚ] and equilibrium[1] consisting of the outer, middle, and inner or sensory ear[2] • eardrum[3] [ʌ] *n* • earlobe[4] [oʊ] *n* • auditory[5] [ɒ:] *adj term* • aural[5] [ɔ:] *adj* • oto-, oro- *comb*
» The rash[6] typically begins at the hairline[7] and behind the ears. One patient had lost a natural ear in an accident.
Use inner[2] / middle[8] / external *ear* • *ear* plugs[9] [ʌ]/ache [eɪk]/ muffs[10] [ʌ]/ drops / wax[11] • cauliflower[12] [ɒ:] *ears* • auditory canal or meatus[13] [ieɪ]/ ossicles[14] / threshold[15] [θreʃʰoʊld] • **aural** discharge[16] / pressure

Ohr
Gleichgewicht[1] Innenohr[2] Trommelfell, Membrana tympani[3] Ohrläppchen[4] (Ge)hör-, auditiv[5] Ausschlag[6] Haaransatz[7] Mittelohr[8] Ohrschutz, Wattepfropf[9] Ohrenschützer[10] Ohrenschmalz, Cerumen[11] Boxerohren[12] Gehörgang, Meatus acusticus[13] Gehörknöchelchen, Ossicula auditus[14] Hörschwelle[15] Ohr(en)fluss, Otorrhoe[16]   15

hair [heɚ] *n usu sing*
  slender threadlike[1] [e] outgrowth [-oʊθ] covering the human scalp[2], face (beard [ɪɚ], mustache[3] [mʌstæʃ]) and body hair; hair loss leads to a receding [i:] hairline[4] and finally to baldness[5] [ɒ:]; artificial hair is called a toupee [tu:peɪ] or wig[6]
  hairy *adj* • hairless *adj* • hairdo *or* hairstyle[7] *n* • haircut *n*
» Drugs can cause diffuse hair loss. This disease favors hairy areas like the scalp. There was a patch[8] of gray-white hair. These patients typically have sparse [ɑ:] axillary and pubic hair[9].
Use to grow/cut/comb *hair* • blond *or* fair [feɚ]/ auburn[10] [ɒ:]/ graying / dry / greasy[11] [i:]/ curly[12] [ɜ:]/ brittle[13] *hair* • *hair* turns gray / falls out • scalp / body / pubic / taste[14] *hair* • *hair* brush / spray / root[15] / shaft / follicle / thinning / growth

Haar
fadenförmig[1] Kopfhaut[2] Schnurrbart[3] Haaransatz[4] Glatzköpfigkeit[5] Haarteil, Perücke[6] Frisur[7] Fleck[8] spärliche Achsel- u. Schambehaarung[9] kastanienbraunes H.[10] fettiges H.[11] gelocktes H.[12] brüchiges H.[13] Geschmacksstiftchen[14] Haarwurzel[15]
                                                              16

9

Unit 9   The Teeth
Related Units: **8** The Head & Neck, **10** Dentition & Mastication, **11** Human Sounds & Speech, Dentistry

tooth [tu:θ] *n*, **teeth** [ti:θ] *pl*   *syn* **dens** *n term*, **dentes** *pl*
  one of the bony structures set in the alveoli [aɪ] of the jaws [dʒɔ:z], used in mastication and assisting in articulation[1]
  dental *adj*
» The tooth may become sensitive to hot or cold, and then severe continuous throbbing pain[2] follows. Oral features [fi:tʃɚz] of vitamin C deficiency include loosening[3] of teeth, swelling, bleeding, ulceration [s] and a burning sensation in the tongue[4] [tʌŋ].
Use *tooth* loss / mobility[5] / surface / socket [ɒ:]/ retention / ache [eɪk]/ position • adjacent[6] [dʒeɪs]/ opposing[7] *teeth* • artificial / natural / poorly aligned[8] [aɪn]/ residual *teeth* • mandibular / maxillary / devitalized *or* non-vital[9] [aɪ]/ tender[10] / spaced *teeth* • pegged[11] / broken *tooth*

Zahn, Zähne; Dens, Dentes
Artikulation, Aussprache[1] pochender / klopfender Schmerz[2] Lockerung[3] Zungenbrennen[4] Zahnbeweglichkeit[5] Nachbarzähne[6] Gegenzähne, Antagonisten[7] Zahnfehlstellung[8] devitale Zähne[9] empfindliche Z.[10] Zapfenzahn[11]
                                                              1

front *or* **anterior** [ɪ] **teeth** *n clin*   opposite **posterior teeth**[1] *n clin*
  the cutting teeth (centrals, laterals, cuspids [ʌ]); the posterior teeth are the bicuspids [aɪ] and molars

Vorder-, Frontzähne
Backenzähne[1]
                                                              2

incisor [sɪ] *or* **incisal tooth** *n term*   *syn* **cutting tooth** *n clin*
  one of the four front teeth–the centrals and laterals–with cutting (incisal) edges in each jaw at the apex [eɪ] of the dental arch [tʃ]
  incisal *adj term*
» A cavity was prepared in the right central incisor. The maxillary right lateral was missing.
Use right / left first *or* central **incisor** *or* **central**[1] • second *or* lateral **incisor** *or* **lateral**[2] • maxillary / mandibular **incisors** • **incisor** crown / area / position / point[3] / contact • **incisal** edge[4] / embrasure[5] [eɪʒɚ]

Schneidezahn, Dens incisivus
linker mittlerer Schneidezahn[1] lateraler / seitlicher S.[2] Inzisalpunkt[3] Schneidekante[4] Einziehung am Schneidezahn[5]
                                                              3

28 BODY STRUCTURES & FUNCTIONS — The Teeth

(tooth) cusp [kʌsp] *n clin*   *syn* **cuspis dentis** *n term*

elevated chewing [tʃuːɪŋ] or tearing [eəʳ] points of the cuspids, bicuspids, and molars
cuspal¹ *adj* • cuspless *adj*
» The cuspal angle² [æŋgl] of the restoration must be increased.
The lingual cusp had to be sacrificed.
Use **cusp** tip³ • **cusp(al)** inclination⁴ • **cusp** -to-fossa relationship • short / distobuccal [ʌ] **cusp**

Zahnhöcker, Cuspis dentis
Höcker-, höckrig¹ Höckerwinkel²
Höckerspitze³ Höckerneigung⁴   4

---

canine [keɪnaɪn] **(tooth)** [eɪ] *n & adj clin*   *syn* **eye tooth** *n inf,*
   cuspid (tooth) *n rare*

one of the corner teeth in the arch next to the laterals identified by a pointed cusp for tearing food
» A fixed prosthesis [iː] extended from the canine to the first molar region.
Use **canine** eminence¹ / alveolus [ɪə]/ guidance² [aɪ]/ mandible • primary [aɪ] **canines**

Eck-, Augenzahn;
Dens caninus
Eckzahnspitze¹ Eckzahnführung²   5

---

premolar [priːmoʊlɚ] *n & adj clin*   *syn* **bicuspid** [aɪ] **(tooth)** *n & adj term*

one of the teeth just behind the cuspids which have two cusps or points
» On statistical average, premolar teeth are retained for a longer period than molar teeth. All molars and the mandibular premolars were missing.
Use mandibular / maxillary **premolar** • first / second **bicuspid** • unrestored / fully erupted¹ [ʌ] **premolars** • at the second **premolar** site

Prämolar, vorderer Backen-,
Stockzahn, Bikuspidat,
D. praemolaris
vollständig durchgebrochene
Prämolaren¹   6

---

molar (tooth) *n & adj clin*   *syn* **cheek** [iː] **tooth** *n inf,* **dens molaris** *n term*

one of the teeth behind the second bicuspids with flattened surfaces and four or five cusps
» The shape and occlusal relation of the denture [dentʃɚ] was similar to natural molars.
Use first or 6-year¹ **molars** • second or 12-year **molars** • premolar-**molar** region • single-**molar** restoration • abscessed lower **molar** • **molar** occlusal force²

Molar, Mahlzahn, großer
Backenzahn, D. molaris
Sechsjahrmolaren¹ molare Kau-
kraft²   7

---

third molar (tooth) *n term & clin*   *syn* **wisdom tooth** *n inf*

one of the most posterior teeth that erupt in late adolescence and have four cusps; their roots are often fused¹ [fjuːzd]
» The incidence of trauma [ɔː] to the mental nerve during removal of third molars is 3-5.5%.
Use impacted² / partially erupted **3rd molar** • **third molar** tuberosity

3. Molar, Weisheitszahn,
D. serotinus
verschmolzen¹ impaktierter / retinierter Weisheitszahn²   8

(dental) arch [ɑːrtʃ] *n term & clin*

(i) horseshoe-shaped¹ ridge supporting the teeth (ii) collectively all upper or lower teeth
» The prosthesis frequently loosened when the patient, who had an atrophic [eɪtrɒːfɪk] dental arch, yawned² [jɒːnd].
Use upper / lower / shortened³ **(dental) arch** • in both **arches** • **arch** width⁴ [wɪdθ]/ length • full **arch** prosthesis⁵ • opposing **arch** impression • U-shaped **arch** form

(i) Zahnbogen (ii) Zahnreihe
hufeisenförmig¹ gähnte² verkürzter
Zahnbogen³ Zahnbogenbreite⁴
Vollprothese⁵   9

---

palate [pælət] *n clin*   *syn* **roof of the mouth** *n clin,* **palatum** [eɪ] *n term*

the bony (hard) and muscular (soft) partition between the oral and nasal cavities; popularly used to refer to the uvula¹ which is also termed pendulous palate¹
palatal *adj term* • palatine [aɪn] *adj* • palato- *comb*
» The boneless soft palate should rise symmetrically when the patient says "ah."
Use soft² / hard³ / high-arched⁴ / cleft⁵ **palate** • **palatine** tonsil⁶ [ɒː]/ arch⁷ • **palatal** wall / vault⁷ [vɔːlt] • **palato**pharyngeal [dʒiːəl] /nasal [eɪ]/glossal

Gaumen, Palatum
Uvula, Zäpfchen¹ weicher G., Gau-
mensegel, Velum palatinum² harter
G., Palatum durum³ Spitz-, Steil-
gaumen, hoher G.⁴ Gaumenspalte⁵
Gaumenmandel⁶ Gaumenbogen⁷
                                     10

---

fren(ul)um [friːnəm ‖ frenjələm] *n term,* **fren(ul)a** or **frenums** *pl*

fold of mucous membranes attaching the lips, cheeks and tongue to the gums
» The lingual frenum¹ may need cutting to increase mobility of the tongue [ʌ].

Frenulum, Bändchen
Zungenbändchen,
Frenulum linguae¹   11

The Teeth

BODY STRUCTURES & FUNCTIONS

gums [gʌmz] *n clin usu pl*   *syn* **gingiva** [dʒɪndʒəvə] *n term*, **gingivae** [iː] *pl*
   epithelial and connective tissues attached to the tooth and alveolar bone
   gingival[1] *adj term* • gingivo-[1] *comb* • gummy[1] *adj jar*
» *The effect of local anesthesia was checked by pricking the gums.*
   There is a band of red, inflamed gingiva along the necks of the teeth.
Use **gingival** tissue / margin[2] [dʒ]/ tenderness • free / attached[3] **gingiva** • marginal **gingivae** • **gingival** gumline[2] / discoloration[4] / massage [ɑː(d)ʒ]/ stippling[5] • receding[6] [iː] **gums** • **gummy** smile[7]

   Note: In the singular *gum* most commonly refers to *chewing gum*.

(dental) alveolus [ælvɪələs] *n term*, **alveoli** [aɪ‖iː] *pl*
                  syn **(tooth) socket** [ɒː] *n clin & inf*
   opening in the maxilla or mandible in which the tooth is attached by the periodontal ligament[1] (abbr PDL)
   alveolar *adj term* • alveolo- *comb*
» *The tooth must be sectioned and atraumatically extracted to preserve socket anatomy. The vertical bite force induces a bending moment as the tooth moves in its alveolus.*
Use **alveolar** process[2] / ridge [dʒ] or crest[3] / bone / socket • extraction[4] **socket**

(dental) crown [kraʊn] *n clin*   *syn* **corona dentis** *n term*
   (i) part of the tooth above the gums covered with enamel (ii) an artificial substitute for that part
» *Decalcification of dental crowns occurs with chronic vomiting[1] (the lingual surfaces of the lower anterior teeth are primarily affected[2]).*
Use artificial[3] / natural (tooth-) **crown**

   Note: The term *crown* more commonly refers to restorations. The expression *dental* or *tooth crown* is used when referring to natural teeth.

(dental or tooth) enamel [ɪnæml] *n clin*   *syn* **enamelum** *n term*
   hard ceramic layer covering the exposed part of teeth
» *These enamel changes range from whitish opaque areas to severe brown discoloration.*
Use **enamel** formation[1] / changes / hypoplasia [eɪʒə]/ powder[2] • saliva-coated [aɪ] **enamel** • **enamel** cuticle[3] [kjuːtɪkl]/ organ

dentin(e) [dentɪn‖dentiːn] *n clin*   *syn* **dentinum** [aɪ] *n term*
   calcium [s] part of a tooth below the enamel containing the pulp chamber [tʃeɪ] and root canals
   dentinal *adj term* • dentino- *comb* • dentinogenesis [dʒe] *n*
» *Caries spreads rapidly in dentin because of its lower mineral content. The pulp is surrounded by hard dentinal walls.*
Use exposed[1] / root[2] / softened **dentin** • **dentin(al)** tubules[3] / surface • **dentinal** pain • **dentino**enamel junction[4] [dʒʌŋkʃ°n] /blasts[5]

cementum [sɪment°m] *n term*   *syn* **(tooth) cement** *n clin*
   layer of mineralized connective tissue covering the dentin of the roots and neck of a tooth
» *Cementum functions as an anchoring substance for the tooth to the alveolar bone. Noncarious teeth can become painful when enamel and cementum do not quite contact each other.*
Use **cementum** deposition • **cemento**enamel junction[1] • **cementum**-like tissue

   Note: Unlike *cementum* the term *cement[2]* also refers to a nonmetallic adhesive [iː] material[3] used for various restorations.

Zahnfleisch, Gingiva
die G. betreffend[1] Zahnfleischrand[2] befestigte G.[3] Zahnfleischverfärbung[4] Zahnfleischtüpfelung[5] Zahnfleischschwund[6] Zahnfleischlächeln, gummy smile[7]

12

Alveole, Zahnfach
Wurzelhaut, Desmodont[1] Alveolarfortsatz[2] Alveolarkamm[3] Extraktionshöhle[4]

13

(Zahn)krone, Corona dentis
Erbrechen[1] betroffen[2] prothetische Krone[3]

14

(Zahn)schmelz, Enamelum
Schmelzbildung, Amelogenese[1] Schmelzpulver[2] Schmelzoberhäutchen[3]

15

Zahnbein, Dentin
freigelegtes D.[1] Wurzeldentin[2] Dentinkanälchen[3] Schmelz-Dentin-Grenze[4] Odonto-, Dentinoblasten[5]

16

Wurzelzement (das), Cementum
Schmelz-Zement-Grenze[1] Zement (der)[2] Befestigungsmaterial[3]

17

BODY STRUCTURES & FUNCTIONS

The Teeth

(dental) pulp [pʌlp] *n clin*   *syn* **pulpa (dentis)** *n term*

soft, spongy [spʌndʒɪ] tissue in the center of the tooth containing blood vessels and nerves
pulpal *adj term* • **pulpless** *adj*

» Teeth with decay[1] [dɪkeɪ] involving the pulp are a potential source of alveolar bone infection.
Use **pulp** chamber [tʃ] *or* cavity[2] / canal • **pulpal** reaction / exposure[3] [-oʊʒɚ] • **pulp** testing[4] / capping[5]

(Zahn)pulpa, Pulpa dentis
Karies[1] Zahnhöhle, Pulpakavum[2] Pulpafreilegung[3] Vitalitäts-, Sensibilitätsprüfung[4] Pulpaüberkappung[5]

18

root (of tooth) [uː] *n clin & term*   *syn* **radix** [eɪ] **dentis** *n term*

part of a tooth below the neck[1]; covered by cementum rather than enamel

» The tooth demonstrated extensive occlusal root caries. The abscess was located at the root apex of a nonvital tooth.
Use **root** apices[2] [eɪpɪsiːz]/ bifurcation [aɪ] • **root canal** filling[3] / treatment[4] (*abbr* RCT) • crown-to-**root** ratio [eɪ] • single-/ two-/ multi[5]-**rooted tooth**

Zahnwurzel, Radix dentis
Zahnhals[1] Wurzelspitzen[2] Wurzelfüllung[3] Wurzelbehandlung[4] mehrwurzeliger Zahn[5]

19

quadrant [kwɒːdrᵊnt] *n term*

the oral cavity is divided anatomically into the upper left and right and the lower left and right quadrants

» The patient had six implants placed per quadrant.
Use mandibular left / opposing[1] / right posterior **quadrant**

Quadrant
Gegenquadrant[1]

20

mesial [miːzɪᵊl] *adj term*   *opposite* **distal**[1] *adj term*

front or forward toward the median [iː] plane [eɪ] following the curvature [kɜːrvətʃɚ] of the dental arch

» The mesial surface of the bicuspid is the portion which is adjacent to[2] [dʒeɪs] the cuspid.

mesial
distal[1] neben, benachbart[2]

21

proximal [ɒː] *adj term*   *sim* **interproximal**[1] *adj term*

denoting the surface between adjacent teeth

» Interproximal caries and periapical [eɪ] lesions [iː] are best visualized [3] by posterior bitewing [aɪ] radiographs[2] [eɪ].
Use **interproximal** space[3] [eɪ]/ surface / brush[4] [ʌ]

proximal
Interdental-, Approximal-[1] Bissflügelaufnahmen[2] Interdentalraum, Approximalbereich[3] Interdentalbürstchen[4]

22

labial [eɪ] *adj term*   *sim* **buccal**[1] [ʌ] *adj, opposite* **lingual**[2], **palatal**[3] *adj term*

towards, referring or adjacent to the lips (labial), cheek [iː] (buccal), tongue [tʌŋ] (lingual) and palate (palatal)
labio- *comb* • **bucco-** *comb* • **linguo-** *comb*

» To restore the labial profile, lip support is obtained from labial denture flanges[4] [dʒ] optimally extended into the vestibule. The maxillary anterior teeth tend to erupt[5] labially.
Use **labial** aspect or surface[6] / gingiva / muscle [mʌsl] • **labio**buccal /palatal /lingual • **bucco**cavity[7] / cusp [ʌ] tip[8] / crown margin [dʒ]/ mucosa • **bucco**alveolar /labial /gingival [dʒ] /lingual • **lingual** nerve[9] / cusp[10] / tipping[11] / to the alveolar crest • **linguo**palatal

labial
bukkal[1] lingual[2] palatal[3] Prothesenrand[4] durchbrechen[5] Labialfläche[6] Mundvorhof[7] bukkale Höckerspitze[8] Lingualnerv, Nervus lingualis[9] Lingualhöcker[10] Lingualkippung[11]

23

occlusal [əkluːzᵊl] *adj term*

referring to the chewing [tʃuːɪŋ] or grinding [aɪ] surface of the bicuspid and molar teeth

» Occlusal and chewing forces were mainly directed in the vertical and horizontal dimensions.
Use **occlusal** plane[1] [eɪ]/ surface[2]

okklusal
Bissebene[1] Kaufläche[2]

24

intraoral [ɔː] *adj term*   *opposite* **extraoral**[1] *adj term*

inside as opposed to (from) outside the mouth

» The intraoral approach has the disadvantage of temporary paresthesia [-θiːʒə] from stretching the mental nerve.
Use **intraoral** anchorage[2] [æŋk]/ environment[3] [aɪ]/ local anesthesia[4] [-θiːʒə]/ camera

intraoral
extraoral[1] intraorale Befestigung[2] Mundmilieu[3] intraorale Leitungsanästhesie[4]

25

Dentition & Mastication | BODY STRUCTURES & FUNCTIONS 31

maxillofacial [mæksɪloʊfeɪʃəl] *adj term*
referring to the dental arches, jaws and face
» An oral-maxillofacial surgeon[1] was consulted because of persistent malocclusion.
Use **maxillofacial** surgery / prosthetics[2] / restoration / defect / augmentation •
maxillopalatine /mandibular /labial /turbinal

Gesicht- u. Kiefer betreffend, maxillofazial
Mund-Kiefer-Gesichtschirurg(in)[1]
Kiefer-Gesichtsprothetik[2]

26

Unit 10   Dentition & Mastication
Related Units: **9** Teeth, **11** Human Sounds & Speech, **2** Food & Drink, Dentistry

dentition [dentɪʃən] *n term*
(i) collective term for the teeth in the dental arch (ii) the teething [tiːðɪŋ] process (from calcification to eruption)
» His dentition is in poor repair[1]. The situation when both deciduous and permanent teeth are present is termed mixed dentition[2].
Use deciduous / permanent / natural / artificial[3] / retarded[4] / precocious[5] [prɪkoʊʃəs] **dentition**

(i) **Gebiss, Dentition**
(ii) **Zahndurchbruch**
in schlechtem Zustand[1] Misch-, Übergangsgebiss[2] Zahnersatz[3] verzögerte D., Dentitio tarda[4] vorzeitige D., Dentitio praecox[5]

1

deciduous [dɪsɪdjʊəs] **teeth** *n term*   *syn* **baby** or **milk teeth** *n clin & inf*
also called primary [aɪ] or temporary (set of) teeth which fall out in childhood and are replaced by the permanent teeth
» The deciduous teeth begin to calcify [s] about the 16th week of prenatal life.
Use to cut[1]/shed[2]/lose **deciduous teeth** • spaced[3] **deciduous teeth**

Milchzähne, -gebiss
Milchzähne bekommen[1] M. fallen aus[2] lückiges Milchgebiss[3]

2

erupt [ɪrʌpt] *vi term*   *syn* **come in** *v phr clin & inf*
(i) when a tooth elongates and breaks the gums (ii) generally, to break through the skin
eruption [ʌ] *n term* • unerupted *adj*
» A significant change in arch width[1] [wɪdθ] occurs with eruption of the permanent teeth.
Use tooth / delayed[2] [eɪ]/ impeded[3] [iː]/ ectopic **eruption** • fully / partially **erupted** • ectopically **erupting** molar

durchbrechen
Zahnbogenbreite[1] verzögerter Zahndurchbruch[2] erschwerter Zahndurchbruch, Dentitio difficilis[3]

3

teething [tiːðɪŋ] *n clin & term*   *syn* **cutting of teeth** *n clin & inf*
process of eruption of the primary teeth normally beginning around the 6th month of life
» Your baby may be teething. Look, he's cut his first tooth. Teething is often associated with excessive drooling[1] [uː] irritability, and biting on hard objects. This problem cannot be ascribed to teething.
Use **teething** problems / process / ring or teether[2] / powders [aʊ]

Zahnen, Zahndurchbruch
Sabbern[1] Beißring[2]

4

exfoliate *vi term*   *syn* **shed** *vt*, **fall out** *vi phr clin & inf*
physiologic shedding of primary teeth in childhood; first the teeth loosen[1] and eventually[2] fall out
exfoliation[3] *n term* • (non)exfoliated *adj*
» The first baby teeth are usually shed when the child is six, but it is not uncommon for them to be retained much longer. By age 9 the permanent incisors reach the dental height [haɪt] of the exfoliated incisors.

(Zähne) verlieren, ausfallen
sich lockern[1] schließlich[2] Zahnwechsel[3]

5

permanent or **secondary teeth** or **dentition** *n term*
adult set of teeth which erupt between about the 6th and 13th year of life
» Once erupted, many permanent teeth do not maintain[1] a fixed position.

bleibende(s) Zähne / Gebiss
beibehalten[1]

6

edentulous [ɪdentʃələs] *adj term*   *syn* **toothless** *adj clin & inf*
having lost all natural teeth
dentulous *adj term* • edentulism *n* • edent(ul)ation[1] *n* • edentulousness *n*
» She received a freestanding prosthesis[2] in each edentulous quadrant [ɒː].
Use partially or semi-/ totally or completely **edentulous** • **edentulous** patient / adult / arch / alveolar ridge[3] [dʒ]/ jaw [dʒɒː]/ maxilla / site

zahnlos
Zahnlosigkeit (durch Zahnentfernung)[1] Freiendprothese[2] Alveolarkamm (nach Zahnverlust)[3]

7

32 BODY STRUCTURES & FUNCTIONS — Dentition & Mastication

denture [dentʃə·] n term syn **plates** [eɪ] n pl, **artificial** or **false teeth** n clin & inf
artificial replacement for some or all natural teeth
» The existing denture was readapted 14 days after fixture installation.
Use full (set of) / partial / upper or maxillary / fixed[1] / removable / temporary or transitional[2] **denture** • **denture** base[3] / satisfaction / wearer [eə·]/-bearing [eə·] area[4] / retention / (in)stability / cleanser[5] [e]/ patient

Zahnprothese, künstliches Gebiss
festsitzende Zahnprothese[1] Interimsprothese[2] Prothesenbasis[3] prothesentragende Fläche[4] Prothesenreiniger[5]   8

salivation [eɪ] n term sim **drooling**[1] [uː] n clin & inf
the secretion of saliva as the mouth waters, e.g. at the sight or smell of tasty food
saliva [səlaɪvə] n term • saliva(to)ry adj • salivate[2] v
» Salivary control was slightly hampered[3] and this led to drooling.
Use **saliva** flow • artificial **saliva** • **salivary** pellicle[4] / gland / secretion / proteins • reduced / increased / profuse[5] **salivation**

Speichelbildung, -fluss, Salivation
Sabbern[1] Speichel produzieren[2] beeinträchtigt[3] exogenes Schmelzoberhäutchen[4] starker / übermäßiger Speichelfluss[5]   9

spit-spit-spit v irr & n inf
(v) to force out the contents of the mouth, usually saliva (n) saliva
spitoon[1] [uː] n term BE
» Rinse[2] and then spit out. Some patients deny production of sputum because spitting is socially unacceptable.
Use **to spit** out • blood **spitting**

(aus)spucken; Spucke
Mundspül-, Speibecken[1]
ausspülen[2]

10

bite-bit-bitten v irr sim **nibble**[1] v clin & inf
to seize [iː] with the teeth or jaws
bite off/through/into[2] v
» The patient was asked to bite as if he was chewing [uː]. Bite into this material.
Use nail[3] **biting** • **bitten** tongue / lips / cheeks [iː]

(zu)beißen
knabbern[1] ab-, durch-, hineinbeißen[2] Nägelbeißen, -kauen[3]

11

bite [baɪt] n clin & term & jar syn **morsel** n inf → U36-12 f
(i) in genE, a mouthful of solid food (ii) forced closure of the jaws or the pressure developed thereby (iii) jargon for various dental terms like interocclusal record[1] and interarch distance
» He only took a bite and then the tooth was loose[2].
Use to take/have a **bite** • **bite** wing[3] / opening[4] / plane / block / force / registration[5] / guard [gɑːrd] / splint[6] / fork /-sized[7] [aɪ] • check**bite**[8]

(i) Bissen, Happen (ii) Biss
Okklusionsbefund, -diagnostik, -analyse[1] locker, lose[2] Bissflügel[3] Bisshöhe[4] Bissnahme[5] Aufbissschiene[6] mundgerecht[7] Checkbiss[8]   12

occlude [əkluːd] v term → U36-7 f
to bring the teeth of both jaws into contact
occlusion n term • malocclusion[1] n • occlusal adj
» As they occlude, all teeth should contact their opponents[2]. The molars occclude normally. The patient was asked to occlude with as much force as possible. First the vertical dimension of occlusion was registered.
Use balanced / in habitual / centric[3] / interfered[4] **occlusion** • **occlusal** contact / force / level / load / plane[5] / surface

okkludieren, Zahnreihen schließen
Okklusionsstörung, Malokklusion[1] Gegenzähne, Antagonisten[2] zentrische Okklusion[3] gestörte Okklusion[4] Okklusionsebene[5]

13

freeway space n term syn **interarch** or **interocclusal distance** n term
gap between the occluding surfaces of opposing teeth with the jaws in physiologic resting position[1]
» The vertical dimension of occlusion should allow for adequate freeway space.
Use anterior / inadequate **freeway space** • excessive **interarch distance**

Interokklusalabstand
Ruhe(schwebe)lage[1]

14

masticate [mæstɪkeɪt] v term syn **chew** [tʃuː], **munch** [ʌ] v clin & inf
chewing food and mixing it with saliva to prepare it for swallowing[1] [ɒː] and digestion [dʒe]
mastication[2] n term • masticatory adj
» While the patient chewed standardized pieces of crispbread, seated upright in a dental chair, recordings of masticatory sequences from start to swallowing were performed.
Use **masticatory** muscles / process[2] / load[3] / mandibular movement / oral mucosa[4] / function / improvement • **masticatory** cycle [saɪkl] / duration[5] / ability / apparatus • mean [iː] **masticatory** force[6] • **masticatory** silent period • **chewing** efficiency[7] [ɪʃ]/ pattern / stroke[8] / ability / contacts / force[6] • **chewing** test food / gum / tobacco

(zer)kauen
Schlucken[1] Kauvorgang[2] Kaubelastung[3] mastikatorische Schleimhaut[4] Kauzyklusdauer[5] mittlere Kaukraft[6] Kauleistung[7] Kaubewegung[8]

15

Dentition & Mastication BODY STRUCTURES & FUNCTIONS 33

gag [gæg] v & n   syn **retch** [retʃ], **heave** [iː] v, sim **choke**[1] [tʃoʊk] v clin & inf
v (i) to retch or cause to retch, e.g. by touching the soft palate[2] (ii) to keep the mouth from closing by placing a mouth prop between the teeth
gag or pharyngeal [-ɪndʒiːəl] reflex[3] n term • gagging adj & n
» He started gagging every time I inserted an instrument. The patient gags reflexively.
Use to experience a **gagging** sensation • a severe **gagger**

(i) würgen, Brechreiz haben
(ii) mit Mundsperrer öffnen; Mundsperrer
(er)würgen; ersticken[1] weicher Gaumen[2] Würg(e)reflex[3]
16

clench [klentʃ] v clin
to squeeze [iː] together tightly [taɪtli], e.g. the upper and lower teeth or the hand to make a fist[1]
teeth clenching[2] n term
» He was encouraged [ɜː] to clench as hard as possible. The patient was a clencher who habitually[3] kept his teeth tightly together.
Use **clenching** force / habit / level / in centric [s] occlusion • nighttime[4] **clenching**

zusammenbeißen, -pressen
Faust ballen[1] Zahnpressen[2] ständig, gewohnheitsmäßig[3] nächtliches Zahnpressen[4]
17

grind [aɪ]-**ground-ground** [aʊ] v irr clin   rel **bruxism**[1] [ʌ] n term
(i) making a grating sound by clenching and rubbing the teeth (ii) to crush food (iii) wearing [eə] away by polishing or abrasion, e.g. to reshape the contour of a tooth
teeth grinding[1] n clin • grinding wheel[2] [iː] n • grinder[3] n jar
» If the patient is a grinder[3] there will be continuous movement of opposing tooth surfaces.
Use **grinding** movement / habit[4] / equipment[5] • **ground** section[6]

(i) knirschen (ii) (zer)mahlen (iii) (ab-, ein)schleifen
(Zähne)knirschen, Bruxismus[1] Schleifstein[2] Knirscher, Schleifmaschine[3] habituelles Knirschen[4] Schleifkörper[5] (ab)geschliffene Fläche[6]
18

attrition n term   sim **demastication**[1], **abrasion**[2] [-eɪʒn] n term
wearing away of the biting surfaces in the process of normal mastication; loss of tooth structure from mechanical wear other than chewing is termed abrasion
abrade[3] [eɪ] v term • abrasive [eɪ] adj & n
» The teeth were replaced because of attrition. With age the biting surfaces become worn[4] (attrition) so that chewing becomes less effective.
Use mechanical [k] **abrasion** • **abrasive** polishing paste[5] / paper[6]/ wear

Attrition, Abrieb
Demastikation, Abkauung[1] Abrasion, Abrieb, -nutzung[2] abreiben, abradieren, abkauen, abtragen[3] abgenutzt[4] Polierpaste[5] Schleifpapier[6]
19

resorption [rɪzɔːrpʃən] n term
removal of bone or tooth structure by pressure; gradual destruction of dentin and cementum of the root, e.g. of the primary teeth prior to shedding
bone resorption[1] n term • bone-resorptive adj • resorb[2]
» Clearly the microdamage induced by the high stresses is one cause of bone resorption.
Use severely **resorbed** edentulous jaws • advanced / extensive / alveolar[3] / (jaw)**bone resorption** • **resorption** of tooth roots[4] • **resorptive** pattern / state [eɪ]/ process / changes

Resorption, Abbau
Knochenabbau[1] resorbieren[2] Alveolarkammabbau[3] Wurzelresorption[4]
20

erosion [ɪroʊʒən] n term   sim **abfraction**[1] n term
loss of tooth structure due to processes not related to bacterial action
erode[2] v term • erosive adj
» Tooth grinding erodes and eventually reduces the height [haɪt] of the dental crowns.
Use **eroded** areas[3] / cement • chemical [k]/ spark[4] **erosion** • **erosive** process

Erosion
Ausbrechen (v. Schmelz, Dentin)[1] abtragen, erodieren[2] usurierte Bereiche[3] Funkenerosion[4]
21

decalcification [dɪkæls-] n term   opposite **calcification**[1] n term
loss of calcium salts from teeth or bone; may be the result of a pathologic process or part of a bone grafting procedure
(de)calcify[2] v term • (de)calcified adj • non-decalcified adj
» Chronic cocaine [koʊkeɪn] snorting[3] may result in widespread decalcification of teeth. Decalcified teeth are more susceptible [se] to decay[4] [dɪkeɪ]. The bone products were freeze-dried, decalcified, and sealed [iː]. As the permanent teeth calcify, the roots of the baby teeth are gradually resorbed.
Use **calcified** tissue / deposits[5] / bone • **decalcified** section / specimen[6] [es] • **decalcifying** solution

Dekalzifikation, -zierung, Entkalkung
Verkalkung, Kalzifikation[1] (ent-,) verkalken[2] Kokainschnupfen[3] kariesanfällig[4] verkalkte Ablagerungen[5] dekalzifiziertes Präparat[6]
22

Unit 11 Human Sounds & Speech
Related Units: 9 The Teeth, 8 The Head & Neck

utter [ʌ] v   sim **articulate**[1] v term

to make a sound with your voice (includes verbal expression[2] but also shouts[3] [aʊ], laughter [læftɚ], cries[4], and other human sounds)

utterance[5] n • articulation[6] n term • (in)articulate[7] adj

» His verbal utterances include unassociated rambling statements[8]. Their speech [spiːtʃ] is well-articulated but has little content. The patient is clear and articulate[9].

Use poor / compensatory / place of **articulation** • compulsive / involuntary / phrase length [leŋθ] **utterances**

äußern, Laute hervorbringen
artikulieren, deutlich (aus)sprechen[1] verbale Äußerung[2] Rufe[3] Schreie[4] Sprechweise, (stimmliche) Äußerung[5] Sprechlautbildung, Artikulation[6] deutlich artikuliert, verständlich[7] unzusammenhängendes Gefasel[8] drückt s. klar u. deutlich aus[9]

1

laugh [læf] v & n   sim **giggle**[1], **snicker**[1], **chuckle**[2] [tʃʌkəl], **roar**[3] [ɔː], **howl**[4] [haʊl] v inf

(v) to smile and make the typical guttural [ʌ] sounds[5] to express amusement or pleasure[6] [eʒ]

laughter[7] n • laughable[8] adj • giggly[9] [ɡɪɡli] adj

» The symptoms include uncontrollably crying and laughter. Coughing[10] [kɒːf-], straining[11] [eɪ], sneezing[12] [iː] and laughing brought on[13] severe [-ɪɚ] headaches.

Use to have to/make sb./be a[14]/raise [reɪz] a[15] **laugh** • belly[16] **laugh** • to **laugh** softly[17] / out loud / one's head off[18] / at[19] sb. or a joke / about sth. • to burst [ɜː] out[3] **laughing** • to **roar** with laughter[20] • roaring / hysterical / nervous **laughter**

lachen; Lachen
kichern[1] kichern, in sich hineinlachen[2] schallend lachen[3] (vor L.) brüllen; heulen[4] Guttural-, Kehllaute[5] Vergnügen, Freude[6] Gelächter[7] lächerlich[8] albern[9] Husten[10] Pressen[11] Niesen[12] verursachte[13] urkomisch sein[14] Gelächter ernten[15] dröhnendes L.[16] leise lachen[17] sich totlachen[18] lachen über[19] vor Lachen brüllen[20]

2

sob [sɒːb] v & n   sim **weep** [iː]-wept-wept[1] v irr, **cry**[1], **whimper**[2], **wail**[3] [eɪ] v

(v) to weep in convulsive [ʌ] gasps[4] with or without shedding tears[5] [tɪɚz]

» The child was sobbing her heart out[6]. She called the ambulance, her voice choked [tʃoʊkd] with sobs[7].

Use to **sob** bitterly[6] / oneself to sleep • to let out a[8] / choking / bitter **sob** • to have a good[9] **weep**

> Note: Mark the two meanings of cry and crying, (i) to break out in tears, and (ii) to shout. → U11-14

schluchzen; Schluchzen
weinen[1] wimmern[2] jammern, klagen[3] krampfartiges Keuchen[4] Tränen vergießen[5] bitterlich / herzzerreißend weinen[6] m. tränenerstickter Stimme[7] aufschluchzen[8] sich ausweinen[9]

3

sigh [saɪ] v & n   sim **moan**[1] [moʊn], **groan**[1] [oʊ] v & n

(v) breathe [briːð] deeply and heavily [e] and exhale audibly[2] [ɒː] to express sadness, boredom[3], etc.

» She sat down with a sigh. The baby's breathing movements resembled[4] a deep sigh. Sighing is a common sign of neurasthenic [nʊɚ-] pain. She woke us up moaning and groaning.

Use to let out/give/heave[5] [iː] **a sigh** • (in)audible[6] **sigh** • **sigh** of relief[7] [iː]

seufzen; Seufzer
stöhnen, klagen; Stöhnen, Ächzen[1] (deutlich) hörbar ausatmen[2] Langeweile[3] ähnlich sein[4] e. Seufzer ausstoßen[5] leiser/lauter Seufzer[6] Seufzer der Erleichterung[7]

4

snore [snɔːr] v & n   rel **snort**[1], **grunt**[2] [ʌ] v & n

(v) to breathe noisily while sleeping due to vibration of the soft palate[3]

» Loud snores were coming from her bedroom. Is there a cure[4] for snoring? An estimated 25% of the adult male population and 15% of the adult female population snore every night. A loud snort accompanies the first breath following an apneic episode.

Use loud / severe / severity [e] of / cyclical [saɪk-]/ habitual / chronic **snoring** • heavy [e] **snorer** • **snore** guard[5] [ɡɑːrd] • **to snort** with laughter

schnarchen; Schnarchen
(wütend) schnauben, prusten; Schnauben[1] knurren, ächzen, brummen, grunzen; Ächzen[2] weicher Gaumen[3] (Heil)mittel[4] Nachtschiene[5]

5

sneeze [sniːz] v & n   rel **cough**[1] [kɒːf] v & n, **to clear one's throat**[2] [θroʊt] phr

to exhale explosively because of a cold, irritants in the nose, etc.

» The pain gets worse with sneezing. Advise the patient to avoid sneezing and blowing his nose[3]. The introduction of allergens into the nose is associated with sneezing, stuffiness[4] [ʌ] and nasal [eɪ] discharge[5] [dɪstʃɑːrdʒ]. Cats make her sneeze. When somebody sneezes you might say 'Bless you'[6].

Use to cause/have a fit or paroxysm of[7] **sneezing** • episodic / violent[8] [aɪə]/ light-induced or photic / irrepressible[9] **sneezing** • **sneezing** fit[7] / reflex[10] / **sneezed** sputum [pjuː] • **sneeze**(-inducing) effect[11] • not to be **sneezed** at[12] • to have/give **a cough** • bad[13] / mild / productive / nonproductive or dry or hacking[14] **cough** • to **cough up** blood / phlegm[15] [flem] • **cough** reflex / syrup

niesen; Niesen
husten, Husten[1] sich räuspern[2] s. die Nase putzen[3] Verstopftsein (d. Nase)[4] Nasensekret[5] Gesundheit[6] Niesanfall (haben)[7] heftiges N.[8] nicht unterdrückbares N.[9] Niesreflex[10] Niesreiz[11] nicht zu verachten[12] starker Husten[13] trockener / unproduktiver H.[14] Schleim aushusten[15]

6

Human Sounds & Speech   BODY STRUCTURES & FUNCTIONS 35

gargle [gɑːrgl] v & n

(v) rinse[1] one's throat with mouthwash[2] and/or make bubbling[3] sounds with the fluid

» *Gargling with saline[4] [eɪ] may remedy[5] a sore throat[6]. In these cases gargles or sprays of lidocaine [eɪ] should be used before intubation.*

gurgeln; Gurgeln, Gurgelmittel
spülen[1] Mundwasser[2] blubbernd[3] Kochsalzlösung[4] helfen bei[5] Halsschmerzen[6]   7

speak [iː] -spoke-spoken v irr   rel **communicate**[1], **vocalize**[2] v

express thoughts in language, e.g. to talk, mention[3] [-ʃən], remark[3], gossip[4], observe, suggest[5] [dʒ], imply[6] [aɪ], state, report, confirm[7] [ɜː], insist (on)[8], hint[9], deny[10] [aɪ], read out loud, etc.
speech[11] [spiːtʃ] n term • communication n • communicative[12] adj
• vocalization[13] n

» *Speech may have a nasal timbre[14] [tæmbɚ] caused by weakness of the palate. Symptoms of confusion, slurred [ɜː] speech[15], ataxia and inappropriate behavior are common.*

Use **to speak** up or louder / fluently[16] / distinctly[17] / coherently[18] [ɪɚ]/ frankly[19] • to deliver[20] **a speech** • **speaking** aids[21] • **speech** development[22] / output / pattern / disturbance[23] / arrest • **speech** center / perception[24] / discrimination / (-language) pathologist[25] / therapist[25] • (un)clear or (un)intelligible [-dʒɪbl]/ clipped or scanning[26] / spontaneous [eɪ]/ disorganized **speech** • purposeful / esophageal[27] [-dʒiːəl]/ absence of **speech** • **language** development / function • spoken / written / body / sign[28] **language** • **communicative** assessment • (non)verbal / level of / to encourage [ɜː] **communication** • **communication** skills[29]

sprechen
kommunizieren, s. verständigen[1] Ausdruck verleihen, vokalisieren[2] erwähnen, bemerken[3] tratschen[4] vorschlagen[5] andeuten, implizieren[6] bestätigen[7] beharren (auf)[8] hinweisen[9] bestreiten, leugnen[10] Sprache[11] mitteilsam, gesprächig[12] Vokalisation[13] Stimmklang, Timbre[14] verwaschene Sprache[15] fließend sprechen[16] deutlich spr.[17] zusammenhängend reden[18] offen/ ehrlich sagen[19] Rede halten[20] Sprechhilfen[21] Sprachentwicklung[22] Sprach-, Sprechstörung[23] Sprachverständnis[24] Logopäde/-in[25] abgehackte Sprechweise, skandierende Sprache[26] Ösophagusstimme[27] Zeichensprache[28] kommunikative Fähigkeiten[29]   8

log(o)- comb   rel **-phasia**[1] [feɪʒ(ɪ)ə], **-arthria**[2] comb

referring to language, speech or words
logopedics[3] [iː] n term • aphasic[4] [eɪz] adj • dysarthric[5] [ɪ] adj

» *Logopedics or speech therapy[3] is the study and treatment of speech defects[6]. Speech output[7] is fluent but paraphasic[8]; comprehension of spoken language is intact. The paraphasic output in conduction aphasia interferes [ɪɚ] with[9] the ability to express meaning.*

Use logorrhea[10] [iːə] • conduction[11] / (non)fluent transcortical / global / anomic[12] / motor[13] **aphasia** • **aphasic** deficit / patient / syndrome • dys[14]/ para**phasia** • **paraphasic** speech • mild / marked / spastic[15] **dysarthria**

Wort-, Sprach-, Sprech-, Logo-
-phasie[1] -arthrie[2] Logopädie[3] aphasisch[4] dysarthrisch[5] Sprach-, Sprechstörungen[6] Sprachproduktion[7] paraphasisch[8] beeinträchtigt[9] Rededrang, Logorrhoe[10] Leitungsaphasie[11] amnestische A.[12] motor. / Broca-A.[13] Dysphasie[14] pyramidale / spastische Dysarthrie[15]
                                                  9

voice n & v   rel **phonation**[1] [eɪ] n term

(n) sound produced by the vocal folds[2] and articulated in the vocal tract
voiced[3] adj • voiceless adj • vocal[4] adj • vocalist[5] n
• phonic[6] adj term • phon(o)-[7] comb

» *Her voice sounded nasal and she had difficulty swallowing[8] [ɒː]. His voice lowered to a whisper. The voice is 'breathy' when too much air passes incompletely apposed vocal cords, as in unilateral vocal cord paralysis.*

Use hoarse[9] [ɔː]/ thick[10] / breathy [breθi]/ low[11] / deep **voice** • high-pitched[12] / hollow-sounding / squeaky[13] [skwiːki] **voice** • harsh[14] / poorly modulated / comforting[15] / (normal) spoken[16] **voice** • to lower[17]/raise/lose **one's voice** • **voice** is shaking or quivering[18] • **voice** box[19] / problem / change • to hear **voices** (within you) • **vocal** apparatus / folds / cords[20] / sounds • **phonic** tic / spasm[21] • **phon**iatrics[22] /ology /etic /etics /eme /asthenia[23] [iː]

Stimme; zum Ausdruck bringen
Stimm-, Lautbildung[1] Stimmlippen[2] stimmhaft[3] Stimm-, vokal[4] Sänger(in)[5] Stimm-, phonisch[6] Laut-, Ton-, phono-[7] beim Schlucken[8] heisere Stimme[9] belegte St.[10] leise St.[11] hohe / schrille St.[12] piepsende St.[13] raue St.[14] beruhigende St.[15] Sprechstimme[16] d. Stimme dämpfen[17] St. zittert[18] Kehlkopf[19] Stimmbänder[20] Stimmritzenkrampf, Laryngospasmus[21] Phoniatrie[22] Phonasthenie, Stimmschwäche[23]   10

BODY STRUCTURES & FUNCTIONS — Human Sounds & Speech

tone [toʊn] **(of voice)** n   *sim* **sound**[1] [saʊnd] n & v
quality (including pitch[2] [tʃ], timbre, loudness or volume, etc.) of a person's voice
intonation[3] n term • overtone[4] n • undertone[5] n
» Suddenly his tone of voice changed. The timbre of the voice depends on the size and shape of the resonating chambers[6] [tʃeɪ-] (mouth, pharynx, nasal sinuses [aɪ], chest, etc.).
Use **in a(n)** harsh[7] / normal / angry / subdued[8] [uː]/ friendly / threatening[9] [e] **tone** • **high-tone** range • **sound** substitution[10] / discrimination[11] • in an[8] **undertone**

Ton(fall,-höhe), Klang, Stimme
Laut, Schall, Ton, Geräusch; klingen, sondieren[1] Tonhöhe[2] Intonation, Sprach-, Satzmelodie[3] Oberton (musik.), Unterton (fig.)[4] Unterton; gedämpft[5] Resonanzkörper[6] in barschem / scharfem Ton[7] m. gedämpfter Stimme[8] m. drohender St.[9] Lautersatz[10] Lautunterscheidung(svermögen)[11]   11

syllable [sɪləbl] n
a unit of language consisting of several phonemes[1] [iː] (vowels[2] [aʊ] or consonants[3])
monosyllabic[4] adj term & clin • syllable-stumbling[5] [ʌ] n
» The form of stuttering[6] [ʌ] in which patients halt[7] [ɒː] before certain syllables they find difficult to enunciate [ʌns] is termed syllable-stumbling or dyssyllabia[5] [eɪ].

Silbe
Phoneme, (Einzel)laute[1] Vokale, Selbstlaute[2] Konsonanten[3] einsilbig; wortkarg[4] Silbenstolpern[5] Stottern[6] stocken[7]   12

pronunciation [ʌ] n   *sim* **phonation**[1], **enunciation**[2] [ʌ] n term
production of sounds in accordance with the phonetic system of a specific language (includes emphasis[3], intonation, and accent[4] [æksənt])
pronounce[5] v • enunciate[6] v term • phonate[7] v • phonetic adj
» The alterations in phonation were due to obstruction. He enunciates each word carefully. She had difficulty segmenting words into pronounceable components.
Use **to pronounce** badly / properly • hard[8] **to pronounce** • correct / word **pronunciation** • normal **phonation** • **phonating** structure • **phonetically** balanced (abbr PB)

> Note: The word pronounced[9] (adj) commonly appears in medical contexts as a synonym for marked[9], e.g. Stiffness was more pronounced in the morning.

Aussprache
Laut-, Stimmbildung[1] Artikulation[2] Betonung[3] Akzent, Tonfall[4] aussprechen; erklären[5] artikulieren[6] Laute bilden, phonieren[7] schwer auszusprechen[8] deutlich, ausgeprägt[9]
   13

shout [ʃaʊt] v & n   *syn* **cry, yell** [jel], **scream** [iː], **holler, shriek** [iː] v & n inf
to raise your voice when talking or utter a loud scream (of protest, anger [ŋg], fear [fɪə], etc)
» During night terrors[1] a child may sit up in bed screaming and thrashing [ʃ] about[2]. A weak or absent cry at birth may suggest [dʒ] vocal cord impairment. In laryngitis [dʒaɪ] vigorous [ɪg] use[3] of the voice (shouting, singing, swearing[4] [eə], roaring[5]) may cause vocal nodules[6].
Use normal hunger / shrill / protracted[7] **cry** • **to shriek** in terror[8] / with laughter

schreien, brüllen, (laut) rufen; Schrei, Ruf, Gebrüll
Nachtangst, Pavor nocturnus[1] (wild) um sich schlagen[2] starke Beanspruchung[3] fluchen[4] brüllen[5] Stimmlippenknötchen[6] langgezogener Schrei[7] vor Angst kreischen[8]   14

murmur [mɜːrmər] v & n   *sim* **mumble**[1] [ʌ], **mutter**[1] [ʌ] v
(v) to speak indistinctly[2] in a low voice (n) constant quiet sound or voice that cannot be heard [ɜː] or understood very well
» She mumbled something about her late husband[3]. She was murmuring to herself.

murmeln, nuscheln; Gemurmel, Raunen
murmeln, nuscheln, brummeln[1] undeutlich[2] verstorbener Ehemann[3]   15

whisper [ʰwɪspər] v & n   *sim* **whispering**[1] n
(v) speaking softly[2] in a low[2] voice without vibration [aɪ] of the vocal cords
» There was impaired [eə] fluency[3] which then resolved[4] into a hoarse whisper. Whispered pectoriloquy[5] is an extreme form of bronchophony in which softly spoken words are readily heard by auscultation [ɒːsk-].
Use **to whisper** into sb's ear • to speak in a / soft[6] **whisper** • **whispered** voice[7] / speech / sounds / bronchophony[5] • **whispered** voice test[8]

flüstern; Geflüster
Flüstern, Getuschel, Gerede[1] leise[2] Redeflussstörung[3] überging in[4] Bronchophonie, Bronchialstimme[5] leises Geflüster[6] Flüsterstimme[7] Flüsterprobe[8]
   16

Human Sounds & Speech   BODY STRUCTURES & FUNCTIONS 37

---

babble v & n   sim **coo**[1] [kuː] v, **lallation**[2] n term

to produce incoherent[3], meaningless sounds, e.g. a baby or like a baby

babbling[4] n • lal(o)- comb • -lalia comb

» By 2 months of age the child's vocalizations[5] include cooing, while babbling begins by 6-10 months of age.
Use **babble** of voices[6] • **lallation** phase[7] • echo[8] [k]/ copro[9]/ rhino[10] [aɪ]/ dys**lalia**[11] • **lalo**phobia[12]

babbeln, plappern; Babbelei, Geplapper
lallen[1] Lallen[2] unverständlich, unzusammenhängend[3] Plappern, Babbelei[4] Sprachäußerungen[5] Stimmengewirr[6] Lallphase[7] Echolalie[8] (zwanghafter) Gebrauch vulgärer Ausdrücke; Koprolalie[9] Näseln, Rhinophonie, -lalie[10] Artikulationsstörung, Dyslalie[11] Sprechangst, Lalophobie[12]   17

---

eloquent [eləkwent] adj   sim **communicative**[1], **talkative**[1] [tɔːk-] adj

very articulate and able to express oneself fluently, clearly, effectively

eloquence[2] n •uncommunicative adj • taciturn[3] [æs] adj

» Profoundly [aʊ] retarded[4] children (IQ < 30) are usually minimally communicative.

wortgewandt, beredt
gesprächig, redselig, mitteilsam[1] Redegewandtheit, Eloquenz[2] schweigsam, wortkarg[3] schwerstbehindert[4]   18

---

ramble v   sim **rant**[1], **chatter**[2] [tʃ], **blab(ber)**[3] v, **go on about sth.**[4] phr

to speak incessantly[5] [se] and in a confused way about unimportant matters

» The patient's language was a rambling monolog. Our new patient keeps ranting on about the melting polar caps. Stop this idle [aɪ] chatter[6], you've got work to do.

faseln, unzusammenhängendes Zeug reden
irres Zeug reden, Tiraden loslassen[1] schwatzen[2] plappern, ausplaudern[3] stundenlang etw. erzählen[4] unaufhörlich[5] leeres Geplapper[6]   19

---

stutter [ʌ] n & v   sim **stammer**[1] [æ] n & v, **pause**[2] [ɔː], **falter**[2] [ɔː] v clin

(n) speech disorder marked by involuntary hesitations[3] and repetitions; mispronunciation and transposition of sounds is referred to as stammering ; esp. in BE usage stutter and stammer are used synonymously

stammerer[4] n • stutterer[4] n • stammering[5] n

» She only stammmers when she is tense[6] or uptight[7] [-taɪt].
Use a severe / nervous **stammer** • to have a[8] **stutter** • syllable[9] **stuttering**

Stottern, Dysphemie; stottern
Stammeln, Dyslalie; stammeln[1] stocken[2] Stocken[3] Stotterer[4] Stottern, Gestotter[5] angespannt[6] nervös[7] stottern[8] Silbenstolpern[9]
                                    20

---

lisp v & n   syn **(para)sigmatism** n term, sim **hiss**[1] v & n

(n) speech defect in which sibilants[2] esp. [s] and [z] are distorted[3] to a hissing sound

» She began lisping when she lost one of her front teeth. Should my 30-month-old see a speech therapist for her lisp? You may even think that your child's lisp sounds cute[4] [kjuːt] now.
Use to speak with/utter with/correct **a lisp** • frontal **lisp**

lispeln; Lispeln, Sigmatismus
zischen; Zischen[1] Zischlaute[2] fehlerhaft gebildet[3] klingt niedlich[4]
                                    21

---

hypernasal [eɪ] adj term   opposite **hyponasal**[1] [haɪpoʊ-] adj term

excessive nasal air emission [ɪʃ] commonly due to velopharyngeal [dʒ] incompetence[2]

» Speech problems including hypernasality and articulation errors[3] are commonly associated with facial [feɪʃəl] clefts[4].
Use hyponasal resonance / voice • **hypernasal** speech[5] • momentary / intermittent[6] hyponasality

hypernasal
hyponasal[1] Insuffizienz d. velopharyngealen Abschlusses[2] Artikulationsstörungen[3] Gesichtsspalten[4] näselnde Sprache, Rhinolalie[5] intermittierende / zeitweilig auftretende Hyponasalität[6]   22

---

aphonia [eɪfoʊnɪə] n term   sim **dysphonia**[1] [dɪs-] n term

inability to vocalize[2] (except for whispered speech) because of disease or injury to organs of speech

» These laryngeal [-dʒɪəl] disorders are commonly associated with hoarseness[3], aphonia, and stridor[4] [aɪ]. Dysphonia refers to any kind of difficulty or pain in speaking.
Use spastic / hysteric **aphonia** • **aphonic** voice[5]

Aphonie, Stimmlosigkeit
Dysphonie, Stimmstörung[1] (laut) aussprechen[2] Heiserkeit[3] Stridor, pfeifendes Atemgeräusch[4] tonlose Stimme[5]
                                    23

11

38 BODY STRUCTURES & FUNCTIONS — Nutrition

Clinical Phrases

The patient spoke in low murmurs. Der/Die Patient(in) murmelte leise vor sich hin. • He has a bad stammer. Er stottert stark. • His voice was breaking much too early. Er hatte viel zu früh den Stimmbruch. • She gave a history of marked difficulty with swallowing and a "hot-potato" voice. Sie klagte über starke Schluckbeschwerden und eine belegte Stimme. • When did you first notice the deepening and coarsening of the voice? Wann ist Ihnen erstmals aufgefallen, dass Ihre Stimme rauer und tiefer wird? • The words are phonetically balanced. Die Sprache ist phonetisch unauffällig. • The patient's spontaneous speech was fluent maintaining appropriate phrase length and melody. Die Spontansprache des Patienten war fließend; Satzlänge und Satzmelodie waren im normalen Bereich.

Unit 12   Nutrition

Related Units: 1 Diet & Dieting, 2 Food & Drink, 10 Dentition & Mastication, Dentistry

nourish [nɜːrɪʃ] v   sim **nurture**[1] [nɜːrtʃɚ] v & n, **feed**[2] [iː] v & n → U1-3

to provide babies or the se̱riously [ɪɚ] ill with food or supply body tissues with nourishing substances [ʌ]

nou̱rishment[3] n • nou̱rishing[4] adj • mal/ overnou̱rishment[5] n term

» Make sure the children are well-nourished[6]. The child's behavior may need to be mo̱dified in order for the parent to be able to appropriately nourish and nurture the baby. Evaluate the patient's state of health, nourishment and physical deve̱lopment. Persistent sepsis and difficulty in nourishing the patient contributed to rapid weight [weɪt] loss.

Use well / poorly[7] / (in)a̱dequately / fully **nourished** • poorly / mal-/ well-**nourished**, abbr W/N patient • **nourishing** oral supplement • **to feed** a baby[2] • to breast[8]- [e]/bottle-/cup-**feed** • o̱ral / IV or drip[9] / enteral **feeding** • **feeding** difficulties

(er)nähren
aufziehen, pflegen; Pflege, Erziehung[1] füttern, ernähren, stillen; Futter, Stillen, Fütterung[2] Nahrung[3] nahrhaft[4] Unter-, Überernährung[5] gut ernährt[6] unterernährt[7] stillen[8] parenterale / künstl. Ernährung[9]

1

nutrient [nuːtriᵊnt] n & adj   sim **nutriment**[1] n

(n) su̱bstance in food that can be meta̱bolized by the o̱rganism to give e̱nergy and build tissue (adj) nourishing

nu̱tritive[2] adj • nutri̱tious[3] [ɪʃ] adj • macronutrient n term

» Nutritional requirements and to̱lerances can be a̱ltered [ɒː] by increased utilization of nutrients, hyper- and malabso̱rption, impaired meta̱bolism of nutrients, and nutrient wastage[4].

Use **nutrient** i̱ntake[5] / u̱ptake[6] [ʌ]/ requirements [kwaɪɚ]/ co̱ntent[7] / delivery / processing / ve̱ssels[8] / solu̱tion[9] / broth[10] • a̱dequate / inge̱sted[11] [dʒ]/ esse̱ntial nutrients / nu̱tritive va̱lue[12] / ra̱tio [eɪʃ] • drug-**nutrient** intera̱ction • **nutritious** diet [aɪə]/ snacks[13]

Nährstoff; nahrhaft
Nahrung(smittel), Nährstoff[1] Nähr-, Ernährungs-[2] nahrhaft[3] Nährstoffverlust[4] Nährstoffzufuhr[5] Nährstoffaufnahme, -resorption[6] Nährstoffgehalt[7] ernährende Gefäße[8] Nährlösung[9] Nährbouillon[10] zugeführte Nährstoff[11] Nährwert[12] nahrhafte Zwischenmahlzeiten[13]

2

nutrition n   syn **alimenta̱tion** n term

(i) process of food uptake and meta̱bolism (ii) study of human food and li̱quid requirements

malnutri̱tion[1] n term • nutri̱tional[2] adj • alimentary[3] adj • nutri̱tionist[4] n

» Dietary i̱ntake and nutritional status were poor. Diet counseling[5] [aʊ] can help improve nutrition. He's a professor of nutrition at Yale.

Use a̱dequate / i̱nfant[6] / total pare̱nteral[7] (abbr TPN) **nutrition** • **nutritional** needs / disorder or disturbance[8] [ɜː]/ asse̱ssment[9] • **nutritional** the̱rapy / suppo̱rt[10] / deficiency [ɪʃ]/ ha̱bits[11] • mi̱ld [aɪ] degree of / seve̱re [ɪɚ]/ chronic / energy protein[12] **malnutrition** • **nutritionally** ba̱lanced diet • artificial[10] [fɪʃ]/ forced[13] **alimentation** • **alimentary** tract or cana̱l[14]

Ernährung(slehre)
Mangel-, Fehlernährung[1] Ernährungs-, nahrhaft[2] alimentär, Nahrungs-, Verdauungs-[3] Ernährungswissenschaft(l)er(in)[4] Ernährungsberatung[5] Säuglingsernährung[6] (totale) parenterale E.[7] Ernährungsstörung[8] Erhebung d. Ernährungszustandes[9] künstliche E.[10] Ernährungsgewohnheiten[11] Protein-Energie-Mangelsyndrom[12] Zwangsernährung[13] Verdauungstrakt[14]

3

Nutrition BODY STRUCTURES & FUNCTIONS **39**

joule [dʒuːl] n, abbr **J**   sim **calorie**[1] [kæləri] n, abbr **cal**

unit of heat or energy content; for referring to food kcal has been replaced by J (4.187 J equals 1 cal).

(non)caloric[2] adj • calorific[3] adj • calorimeter n

» Excess [ɪksɛs] calories[4] are stored in the body as fat. Every effort should be made to provide sufficient [ɪʃ] amounts of carbohydrate [aɪ] and calories.

Use to burn[5]/count **calories** • empty / large or kilo**calories** • **calorie**-conscious[6] [ʃ] / content • **caloric** intake / expenditure[7] [tʃɚ]/ restriction / requirement[8] / deficiency • high / low[9]-**calorie diet** • **caloric** excess / deficit / recommendation[10] / value[11]

Joule
Kalorie[1] kalorisch, Kalorien-[2] wärmeerzeugend[3] überschüssige Kalorien[4] K. verbrauchen / -brennen[5] kalorienbewusst[6] Kalorienverbrauch[7] Kalorienbedarf[8] kalorienarme Kost[9] empfohlene Kalorienzufuhr[10] Brennwert, kalorischer Wert[11]

4

carbohydrates [aɪ] n term   syn **carbs** n jar, rel **starch**[1] [stɑːrtʃ] n clin

main ingredients[2] [iː] in many foods including sugar compounds[3], starches, glycogen [glaɪkədʒ°n], and cellulose polysaccharides; starch is built up of glucose residues[4] and converted[5] into dextrin, glucose, and maltose

starchy[6] adj • carbohydrate-rich adj

» Much of the carbohydrate we ingest is in the form of starch. A diet with excessive nonprotein calories from starch or sugar but deficient in total protein and essential amino acids eventually results in protein-energy malnutrition. Carbohydrate-rich meals are advisable [aɪz].

Use **carbohydrate** (mal)absorption / metabolism / oxidation / stores[7] • rich in / simple / complex / easily digestible[8] [daɪdʒ-] **carbohydrates** • to hydrolyze[9] [aɪ]/ soluble / corn[10] / potato **starch** • **starch** solutions / sugar[11] / intolerance • **starchy** food / vegetables

Kohlenhydrate (KH)
Stärke[1] Bestandteile[2] Zuckerverbindungen[3] Glukosereste[4] aufgespalten[5] stärkehaltig[6] KH-Depots[7] leicht verdauliche KH[8] Stärke abbauen / spalten[9] Maisstärke[10] Stärkezucker[11]

5

saccharides [sækəraɪdz‖ɪdz] n pl   syn **sugars** [ʃʊgɚz] n

saccharides are classified as mono- [daɪ], tri- [traɪ], and polysaccharides according to the number of monosaccharide groups they are composed of

saccharin(e)[1] n & adj • saccharo- comb • sacchariferous[2] adj term

» Nonabsorbable saccharides (e.g. sorbitol) help promote the evacuation of stools[3]. The nonnutritive sweetener saccharin is considered safe for consumption [ʌ] by all people with diabetes [daɪəbiːtɪz].

Use (un)split di[4]/ lipopoly/ mucopoly**saccharides** • **high-sugar** dessert[5] • **sugar-containing** beverages[6] • fasting blood[7] (abbr FBS) / milk[8] / fruit **sugar** • simple / complex / triple[9] [ɪ]/ starch **sugars** • **sugar-free** gum

Saccharide, Zucker
Saccharin, Süßstoff; Zucker-[1] zuckerhaltig[2] Stuhlgang fördern[3] (un)aufgespaltene Disaccharide[4] stark gesüßte Nachspeise[5] zuckerhaltige Getränke[6] Nüchternblutzucker[7] Milchzucker, Laktose[8] Dreifachzucker[9]

6

glucose [gluːkoʊs] n term   syn **dextrose** n term

simple sugar found in certain foods; fructose and other monosaccharides are converted into glucose which is the chief source of energy for the body; its metabolism[1] is controlled by insulin; excess glucose is stored in the form of glycogen[2] [glaɪkədʒ°n] or converted into fat (adipose tissue)

gluco- comb • gluconate[3] [eɪ] n term • glucosamine[4] [iː] n

» Unlike other organs, the brain relies mainly on[5] glucose to supply its energy requirements.

Use liquid **glucose** • **glucose** load[6] / threshold[7] [θrɛʃoʊld]/ tolerance factor (abbr GTF) • **glucose** tolerance test / administration[8] / feeding / metabolism / blood / CSF[9] / urine / postprandial[10] / fasting plasma[11] **glucose level** • **glucose**-nitrogen [aɪ] ratio [eɪʃ]/ assimilation / carrier[12] • **gluco**kinase [kaɪneɪz]/genesis [dʒen]/corticoid / suria[13]

Glukose, Traubenzucker, Dextrose
Stoffwechsel, Metabolismus[1] Glykogen[2] Glukonat[3] Glukosamin[4] abhängig sein von[5] Glukosebelastung[6] Glukoseschwelle[7] Glukosegabe[8] Liquorzucker(spiegel)[9] Glukosespiegel nach Nahrungszufuhr[10] Nüchternblutzucker[11] Glukosetransporter[12] Glukosurie[13]

7

lactose [læktoʊs] n term   syn **milk sugar** n clin, **lactin** n term rare

disaccharide in mammalian [eɪ] milk[1] used in modified milk preparations and food for infants

lacto-[2] comb • lactosuria[3] n term • lactose-free /-containing adj

» The drug reduces the rate of absorption of most carbohydrates such as starches, dextrins, maltose, and sucrose (but not lactose). Hereditary lactase deficiency[4] [fɪʃ] causes lactose intolerance.

Use (non)metabolized / (un)hydrolized[5] [aɪ] **lactose** • **lactic** acid[6] • **lactose** content / ingestion / assay [æseɪ] or tolerance test[7] / intolerance[8] / (mal)absorption • **lacto**ferrin /genic /vegetarian

Laktose, Milchzucker
Säugetiermilch[1] lakto-, Milch-[2] Laktoseausscheidung i. Harn, Laktosurie[3] angeborener / kongenitaler Laktasemangel[4] aufgespaltene Laktose[5] Milchsäure[6] Laktosebelastung[7] Laktoseintoleranz[8]

8

protein [prouti:n] n

compounds of one or more polypeptides [aɪ] involved in many essential body structures and functions (hormones, enzymes [zaɪ], muscle contraction, blood clotting[1] immunological response)

proteo- *comb* • proteinuria[2] *n term* • proteolytic[3] [ɪ] *adj*

» Reduction in physical activity results in a decrease in both energy and protein requirements.

Use **protein** balance[4] / concentration / deficiency / biosynthesis [sɪn]/ efficiency ratio • structural[5] / soy [sɔɪ]/ whey[6] [weɪ]/ egg **protein** • basic / foreign[7] [ɒː]/ native [eɪ] or natural[8] / C-reactive (*abbr* CRP) **protein** • **protein**-bound iodine[9] [aɪədɪn] (*abbr* PBI) / binding / denaturation[10] / kinase [aɪ] • **proteolytic** enzyme[11] • **proteo**glycans[12] [aɪ]/lysis

Protein, Eiweiß

Blutgerinnung[1] Proteinurie[2] eiweißabbauend, proteolytisch[3] Proteinbilanz, -haushalt[4] Strukturprotein, Gerüsteiweiß[5] Molkeeiweiß[6] Fremdprotein[7] natives P.[8] proteingebundenes Iod[9] Proteindenaturierung[10] Protease, proteolytisches Enzym[11] Proteoglykane[12]

9

---

amino acids [æminoʊ æsɪdz] *n*   *abbr* **AA,** *syn* **aminos** *n jar*

nitrogen-bearing[1] [naɪtrədʒ⁀n] organic acids absorbed in the gut[2] [ʌ] that are the building blocks of the body's own protein

aminoacidemia[3] [iː] *n term* • aminoaciduria[4] *n term*

» The 9 essential amino acids (among them leucine [luːsiːn], tyrosine [aɪ], valine [eɪ‖æ], threonine [iː], lysine [aɪ]) cannot be produced by the body and must be absorbed from the diet.

Use (non)essential[5] (*abbr* EAA and NEAA) / basic[6] [eɪ]/ acidic [sɪ]/ **amino acid** • neutral [uː]/ aromatic / branched chain[7] (*abbr* BCAA) / BCAA-enriched **amino acid** • **amino acid** metabolism / content / composition / solution[8] / infusion / imbalance

Aminosäuren

stickstoffhaltig[1] Darm[2] Aminoazidämie[3] Aminoazidurie[4] (nicht) essentielle Aminosäure[5] basische A.[6] verzweigtkettige A.[7] Aminosäurelösung[8]

10

---

fat [fæt] *n & adj*   *syn* **lipid** [lɪpɪd] *n & comb term*

n (i) the triglycerides [traɪglɪs-] in greasy [iː], oily and waxy substances that are insoluble[1] in water (ii) adipose or fatty body tissue; adj (i) containing or composed of fat (ii) impolite expression for being big, overweight or obese[2] [iː]

fatty[3] *adj* • lip(o) *comb* • lipoid[4] *adj*

» You should reduce the amount of fat in your diet. Try vegetable fats[5] such as palm [pɑːm] oil instead of butter, meat or cheese. Polyunsaturated fat is a triglyceride composed of fatty acids that contain 2-4 double bonds[6].

Use **fat** absorption /-free / deposits[7] / pad[8] / exchange / embolism • saturated [sætʃɚ-]/ (mono/poly)unsaturated[9] **fatty acids** • long-/medium-chain[10] / free / triglyceride **fatty acids** • **fatty** meal / foods / tissue[11] / stool[12] / brown[13] / depot **fat** • simple / compound[14] **lipid** • **lipo**protein /tropic • **lipid**emia [iː]/osis

Fett, Lipid; fett(haltig), -süchtig, -leibig

unlöslich[1] fettleibig[2] fetthaltig, Fett-[3] fettartig, lipoid[4] pflanzliche Fette[5] Doppelbindungen[6] Fetteinlagerungen[7] Fettpolster[8] mehrfach ungesättigte Fettsäuren[9] mittelkettige F.[10] Fettgewebe[11] Fettstuhl, Steatorrhoe[12] braunes F.[13] komplexes Lipid[14]

11

---

essential [ɪsenʃᵊl] **fatty acid** [æsɪd] *n term*   *abbr* **EFA**

EFAs cannot be synthesized [sɪnθəsaɪzd] by the body and must be supplied in the diet; they include linoleic [lɪnəliːɪk] acid[1], omega-3 fatty acids [2], and monounsaturated fats[3]

» Deficiencies in EFAs can develop quickly in the infant of very low birth weight [weɪt], who has little body stores of essential fatty acids at the time of birth.

essentielle Fettsäure

Linolsäure[1] Omega-3-Fettsäuren[2] einfach ungesättigte Fette[3]

12

---

vitamin [aɪ‖ɪ] *n*   *sim* **multivitamin, provitamin** *n*

organic substances present in small amounts in natural foodstuffs; essential to normal metabolism; insufficient amounts in the diet can cause deficiency diseases[1]

» Disorders of vitamin excess[2] may now be more common than vitamin deficiency[3]. Retinol (vitamin A) is important for healthy skin, teeth and bones. The vitamin B complex includes thiamin [θaɪəmɪn] (B-1), riboflavin [raɪboʊfleɪvɪn] (B-2), and pyridoxine [pɪrᵊdɒːksɪn] (B-6).

Use **vitamin** preparations[4] / level / B-12 deficiency / supplement[5] / absorption • fat soluble / water soluble[6] / high potency **vitamin** • excess intake / synthetic analogues[4] **of vitamins** • **vitamin** A precursor[7] [ɜː]/ derivative[8] / toxicity

Vitamin

Mangelkrankheiten[1] Hypervitaminosen[2] Vitaminmangel[3] Vitaminpräparate[4] Vitaminzusatz, -anreicherung[5] wasserlösliches V.[6] Provitamin A[7] Vitaminderivat[8]

13

Nutrition BODY STRUCTURES & FUNCTIONS 41

folic acid [foʊlɪk æsɪd] *n term* *syn* **folacin** [foʊləsɪn],
sim **folate**[1] [foʊleɪt] *n term*

a member of the vitamin B complex necessary for the production of red blood cells and in pregnancy

» Folic acid can also be produced synthetically. Vitamins A, B6, B1 and B3 as well as folate (folacin or folic acid) may be deficient in apparently [eɚ]well-nourished alcoholics.

Use **folic acid** deficiency anemia[2] [iː]/ supplementation[3] / antagonist / synthesis inhibitor[4]

Folsäure

Folat, Folsäuresalz[1] Folsäuremangelanämie[2] Folsäuresupplementierung[3] Folsäuresynthesehemmer[4]

14

ascorbic [əskɔːrbɪk] **acid** *n term* *syn* **vitamin C** *n clin*

a water-soluble antioxidant[1] and detoxifier[2] which must be supplemented[3] [ʌ] regularly as it cannot be stored

» Vitamin C functions primarily in the formation of collagen [kɒlədʒᵊn], the body's chief protein substance and aids in[4] the absorption of iron.

Use L-**ascorbic acid** deficiency / level • **vitamin C**-deficient patients • to replenish[5] / total-body pool of[6] / long-term use of[7] **vitamin C**

Ascorbinsäure, Vitamin C

Antioxidans[1] Entgiftungsmittel[2] ergänzt, zugeführt[3] fördert[4] Vit. C ergänzen[5] Vitamin C Gesamtmenge i. Körper[6] Vitamin C-Langzeittherapie[6]

15

(dietary) fiber [daɪəteri faɪbɚ] *n sing, BE* **fibre** *syn* **roughage** [rʌfɪdʒ] *n espBE*,
sim **bulk**[1] [ʌ] *n clin*

largely indigestible material, e.g. bran[2] [æ], cereals [sɪɚ] and vegetable fibers serving as a stimulant of intestinal peristalsis[3]

bulky[4] *adj* • bulkage[5] *n* • bulkiness[6] *n*

» If you ingest a diet higher in roughage, you will produce more frequent and bulkier stools[7]. Pectin is a soluble fiber found in the skins of fruits and vegetables thought to slow digestion and keep food in the stomach longer. Enhanced fiber intake increases fecal [fiːkᵊl] bulk[8].

Use intake of **dietary fiber** • low / high[9] **roughage diet** • **high-fiber** diet[9] / content / intake • **fiber** supplementation / supplement • dietary[10] / intestinal / muscle[11] [mʌsl] **bulk** • **bulk**-producing agent / forming laxatives[12] • **bulky** food[9] / tumors

Ballaststoffe

Ballaststoffe; Menge, Masse, Volumen[1] Kleie[2] Darmtätigkeit, Peristaltik[3] voluminös, raumfüllend[4] Füllmaterial (Darm)[5] Volumen; Beliebtheit[6] voluminösere Stühle[7] Kotmasse[8] ballaststoffreiche Nahrung[9] Ballaststoffe[10] Muskelmasse[11] Füllmittel, Quellstoffe[12]

16

trace [treɪs] **element** *n term* *sim* **trace mineral**[1], **trace metal**[2], **micronutrients**[3] [uː] *n term*

inorganic molecules in food (e.g. iron[4] [aɪɚn], iodine[5] [aɪə], copper[6], fluorine[7] [iːǁɪ], manganese[8] [iː], selenium[9] [iː], zinc[10] [z], silicon[11]) required in minute[12] [maɪnuːt] amounts (less than 1 mg/d) which are essential nutritionally and in metabolism

trace[13] *v* • traceable[14] *adj* • (radio)tracer *n*

» The functions of trace elements and of more abundant[15] [ʌ] metals (calcium[16] [kælsɪəm], phosphorus, potassium[17], sodium[18] [oʊ], chloride[19] [aɪ], and magnesium [iː]) are determined, in part, by their charges[20] [tʃɑːrdʒɪz], mobilities, and binding constants to biological ligands[21] [aɪ].

Use disturbance in / absorption of **trace elements** • **trace** amounts[22] / component / concentration / metal deficiency / impurity[23] [pjʊɚ] • to be found in **traces**[24] • to be **traceable** to sth[25]

> Note: Mark the difference between *silicon* and *silicone*[26] and between *manganese* and *magnesium*.

Spuren-, Mikroelement

mineralisches Spurenelem.[1] metallisches Sp.[2] essentielle Mikroelemente[3] Eisen[4] Iod[5] Kupfer[6] Fluor[7] Mangan[8] Selen[9] Zink[10] Silizium[11] sehr kleinen[12] aufspüren[13] nachweis-, auffindbar[14] reichlich vorhanden[15] Kalzium[16] Kalium[17] Natrium[18] Chlorid[19] Ladungen[20] Liganden[21] geringste Mengen[22] minimale Verunreinigung[23] in Spuren (vorkommen)[24] zurückzuführen auf[25] Silikon[26]

17

Unit 13 General Pathology
Related Units: 3 Injuries, 16 Pain, 17 Fractures, Dentistry

pathologic(al) [pæθəlɒːdʒɪk] *adj term*

related to the causes [ɔː], development, and nature of abnormal conditions, to the resulting structural and functional changes, or to pathology as a medical science and specialty

pathology[1] *n term* • pathologist[2] *n* • pathogen[3] *n* • patho-, -opathy *comb*

» This condition is characterized pathologically by diffuse inflammatory changes. Psychoses [saɪkoʊsiːz] are manifested by pathology in all areas of mental function.

Use **pathologic** anatomy / histology / feature[4] [fiːtʃɚ]/ changes / abnormality / condition • **pathologic** finding[5] / appearance [ɪɚ]/ structure / confirmation • **pathologic** entity[6] / examination / diagnosis / staging • anatomical / cellular[7] / clinical / comparative / functional / humoral / medical / molecular / surgical **pathology** • underlying[8] / characteristic / dental / endocrine [ɪ‖aɪ]/ bladder / bowel [aʊ]/ speech / negative for[9] **pathology** • (no) evidence[9] / site / type **of pathology** • cyto/ histo[10]/ neuro [ʊɚ]/ immuno**pathology** • (lymph)aden/ arthr/ coagul[11]/ nephr/ encephalo**pathy** • **patho**genic[12] [dʒe] /genesis /physiology /psychology [-saɪk] • cyto [saɪ-]/ neuro**pathogen**

pathologisch, krankhaft
Pathologie, path. Prozess / Befund[1] Pathologe/in[2] (Krankheits)erreger[3] path. Merkmal[4] p. Befund[5] p. Einheit[6] Zell-, Zytopathologie[7] Grundleiden, -krankheit[8] kein path. Befund[9] Histopathologie[10] Koagulopathie, Gerinnungsstörung[11] pathogen, krankheitserregend[12]

1

morbid [ɔː] *adj term* → U18-12, U14-9   *syn* **diseased** [iː] *adj clin*

related to physical or mental diseases or pathologic conditions

morbidity[1] *n term* • comorbidity[2] *n* • dys-[3] [dɪs], mal-[3] *comb*
• -osis, -iasis [aɪ] *comb*

» Hypernatremia [iː] in the elderly is a heterogeneous [dʒiː], morbid, and iatrogenic [aɪæ-] entity. In most cases there is little clinical morbidity or deterioration[4] [ɪɚ] of global ventricular function.

Use **morbid** mood[5] / depression / obesity[6] [iː]/ fear / jealousy[7] [dʒel-]/ anatomy[8] *(BE)*
• cardiovascular / drug-related / fetal [iː] **morbidity** • **dys**function(al) /plasia [eɪʒ] / peptic • tubercul/ acid/ cirrh [sɪr-]/ leukocyt**osis** [uː] • ameb/ cholelith[9] [k] / psor[10] [s]/ candid**iasis** • mal**formation**[11] /function(ing) /position[12]

krank(haft), pathologisch, morbid
Morbidität, Krankheitshäufigkeit[1] Komorbidität, Begleiterkrankung[2] Dys-, Fehl-, gestört[3] Verschlechterung[4] Verstimmung[5] Fettsucht, Adipositas[6] krankhafte Eifersucht[7] patholog. Anatomie[8] Cholelithiasis, Gallensteinleiden[9] Psoriasis, Schuppenflechte[10] Missbildung[11] Lageanomalie[12]

2

focus *term, pl* **-i** [foʊsaɪ]   *sim* **lesion**[1] [liːʒən] *n term* → U3-5

center or starting point of a pathologic process or change in the tissues; the term lesion is often used to refer to one of the sites of a multifocal disease

focal[2] [foʊkəl] *adj term* • multifocal *adj*

» Lesions may be localized, circumscribed[3] [aɪ], discrete[4] [iː], linear, poorly demarcated[5], diffuse or generalized in distribution. Were you able to determine the initial [ɪʃ] focus of infection?

Use **lesions** consist of / contain / are composed of / are confined [aɪ] to[6] / are clustered [ʌ] in • **lesions** are centered around / begin as / spread [e] to[7] / are associated [oʊʃ] with[8] • carious[9] / upper GI tract bleeding / primary [aɪ]/ solitary[4] / elevated[10] / genetic **lesion** • inflammatory / chronic / pre-existing / (intracranial [eɪ]) / mass[11] / obstructive / palpable[12] / painless **lesion** • **focus of** inflammation[13] • principal / contiguous[14] [-ɪgjʊəs]/ external **focus** • multiple / metastatic[15] **foci** • **focal** abscess / infection[16] / hemorrhage / infiltrate / neurologic deficit

(Krankheits)herd, Fokus
Läsion, Schädigung, Verletzung, Tumor[1] herdförmig, fokal[2] umschrieben[3] einzelstehend, solitär[4] schlecht abgegrenzt[5] sind beschränkt auf[6] breiten sich aus[7] gehen einher mit[8] kariöse Läsion[9] erhabene L.[10] intrakranielle Raumforderung[11] tastbare L.[12] Entzündungsherd[13] Nachbarherd[14] Metastasenherde[15] Fokal-, Herdinfektion[16]

3

affect *vt clin*   *syn* **involve** *vt, sim* **compromise**[1] [-maɪz], **impair**[2] [eɚ] *vt clin*

(i) to have a morbid, incapacitating[3], or otherwise damaging impact (ii) to influence in some way

(un)affected *adj term* • (un)involved *adj* • involvement[4] *n* • impairment[5] *n*

» Males and females are equally affected. Many antibiotics impair renal function.

Use **to affect** adults / the bowel • adversely[6] / most commonly **affected** • **affected** joints / area / limb[7] [lɪm]/ eye / boys / first-degree relatives • **impaired** function / perfusion / vision[8] [ʒ] • hemodynamically / immuno[9]/ acutely **compromised** • cognitive / transient[10] / irreversible / neurologic **impairment** • nodal[11] [oʊ]/ pleural [ʊɚ]/ intestinal / systemic / metastatic[12] / secondary / concomitant renal[13] **involvement**

(i) befallen, angreifen
(ii) betreffen
beeinträchtigen, gefährden[1] einschränken, schwächen, schädigen[2] behindernd, arbeitsunfähig machend[3] Befall, Beteiligung[4] Störung, Schwächung, Schädigung[5] geschädigt, angegriffen[6] betroffene Extremität[7] eingeschränktes Sehvermögen[8] abwehrgeschwächt[9] vorübergehende Beeinträchtigung[10] Lymphknotenbefall[11] Metastasierung[12] gleichzeitige Nierenbeteiligung[13]

4

General Pathology | MEDICAL SCIENCE 43

anomaly n term   syn **abnormality** n, sim **mal/deformation**[1] n term

deformity[1], impairment, dysfunction or deviation[2] [iː] from the average or norm · anomalous[3] adj term · abnormal[3] adj · de-/malformed adj

» Occlusion may occur as a result of an anomalous course[4] of the artery. This leads to anomalies involving the eyes, brain, and kidneys.

Use congenital[5] / chromosome / fetal / vertebral / genital / developmental **anomaly** · **malformed** fetus[6] [iː]/ teeth · **deformed** joint / heart [ɑː] / valves[7] [æ]/ nail / ear

Anomalie, Fehlbildung

Missbildung, Deformierung, Deformität[1] Abweichung[2] abnorm, anomal[3] abnormer Verlauf[4] angeborene Fehlbildung[5] missgebildeter Fetus[6] deformierte Herzklappen[7]

5

congenital [dʒen] or **inborn** adj term   opposite **acquired**[1] [əkwaɪə·d] adj term

diseases, malformations, anomalies, mental or physical traits[2] [eɪ] existing at birth hospital-[3]/ community-/ household-/ transfusion-acquired adj term

» Rubella causes a variety [aɪə] of congenital defects, e.g. deafness[4] [defnəs] and mental retardation.

Use **congenital** disorder / absence of the eye[5] / malformation / deficiency / infection / heart disease[6] / deafness · to occur on a **congenital** basis · **inborn** error of metabolism[7] · perinatally [eɪ]/ nosocomially / venereally [ɪɚ] or (hetero)sexually[8] / occupationally[9] [eɪʃ]/ domestically / acutely **acquired**

angeboren, kongenital

erworben[1] Merkmale, Eigenschaften[2] nosokomial[3] Taubheit[4] Anophthalmus congenitus[5] angeborener Herzfehler[6] genet. Stoffwechseldefekt[7] durch Sexualkontakt erworben[8] berufsbedingt, Berufs-[9]

6

hereditary or **inherited** adj term   sim **familial**[1] adj term

transmitted from parent to offspring[2] in an ancestral [se] line of descent[3] [dɪsent] inherit (from)[4] v · inheritance[5] n term · heredity[5] n · inheritable[6] adj · heredo- comb

» Synovitis [aɪ] is frequently seen in familial forms with early onset[7]. The ancestral history[8] showed dominant inheritance of susceptibility[9] [sep] to retinoblastoma. Both disorders are inherited as autosomal [ɒː] inherited traits[10].

Use **hereditary** syndrome · **inherited** clotting [ɒː] disorder[11] / trait / genetic defect · mode of / maternal[12] / Mendelian **inheritance** · familial / autosomal / dominant[13] / recessive / x-linked[14] **inheritance pattern** · **familial** x-linked trait / tendency / (pre)disposition or susceptibility[9] · **familial** transmission / syndrome / pattern / clustering [ʌ] or aggregation[15] · **familial** occurrence[16] [ɜː]/ incidence / polyposis · x-linked[14] **heredity** · **heredo**familial /pathology

Note: Do not confuse familial and familiar as in to be familiar with[17].

erblich, hereditär, Erb-

familiär[1] Kind, Nachkomme[2] von einer Generation auf die nächste[3] erben[4] Vererbung, Heredität[5] erblich, vererbbar[6] Beginn, Ausbruch[7] Ahnengeschichte[8] (fam. Prä)disposition[9] autosomal vererbte Merkmale[10] angeborene Koagulopathie / Gerinnungsstörung[11] maternale Vererbung[12] dominante V.[13] X-chromosomaler Erbgang[14] fam. Häufung[15] f. Auftreten[16] vertraut sein mit[17]

7

idiopathic [ɪdɪoʊpæθɪk] adj term

referring to a disease of unknown cause or etiology[1] [iː]

» The majority of cases are idiopathic in origin.

Use **idiopathic** pericarditis [aɪ]/ vitiligo [aɪ‖ɪ] · **chronic idiopathic** jaundice[2] [dʒɒːndɪs] / diarrhea [daɪəriːə]

idiopathisch, genuin, essentiell

Ätiologie, (Krankheits)ursache[1] chronische(r) idiopathische(r) Gelbsucht / Ikterus[2]

8

iatrogenic [aɪætrədʒenɪk] adj, **-ically** adv term → U19-15

induced by an unfavorable[1][eɪ] response to medical or surgical treatment

» Pneumothorax [nuː-] may be classified as spontaneous [eɪ], traumatic, or iatrogenic, depending on the cause. Many renal infections are iatrogenic, i.e. introduced at the time of stone manipulation.

Use **iatrogenic** factor / infection / trauma [ɒː]/ complication · **iatrogenically** induced / triggered[2] / compromised[3]

iatrogen, durch d. Arzt verursacht

ungünstig, unerwünscht[1] iatrogen[2] durch ärztliche Maßnahmen beeinträchtigt[3]

9

irritation [ɪrɪteɪʃ°n] n term → U16-3

(i) itching[1] [ɪtʃ], painful, or incipient[2] [sɪp] inflammatory reaction (ii) overexcitation[3] [ksaɪ] or excessive sensitivity[4]

irritate v term · irritative or -able[5] adj · irritability[6] n · irritant[7] n

» All penicillins are irritating to the CNS. There was some local irritation at the site of injection.

Use nerve root[8] / meningeal [-dʒɪəl] / gastric[9] / chronic / chemical **irritation** · (generalized/focal) nervous / neuromuscular / reflex / gastric (outlet) **irritability** · **irritative** reaction / lesion / voiding symptoms[10] · **irritable** mood[11] [uː]/ and tense patient[12] / bladder[13] / colon or bowel syndrome[14]

Reizung, Irritation

juckende[1] beginnende[2] Überreizung[3] Überempfindlichkeit[4] reizbar, Reiz-[5] Reizbarkeit, Irritabilität[6] Irritans, Reizmittel[7] Nervenwurzelreizung[8] Magenreizung[9] Reizblasen-Syndrom, irritative Blasenentleerungsstörung[10] gereizte Stimmung[11] reizbare(r) und nervöse(r) Patient(in)[12] Reizblase[13] Reizkolon[14]

10

inflammation [ɪnfləmeɪʃᵊn] *n term*

dynamic cytologic and histologic reactions in response to injury or abnormal stimulation caused by physical, chemical, or biologic agents; includes local reactions and the resulting morphologic changes, destruction or removal of injurious[1] [dʒuɚ] materials, and responses leading to repair and healing

inflamed[2] [eɪ] *adj term* • -itis [aɪtɪs] *comb* • (non-/ anti-)inflammatory[3] [æ] *adj*

» *Inflammations of mucous membranes with free discharge[4] [-tʃɑːrdʒ] are called catarrh. The so-called cardinal signs of inflammation[5] are redness, heat, swelling, pain, and inhibited function.*

Use (sub)acute / chronic / exudative[6] [uː]/ catarrhal / adhesive[7] [iː] **inflammation** • allergic [ɜː]/ atrophic / degenerative **inflammation** • focal[8] / fibrinous [aɪ]/ fibroid / granulomatous **inflammation** • hyperplastic *or* proliferative[9] / interstitial [ɪʃ]/ necrotic[10] **inflammation** • productive [ʌ]/ sclerosing / serous[11] [ɪɚ]/ serofibrinous / purulent [pjʊ] *or* suppurative[12] [ʌ] **inflammation** • **inflammatory** process / reaction / eruption[13] / bowel disease / exudate / infiltrate • **anti-inflammatory drugs**[14]

▪ **Note:** All terms for inflammations end in **-itis**, e.g. gastritis, bronchitis [k], etc.

pus [pʌs] *n term*

a protein-rich liquid inflammation product comprised of leukocytes [uː], a thin fluid, and cellular debris[1]

purulent[2] [pjʊᵊrᵊlᵊnt] *adj term* • pyo- [paɪoʊ] *comb* • purulence[3] *n*

» *An abscess is a localized collection of pus in a cavity formed by the disintegration of tissue[4].*

Use to release [iː] *or* discharge[5]/contain **pus** • sterile / foul-smelling[6] [aʊ]/ gross[7] [oʊ]/ frank[8] / localized / loculated **pus** • aspiration / drainage[9] / evacuation *of* **pus** • **pus** collections[10] /-forming[11] / formation / cells • **pus** from an abscess • **purulent collections**[10] / effusion[12]

consolidation *n term*   *rel* **infiltration**[1] *n term*

(i) solidification[2] into a firm dense mass; esp. inflammatory changes of the lung due to the presence of cellular exudate in the air spaces (ii) stage in healing, e.g. in fractures when the callus changes into bone

consolidate[3] *v term* • consolidated *adj* • infiltrate[4] *v & n* • infiltrative[5] *adj*

» *Chest x-rays show consolidation in several pulmonary segments. The normal sound of underlying air-containing lung is resonant, while consolidated lung or a pleural [ʊɚ] effusion[6] sounds dull[7] [ʌ].*

Use to undergo[3] **consolidation** • areas[8] / (x-ray) signs[9] *of* **consolidation** • pulmonary[10] / (multi)lobar / diffuse / focal[11] / segmental **consolidation** • massive / patchy[12] / parenchymal / air space **consolidation** • **consolidated** pulmonary infiltrate • organ / pulmonary / metastatic / tumor / bone marrow[13] **infiltration** • nodular / diffuse / pulmonary / cellular / inflammatory[14] / interstitial [ɪʃ] **infiltrate** • **infiltrative** tumor / lung disease / process

induration *n term*

(i) pathological process of becoming extremely firm or hard (ii) focus of indurated tissue

indurated *adj* • indurate[1] *v* • indurative *adj*

» *The rash[2] tends to be associated with muscular pain, tenderness, and induration. After rupture the tissues surrounding the ulcer [ʌlsɚ] often become indurated, reddened and tender[3].*

Use localized / extensive / focal / painful / palpable / leathery [e] *or* brawny[4] [ɒː] / red / gray / doughy[5] [doʊi] **induration** • area / degree *of* **induration** • **indurated** borders / edges / nodules[6] / inflammatory tissue / plaque / ulcer

---

Entzündung

schädlich, schädigend[1] entzündet[2] entzündlich[3] (Flüssigkeits)absonderung[4] klassische Entzündungszeichen[5] exsudative E.[6] Adhäsion infolge v. E.[7] fokale E.[8] proliferative E.[9] nekrotisierende E.[10] seröse E.[11] eitrige E.[12] entzündl. Exanthem[13] entzündungshemmende Mittel, Antiphlogistika[14]

11

Eiter, Pus

Zelltrümmer[1] eitrig, purulent[2] Eiterung, Eiterbildung[3] Gewebeeinschmelzung[4] Eiter absondern[5] übelriechender Eiter[6] makroskop. sichtbare Eiterung[7] klin. manifeste Abszedierung[8] Eiterableitung[9] Eiteransammlungen[10] eiterbildend[11] eitriger Erguss[12]

12

(i) Verdichtung (ii) (Ver)festigung, Ausheilung

Infiltration[1] Hart-, Festwerden[2] verdichten[3] infiltrieren; Infiltrat[4] infiltrativ[5] Pleuraerguss[6] gedämpft[7] Verdichtungsareale[8] (radiolog.) Verschattung[9] pulmonale Verdichtung[10] Verdichtungsherde[11] intrapulm. Verdichtungsbezirke[12] Knochenmarkinfiltration[13] entzündliches Infiltrat[14]

13

Induration, Verhärtung

verhärten, indurieren[1] Ausschlag, Exanthem[2] (druck)schmerzempfindlich[3] Gewebeverhärtung[4] teigige Induration[5] indurierte Knoten[6]

14

General Pathology

hypertrophy [haɪpɜːrtrəfi] *n term*   *sim* **hyperplasia**[1] [-eɪʒ(ɪ)ə] *n term*
  increase in bulk[2] [ʌ] (through increase in size not in number of cells) of an organ or tissues not due to tumor formation
  hypertrophic[3] *adj term* • hypertrophied[4] *adj* • hyperplastic[5] *adj*
» The patient presents with marked hypertrophy of the left ventricle, involving in particular the interventricular septum of the left ventricular outflow tract.
Use cardiac[6] / left ventricular[7] (*abbr* LVH) / gastric / glomerular / benign [-aɪn] prostatic[8] (*abbr* BPH) / compensatory[9] **hypertrophy** • **hypertrophic** scar[10] / gastritis[11] / cardiomyopathy[12] • **hypertrophied** muscle / ventricle

> **Note:** Although different in meaning, *hypertrophy* and *hyperplasia* are often (incorrectly) used synonymously.

nodule [nɒːdjʊl] *or* **-lus** *n term*   *sim* **swelling**[1], **tumor**[1] [tjuːmɚ] *n term*,
                                              lump[1] [ʌ], **mass**[1] *n jar & clin*
  (i) a small, palpable mass of solid pathologic tissue (ii) rarely also a node of normal tissue
  nodosity[2] *n term* • nodular *or* nodose[3] [noʊdoʊs] *adj* • nodulation[4] *n*
» Most multinodular goiters[5] are benign, while a solitary[6] thyroid [aɪ] nodule tends to be malignant.
Use pulmonary / rheumatoid[7] [uː] / gouty[8] [aʊ] / solitary *or* discrete[9] **nodule** • subcutaneous [eɪ] / calcified [s] / ulcerated / mobile[10] [ə‖aɪ] / metastatic **nodules** • **nodular** aggregations[11] / lesion / hyperplasia • breast [e] / painless[12] / firm **lump** • axillary / abdominal / asymptomatic / palpable **mass**

> **Note:** Even though the term *tumor* is generally used for any morbid enlargement or swelling, patients are more likely to associate this word with its second meaning, i.e. *neoplasia*. Therefore, the expressions *swelling*, *mass*, and *lump* should be preferred when talking to patients.

ulcer [ʌlsɚ] *n term & clin*   *sim* **sore**[1] [sɔːr] *n & adj clin*,
                                   rel **erosion**[2] [ɪroʊʒ³n] *n term*
  lesion on the surface of the skin or mucosa caused by loss of superficial[3] [ɪʃ] tissue (esp due to inflammation)
  ulcerative[4] *adj term* • ulcerated *adj* • ulceration[5] *n* • erosive *adj*
» A wound [uː] with superficial loss of tissue from trauma is not primarily an ulcer, but may become ulcerated if infection occurs.
Use **ulcer** crater[6] [eɪ] / gastric[7] / peptic[8] / decubitus[9] / symptomatic / penetrating / inflamed / perforated[10] **ulcer** • varicose[11] / aphthous[12] [æfθəs] / venereal *or* soft[13] / rodent[14] [oʊ] / / hard[15] **ulcer** / groin[16] / marginal[17] [dʒ] / chronic / indolent[18] / sloughing [ɒːf] *or* perambulating[19] **ulcer** • healed / herpetic / serpiginous [ɪdʒ] *or* creeping[20] **ulcer** • dendritic [ɪ] / diphtheritic / distention / undermining [aɪ] **ulcer** • **ulcer of the** foot / cornea • bed *or* pressure[9] / running[21] / cold[22] / oriental[23] / plaster[24] **sore**

MEDICAL SCIENCE 45

Hypertrophie, Vergrößerung
Hyperplasie[1] Größe[2] hypertroph[3] vergrößert[4] hyperplastisch[5] Herzhypertrophie[6] Linksherzhypertrophie[7] benigne Prostatahyperplasie[8] kompensat. / vikariierende Hypertrophie[9] hypertrophe Narbe[10] Ménétrier-Syndrom[11] hypertroph. Kardiomyopathie[12]

15

Nodulus, Knoten, Knötchen
Schwellung, Geschwulst, Tumor, Knoten[1] Knoten(bildung), Nodositas[2] knotig, knotenförmig[3] Knotenbildung[4] Kropf, Struma[5] solitär[6] Rheumaknoten, N. rheumaticus[7] Gichtknoten, Tophus arthriticus[8] Solitärknoten[9] bewegliche K.[10] Knotenansammlungen[11] indolenter Knoten[12]

16

Ulkus, Ulcus, Geschwür
wunde Stelle, Hautläsion, Geschwür; wund[1] Erosion[2] oberflächlich[3] ulzerös, ulzerierend[4] Geschwürbildung, Ulzeration[5] Ulkuskrater[6] Magengeschwür, U. ventriculi[7] Ulcus pepticum[8] Dekubitalgeschwür[9] perforiertes U.[10] U. varicosum, Unterschenkelgeschwür[11] Aphthe[12] weicher Schanker, U. molle venereum[13] U. rodens, exulzerierend wachsendes Basaliom[14] U. durum, harter Schanker[15] Granuloma inguinale[16] Randulkus[17] nicht heilendes Geschwür[18] U. phagedaenicum[19] kriechendes G.[20] eiternde Wunde[21] Herpes simplex[22] kutane Leishmaniase, Orientbeule[23] Druckstelle d. Gipsverband[24]   17

46 MEDICAL SCIENCE — General Pathology

obstruction [ʌ] n term   sim **occlusion**[1], **obturation**[2] n, rel **obliteration**[3], **atresia**[4] [-iːʒ(ɪ)ə] n term

blockage or clogging[2] of vessels, ducts, and body passages, e.g. by occlusion, obturation or stenosis

obstruct[5] v term • (non)obstructive[6] adj • obstructing[6] adj • occlude[7] v • occlusive adj • atretic [e] or imperforate[8] adj

» Barium enema[9] demonstrated an obstructing lesion in the colon. Simple mechanical [k] obstruction of the colon may develop insidiously[10].

Use to produce/cause/demonstrate/relieve **obstruction** • strangulating / pyloric [aɪ]/ intestinal / airway(s)[11] / nasal / extrahepatic / biliary[12] [ɪ] **obstruction** • bladder outlet[13] / cardiac outflow / fixed coronary / membranous **obstruction** • recurrent[14] / prolonged / pronounced[15] / partial **obstruction** • **obstructed** airway / vessels • **obstructing** foreign [fɔːrɪn] body / tumor / calculi [aɪ] • **obstructive** process / lung disease / shock / uropathy[16] • intestinal / choanal[17] [koʊənʲl]/ biliary[18] **atresia** • **atretic** duct [ʌ] • **imperforate** hymen[19] [aɪ]/ anus[20] [eɪ]

Obstruktion, Verlegung, Abflussstörung
Okklusion, Verschluss[1] Verlegung[2] Obliteration, Verödung[3] Atresie[4] obstruieren, verlegen[5] obstruktiv, obturierend[6] verstopfen, -schließen[7] atretisch[8] Bariumeinlauf[9] schleichend[10] Atemwegsobstr.[11] Gallengangobstr.[12] Blasenhalsobstr.[13] rezidivierende O.[14] ausgeprägte O.[15] Harnwegsobstruktion[16] Choanalatresie[17] Gallengangatr.[18] hymenale A., Hymen imperforatus[19] Analatresie[20]

18

stricture [strɪktʃɚ] n term   sim **stenosis**[1] [oʊ] n term, pl -ses

abnormal narrowing of a tube or duct due to contracture[2] [-æktʃɚ] or deposition of tissue

constrict[3] v term • constriction[4] n • constrictive adj • strictured adj

» Crohn's disease may produce gastric ulceration and/or scarring[5] with stricture formation. Peptic esophageal [dʒɪəl] ulcers heal slowly, tend to recur, and leave a stricture upon healing.

Use biliary / urethral[6] [iː]/ rectal / peptic / short / annular[7] / anastomotic[8] **stricture** • contractile / bridle[9] [aɪ]/ functional **stricture** • nondilatable [aɪleɪt]/ intrinsic / spasmodic[10] / permanent / temporary / recurrent **stricture** • **stricture** dilation[11] • **constrictive** pericarditis / edema[12]

Striktur, (hochgradige) Verengung
Stenose, Verengung[1] Kontraktur[2] verengen[3] Ein-, Verengung, Einschnürung, Konstriktion[4] Narbenbildung[5] Harnröhrenstriktur[6] anuläre Verengung[7] Anastomosenstr.[8] Bridenstriktur[9] spastische / funktionelle Str.[10] Bougierung[11] Stauungsödem[12]

19

stenosis [stənoʊsɪs] n term, pl -ses

narrowing or constriction of a heart valve, blood vessel, or other body passages

stenose[1] v term • stenotic or stenosed adj • stenosing[2] adj

» One of the arteries to the brain is markedly stenosed. The success rate in treating stenoses of small vessels are better than for complete occlusion.

Use valvular[3] / mitral [aɪ]/ aortic[4] [eɪ]/ tracheal [k]/ artherosclerotic / carotid / ureteral[5] / pyloric[6] [aɪ]/ anal [eɪ] **stenosis** • partial[7] / high-grade[8] / short / degree or severity of **stenosis** • **stenosed** aortic valve / Eustachian [juː] tube • **stenotic** lesion / segment • **stenosing** tenosynovitis

Stenose, Verengung
stenosieren, eng werden[1] verengend[2] (Herz)klappenstenose[3] Aortenstenose[4] Harnleiterstenose[5] Pylorusstenose[6] inkomplette S.[7] hochgradige S.[8]

20

calculus n term, pl **-i** [aɪ]   syn **stone, concretion** [iː] n term

concretion usually composed of salts of inorganic or organic acids forming in body passages, most commonly in the biliary and urinary tracts

(a)calculous[1] adj term • -lith(o)- comb • stone-free[2] /-forming[3] adj

» Calculi less than 1cm in diameter may be approached endoscopically. If a stone has previously been passed or if one is recovered, its chemical composition should be analyzed.

Use salivary[4] / biliary / urinary[5] / vesical[6] / preputial[7] [uːʃ] **calculus** • uterine [aɪ‖ɪ]/ arthritic [ɪ]/ bronchial / cerebral **calculus** • lacrimal[8] / mammary[9] / intestinal[10] / pancreatic **calculus** • pleural [ʊɚ]/ dental[11] / pulp [ʌ]/ subgingival [dʒ] **calculus** • staghorn[12] / apatite [aɪ]/ struvite [-uːvaɪt]/ oxalate [eɪ]/ coral[13] / cystine [sɪ]/ fibrin / weddellite[14] / hematogenetic / encysted / pocketed[15] / dislodged[16] [ɒːdʒ]/ renal[17] **calculus** • common duct[18] / gall[19] / kidney[17] **stone** • **stone** disease[20] / clearance[21] / impaction[22] / extraction / former[23] / gastric[24] / calcium [s] **concretion** • **litho**tomy /tripsy[25] /tripter • uro/ nephro/ chole**lithiasis**

Stein, Konkrement
(nicht) steinbedingt, Stein-[1] steinfrei[2] steinbildend[3] Speichelstein, Sialolith[4] Harnstein[5] Blasenst.[6] Balanolith, Präputialstein[7] Dakryolith[8] Milchgangst.[9] Kotst.[10] Zahnst.[11] Ausgussst.[12] Korallenst.[13] Weddellitst.[14] eingekapselter Blasenst.[15] abgegangener S.[16] Nierenstein[17] Choledochusstein[18] Gallenstein[19] Steinleiden[20] Abgang d. Steines[21] Steinimpaktion, -einklemmung[22] Steinbilder[23] Gastrolith, Magenstein[24] Lithotripsie, Steinzertrümmerung[25]

21

prolapse [n proʊlæps‖v -læps] n & v term   sim **ptosis**[1] [toʊsɪs] n term

(n) displacement or sagging[2] of an organ or structure, esp at a natural or artificial orifice

ptotic adj term • prolapsing adj • prolapsed adj

» A long pedunculated [ʌ] polyp[3] had prolapsed through the anus. Ptosis, i.e. a droopy[4] [uː] upper eyelid, may be congenital or acquired.

Use mitral valve[5] /mucosal / rectal[6] / uterine / intervertebral disk[7] **prolapse** • partial / first-degree / complete[8] / postpartum **prolapse** • fluctuating[9] / myo/ nephro/ neurogenic / progressive **ptosis**

Vorfall, Prolaps
Ptose, Senkung[1] Senkung[2] gestielter Polyp[3] herabhängend[4] Mitralklappenprolaps[5] Rektumprolaps, Mastdarmvorfall[6] Diskushernie, Bandscheibenvorfall[7] Totalprolaps[8] intermittierende Ptose[9]

22

General Pathology | **MEDICAL SCIENCE** **47**

hernia [hɜːrnɪə] *n term*   *rel* **rupture**[1] [rʌptʃɚ] *n & v term* → U3-18

protrusion[2] of a structure through the tissues normally enclosing it

herniate[3] *v term* • herniation[4] *n* • hernial *adj* • hernio- ,-cele [siːl] *comb*

» Surgery is indicated if the hernia has incarcerated[5]. The hernia sac[6] was excised [aɪ]. A ureterocele is a ballooning[7] [uː] of the distal submucosal ureter into the bladder.

Use **hernial** sac[6] / canal[8] / defect • abdominal / hiatal or hiatus[9] [aɪeɪ]/ inguinal[10] / scrotal [oʊ]/ direct **hernia** • umbilical[11] [ʌ]/ diaphragmatic / orbital / cerebral **hernia** • epigastric / sciatic[12] [saɪætɪk]/ obturator / incisional[13] [sɪʒ] **hernia** • lumbar [ʌ]/ sliding or slipped[14] / double loop [uː]/ (ir)reducible[15] / strangulated[16] **hernia** • complete / concealed[17] [siː]/ retrograde / synovial [aɪ] **hernia** • **hernia** repair[18] / defect • **hernia of the** broad ligament of the uterus • **herniated** intervertebral disk[19] / bowel / material or mass[20] • lumbar disk / brain[21] / internal **herniation** • **hernio**plasty[18] /rrhaphy • recto/ varico/ cysto[22]/ meningo/ hydro**cele**

cyst [sɪst] *n term*   *sim* **pseudocyst**[1] [suːdoʊsɪst] *n term*

abnormal sac containing gas, fluid or semisolid material which has a membranous lining[2] [aɪ]

cystic[3] *adj term* • cyst(o)- *comb* • cyst-like *adj* • cystitis[4] [sɪstaɪtɪs] *n*

» The contents of the encapsulated cyst[5] ruptured into the bronchioles.

Use jaw[6] / ovarian / sebaceous[7] [eɪ]/ calcified / ruptured / multilocular[8] / solitary / sequestration[9] **cyst** • **cyst** fluid / leakage[10] [liːkɪdʒ]/ wall / cavity • **cystic** disease / lesion / fibrosis[11] [aɪ]/ dilation • **cystic** duct[12] / spaces / kidney[13] /degeneration [dʒ] • **cysto**urethrography[14] /gram /cele /sarcoma /scopy • pancreatic **pseudocyst**

fistul(iz)ation *n term* → U35-21

pathologic or therapeutic [pjuː] formation of an abnormal passage from one epithelialized [iː] surface to another

fistula[1] *n term, pl* -as *or* -ae [iː] • fistulated *adj* • fistulous[2] *adj* • fistulo- *comb*

» Fistulas to the bladder or vagina [dʒ] produce recurrent infections.

Use arteriovenous[3] [iː]/ bronchopleural [ʊɚ]/ pancreatic / perilymph / (peri)anal / vesical[4] / tracheoesophageal[5] [-dʒɪəl] **fistula** • draining[6] / internal[7] / blind[8] / long-standing **fistula** • **fistulous** tract[9] / opening[10] / communication[11] / anomaly • **fistul**otomy /graphy

hematoma [hiːmətoʊmə] *n term, pl* -**as**
                rel **hemorrhage**[1] [hemərɪdʒ] *n & v term* → U3-13

localized mass of extravasated[2] blood confined [aɪ] in tissue spaces, e.g. a bruise[3] [bruːz] or a black eye[4]

hemorrhagic *adj term* • bleeding[1] [iː] *n* • bleed[5] *v* • ooze[6] [uːz] *v*

» Some hematomas will resorb, but those that become encapsulated usually require surgical treatment. In hematomas the blood is usually clotted and may manifest various degrees of organization and discoloration. Incidentally discovered[7] aneurysms [ænjɚ-] that have not previously [iː] hemorrhaged have a 2-3% annual risk of bleeding.

Use (intra)cerebral / superficial [ɪʃ]/ (intra)cranial[8] [eɪ]/ epi- or extradural / subdural **hematoma** • to control or arrest[9] *a hemorrhage* • to stop[9] *a bleeding* • subarachnoid [æk] / intraventricular **bleeding** • postpartum[10] / nasal / retinal / gastric / splenic [e]/ pelvic / subungual [ʌ] or splinter[11] **hemorrhage** • punctate[12] [ʌ]/ oozing[13] / occult / spurting[14] [ɜː]/ intermediate / internal[15] **hemorrhage** • primary / secondary[16] / serous [ɪɚ]/ unavoidable **hemorrhage** • **hemorrhagic** rash[17] / fever [iː]/ cystitis / shock / infarction / stroke[18] / necrosis

Hernie, Bruch
Ruptur, Riss; reißen, platzen[1] Hervortreten[2] austreten[3] Einklemmung, Herniation[4] inkarzeriert, eingeklemmt[5] Bruchsack[6] ballonförmige Auftreibung[7] Bruchpforte[8] Hiatushernie[9] Leistenbruch[10] Nabelbruch[11] Hernia glutealis / ischiadica[12] Narbenbruch[13] Gleithernie[14] (ir)reponible H.[15] inkarzerierte H.[16] nicht palpierbare H.[17] Bruchoperation, Hernioplastik[18] Bandscheibenvorfall[19] Bruchinhalt[20] zerebrale Herniation[21] Zystozele[22]   23

Zyste
falsche Z., Pseudozyste[1] epitheliale Auskleidung[2] zystisch; Blasen-[3] Zystitis, Blasenentzündung[4] eingekapselte Zyste[5] Kieferzyste[6] Atherom, Talgzyste[7] mehrkammerige / multilokuläre Z.[8] Sequesterzyste[9] Austritt v. Zystenflüssigkeit[10] zyst. Fibrose, Mukoviszidose[11] Gallenblasengang, D. cysticus[12] Zystenniere[13] Miktionszystourethrographie[14]   24

**Fistelbildung;
Anlegen einer Fistel**
Fistel[1] fistelartig, Fistel-[2] aterio-venöse Fistel[3] Blasenfistel[4] Ösophagotrachealfistel[5] ableitender Fistelgang[6] innere Fistel[7] blind endende F.[8] Fistelgang[9] Fistelmaul, -mund[10] fistelartige Verbindung[11]
                                25

Hämatom, Bluterguss
Blutung, Hämorrhagie; bluten[1] (aus d. Gefäßen) ausgetreten[2] blauer Fleck, Bluterguss[3] blaues Auge[4] bluten[5] (Blut) sickern[6] zufällig entdeckt[7] intrakranielles Hämatom[8] Blutung stillen[9] Nachgeburtsblutung[10] subunguale Blutung[11] punktförm. / petechiale Blutung[12] Sickerblutung[13] pulssynchron spritzende B.[14] innere B.[15] Nachblutung[16] hämorrhagisches Exanthem[17] häm. Insult[18]
                                26

MEDICAL SCIENCE — General Pathology

petechia [pɪtekɪə] *n term, usu pl* **-ae** [iː]
    sim **ecchymosis**[1] [ekɪmoʊsɪs] *n term, pl* **-ses** [siːz]
punctate purpuric[2] [pɜːrpjʊərɪk] lesion due to extravasation of blood into tissues differing from ecchymosis only in size
petechial *adj term* • ecchymotic *adj* • micropetechiae *n*
» The rash of scarlet fever[3] blanches[4] on pressure, may become petechial, and fades[5] [eɪ] in 2-5 days. Signs of coagulopathy include hematuria, easy bruising[6], hematemesis, petechiae, and oozing at sites of venipuncture. Purpura and ecchymoses may also be present.
Use palatal / discrete[7] [iː]/ linear / scattered[8] **petechiae** • **petechial** hemorrhage / lesion / rash • **petechially** confluent[9]

Petechie, punktförmige Hautblutung
Ekchymose, flächenhafte Hautblutung[1] purpuraartig[2] Scharlach[3] blass werden[4] verblassen, -schwinden[5] Neigung z. Hämatomen[6] einzelne P.[7] disseminierte P.[8] mit konfluierenden P.[9]

27

ischemia [ɪskiːmɪə] *n term*   *opposite* **hyperemia**[1] [aɪ] *n term BE* **-aemia**
local deficiency of blood due to functional constriction or mechanical obstruction of vessels
(anti-)ischemic[2] *adj term* • hyperemic[3] *adj* • ischemia-induced *adj*
» At laparoscopy the terminal ileum appeared hyperemic and boggy[4]. Obstruction was related to hyperemia and engorgement[5] [dʒ] of the microvasculature.
Use to precipitate[6] [sɪ]/produce/develop[7] **ischemia** • cerebral / myocardial [aɪ]/ intestinal / peripheral **ischemia** • end-organ / limb[8] [lɪm]/ digital [dʒ] **ischemia** • exercise-induced / postural[9] [tʃɚ]/ focal / local / tourniquet[10] [tɜːrnɪkət] **ischemia** • irreversible / persistent / transient / silent / recurrent / profound[11] [aʊ]/ relative **ischemia** • active / passive / conjunctival [aɪ]/ pulp / congestive[12] [dʒe] **hyperemia** • **hyperemic** mucosa

Ischämie, Blutleere
vermehrte Blutfülle, Hyperämie[1] ischämisch[2] hyperämisch[3] aufgequollen[4] Anschwellen[5] Ischämie auslösen[6] ischämisch werden[7] Extremitätenischämie[8] lagebedingte I.[9] Esmarch-Blutleere[10] absolute / totale I.[11] Stauungshyperämie[12]

28

degenerative [dɪdʒenərətɪv] *adj term*   *rel* **atrophic**[1] [eɪtrɒːfɪk] *adj term*
marked by gradual deterioration[2] [ɪɚ] of cells and organs with concomitant[3] loss of function
degeneration[4] *n term* • degenerate *v* • degenerating *adj* • atrophy[5] [ætrəfi] *n & v*
» Atrophy is a wasting [eɪ] of tissues[6] due to necrosis and resorption of cells, diminished cellular proliferation, pressure, ischemia, malnutrition, lessened function, hormonal changes, etc. At endoscopy, atrophic degeneration and scalloping[7] of the duodenal folds were observed.
Use cerebellar / macular[8] / hyaline [haɪəlɪn] / arthritic / fatty / cheesy[9] [iː]/ progressive **degeneration** • **degenerative** lesion / changes / joint disease[10] • **atrophic** age-related macular degeneration / gastritis / skin • degenerative / scar / gingival[11] [dʒ]/ muscle *or* muscular **atrophy** • disuse *or* inactivity[12] / senile[13] [siːnaɪl]/ optic[14] **atrophy**

degenerativ
atrophisch[1] allmähliche Verschlechterung[2] bei gleichzeitigem[3] Degeneration, Entartung[4] Atrophie; verkümmern, atrophieren[5] Gewebeschwund[6] Fältelung[7] Makuladegeneration[8] Verkäsung[9] degen. Gelenkerkrankung, Arthrose[10] Gingivaatrophie[11] Inaktivitätsatrophie[12] Altersatrophie[13] Sehnerven-, Optikusatrophie[14]

29

necrosis [nekroʊsɪs‖nɪ-] *n term*   *syn* **cell death** *n, rel* **gangrene**[1] [iː] *n term*
localized death of cells as a result of irreversible damage (e.g. shrinkage of tissue[2])
necrotic[3] *adj* • necrose[4] [oʊs] *v* • necrotizing *adj* • gangrenous[5] *adj*
» The outlines of individual necrotic cells are indistinct, and cells may become merged[6] [ɜːrdʒ], sometimes forming a focus of coarsely[7] [ɔː] granular[7], amorphous, or hyaline [aɪ] material. Swelling, edema, and then frank necrosis of the scrotal wall progressing to gangrene may occur, resulting in fever and toxemia [iː].
Use to undergo **necrosis** • tissue[8] / aseptic / avascular / fat / caseation *or* caseous[9] [eɪ] **necrosis** • central / focal[10] / total / coagulation / bridging[11] / cystic **necrosis** • epiphyseal [fɪs]/ fibrinoid [aɪ]/ laminar / cortical / renal papillary / acute tubular **necrosis** • progressive / pressure[12] / hemorrhagic / radiation[13] / hepatic[14] / suppurative[15] [ʌ] **necrosis** • **necrosis** of the newborn • tumor **necrosis** factor, *abbr* TNF • to be/become/appear **necrotic** • **necrotic** debris[16] [debriː]/ foci [foʊsaɪ] / tissue • dermal / venous [iː]/ emphysematous [iː] *or* gas[17] **gangrene** • (non)traumatic / distal / wet[18] / dry / incipient[19] [sɪ] **gangrene**

Nekrose, Zell-, Gewebstod
Gangrän, Brand[1] Gewebeschrumpfung[2] nekrotisch[3] absterben, nekrotisieren[4] gangränös[5] verschmolzen[6] grobkörnig[7] Gewebstod[8] verkäsende N.[9] fokale N.[10] nekrotisierender Verbindungsgang[11] Drucknekr.[12] Strahlennekr.[13] Lebernekr.[14] eitrige N.[15] nekrot. Gewebetrümmer[16] Gasbrand, -ödem[17] feuchte Gangrän[18] beginnende G.[19]

30

Unit 14 Medical Statistics
Related Units: **15** Medical Studies & Research

statistics [stətɪstɪks] *n term usu pl*

collection of values, facts or other items [aɪ] of information which are then numerically analyzed, particularly with regard to the probability[1] that the resulting empirical findings are due to chance[2]

statistical *adj term* • biostatistics[3] [aɪ] *n* • statistician [-tɪʃᵊn] *n*

» Current [ɜː] **statistics** for amputation show improved disease-free survival rates. The statistical risk of recurrence [ɜː] is 50%. The dismal statistics[4] of out-of-hospital cardiac arrest patients may be significantly improved by newer and more aggressive interventions.

Use to interpret **statistics** • inferential[5] • descriptive / vital[6] [aɪ] **statistics** • health / cancer / outcome / mortality[7] / survival[8] / five-year **statistics** • **statistical** analysis / study / evidence[9] / comparison / difference / likelihood[1] [ʊ]/ power[10] / genetics • to approach [oʊtʃ]/achieve [tʃiː] *or* reach[11]/be evaluated for **statistical significance**

Statistik
(stat.) Wahrscheinlichkeit[1] Zufall[2] Biostatistik[3] schlechte Statistik[4] Inferenzstatistik[5] (Bevölkerungs)statistik[6] Mortalität(sstatistik)[7] Überleben(sstatistik)[8] stat. Nachweis[9] stat. Teststärke, Power[10] statistische Signifikanz erreichen[11]

1

subject [sʌbdʒekt] *n term*   *sim* **individual** [-vɪdʒʊəl], **patient** [peɪʃənt], **case**[1] [eɪ] *n term*

object of research, treatment, observation, experimentation, or dissection[2]

» This complication was not seen in young subjects. 41% of subjects were lost to followup[3]. This is the first reported case of increased Tc 99m uptake due to thyroid [aɪ] follicular carcinoma.

Use asymptomatic *or* healthy *or* normal / severely [ɪɚ] ill / human / clinical research **subjects** • well-motivated / (non)obese[4] [iːs] elderly / control[5] **subjects** • **subject** status[6] [eɪ] • affected[7] / otherwise healthy [e]/ high-risk[8] **individuals** • infected / susceptible[9] [sep]/ untreated [iː] **individuals** • **individual case** management / screening [iː] • **case** study[10] / report / series [sɪɚːz]

Proband, Testperson, Untersuchungsobjekt
Fall[1] Sektion, Obduktion[2] konnten nicht weiter kontrolliert werden[3] fettleibige Probanden[4] Kontrollpersonen[5] Probandenstatus[6] betroffene Personen[7] Risikopersonen[8] anfällige P.[9] Fallstudie, Kasuistik[10]

2

population *n term*   *sim* **cohort**[1], **series**[2] [sɪɚːz] *sing & pl*, **(sub)group** [ʌ], **subset** *n term*

set of objects, events[3], or subjects in a particular class from which a sample is drawn

» A contemporary[4] watchful waiting[5] population was selected as a control.

Use **population**-based[6] [eɪ] • (non)white / ag(e)ing [eɪdʒɪŋ]/ age-matched[7] / community-based / cell **population** • eligible[8] [dʒ]/ female [iː]/ general[9] / normal / pediatric [iː]/ patient / study **population** • placebo[10] [siː]/ prospective / screening / 1930 birth **cohort** • controlled / prospective / small / large / consecutive[11] / autopsy [ɒː] **series**

> Note: *Series* is both a singular and plural noun and can be used with a singular verb and the indefinite article, e.g. *a large series is/was ...*

Population
Kohorte[1] Reihe[2] Ereignisse[3] gleichaltrig[4] mit Surveillance[5] bevölkerungsbasiert[6] in d. gleichen Altersgruppe[7] d. Einschlusskriterien erfüllende P.[8] Allgemeinbevölkerung[9] Placebogruppe[10] konsekutive Patientenserie[11]

3

sample [æ] *n & v term*   *rel* **sampling**[1] *n term*

representative portion of a population selected for research to achieve statistically significant results

» Selection of low-risk subsets resulted in inadequate sample size[2] [saɪz]. When sample size is calculated, the frequency of the condition to be prevented, the anticipated[3] [tɪs] effectiveness of the treatment thought to be clinically relevant, and variables such as predicted dropouts[4] and crossovers[5] must be taken into account.

Use to draw[6] [ɔː] **a sample** • random[7] [æ]/ big / small / representative / (un)biased[8] [aɪ] **sample** • **sample** size • estimated **sample** size[9] • **sampling** error / method[10] / with(out) replacement[11] • (quasi-)random [kweɪzaɪ]/ single or basic[12] / cluster[13] [ʌ]/ stratified[14] / quota [kwoʊ] **sampling**

Stichprobe; S. erheben / ziehen
Stichprobenerhebung, -entnahme[1] Stichprobengröße, -umfang[2] erwartete[3] Ausfälle, Therapieabbrecher[4] Therapiewechsler[5] S. ziehen[6] Zufallsstichprobe[7] (un)verzerrte S.[8] geschätzter Stichprobenumfang[9] Stichprobenverfahren[10] Stichprobenerhebung mit/ohne Zurücklegen[11] Ziehen e. einfachen Zufallsstichprobe[12] Z. e. Klumpen- / Cluster-Stichprobe[13] Z. e. geschichteten / stratifizierten Stichprobe[14]

4

Medical Statistics

parameter n term   syn **variable** n term, sim **trait**[1] [eɪ], **(co)factor**[2], **phenomenon**[3], **indicator**[4], **index**[5] n term

a characteristic[1] of a population

uni/ multivariate[6] adj term • multifactorial adj • variable[7] adj inf

» In prostate cancer disease-specific variables are poor discriminants[8] of general quality of life. Nodal involvement was predictable preoperatively by clinical and histological parameters.

Use biochemical / prognostic or predictive / gross [oʊ] neurological[9] **parameter** • serologic [ɪɚ]/ laboratory / sensitive / suitable [uː]/ single **parameter** • random or chance / (in)dependent[10] / stochastic [kæ]/ baseline clinical **variable** • outcome / binomial [aɪ] or dichotomous[11] [daɪkɒːt-]/ ordinal / discrete [iː] **variable** • continuous[12] / intervening [iː]/ quantitative **variable** • growth / prognostic / risk[13] / predisposing[14] [iː] **factor** • etiologic [iː]/ contributing / complicating **factor**

Parameter, Kenngröße, Variable
Merkmal[1] (Ko)faktor[2] Phänomen[3] Indikator[4] Index, Kennziffer[5] uni-/multivariat[6] variabel, veränderlich[7] Unterscheidungsparameter[8] makroskopische neurolog. Variable[9] (un)abhängige V.[10] dichotome Variable, V. mit 2 Ausprägungen[11] stetige V.[12] Risikofaktor[13] Prädispositionsfaktor[14]

5

scale(d) [skeɪld] or **standard score** n term
                              opposite **raw score**[1] [rɒː skɔːr] n term

statistically referenced score representing the deviation of a raw score from its mean [iː] in standard deviation units

score[2] v term • score[3] n • scoring n • scale[4] n

» The study group started at a lower pretreatment score than did the placebo arms. Score the findings on a scale of 0-2. This is an objective score comprising 5 urodynamic parameters.

Use to assign [əsaɪn] a **score** • age-equivalent / clinical performance **score** • initial prognostic / point or numerical[5] / percentile rank **score** • symptom / (Gleason) tumor / IQ / achievement [tʃiː] **score** • Apgar[6] / trauma / Glasgow Coma **score** • **raw score** table (comparison) / grouping / method • **scoring** system[7] • color / numerical[7] / self-rating **scale** • **scale** down

Standardwert(e), Z-Wert(e)
Rohwert(e)[1] verzeichnen, erzielen[2] Wert, Score, Ziffer[3] Skala, Maßstab, Schema[4] Punktezahl[5] Apgar-Wert, -Score[6] Punktsystem, -schema[7]

6

incidence [ɪnsɪdəns] n term   sim **prevalence**[1] [prevələns] n term

the number of new cases of a disease in a defined population over a specific period of time

» It is associated with a 15% incidence of fetal [iː] bradycardia. The number of cases of a disease existing in a given population within a specific period [ɪɚ] of time is termed period prevalence[2]. In low-prevalence populations the ELISA test was less accurate.

Use age-adjusted[3] [dʒʌ]/ age-specific / annual / cumulative / cancer **incidence** • increase in / fall in / peak [iː]/ overall[4] / reported / true[5] / worldwide **incidence** • **incidence** rate • estimated / HIV / population / smoking / point[6] **prevalence** • prevalence index / rate[7]

Inzidenz, Neuerkrankungsrate
Prävalenz[1] Periodenprävalenz[2] altersadjustierte I.[3] Gesamtinzidenz[4] wahre I.[5] Punktprävalenz[6] Prävalenzrate[7]

7

rate [reɪt] n term   sim **ratio**[1] [reɪʃ(ɪ)oʊ], **percentage**[2] [pɚsentɪdʒ], **proportion**[3], **preponderance**[4] n term

proportion per 1,000 (or 100,000) of the population, e.g., number of births per 1,000 residents[5]

» Alpha interferon has had a 15–20% response rate. Men outnumber women [wɪmɪn] by a 3:1 ratio. The ratio of helper to suppressor (H/S) cells in healthy individuals is about 1.6 to 2.2. This is a sizeable[6] [aɪ] percentage of cases.

Use crude[7] [uː]/ standardized / adjusted[8] **rate** • birth / pregnancy / complication / cure[9] / death / failure **rate** • recurrence[10] / retreatment / success / 5-year actuarial[11] **rate** • odds[12] (abbr OR) / likelihood / risk-benefit / birth-death **ratio** • **percentage** points • calculated / fixed high / large / small **percentage** • male-to-female[13] [fiːmeɪl] **preponderance**

Rate
Quotient, Verhältnis[1] Prozentsatz[2] Verhältnis[3] Überwiegen, -hang, -gewicht[4] Einwohner[5] beträchtlich[6] rohe Rate[7] adjustierte R.[8] Heilungsrate[9] Rezidivrate[10] 5-Jahresrate[11] Chancenverhältnis, Odds Ratio[12] Überhang bei Männern[13]

8

Medical Statistics   MEDICAL SCIENCE

morbidity (rate) n term   rel **mortality (rate)**[1] n term

proportion of patients in a given population who have a particular disease at a given time

» During colonoscopy polyps can usually be excised with a lower morbidity rate. The mortality rate is the number of deaths divided by the population in which they occur. They assessed mortality adjusted for age[2] and severity [e] of comorbidity[3] at the time of surgery.

se to predict/reduce/minimize[4]/cause[5]/produce[5]/carry[5]/influence **morbidity** • alcohol-related / asthma [z]/ cardiac / fetal [iː]/ childhood **morbidity** • (peri)operative / long-term / significant or severe [ɪəʳ] or major [meɪdʒəʳ] **morbidity** • minor [aɪ] or low / minimal associated [oʊʃ]/ trivial **morbidity** • crude /5-year / specific / hospital / conditional / infant[6] / perinatal [eɪ] **mortality rate** • standardized **mortality** rate or ratio[7] (abbr SMR)

Morbidität(srate)
Mortalität(srate), Sterblichkeit[1] altersadjustierte Mortalität[2] Grad der Komorbidität / Zweiterkrankung[3] Morbidität gering halten[4] verbunden sein mit einer Morbidität[5] Säuglingssterblichkeitsrate[6] standardis. Mortalitätsquotient[7]

9

mean [miːn] n sing & adj term   sim **median**[1] [ˈmiːdɪən] n & adj term

(n) average[2] [ˈævərɪdʒ] value (usually the arithmetic mean[3] unless otherwise specified) of a sample or population

» Mean time of narcotics use postoperatively was 4.3 days; 72 patients were considered cured [kjʊəd] after a mean of 18 sessions. The median value divides the probability distribution of a random variable in half.

Jse sample / population / geometric[4] **mean** • **mean** age / concentration / decrease [iː] • standard error of the[5] **mean** (abbr SEM) • **median** followup period[6] / hospital stay

Mittel(wert); mittlere(r)
Median, Zentralwert; median(e)[1] durchschnittlich[2] arithmetischer Mittelwert[3] geometrischer M.[4] Standardfehler d. Mittelwerts[5] medianer Nachuntersuchungszeitraum[6]

10

percentile [pəˈsentaɪl] n term   sim **quartile**[1] [kwɔːr-], **fractile**[2], **decile**[3] [es] n term

rank position of an individual in a serial [ɪə] array[4] [əreɪ] of data stated in terms of what percentage of the group (s)he equals [iː] or exceeds [iː]

» About 30% of these children are below the third percentile for height[5] [haɪt]. The men in the quartile with the highest values had a 3 times higher risk of stroke than those in the lowest quartile.

Jse above/below the 5th / 95th / growth / age-matched[6] **percentile** • **percentile** curve [ɜː]/ level / rank[7] / for age and sex[8]

Perzentil(e)
Quartil(e)[1] Fraktil(e)[2] Dezil(e)[3] nach Größe geordnete Reihe[4] (Körper)größe[5] altersentsprechende P.[6] Perzentilenrang[7] Alters- u. Geschlechtsperzentile[8]

14

11

frequency [iː] **distribution** [-bjuːʃən] n term   rel **outlier**[1] [aʊtlaɪəʳ] n term

statistical description of raw data in terms of the number or frequency of items [aɪ] characterized by each of a series or range of values of a continuous variable

» The distribution of the ratios was non-Gaussian. A reading[2], value or measurement [eʒ] far outside the central range of the data is termed an outlier and is considered to be in error[3].

Jse normal or Gaussian[4] / standardized normal / binomial [aɪ]/ probability[5] **distribution** • even[6] [iː]/ linear / Student's or t-[7] / Poisson / sex / female-to-male [iː] **distribution** • randomly / uniformly[8] **distributed** • **distribution** curve [ɜː]/ coefficient[9] [ɪʃ]/ free test[10]

Häufigkeitsverteilung
Ausreißer[1] Messwert[2] falsch, fehlerhaft[3] Gauß-, Normalverteilung[4] Wahrscheinlichkeitsvert.[5] gleichmäßige V.[6] Student-, t-V.[7] gleichverteilt[8] Verteilungskoeffizient[9] verteilungsunabhängiger Test[10]

12

deviation [diːvɪeɪʃən] n term   sim **skew(ness)**[1] [skjuːnəs] n term

(i) departure[2] [-tʃəʳ] from symmetry of a frequency distribution
(ii) shift[3] away from the normal course or site

deviate[4] [diːvɪeɪt] v term • skew v

» The standard deviation is the statistical index of the variability within a distribution (the square [skweəʳ] root [5] [uː] of the average of the squared deviation from the mean). The median, range, upper quartile and the skewness of chain code variance were most predictive of recurrence [ɜː].

Use standard[6] **deviation** (abbr SD) / of the mean (abbr SDM) • measure of **skewness** • **skew** distribution[7]

Abweichung
Schiefe[1] Abweichung[2] Verschiebung[3] abweichen[4] Quadratwurzel[5] Standardabweichung[6] schiefe Verteilung[7]

13

variance [vɛriəns] n term sim **variation**[1] [vɛrieɪʃ°n] n term
(i) variation found between a set of observations (ii) state of being variable, different, divergent[2] [daɪvɜːrdʒənt]
variant[3] adj & n • variability[4] n • covariance[5] n term
» Variance is calculated as the square of the standard deviation. Mean pressure responses and measures of variance were calculated. These findings are at variance with[6] those of Bell.
Use analysis of[7] **variance**, abbr ANOVA • coefficient [fɪʃ] of **variation**[8] (abbr CV) • intra-/ inter-observer[9] **variance**

Varianz
Variation[1] unterschiedlich[2] abweichend; Abart, Variante[3] Variabilität[4] Kovarianz[5] weichen ab von[6] Varianzanalyse[7] Variationskoeffizient[8] Intra-/ Inter-Beobachter-Varianz[9]

14

range [reɪndʒ] n term
statistical measure [eɜ] of the variation of values determined by the endpoint values[1]
long-range[2] adj term • range[3] v
» The clinical spectrum of the disease ranges from mild to life-threatening[4] [e]. The plasma concentrations exhibit[5] episodic increases, with values ranging up to 4 pmol/L.
Use broad [ɒː]/ wide [aɪ]/ narrow / in the 80–90% / age / reference[6] / therapeutic[7] [pjuː] **range** • **to range** from A to B / between A and B

Spannweite, Bereich
Extremwerte[1] langfristig[2] liegen, schwanken[3] lebensgefährlich[4] weisen auf[5] Referenzbereich[6] therapeutische Breite[7]

15

degrees of freedom n term   abbr **df**
the number of observations (subjects, test items and scores[1], trials[2] [aɪ], conditions, etc.) minus the number of independent restrictions[3] in the sampling undertaken
» Patients with stress incontinence had a leak [iː] point pressure[4] of 42 cmH$_2$O (P=0.126, df=10).

Freiheitsgrade, FG
Werte, Scores[1] Versuche, Untersuchungen[2] Einschränkungen, Restriktionen[3] Blasendruck bei unwillkürlichem Harnabgang[4]

16

confidence interval n term   abbr **CI** n term
statistical measure for the range of uncertainty about the probability of an outcome
» Actuarial disease-specific survival rates and associated 95% confidence intervals were calculated using the Kaplan-Meier method[1].
Use **confidence** limit[2] / band / level[3] • disease-free / follow-up **interval**

Konfidenzintervall, Vertrauensbereich
Kaplan-Meier Schätzung / Methode[1] Konfidenzgrenze[2] Konfidenzniveau[3]

17

bias [baɪəs] n term   syn **systematic error, distortion** [dɪstɔːrʃ°n] n, rel **confounder**[1] [aʊ] n term
deviation [diːvieɪʃ°n] of results from the truth or mechanisms [k] leading to such deviation, e.g. analysis bias, measurement bias, selection bias, withdrawal [-ɒːəl] bias[2], etc.
biased[3] adj • unbiased[4] adj • confounding adj
» The common biases of screening are length, lead-time [iː] and selection biases. Lead-time bias[5] occurs when the patient is merely [ɪɚ] diagnosed at an earlier time but life expectancy[6] remains unchanged. An extreme [iː] form of length bias is overdiagnosis. The data may be biased.
Use to minimize/be prone [oʊ] to[7]/reflect **bias** • selection / gender [dʒ]/ information / length / confounding / recall **bias** • **biased** study / sample[8] [æ] • to be **biased** toward children[9] / by personal involvement / related to patient selection • **unbiased** estimator[10] • sampling / standard[11] / systematic / false-positive [ɔː]/ false-negative error • confounding variable[1]

Bias, systemat. Fehler / Verzerrung
Störgröße, verzerrender Faktor[1] Verzerrung durch abgebrochene Beobachtungen[2] verzerrt[3] unverzerrt[4] Lead-time Bias[5] Lebenserwartung[6] Bias-anfällig sein[7] verzerrte Stichprobe[8] gegenüber Kindern befangen / voreingenommen sein[9] erwartungstreue Schätzfunktion[10] Standardfehler[11]

18

event [ɪvent] n term
experience, incident[1], trait, or clinical condition defined by a binary [aɪ] outcome measure[2]
» It is not relevant when the underlying event[3] took place. Ovulation or some other natural event causing mild discomfort may be experienced as an abdominal catastrophy.
Use **event** rate / -driven data[4] / analysis / recorder • simple / certain[5] / (non-)excluding[6] / impossible / complementary **event** • clinical / random[7] / initial [ʃ]/ recurrent[8] / stressful / reportable **event** • perinatal [eɪ]/ negative life / traumatic / precipitating[9] [sɪp]/ isolated [aɪ] **event** • work-related / multicasualty[10] [-ʒ(ʊ)əlti]/ (pre)terminal [ɜː] **events**

Ereignis
Vorfall[1] dichotomer Parameter[2] ursächliches E.[3] ereignisabhängige Daten[4] sicheres E.[5] (nicht) ausschließendes E.[6] zufallabhängiges E.[7] wiederkehrendes E.[8] auslösendes E.[9] Naturkatastrophen[10]

19

Medical Statistics

endpoint *n term*   *syn* **primary** [aɪ] **outcome** *or* **event** *n term*
outcome variable used to judge[1] [dʒʌdʒ] the effectiveness of treatment
» In terms of major endpoints the test drug did not prove superior [ɪɚ] to[2] placebo [siː]. Endpoints examined were semen [iː] analyses, sperm [ɜː] functional assessments[3], and pain scores.
▌se hard[4] / soft[5] / study / valid[6] / primary / secondary / multiple **endpoints** • **endpoint** analysis • clinical / treatment / quality-of-life[7] / overall / long-term[8] **outcome** • favorable [eɪ]/ poor / adverse [ɜː]/ fatal[9] [eɪ] **outcome**

Endpunkt, Zielgröße
beurteilen[1] sich als besser erweisen als[2] Spermiogramme[3] harte Endpunkte[4] weiche E.[5] valide E.[6] Ergebnis einer Lebensqualitätsstudie[7] Langzeitergebnis[8] letaler Ausgang[9]

20

statistically significant *adj term*   *opposite* **insignificant**[1] *adj term*
the statistical probability (must be <5%) that a finding is very unlikely the result of chance alone
significance[2] *n term*
» Raised [eɪ] alkaline phosphatase was of no prognostic value, while creatinine reached marginal [dʒ] significance[3]. The factor was found to be of significance for tumor recurrence.
▌se highly **significant** • statistically **insignificant** • least **significant** difference[4] (*abbr* LSD) • **significance** level[5] • p-value[6] • prognostic / clinical / borderline[3] **significance**

statistisch signifikant
nicht signifikant[1] Signifikanz[2] grenzwertige S.[3] Grenzdifferenz[4] Signifikanzniveau[5] p-Wert[6]

21

false [ɔː] **positive** *adj & n term*   *opposite* **false negative**[1] *adj & n term*
test result which wrongly indicates the presence of a disease, condition or finding
» No false positives were found in the control group[2]. The two false negative results were obtained in normotensive patients[3].
▌se **false positive** error[4] / result [ʌ]/ rate / scan / test / cultures [ʌ] • true[5] **positive** / **negative**

falsch-positiv(er Wert)
falsch-negativ(er Wert)[1] Kontrollgruppe[2] bei Normotonikern[3] falsch positiver Fehler[4] richtig positiv / negativ[5]

22

sensitivity *n term*   *rel* **specificity**[1] [spesɪfɪsəti] *n term*
proportion of individuals with a positive test result for the disease that the test is intended to reveal [iː]
» The reliability[2] [aɪə] of a diagnostic test is measured by its sensitivity and specificity. The specificity of a screening test is the number of true negative results as a proportion of the total of true negative and false-positive results. The test has a sensitivity of 75% and a specificity of 95%.
▌se 95% / high / moderate / low / lack of[3] **sensitivity** • to increase[4] [iː]/enhance[4] [æ]/ diagnostic **specificity**

Sensitivität
Spezifität[1] Reliabilität, Zuverlässigkeit[2] mangelnde Sensitivität[3] die Spezifität verbessern[4]

23

cut-off *or* **cutoff (point** *or* **value)** *n term*   *syn* **cut-point,**
                          threshold [θreʃould] *n term*
point or value in an ordered sequence [iː] used to separate these values into two subgroups
» Test sensitivity and specificity depend on the reference range used, i.e. the cutoff point above which a test is interpreted as abnormal. Many programs use age cutoffs[1] to select potential transplant recipients[2] [sɪp].
▌se sharp[3] / low / subgrouping **cutoff** • a **cutoff** value of 4 ng/mL

Schwellenwert, Grenzwert, Cutoff
Altersgrenzen[1] Transplantatempfänger[2] exakter Grenzwert[3]

24

survival [sɚvaɪvᵊl] *n term*   *sim* **survivorship**[1] *n term*
period between the institution or completion of any procedure and death
survive[2] *v* • survivor[3] *n*
» The limiting factor for survival was the tumor, not age. Children with Hodgkin's disease have a 75% overall survival rate at more than 20 years' followup. Median survival was 11 months.
▌se **survival** rate[4] / time or period[5] / probability / curve / benefit[6] / trial / analysis[7] • **survival** to adulthood[8] / to the 6th decade / to age 50 • **survival** from colon cancer / following bypass surgery / at 1 year • median or mean / disease-free / event-free[9] / cumulative **survival** • infarct / expected graft[10] / improved / lower **survival** • long-term / childhood cancer **survivor**

Überleben(szeit)
Überleben, Gruppe der Überlebenden[1] überleben[2] Überlebende(r)[3] Überlebensrate[4] Überlebenszeit[5] Überlebensvorteil[6] Überlebenszeitanalyse[7] Ü. bis ins Erwachsenenalter[8] ereignisfreies Ü.[9] erwartete Transplantatlebensdauer[10]

25

life-table analysis [əˈnæləsɪs] *n term*   **syn survival analysis** *n term*

a method of analysis that relies [aɪ] on a count of the number of events (e.g. death) observed and the time points at which those events occurred [ɜː], relative to some zero [ɪə] point[1]

» In life-table analysis for clinical trials the time to an event for a patient is usually measured from the time of randomization and treatment effects are assessed by comparing event rates in the different treatment groups. Lifetable analysis to 15 years failed to yield a deterioration[2] [ɪɚ] in graft outcome for these patients.

Use to run *a life-table analysis* • to generate [dʒen-]/prepare/create [ieɪ] *a life table* • period / abridged[3] [ɪdʒ]/ survivor analysis / cohort[4] *life table* • *life-table* methods / event rates / survivorship

Überlebenszeitanalyse, -statistik
Nullzeitpunkt[1] Verschlechterung aufzeigen[2] abgekürzte Sterbetafel[3] Kohortensterbetafel[4]

26

table *n term*   **sim diagram**[1] [aɪə], **graph**[1] *n*, **chart**[1] [tʃ], **plot**[1] *n & v term*

data arranged in parallel rows [rouz] and columns[2] to display the essential facts in an easily appreciable[3] [iːʃ] form

tabulation[4] *n term* • tabulated[5] *adj* • plotter[6] *n* • -gram *comb*

» Surface area, like metabolic rate, is not a linear function of weight [weɪt] and requires the use of a table or nomogram. The postoperative results are summarized in the table. The pressure was plotted against the flow rate. This increase was evidenced by[7] a larger area under the curve (abbr AUC) in the receiver [iː] operating characteristic (abbr ROC) plot.

Use tabulated results • contingency[8] [ɪndʒ]/ (cohort) life *table* • bar[9] / scatter[10] / block[11] / vector *diagram* • pie[12] [aɪ]/ bar[9] / flow[13] *chart* • ROC / Kaplan-Meier[14] / scatter[10] *plot* • *to plot* X against Y[15] • acid-base *nomogram* • histogram

Tabelle, Tafel
Diagramm, Graph, graphische Darstellung; (i. Graph) eintragen, plotten[1] Spalten[2] übersichtlich[3] tabellarische Darstellung[4] tabellarisch[5] Kurvenschreiber[6] belegt durch[7] Kontingenztafel[8] Säulen-, Balkendiagramm[9] Streudiagr.[10] Blockd.[11] Kreis-, Tortendiagramm[12] Flussd.[13] Kaplan-Meier Diagramm[14] X gegen Y auftragen[15]

27

multivariate [-ɪɪt‖ɪeɪt] **analysis** *n term*   **syn multivariable analysis** *n term*

statistical model in which more than one dependent variable is simultaneously [eɪ] predicted

» Data from the Mayo Clinic using multivariate analysis indicate that only the presence of a locally advanced lesion [iːʒ] was independently predictive of recurrence and ultimate [ʌ] death from disease.

Use *multivariate analysis* of variants (abbr MANOVA) • *multivariate* relative risk model • frequency / univariate / bivariate[1] / covariance[2] *analysis* • factor / interim / cluster[3] / correspondence / discriminant[4] *analysis*

multivariate / mehrdimensionale Analyse
bivariate A.[1] Kovarianzanalyse[2] Cluster-Analyse[3] Diskriminanzanalyse[4]

28

prediction [prɪdɪkʃ°n] *n term*   **sim estimation**[1] [estɪmeɪʃ°n] *n term*

statement anticipating[2] [tɪs] or forecasting[3] [æ] a future event or prognosis

predictive *adj term* • predict *v* • predictor[4] *n* • estimate[5] *n & v*

» A positive biopsy finding has a predictive value of about 90%. Location and thickness of primary melanoma are the most accurate predictors of prognosis.

Use positive[6] / negative *predictive value* • actuarial[7] *estimation* • *estimation* of a proportion

Vorhersage, Prädiktion
Schätzung[1] vorhersehen[2] voraussagen[3] prädiktiver Parameter[4] Schätzwert; schätzen[5] positiver Vorhersagewert[6] (Sterbe)tafelmethode[7]

29

reliability [rɪlaɪəbɪləti] *n term*   **rel reproducibility**[1], **validity**[2] *n term*

measure [eʒ] of the consistency of statistical data (i.e. results are reproducible on retesting)

validation[3] *n term* • validate[4] *v* • valid[5] [vælɪd] *adj* • (un)reliable[6] *adj*

» Cancers can be detected with a high degree of reliability with colonoscopy. Suboptimal effort limits the validity of lung volume calculations derived [aɪ] from[7] spirometry [aɪ].

Use test-retest[8] / interjudge[9] [-dʒʌdʒ] *reliability* • *reliable* indicator / marker / test • internal / external / predictive *validity* • protocol *validation*

Reliabilität, Zuverlässigkeit
Reproduzierbarkeit[1] Gültigkeit, Validität[2] Gültigkeitsprüfung[3] validieren[4] gültig[5] (un)zuverlässig[6] basierend auf[7] Retest-Stabilität[8] Inter-Beobachter-Reliabilität[9]

30

probability *n term*   **syn likelihood** [laɪklihʊd] *n genE*

statistical measure indicating how likely[1] a specific event is to occur [ɜː]

(im)probable[2] *adj* • to be (un)likely to happen[2] *phr*

» Prosthetic replacement has the greatest probability of preventing recurrence. The probability of obtaining[3] a given outcome due to chance is expressed by the P value (a significance of p < 0.05 means that up to 5 times out of 100 the result could have occurred by chance).

Use *probability* interval / curve [ɜː]/ distribution[4] / density[5] • low / high / greater / calculation of / conditional[6] *probability* • posttest / pretest / prior [praɪɚ]/ 1% / long-term *probability* • lifetime[7] / cumulative [kjuː] survival[8] *probability* • **high-probability** lung scan

Wahrscheinlichkeit
wahrscheinlich[1] (un)wahrscheinlich[2] erzielen[3] Wahrscheinlichkeitsverteilung[4] Wahrscheinlichkeitsdichte[5] bedingte W.[6] Lebenszeitw.[7] kumulative Überlebenswahrscheinlichkeit[8]

31

Medical Studies & Research

MEDICAL SCIENCE

correlation *n term*   *sim* **association**[1], **relation(ship)**[2], **link**[3] *n term*

degree of relationship (positive or negative) between two sets of paired [eə·] measurements[4] of traits [eɪ] or events

(un)**correlated**[5] *adj term* • **correlate** *v* • **correlative**[6] *adj*

» *There is a strong correlation with the presence of HLA-B27 antigen. The reliability of the index was high, with a test-retest correlation coefficient of r = 0.93.*

Use Spearman's rank[7] / Pearson's **correlation coefficient** • cross-[8]/ auto**correlation** • **to correlate** with / well / better / poorly[9] / closely / strongly • **to correlate** directly / positively / negatively / inversely[10] [ɜː] • **to be correlated** with • **correlation** between A and B / of A and/with B • **correlative** study • causal [kɒːl] close / inverse linear[11] **relationship** • to be **associated** with[12]

Korrelation

Zusammenhang[1] Beziehung[2] Verbindung[3] zwei Wertepaare[4] (un)korreliert[5] Korrelations-[6] Spearman'scher Rangkorrelationskoeffizient[7] Kreuzkorrelation[8] schwach korrelieren[9] gegensinnig k.[10] gegensinnig lineare K.[11] in Zusammenhang stehen[12]

32

regression [rɪɡreʃ⁽ə⁾n] *n term*   *rel* **slope**[1] [sloʊp] *n term*

functional relationship between a dependent and one or more independent variables

» *Prediction of mortality was performed by logistic [dʒ] regression analysis[2].*

Use **regression** coefficient[3] / line[4] / curve • univariate[5] / bivariate [aɪ]/ linear [ɪ]/ multiple [ʌ] **regression**

Regression

Steigung[1] logistische Regressionsanalyse[2] Regressionskoeffizient[3] Regressionsgerade[4] univariate Regression[5]

33

chi-square(d) [kaɪ-] **test** *n term*   *rel* **t-** or **student's test**[1] *n term*

statistical technique [iːk] whereby variables are categorized to determine[2] whether a distribution of scores is due to chance or experimental factors

» *The chi-square test and ROC curves[3] were used for statistical analysis.*

Use significance[4] / binomial / log-rank[5] / parametric **test** • **chi-square** analysis • Pearson **chi-square analysis** • partition [ɪʃ] of the[6] **sum of squares**, *abbr* SS • chi-**squared** • nonparametric or distribution free[7] / Wilcoxon's rank sum[8] / Mann-Whitney U[9] **test** • **test of** independence / fit / significance[4]

Chi²-Test, χ² Test

t-Test[1] feststellen[2] ROC (Receiver-Operating-Characteristic) Kurven[3] Signifikanztest[4] Logrank-Test[5] Zerlegung der Quadratsummen[6] parameterfreier T.[7] Wilcoxon (Rangsummen)test[8] U-Test nach Mann und Whitney[9]

34

proportional [ɔːrʃ] **hazard model** *n term*

syn **Cox (regression** [eʃ]**) model** *n term*

regression method for modelling censored survival data which assumes the ratio of the risks (hazard ratio)

» *The present study is aimed at updating prognosis in primary biliary cirrhosis [sɪr-] using a time-dependent Cox regression model. Cox regression uses the maximum likelihood method rather than the least [iː] squares method.*

Use linear regression[1] **model** • **proportional** odds model[2] / censorship [sen-]

Cox Regression

lineares Regressionsmodell[1] Modell m. proportionalen Ja-Nein Quotienten[2]

35

Unit 15   Medical Studies & Research
Related Units: 14 Medical Statistics

study [stʌdi] *n & v term*   *sim* **clinical trial**[1] [traɪ⁽ə⁾l] *n term*

(i) research activities involving the collection, analysis, or interpretation of data
(ii) project involving several investigations or a clinical trial
(iii) diagnostic investigations (biochemical [k], imaging studies[2], etc.)

» *A prospective study is under way[3] to evaluate these two treatment options.*

Use to perform/carry out/make/undertake/launch[4] [ɒː] **a study** • to be under **study**[5] • longitudinal[6] / (quasi-)experimental / non-experimental research / cross-sectional *or* prevalence[7] / follow-up[8] / prospective[9] / retrospective **study** • interventional[10] / observational[11] / historical / epidemiological / parallel cohort / case-control(ed)[12] / feasibility [iː] *or* pilot[13] [aɪ] **study** • **study** participant / population / protocol / manual • randomized / (un)controlled / triple-blinded [ɪ]/ single-blind[14] / multicenter **(clinical) trial** • phase I / II / III / IV / open label[15] [eɪ] **trial**

Studie, Untersuchung; untersuchen

klinische Studie / Untersuchung[1] bildgebende Verfahren[2] im Gange[3] Studie beginnen[4] wird zur Zeit untersucht[5] Longitudinal-, Längsschnittstudie[6] Prävalenz-, Querschnittstudie[7] Verlaufsuntersuchung[8] prospektive Studie[9] Interventionsst.[10] Beobachtungsst.[11] Fall-Kontroll-Studie[12] Pilotstudie[13] einfach blinde St.[14] offene Studie[15]

1

56 MEDICAL SCIENCE — Medical Studies & Research

investigation [-geɪʃən] n term · sim **research**[1] [n riː-, v rɪsɜːrtʃ] term

(i) a thorough[2] [θɜːrə] and systematic examination or study of unknown issues[3]
(ii) a clinical study or trial

investigator[4] n term • investigate v • investigational[5] adj • investigative[5] adj • researcher[6] n

» These observations warrant[7] [ɔː] further investigation into the effects of different management approaches. Laboratory investigations revealed microhematuria [iː].

Use to do **research**[1] on / into • **research** fellow[8] / worker[6] • clinical / preliminary[9] / longitudinal / (non-)invasive [eɪ] / multidisciplinary / parallel group **investigation** • principal **investigator** • **investigational** treatment[10] / new drug application[11] (abbr INDA or IND) / device [dɪvaɪs] exemption[12] (abbr IDE) • in an **investigative** stage[13] [steɪdʒ] • to be under **investigation**

(i) (wissenschaftliche) Untersuchung (ii) klinische Studie
(Er)forschung, (er)forschen[1] gründlich[2] Zusammenhänge, Fragen[3] Untersucher[4] Test-, Forschungs-, Untersuchungs-[5] Forscher(in), Wissenschafter(in)[6] rechtfertigen[7] Forschungsstipendiat(in)[8] vorläufige U.[9] experimentelle Behandlung[10] Einsatz e. neuen Testmedikaments[11] Sondergenehmigung f. neues Medizinprodukt[12] im Forschungsstadium[13]
2

---

objective [dʒek] n term · syn **aim** [eɪm], sim **purpose**[1] [pɜːrpəs] n

research papers[2] about medical studies are usually structured as follows: title, abstract, introduction and objectives, materials and methods, results, discussion, and conclusion(s)

aim (at)[3] v

» The objective of the present study[4] was to assess[5] the response of BPH patients to doxazosin.

Ziel, Zielsetzung
Zweck[1] wissensch. Arbeiten / Publikationen / Vorträge[2] abzielen auf, anstreben[3] vorliegende Studie[4] untersuchen[5]
3

---

patient recruitment [uːt] n term · sim **enrollment**[1], **assignment**[2] [aɪn], **allocation**[2] n term

selecting and obtaining informed consent[3] from patients (subjects) to participate in clinical trials

recruit [uːt] v term • enroll in(to)[4] v • enrollee[5] [iː] n • allocate v • assign v

» It is recommended that children with brain tumors be enrolled in multicenter protocols. The study was inconclusive owing [oʊɪŋ] to problems in recruitment and low subject enrollment.

Use **patient recruitment** goal [oʊ] • **enrollment** criteria[6] [kraɪtɪrɪə] • time of / at / prior [aɪ] to[7] **enrollment** • uniform or equal [iː] treatment / stratified **allocation**[8] • fixed / adaptive **allocation design** • randomly **allocated** to treatment[9]

Patientenrekrutierung
Aufnahme[1] Zuteilung[2] aufgeklärte Einwilligung einholen[3] i.d. Studie aufnehmen[4] Studien-, Versuchsteilnehmer[5] Aufnahmekriterien[6] vor der A.[7] stratifizierte Zuteilung[8] randomisiert der Behandlung zugeteilt[9]
4

---

randomization [rændəmaɪzeɪʃən] n term

(i) a chance[1] [tʃæns] assignment of treatments in an experiment (ii) a statistical selection process in which all subjects or samples presumably have the same chance of being selected[2]

random[1] adj term • randomize[3] v • (non)randomized adj • randomizer[4] n

» Altogether 512 patients were randomized to chemotherapy [kiː-]. The visit where a participant is randomly assigned[5] to treatment groups of a clinical trial is termed randomization visit.

Use **random** number[6] / variable / process / allocation[7] / population / biopsy [aɪ] • **randomized** clinical trial[8] / controlled study / blocking[9] / prospective series • **randomization** visit / process • at[1] **random** • in a **random** fashion[1]

Randomisierung, Zufallszuteilung
zufällig[1] Rekrutierungschance[2] randomisieren[3] Zufallsgenerator[4] zugeteilt[5] Zufallszahl[6] Zufallszuteilung[7] randomis. klinische Studie[8] blockweise Randomisierung[9]
5

---

prospective adj term · opposite **retrospective**[1] adj term

subjects with a specific trait [eɪ] or parameter are identified and then observed for the occurrence[2] [ɜː] of the outcome

» This prospective two-part trial comprised[3] [aɪ] a pilot study of 10 men.

Use **prospective** study / survey[4] [ɜː] / clinical trial / series[5] [ɪə] • **prospective** evaluation / observation protocol / data [eɪ] • **prospective** blood donor[6] [oʊ] / recipient[7] [sɪ] • **retrospective** analysis / chart [tʃ] / review[8] [iː]

prospektiv
retrospektiv[1] Eintreten[2] bestand aus[3] prospektive Erhebung[4] p. Versuchsserie[5] potentieller Blutspender(in)[6] prosp. Empfänger(in)[7] retrospektive Analyse von Krankengeschichten[8]
6

---

protocol n term · sim **study manual of operations**[1] n term

(i) precise plan for a clinical trial or a therapeutic [pjuː] regimen[2] [redʒ-]
(ii) guidelines (iii) official notes (e.g. at autopsy [ɔː])

» Fifty patients were on a surveillance [səveɪləns] protocol[3] after orchiectomy [k] alone. Treatment audits[4] [ɔː] were performed for adherence [ɪə] to protocols[5]. Patients who desire more aggressive treatment should be referred[6] for experimental protocol therapy.

Use **protocol** trial / design[7] • study / treatment / testing / chemotherapeutic [kiː-] **protocol** • three-drug / transfusion / field[8] / formal **protocol** • well-designed / followup / watchful waiting[3] / FDA-approved[9] / short-stay **protocol**

(Studien)protokoll
Studienanleitungen[1] Behandlungsplan[2] Surveillance, Beobachtungsstrategie[3] Therapiekontrollen[4] Einhaltung d. Behandlungsprotokolle[5] überwiesen[6] Studiendesign[7] Studienprot. f. Feldversuch[8] v. d. U.S. Gesundheits- u. Lebensmittelbehörde genehmigtes Studienprotokoll[9]
7

15

Medical Studies & Research   MEDICAL SCIENCE 57

placebo [pləsiːboʊ] *n term*   *sim* **inactive control** *or*
                                         sham [ʃæm] **treatment**[1] *n term*

(i) inert[2] [ɜː] substance (a sugar pill) identical in appearance with the drug studied which is administered under the pretense of real treatment; used in clinical trials to distinguish between the actual efficacy [-kəsi] of an experimental drug and its suggestive [dʒe] effect (ii) more generally, any ineffective treatment (usually prescribed to meet a patient's demands)

» Eighty percent of the patients who received a placebo became asymptomatic. Prokinetic agents were superior [ɪɚ] to[3] placebo. Those initially on placebo were switched [tʃ] to drug at the end of the 4th week of the trial.

Use **placebo** effect / control group / responder[4] / relief [iː]/ therapy /-treated patient /-controlled trial • nonmedicine **placebo** • **sham**-treated controls / group / feeding[5] [iː]/ lavage [ɑː3]

Plazebo, Leer-, Scheinmedikament
Scheinbehandlung[1] inaktiv, unwirksam[2] wirksamer, besser[3] Placeboresponder[4] Scheinfütterung[5]

8

blind [blaɪnd] *adj term*   *syn* **blinded** *adj term*

(adj) keeping study participants and/or investigators from knowing which subjects are assigned to the treatment and the placebo group in order to keep biases[1] [baɪəsɪz] or expectations from influencing the results

blind[2] *v term* • unblind[3] *v*

» Our randomized double-blind study shows that administration of alpha-blockers is effective.

Use single[4]-/ double[5]-**blind study** • partially [ʃ] **blinded** • **blind(ed) study**[6] / sham controlled study / placebo trial / procedure

blind
verfälschende Faktoren, Verzerrungen[1] verblinden[2] offenlegen[3] einfacher Blindversuch[4] Doppelblindversuch[5] Blindversuch[6]

9

control group *n term*   *opposite* **treatment** *or* **experimental group**[1] *n term*

subjects [ʌ] (e.g. healthy individuals or normals) participating in the same experiment as the treatment group but not exposed to[2] the test medication or the variable under investigation[3]

(case-)controlled *adj term* • control *v* • controls[4] *n pl*

» There was no difference in survival between control and study groups[1]. The results were compared to normals[5] for patient age. Healthy [e] volunteers[6] served as controls.

Use **control** animals / patients / population / samples • healthy *or* normal / age-matched / untreated / nonoperative[7] / unexposed / own / historical[8] **controls** • (in)active **control treatment** • **controlled** clinical trial[9]

Kontrollgruppe
Test-, Behandlungsgruppe[1] nicht exponiert bzgl.[2] Prüfvariable[3] Kontrollpersonen[4] Gesunde[5] gesunde Freiwillige[6] nicht operierte Kontrollpersonen[7] historische K.[8] kontrollierte klin. Studie[9]

10

treatment block *n term*   *sim* **blocking**[1] *n*, **series**[2] [sɪɚiːz] *n sing & pl*,
                                          cohort[3] *n term*

prespecified[4] number of patients enrolled in a study and assigned to the various study treatments in such a way so as to satisfy a preset[4] allocation ratio [reɪʃ(ɪ)oʊ]

Use **treatment block** size • **block** design[5] • hospitalized[6] **cohort** • **cohort** members / study[7] • *a* published [ʌ]/ small / large / consecutive[8] **series**

Therapieblock
Blockbildung, blockweise Zuteilung[1] Patientenreihe, -serie[2] Kohorte[3] (vorher) festgelegt[4] Blockanlage[5] stationäre Kohorte[6] Kohortenstudie[7] konsekutive Patientenreihe[8]

11

treatment arm *n term*

term sometimes used in place of study treatment, or study group

» Ten patients were randomized[1] to each arm of the study.

Use chemotherapy [kiː-]/ therapeutic [pjuː]/ no drug / control **arm**

Therapiearm
nach dem Zufallsprinzip zugeteilt, randomisiert[1]

12

factorial design [dɪsaɪn] *n term*

treatment structure in which one study treatment is used in combination with at least one other study arm in a trial, or where multiples of a defined dose of a specified treatment are used in the same trial

Use partial [ʃ]/ full **factorial design** • adaptive / parallel group / group sequential[1] [sɪkwɛnʃəl]/ crossover **design** • **factorial** treatment structure

faktorielles Design
gruppensequentielles Design[1]

13

(treatment) crossover *n term*

planned (e.g in a crossover trial) or unplanned switch[1] of study treatments for a patient in a clinical trial

noncrossover[2] *adj term*

» Unplanned crossovers are called "drop out"[3] and "drop in[4]."

Use **crossover** trial[5] • **crossed** treatments

Therapiewechsel, Crossover
Wechsel[1] ohne Therapiewechsel[2] Ausfall, Therapieabbrecher[3] Zugang, Therapiewechsler[4] Crossover-Studie[5]

14

15

MEDICAL SCIENCE

data [deɪtə] n term pl only   rel **information**[1], **documentation**[2] n term sing only
collection of facts on a specific patient or set of patients from which conclusions may be drawn
d**o**cument[3] v & n term • (un)d**o**cumented adj • informative adj
» There are only few data available for comparison.
Use to obt**ai**n [eɪ]/collect[4]/retrieve[5] [iː]/store/evaluate/analyze/pr**o**cess[6]/compare/confirm[7] *data* • scanty[8] [sk]/ab**u**ndant[9] [ʌ] *data on* sth. • **o**rdinal / n**o**minal / interval / hist**o**rical *data* • baseline[10] [eɪ]/ (un)c**e**nsored [s]/ anat**o**mic *data* • *data* item [aɪ]/ field / form[11] / entry / base[12] / file[13] [aɪ] • *data* editing / prot**e**ction[14] / and safety m**o**nitoring board, abbr DSMB • well/poorly *documented* • *information* retrieval / on sth. / about sth.

Daten(material), (Mess)werte, Angaben
Fakten, Informationen[1] Dokumentation, Unterlagen[2] dokumentieren, belegen; Dokument[3] Daten erheben[4] D. abrufen[5] D. verarbeiten[6] D. bestätigen[7] spärliche D. über[8] zahlreiche D.[9] Ausgangswerte[10] Datenerhebungsblatt[11] Datenbank[12] Datei[13] Datenschutz[14]   15

case report form n term, abbr **CRF**   syn **case record form** n term
standardized data entry form for all information collected and used in a clinical trial
» Even in circumstances where there is other documentation in addition to CRFs (e.g. lab slips[1]), generally all key [kiː] values[2] that will be analyzed appear on the CRF.

Patientenerhebungsbogen
Laborberichte[1] Schlüsselwerte[2]
   16

evidence n & v term   sim **confirmation**[1], **proof**[2] [uː], **verification**[3] n term
(n) observations or findings which indicate, support or confirm [ɜː] assumptions[4] [ʌ] or conclusions [uː]
evident[5] adj term • (un)confirmed adj • verify[6] v
» A growing body of evidence[7] supports our theory. There is no evidence of recurrent [ɜː] disease.
Use to seek [iː]/provide[8]/exhibit[8]/reveal[8] [iː]/search for *evidence* for / in favor of / in support of / against • strong[9] / clear(-cut)[10] / conclusive[11] [uː]/ overwhelming[12] / experimental / anecdotal[13] *evidence* • clinical / gross[14] [oʊ]/ radiographic *evidence*

Nachweis, Beweis, Beleg; belegen, beweisen
Bestätigung[1] Beweis[2] Verifizierung[3] Annahmen bestätigen[4] offensichtlich, evident[5] überprüfen, verifizieren[6] Beweismaterial[7] Be- / Nachweis liefern[8] viele / gute B.[9] eindeutige B.[10] schlüssige B.[11] schlagender B.[12] vereinzelte Belege[13] makroskopischer Nachweis[14]   17

in vitro [iː] phr term   opposite **in vivo**[1] [iː] phr term
in an artificial [fɪʃ] environment [aɪ] e.g. a test tube[2] or culture [ʌ] media [iː] rather than[3] in the living body
» These agents inhibit cellular proliferation[4] in prostate [ɒː] cancer [æ] both in vitro and in vivo.
Use *in vitro* techniques [iːk]/ model / analysis / fertilization[5] •
in vivo administration / experiment

in vitro
in vivo[1] Reagenzglas[2] anstatt[3] Zellwachstum[4] künstliche Befruchtung[5]
   18

alternative hypothesis [haɪpɒːθəsɪs] n term, pl -**ses** [iːz]
opposite **null** [ʌ] **hypothesis**[1] n term
assumption [ʌ] that the study will yield[2] [jiːld] observations, results, differences in outcome measures [eʒ] between study groups that are not the result of chance alone
hypothesize[3] v term • postulate[4] v & n • hypothetical adj
» Some authors hypothesize that a more virulent [ɪ] clone must be responsible.
Use to advance[3]/develop/propose[3]/postulate *a hypothesis* • to put forward[3]/confirm/ support/reject[5] [rɪdʒekt]/accept *a hypothesis* • null treatment / working[6] / (un)tenable[7] [e] *hypothesis* • one-tailed [eɪ] or one-sided / two-tailed or two-sided[8] *alternative hypothesis*

Alternativhypothese
Nullhypothese[1] ergeben[2] eine H. aufstellen[3] postulieren, Postulat aufstellen; Postulat[4] H. widerlegen[5] Arbeitshypothese[6] unhaltbare H.[7] zweiseitige Alternativhypothese[8]
   19

intention-to-treat analysis [ənæləsɪs] n term   syn **analysis by intention** [ʃ] **to treat** n term
data analysis in which the primary outcome data are analyzed by assigned treatment and irrespective of treatment adherence[1] [ɪə] (analysis by treatment administered)
» The endpoint of the study was analyzed according to the intention-to-treat principle.

Intention-to-treat Analyse
unabhängig von der Therapietreue[1]
   20

treatment lag [læg] n term
time required (or thought to be required) for a therapy to exert[1] [ɜː] its full effect
» The time lag[2] for a successful response may be 6-8 weeks.
Use **lag** period / phase [feɪz] • **to lag** behind[3] / jet[4] / lid *lag* • *treatment* interaction[5] / effect / compliance[6] [aɪ]/ difference / failure[7] [feɪlɚ]

Wirkungsverzögerung
entfalten[1] zeitliche Verzögerung[2] sich verzögern[3] Zirkadian-, Jet-Lag-Syndrom[4] Wechselwirkung von Wirkstoffen[5] Compliance[6] Therapieversager[7]   21

Medical Studies & Research MEDICAL SCIENCE 59

expanded [æ] **access** [æksɛs] *n term*

broad term for methods of distributing experimental drugs to patients who are unable to participate in ongoing clinical efficacy [ɛfɪkəsi] trials and have no other treatment options[1]

» These drugs are available to selected patients via expanded access. Types of expanded-access mechanisms [k] include parallel track, IND treatment[2], and compassionate use.

Use **expanded access** program / trial

erweiterter Therapiezugang
Behandlungsmöglichkeiten[1] experimentelle medikamentöse Behandlung[2]

22

compassionate [kəmpæʃənət] **use** *n term*

providing unapproved drugs to very sick patients who have no other treatment options for which case-by-case approval[1] [uː] must usually be obtained[2] [eɪ] from the FDA (Food and Drug Administration)

» Because of toxicity, some agents have been withdrawn [ɔː] from the market[3] but are still available for compassionate use.

Use **compassionate use** protocol / program / group / arm of the study

Verabreichung von nicht zugelassenen Testmedikamenten
Bewilligung[1] eingeholt[2] aus dem Verkehr gezogen[3]

23

institutional review [rɪvjuː] **board** [ɔː] *n term*   *abbr* **IRB**,
                              syn **hospital ethics** [ɛθɪks] **committee** *n term*

a committee of physicians [fɪzɪʃ°nz], statisticians [ɪʃ], community advocates, and others which must first approve[1] [uː] a clinical trial and ensure[2] [-ʃʊɚ] that it is ethical and that the rights of the study participants are protected

Ethikkommission
genehmigen[1] sicherstellen[2]

24

steering [stɪɚ-] **committee** *n term*   *abbr* **SC**

(i) broadly, the committee responsible for directing the activities of a designated[1] project
(ii) key committee in the organizational structure of a multicenter clinical trial

» The SC is responsible for conduct[2] of the trial and gets the reports from all other committees, except the Adverse Experience Committee[3] and Data and Safety Monitoring Board and the Advisory Review and Treatment Effects Monitoring Committee.

Use publications / research ethics[4] (*abbr* REC) / infection control[5] (*abbr* ICC) / standing[6] / joint[7] [dʒ]/ advisory[8] [aɪ] **committee**

Studienbegleitkommission
festgelegt[1] Durchführung[2] Beschwerdeausschuss[3] Ethikkommission[4] Arbeitsgruppe f. Seuchenbekämpfung[5] ständiger Ausschuss[6] gemeinsamer A.[7] Beratungskomitee[8]

25

efficacy [ɛfɪkəsi] *n term*   *syn* **effectiveness**, *sim* **efficiency**[1] [ɛfɪʃ°nsi] *n term*

capacity or power of a procedure [iː], drug etc. to produce a desired effect

effect[2] *n & v* • effective[3] *adj* • efficacious[3] [keɪʃ] *adj* • (in)efficient[4] [ɪʃ] *adj*

» Our study confirms the efficacy of patient-controlled analgesia [dʒiː]. Corticosteroid [ɪɚ‖er] therapy alone is considered to be less efficacious than major endocrine [aɪ‖ɪ] ablation [eɪʃ].

Use to be of/show/demonstrate **great efficacy** • long-term / documented / overall / therapeutic **efficacy** • cost-**efficient** • to have an / carry-over[5] / beneficial[6] [fɪʃ] **effect** • desired[7] [aɪ]/ favorable[8] [eɪ]/ profound [aʊ]/ systemic **effect** on

Wirksamkeit, Effektivität
Leistungsfähigkeit, Effizienz[1] Wirkung; (be)wirken[2] wirksam, effektiv[3] (un)wirksam, (in)effizient[4] Nachwirkung[5] wohltuende / günstige Wirkung[6] erwünschte W.[7] günstige Wirkung[8]

26

outcome [aʊtkʌm] *n term*

condition of a patient following therapeutic intervention[1]

» Nutrition recommendations were developed to meet treatment goals[2] and desired outcomes[3]. Intracranial [eɪ] bleeding (sometimes fatal [eɪ] in outcome) occurred following hypertensive crisis.

Use to affect[4]/alter [ɒː]/improve [uː] **outcome** • **outcome** criteria [aɪ]/ data / statement • treatment / clinical / surgical[5] / primary **outcome** • 3-year / long-term / censored[6] / maternal-fetal [iː] **outcome** • fatal[7] / (un)favorable[8] / poor[9] **outcome** • multiple [ʌ] **outcomes** • binary[10] [aɪ] **outcome measure**

Therapieergebnis, Resultat, Folge
therapeutischer Eingriff[1] Behandlungsziele erreichen[2] angestrebte Behandlungsergebnisse[3] Behandlungsergebnis beeinflussen[4] Operationsergebnis[5] zensiertes E.[6] Tod, Exitus[7] (un)günstiges Ergebnis[8] schlechtes E.[9] binärer Ergebnisparameter[10]

27

censoring [sɛnsərɪŋ] *n term*

term used mainly in survival [aɪ] analyses[1] to denote an individual who has not experienced the event of interest at a specific point, e.g. at the time of interim analysis, end of study, or of lost to followup[2]

» The process by which patient outcome data cannot be obtained beyond a specific point in time is termed censoring.

zensierte Beobachtung
Überlebenszeitanalysen[1] nicht mehr zur Verlaufskontrolle erscheinen, nicht mehr zur Verfügung stehen[2]

28

withdrawal [wɪθdrɔː'l] *n term*   *sim* **drop-out** *or* **dropout**[1] *n jar*

removing an individual from a study because of unwillingness or inability to return for follow-up

withdraw[2] *v term* • drop out[2] *v inf*

» *Withdrawals were mainly due to side effects of treatment; 12 pts. withdrew* [uː] *during treatment, 2 dropped out because of* intercurrent [ɜː] *disease[3], and 3 were lost to follow-up. Patients had the option of dropping out of the study at any time. There was a steady* [e] *dropout of patients.*

Use **withdrawal** from treatment / from the study / rate • patient / systematic **drop-out** • **drop-out** rate[4]

Studienabbruch, abgebrochene Beobachtung
Drop-out, Studienabbrecher(in); Ausfall[1] ausscheiden, ausfallen[2] interkurrente Erkrankung[3] Ausfallsrate, Drop-out Rate[4]

29

stopping rule [uː] *n term*   *sim* **termination**[1], **stop condition**[2] *n term*

rule usually set prior [aɪ] to patient recruitment [uː] that specifies[3] a limit for the observed test-control treatment difference for the primary outcome, which, if exceeded [iː], leads to termination of the test or control treatment, depending on the direction of the observed difference

» *A stop condition is encountered[4]* [aʊ] *when a patient enrolled* [oʊ] *in a trial, requires or permits clinic personnel to take some action related to that patient, such as instituting a change in treatment or terminating[5] follow-up of that patient.*

Use early **stopping** • premature[6] [priːmətʊɚ] ***termination*** • ***termination*** stage / of the procedure

Studienabbruchbestimmung
Beendigung, Abbruch[1] Studienabbruchbedingung[2] festlegen[3] liegt vor[4] abbrechen, beenden[5] vorzeitige Beendigung[6]

30

Unit 16 Pain
Related Units: **47** Basic Terms in Anesthesiology, **48** Types of Anesthesia & Anesthetics, **3** Injuries, **13** General Pathology

discomfort n

sligthly painful feeling, e.g. after a minor injury[1] or being in an uncomfortable[2] position; often used as a clinical understatement

(un)comfortable[3] adj • comfort[4] n & v

» Does this cause any discomfort? There was some discomfort but no real pain.
Use to cause/feel/experience[5]/tolerate[6]/control/aggravate[7]/ameliorate[8] [iː]/ minimize **discomfort** • migratory [aɪ]/ postprandial / vague [veɪɡ] **abdominal discomfort** • aching / acute / mild / chest / pelvic / epigastric / postural[9] [pɒːstʃərəl]/ local / residual[10] **discomfort**

(leichte körperliche) Beschwerden, Unpässlichkeit
leichte Verletzung[1] unbequem, unangenehm[2] angenehm[3] Trost, Beruhigung, Bequemlichkeit; trösten[4] sich unwohl fühlen[5] B. ertragen[6] B. verstärken[7] B. lindern[8] haltungsbedingte B.[9] Restbeschwerden[10]   1

distress n & v clin   sim **suffering**[1] [ʌ] n clin

(i) being affected by worries, extreme sadness, pain (ii) to be in danger or in urgent [ɜːrdʒənt] need of help

distressed[2], -ing, -ful adj •suffer (from)[3] v • sufferer[4] n

» The patient was in acute distress because of central chest pain. Distress mostly refers to emotional suffering. He is suffering from severe malnutrition. He did not suffer at all and died peacefully. For some death may represent an escape from unbearable [eə] suffering[5].
Use **to be in** (no) acute[6] / minimal **distress** •signs of **distress** • emotional / physical / family[7] / respiratory[8] / fetal [iː] **distress** • **distressing** experience / symptom[9] • **distressed** child / family[10] • hay [heɪ] fever[11] [iː]/ chronic tinnitus **sufferer**

> Note: Mark the difference between to suffer from[12] an illness and to suffer a stroke[13], a heart attack, an injury, etc.

Not(lage), Leid, Kummer; bedrücken, beunruhigen
Leid(en)[1] notleidend, bekümmert[2] (er)leiden[3] Leidende(r), Patient(in)[4] unerträgliche(s) Leiden[5] dringend Hilfe benötigen[6] familiäre Sorgen[7] Atemnot[8] beunruhigendes Symptom[9] besorgte Familienangehörige[10] Heuschnupfenpatient(in)[11] leiden an[12] Schlaganfall erleiden[13]   2

hurt-hurt-hurt [hɜːrt] v irr & adj   sim **irritate**[1], **bother**[2] [ɒː] v

v (i) to feel physical or emotional pain (ii) injure oneself or sb. else or be injured → U3-1

to get/be hurt phr • irritating[3] adj • irritation[4] n • bothersome[5] adj

» Where does it hurt most? The light hurts my eyes. Are you hurt? I was deeply hurt by his remarks. His irritating rash[6] [æ] has become extremely bothersome. It does not bother me that much.
Use to cause/avoid **irritation** • skin / mucosal[7] / gastric / local **irritation** • to (be) **bother(ed)** about sth.[8]

schmerzen, weh tun; (sich) verletzen; verletzt
irritieren, stören[1] zu schaffen machen, stören[2] unangenehm, störend[3] Irritation, Reizung[4] lästig, beeinträchtigend[5] Hautirritation[6] Schleimhautreizung[7] sich Sorgen machen[8]   3

ache [eɪk] v & n & comb

(v) to hurt constantly (n) a continuous, not very intense, often not precisely localized pain

headache[1] n • toothache[2] n • earache n • aching[3] adj

» My arm is giving me much less pain but still aches when I carry something heavy. Low abdominal pain is usually crampy[4] or colicky but may be a dull constant ache.
Use dull[5] [ʌ]/ vague / mild / generalized [dʒen-]/ deep-seated[6] **ache** • muscle / stomach-[7] [k]/ belly**ache**[8] • throbbing[9] head**aches** • **aching** feet / pains[10] • to be **aching** all over[11]

schmerzen, weh tun; Schmerz(en); -weh, -schmerzen
Kopfschmerzen[1] Zahnschmerzen[2] schmerzhaft[3] krampfartig[4] dumpfer S.[5] tiefsitzender S.[6] Magenschmerzen[7] Bauchschmerzen[8] klopfende/pochende Kopfschmerzen[9] Schmerzen am ganzen Körper, Wehwehchen[10] alles tut weh[11]   4

aches and pains phr   sim **aching pains**

refers to minor pains all over the body, esp. in muscles or joints, after excessive exercise

» Prostration[1] and generalized aches and pains are commonly the first manifestations of influenza. It's no problem – just the aches and pains of old age[2].
Use vague / widespread [e]/ disseminated / generalized[3] **aches and pains** • growing[4] **pains**

Gliederschmerzen, S. am ganzen Körper, Wehwehchen
Erschöpfung(szustand), Prostration[1] Altersbeschwerden, -wehwehchen[2] Schmerzen am ganzen Körper[3] Wachstumsschmerzen[4]   5

pain n usu sing syn **dolor** n term rare

(i) unpleasant sensation¹ [eɪ] related to tissue damage, conveyed² [eɪ] to the brain by nerve fibers where its conscious appreciation³ [iːʃ] may be modified by various factors (ii) painful uterine contraction in childbirth (usu pl)

painful⁴ adj • pained⁵ adj • painless, pain-free adj • indolent⁶ adj

» How long have you had this pain? You won't feel any pain. This is a completely painless procedure.

Use to cause or arouse [aʊ] or evoke or give rise to⁷/aggravate **pain** • **pain** arises / spreads / persists⁸ / recurs • to be in/feel **pain** • to have a **pain** in the chest • a pained face⁹ / expression • **pain-free** intervals • **pain** therapy • **pain on** palpation / coughing¹⁰ [kɒːfɪŋ] / urination • menstrual or period / labor¹¹ [eɪ] **pains** • (in)sensitivity to **pain**¹² • painful stimuli [aɪ]/ sensation / joints / swallowing¹³ / lesion • painless swelling / mass¹⁴ • indolent ulcer¹⁵ [ʌlsɚ]

> Note : Pain is normally singular. When used in the plural it refers to the pain related to menstruation or childbirth or to show that it recurs. It can also mean to try very hard , e.g. in painstaking¹⁶ and to take or go to great pains¹⁷.

character or **nature of pain** n clin

» What kind of pain is it? Ulcer pain is typically described as "aching discomfort". Colicky pain¹ is usually promptly alleviated² [əliːvɪeɪt-] by analgesics. Tearing [eɚ] pain is characteristic of a dissecting aneurysm³ [-vɚɪzm].

Use **pain** of a colicky nature¹ • burning / crampy / cutting / lancinating⁴ / stabbing or piercing⁵ / shooting⁶ [uː]/ boring⁷ **pain** • stinging⁵ / gnawing⁸ [nɒːɪŋ] / dragging or tearing⁹ **pain** • disabling¹⁰ / psychogenic [saɪkoʊdʒenɪk]/ hunger¹¹ / rest¹² **pain**

duration [eɪ] and **periodicity of pain** n clin

» When did you first notice this pain? How long did it last? The episodes of pain became more frequent, remissions¹ became shorter, and a dull ache persisted between the episodes of stabbing pain.

Use fleeting² [iː]/ intermittent / chronic / steady [e] or persistent³ **pain** • lingering³ [ŋg]/ unremitting or stubborn⁴ [ʌ]/ nagging⁵ [æ]/ night / delayed⁶ [eɪ]/ postprandial **pain**

intensity of pain n clin

» Doctor, this pain is killing me. Does anything make it worse? How do you get relief? Lidocaine is ineffective for prevention or relief of this intense pain. Agonizing pain is a sign of serious [ɪɚ] or advanced disease.

Use mild¹ [aɪ]/ dull² [ʌ]/ moderate / intense or sharp³ / acute **pain** • intractable⁴ / severe³ / intolerable⁵ / violent [aɪə] or killing⁶ / excruciating [uːʃ] or exquisite or agonizing⁷ [aɪz] **pain**

site [saɪt] or **loc(aliz)ation of pain**

» Could you point to the spot where it hurts most. A history of renal stones might be a cause of referred back pain.

Use deep(-seated)¹ / superficial² / (poorly) localized³ / diffuse / radiating⁴ [eɪ] **pain** • spreading [e]/ migratory⁵ [aɪ]/ generalized / non-specific / referred⁶ [ɜː] **pain** • chest / flank⁷ / phantom limb⁸ [lɪm]/ joint / suprapubic [pjuː]/ upper abdominal / epigastric / low(er) back⁹ **pain**

tender adj clin sim **sore**¹ [sɔːr], **painful** adj inf & clin

sensitive² or painful as a result of pressure or contact which normally does not cause discomfort

tenderness³ n clin • soreness, painfulness n rare

» The cardinal manifestations are fever, pain (continuous, stabbing, or pleuritic [ʊɚ]) and an enlarged and tender liver. Bursitis [-aɪtɪs] is likely to cause focal tenderness⁴ and swelling.

Use **tender** point / swelling / mass⁵ • **tender(ness)** to palpation / to motion⁶ / over the injury • abdominal / costovertebral angle [ŋg]/ exquisite⁷ **tenderness** • diffuse / point or pencil⁸ / localized⁴ / rebound⁹ **tenderness** • **sore** throat¹⁰ [oʊ]/ muscles¹¹ / nipples¹²

(i) Schmerz(en) (ii) Wehen
Empfindung¹ übertragen² bewusste Wahrnehmung³ schmerzhaft⁴ schmerzerfüllt⁵ langsam heilend, schmerzlos, indolent⁶ S. verursachen⁷ S. halten an, persistieren⁸ schmerzverzerrtes Gesicht⁹ S. beim Husten¹⁰ Wehen¹¹ Schmerzunempfindlichkeit¹² Schluckbeschwerden¹³ indolenter Tumor¹⁴ schlecht abheilendes / indolentes Geschwür¹⁵ sorgfältig, gewissenhaft¹⁶ sich Mühe geben¹⁷

6

Schmerzqualität
kolikartige Schmerzen¹ gelindert² Aneurysma dissecans³ lanzinierender S.⁴ stechender S.⁵ plötzlich einschießende S.⁶ bohrender Schmerz⁷ nagender S.⁸ ziehende Schmerzen⁹ starke (arbeitsunfähig machende) S.¹⁰ Nüchternschmerz¹¹ Ruheschmerz¹²

7

Schmerzdauer
Remissionen, Besserung¹ flüchtiger Schmerz² anhaltende Schmerzen³ hartnäckige S.⁴ dumpfe S.⁵ Spätschmerz⁶

8

Schmerzintensität
leichte Schmerzen¹ dumpfer Schmerz² heftige / starke S.³ therapierefraktäre S.⁴ unerträgliche S.⁵ rasende S.⁶ qualvolle Schmerzen⁷

9

Schmerzlokalisation
Tiefenschmerz¹ oberflächl. S.² schwer abgrenzbarer S.³ ausstrahlende S.⁴ wandernder S.⁵ Synalgie, übertragener S.⁶ Flankenschmerz⁷ Phantomschmerz⁸ Kreuzschmerzen⁹

10

(druck)schmerzhaft, druckempfindlich
wund, entzündet¹ empfindlich² Druckschmerz, Schmerzhaftigkeit³ lokalisierter Schmerz⁴ schmerzhafter Knoten⁵ Bewegungsschmerz⁶ überaus starke Schmerzen⁷ Punktschmerz⁸ Loslassschmerz⁹ Halsschmerzen¹⁰ Muskelschmerzen, -kater¹¹ empfindliche Brustwarzen¹²

11

Kundenservice

Bitte informieren Sie mich zukünftig regelmäßig über folgende Themen:

- ☐ Allgemeinmedizin
- ☐ Anästhesie
- ☐ Arbeitsmedizin
- ☐ Arzneimitteltherapie
- ☐ Chirurgie
- ☐ Dermatologie
- ☐ Geriatrie
- ☐ Gesundheitsökonomie
- ☐ Gynäkologie/Geburtshilfe

- ☐ HNO
- ☐ Krankenpflege
- ☐ Innere Medizin
- ☐ Intensivmedizin
- ☐ Neurologie
- ☐ Notfallmedizin
- ☐ Ophthalmologie
- ☐ Orthopädie
- ☐ Pädiatrie

- ☐ Palliativmedizin
- ☐ Pharmakologie
- ☐ Psychiatrie
- ☐ Psychotherapie
- ☐ Radiologie
- ☐ Schmerztherapie
- ☐ Ultraschall
- ☐ Urologie
- ☐ Zahnmedizin

Meine Schwerpunkttätigkeiten:

- ☐ Kieferorthopädie
- ☐ Orale Chirurgie
- ☐ Implantologie
- ☐ MKG-Chirurgie

- ☐ Konservierende Zahnheilkunde
- ☐ Prothetik
- ☐ Parodontologie
- ☐ Endodontie

Ja, bitte senden Sie mir ein kostenloses Probeheft der Zeitschrift ZWR:

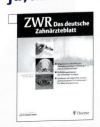

- informiert kompetent über aktuelle Entwicklungen in der Zahnheilkunde
- liefert im Fortbildungsteil praktische Tipps und konkrete Hinweise für das gesamte zahnmedizinische Behandlungsspektrum

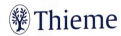

Antwortkarte

Georg Thieme Verlag KG
Kundenservice
Postfach 30 11 20
70451 Stuttgart

Bitte frankieren falls Marke zur Hand

Meine Anschrift

Name/Vorname

Straße

Land/PLZ/Ort

Tel./FAX

Facharztbezeichnung

☐ Ja, bitte informieren Sie mich künftig auch per e-mail.

e-mail Adresse

Meine Anschrift: ☐ dienstlich ☐ privat
Tätigkeitsort: ☐ Klinik ☐ Praxis

Pain **GENERAL CLINICAL TERMS** 63

---

wince [wɪns] *v & n*   *syn* **flinch** [flɪntʃ] *v rare*
to move back, tighten[1] [aɪt] the muscles because of pain or make a pained face[2]
» The boy watched me stick in the needle without wincing. "Ouch[3]," [aʊtʃ] he said with a wince. The pain may be so intense that the patient winces, hence[4] the condition is termed tic[5].

(vor Schmerz) zusammen- zucken; Zucken
anspannen[1] schmerzverzerrtes Gesicht[2] au (weh)[3] daher[4] Tic(k), Muskelzucken[5]   12

---

stitch [stɪtʃ] *n & v*   *syn* **twinge** [twɪndʒ] , **pang** *n*
sharp pain of short duration, e.g. a stitch in the side[1] which is due to excessive physical exercise
» Suddenly I felt this slight twinge in my hamstring[2] again. If you are prone [oʊ] to[3] stitches[1] do your exercise with an empty stomach[4].
Use breast[5] [e]/ hunger **pang**

Stich, (kurzer) stechender Schmerz; stechen
Seitenstechen[1] Oberschenkelbeuger[2] neigen zu[3] mit leerem Magen, nüchtern[4] stechender Brustschmerz[5]   13

---

paroxysm [pærəksɪzᵊm] *n*   *sim* **attack**[1] *n*
recurrent bouts[2] [aʊ] of sharp pain or symptoms such as chills[3] [tʃ], colics or cramps that are sudden in onset[4]
• paroxysmal[5] *adj*
» Certain maneuvers [uː] triggered paroxysms of pain. His infection was characterized by paroxysms of chills, fever, and sweating [e]. A transient, paroxysmal disturbance of cardiac rhythm [ɪ] was suspected.
Use **paroxysmal** pain[6] / symptoms / tachycardia[7] [k]/ cough[8] [kɒːf] / nocturnal dyspnea [dɪspniːə] (*abbr* PND) / vertigo[9] [ɜː]/ hypertension • spasmodic[10] **paroxysm**

Anfall, Paroxysmus
Anfall, Attacke[1] wiederkehrende Anfälle[2] Schüttelfrost[3] plötzlich auftretend[4] anfallsartig, paroxysmal[5] Schmerzattacken[6] paroxysmale Tachykardie[7] Hustenanfälle[8] Schwindelanfälle[9] anfallsartiger Muskelkrampf[10]   14

---

colic [kɒlɪk] *n clin*
paroxysmal pain in the abdomen typical of gastrointestinal disorders, stone disease[1], and in infants
colicky[2] *adj clin*
» He complained of colicky flank pain[3] radiating to the groin[4]. Biliary colic[5] may be precipitated[6] by eating a fatty meal. She was a colicky baby[7] who had 3-6 loose stools[8] [uː] per day.
Use gastric / biliary [bɪliəri] or hepatic[5] / renal[9] [iː]/ menstrual / pancreatic / tubal **colic**

Kolik
Steinleiden[1] kolikartig[2] Flankenschmerz[3] Leiste(nbeuge)[4] Gallenkolik[5] ausgelöst[6] von Bauchkrämpfen geplagtes Baby[7] breiige Stühle[8] Nierenkolik[9]   15

---

lumbago [lʌmbeɪɡoʊ] *n term*   *sim* **sciatica**[1] [saɪætɪkə] *n term & clin*
lower back pain[2] caused by muscle strain[3] [eɪ], arthritis [aɪ] or a ruptured intervertebral disk[4]
sciatic[5] [saɪætɪk] *adj clin*
» Sciatica is characterized by low back pain radiating [eɪ] down[6] the buttock[7] [ʌ] and down the knee [niː].
Use **sciatic** pain / nerve (distribution)

Lumbago, Hexenschuss
Ischias(syndrom)[1] Kreuzschmerzen[2] Muskelhartspann, -verspannung[3] Bandscheibenvorfall[4] Ischias-[5] ausstrahlen[6] Gesäß[7]   16

---

paresthesia(s) [pæresθiːʒə] *n term*   *rel* **pins-and-needles**[1] *phr clin*
abnormal sensation such as tingling [ŋɡ] pain[2], numbness[3] [nʌmnəs], prickling[4] or burning
paresthetic [e] *adj term* • dysesthesia *n* • hyperesthesia *n*
» Severe pain, numbness, paresthesia and coldness developed.
Use general / perioral / distal limb / painful **paresthesia**

subjektive Missempfindung, Parästhesie
Kribbeln, Ameisenlaufen[1] schmerzhaftes Brennen[2] taubes Gefühl[3] Prickeln[4]   17

---

pain threshold [θreʃʰoʊld] *n term*   *rel* **pain tolerance**[1] *n*
the threshold of pain refers to the smallest intensity of pain the patient is able to appreciate[2] [iːʃ], while pain tolerance is the maximum (s)he can endure[3]; the unit of pain intensity is dol
» Assess[4] joint swelling and functional activity and the patient's pain tolerance.
Use low / high **pain threshold** • to appreciate/induce[5]/produce[5] pain • to bear[3] [beɚ]/endure/put up with[6] **pain**

Schmerzschwelle
Schmerztoleranzgrenze[1] empfinden[2] ertragen[3] abklären[4] Schmerzen verursachen[5] s. mit den Schmerzen abfinden[6]   18

16

64 GENERAL CLINICAL TERMS Pain

pain relief [rɪliːf] *n clin* *sim* **palliative therapy**[1] *n term*

to deaden pain[2] [e] and obtund [ʌ], dull [ʌ] or blunt [ʌ] sensation[3]
relieve[4] *v clin* • palliate[4] *v term* • palliation[5] *n* • palliative[6] *adj & n*

» *How do you get relief? The pain was well controlled. Radiotherapy for palliation of pain significantly improves the quality of life of patients suffering from incurable malignancies. The drug failed to relieve suffering.*

Use to relieve [-iːv] *or* ease [iːz] *or* soothe [suːð] *or* alleviate [iː] *or* mitigate[7] / abolish / suppress **pain** • **pain** subsides [aɪ] *or* resolves[8] • **palliative** needs / home care / drug[9] / measures [eʒ]/ surgery[10]

Schmerzlinderung, -beseitigung
Palliativtherapie[1] Schmerz stillen[2] Sensibilität herabsetzen[3] mildern, lindern[4] Linderung[5] palliativ, lindernd; Palliativum[6] Schmerz lindern[7] S. lässt nach[8] Palliativum[9] Palliativoperation[10]

19

analgesic [ænəldʒiːzɪk] *n & adj* *syn* **pain killer** *n inf & jar*

(n) drug to render a patient pain-free[1] without clouding [aʊ] of consciousness[2]
(adj) deadening pain sensation
analgesia[3] [ænəldʒiːzɪə] *n term* → U47-7

» *Will this kill the pain, doc? The patient required very large amounts of analgesics for relief.*

Use to obtund / dull / blunt **pain sensation** • **pain** receptor / sensitive pathways[4] • **pain**-transmission neurons [ʊɚ] • **analgesic** receptor / nephropathy[5]

schmerzstillendes Mittel, Analgetikum; schmerzstillend, analgetisch
Patient(in) schmerzfrei machen[1] Bewusstseinstrübung[2] Aufheben der Schmerzempfindung, Analgesie[3] Schmerzbahnen[4] Analgetika-Nephropathie[5]

20

-algia [ældʒə] *comb* *syn* **-(o)dyn(o)** [dɪn] *comb*

refers to pains all over the body, esp in muscles or joints or after excessive exercise

» *Acute jaw* [dʒɔː] *or throat pain after therapy may be due to glossopharyngeal* [-færɪndʒiːəl] *neuralgia* [nʊəældʒə]*.*

Use my[1] [aɪ] / (trigeminal) [aɪdʒe] neur[2] / ot/ caus/ arth**algia** • prostato[3]/ pleuro [ʊɚ]/ teno**dynia**[4] [tenədɪnɪə]

-schmerz
Muskelschmerzen, Myalgie[1] Trigeminusneuralgie[2] Prostatodynie[3] Sehnenschmerz, Ten(d)odynie, Tenalgie[4]

21

Clinical Phrases

Doctor, I have an awful pain in my shoulder. Herr Doktor, ich habe schreckliche Schmerzen in der Schulter. • When did you first notice this pain? Wann traten diese Schmerzen erstmals auf? • What brings it on? Wodurch werden sie ausgelöst? • Did it come on suddenly? Sind die Schmerzen plötzlich aufgetreten? • Does anything make it worse? Werden sie durch irgendetwas verstärkt? • Did you notice pins and needles? Spürten Sie ein Kribbeln? • He won't feel the pain. Er wird keine Schmerzen haben. • I've had this pain on and off for the past three months. Ich hatte diese Schmerzen immer wieder in den letzten 3 Monaten. • How much are you bothered by the urinary symptoms? Wie sehr fühlen Sie sich durch die Beschwerden beim Harnlassen beeinträchtigt? • Take care to avoid any skin irritation. Hautreizungen sollten Sie nach Möglichkeit vermeiden. • He went on to suffer multiple relapses. Er hatte immer wieder einen Rückfall. • She continued to suffer from stiffness and joint pain for several years. Sie litt noch mehrere Jahre lang an Gelenkschmerzen und Steifigkeit. • I usually drink a glass of milk to soothe the pain. Normalerweise trinke ich zur Schmerzlinderung ein Glas Milch. • She is without pain now. Sie ist jetzt schmerzfrei. • Freedom from pain was achieved on postoperative day 5. Schmerzfreiheit bestand ab dem 5. postoperativen Tag.

Unit 17 Fractures

Related Units: 3 Injuries, 46 Radiology, 29 Fracture Management, 45 Maxillofacial Surgery

fracture [fræktʃɚ] v term → U3-20   syn **break** [eɪ]-broke-broken v irr,
    sim **crack¹** v & n clin

to cause a break in the continuity of a bone

fracture² n term, abbr Frx • refracture³ v & n • fractured⁴ adj

» Direct root [uː] compression may be relieved by reduction⁵ [ʌ] of the dislocation or by removal of fractured bone or disrupted disk. Most fractures of the clavicle occur in the middle third. Oblique [-iːk] views may also help identify and evaluate fractures of the tibial plateau⁶ [oʊ].

Use **to fracture** a bone / one's shin⁷ • simple / closed⁸ / isolated [aɪ]/ (in)complete⁹ / subperiosteal / pathologic¹⁰ / spiral¹¹ [aɪ] **fracture** • (radial [eɪ]) neck / (femoral [e]) shaft / transverse¹² / oblique¹³ **fracture** • (sub)trochanteric [k]/ supracondylar / growth plate or epiphyseal [ɪ]/ articular¹⁴ / (un)stable [eɪ] **fracture** • nasal / pelvic **fracture** • **fracture of the** patella • micro**fracture** • exposure of / motion at / separation at **the fracture site** • **fracture** healing¹⁵ [iː]/ cleft¹⁶ • **fractured** pelvis / rib / clavicle / tooth¹⁷ / nose / base of skull¹⁸

(Knochen) brechen / frakturieren
(zer)brechen; e. Sprung bekommen; Riss, (Knochen)fissur¹ (Knochen)fraktur, -bruch,² erneut brechen; Refraktur³ gebrochen, frakturiert⁴ Einrichtung, Reposition⁵ Tibiakopf⁶ s. d. Schienbein brechen⁷ geschlossene Fraktur⁸ (un)vollständige / (in)komplette F.⁹ pathol. F., Spontanfraktur¹⁰ Dreh-, Spiralbruch, Torsionsfraktur¹¹ Querfraktur¹² Schrägfraktur¹³ Gelenkfraktur¹⁴ Knochenbruch-, Frakturheilung¹⁵ Bruchspalt¹⁶ Zahnfraktur¹⁷ Schädelbasisbruch¹⁸   1

fragment n term   sim **chip¹** [tʃɪp] n, **splinter²** n & v clin

fragmentation³ n term • fragment⁴ v • to chip (off)⁵ v clin

» A displaced free fragment may tear [teɚ] the overlying lateral meniscus. A cartilage [-ɪdʒ] was chipped and fragments floated in the joint. If the bones are fragmented the fracture is said to be comminuted.

Use (nasal) bone / fracture / cartilage⁶ / osteochondral [kɒ] **fragment** • articular / butterfly⁷ / styloid [aɪ]/ (extruded) disk / femoral head **fragment** • devascularized / necrotic / displaced⁸ / free **fragment** • (cancellous [kæns-]) bone⁹ / grafted **chips** • **chip** fracture¹⁰ • **chipped** ankle / cartilage / knee [niː] • buried¹¹ [e]/ wood **splinter**

(Knochen)fragment, Bruchstück
(Knochen)splitter, -fragment¹ Splitter; (zer)splittern² Fragmentation, Zersplitterung³ in Stücke brechen, fragmentieren⁴ absplittern, -sprengen⁵ Knorpelfragment⁶ Biegungskeil⁷ verschobenes / disloziertes F.⁸ Spongiosaspäne⁹ Absprengungs-, Abrissfraktur¹⁰ verschobener Splitter¹¹   2

closed fracture n term   sim **simple fracture¹**,
    opposite **open** or **compound** [aʊ] **fracture²** n term

bone fracture that is not associated with a break or laceration³ [s] in the overlying skin

» Open fractures require operative reduction, but closed fractures should be managed with a posterior plastic splint⁴. As occult [ʌ] fracture⁵ is a common underlying cause, arthrocentesis for posttraumatic joint effusions might result in a compound fracture.

Use **closed** (Colles'/uncommmimuted) fracture / disruption / (head) injury⁶ / reduction or manipulation⁷ • **open** (tibial/forearm/contaminated/comminuted) fracture⁸ / dislocation⁹ • **compound** dislocation⁹ / depressed skull fracture¹⁰ / wound¹¹ [uː]

geschlossener Bruch
einfacher Bruch¹ offener B.² Zerreißung³ Schiene⁴ i. Röntgen nicht nachgewiesene F.⁵ stumpfe (Schädel)verletzung⁶ geschlossene Reposition / Einrichtung⁷ offene Trümmerfraktur⁸ offene Luxation⁹ Schädelimpressionsfraktur¹⁰ offene Wunde¹¹   3

(sub)luxation [ʌ] or **dislocation** n term   rel **displacement¹**,
    angulation² n term → U3-20

displacement of a bone from its articulation

luxate³ [ʌ] v term • dislocate⁴ v • subluxated⁵ adj • redisplacement⁶ n • angulate⁷ v • angular⁸ adj

» Small elevators⁹ were used to carefully luxate¹⁰ the teeth to be extracted. Unstable fracture-dislocations of the middle and upper thirds of the ulnar shaft complicated by dislocation of the radial head are termed Monteggia [-edʒə] fracture.

Use fracture-¹¹ / partial¹² [ʃ]/ closed / complete / habitual¹³ / pathologic¹⁴ [ɒːdʒ]/ obturator **dislocation** • **dislocation of the** hip (joint) / radial head / distal fragment • fracture / congenital [dʒe] (hip)¹⁵ / elbow / (posterior) facet¹⁶ [fæset]/ atlanto-axial **subluxation** • **subluxated** digit [dɪdʒɪt] • **displaced** fracture¹⁷ • (in)significant / (un)acceptable¹⁸ / 10-degree / late **angulation** • **angulated** radial [eɪ] neck fracture¹⁹ / lesion [iːʒ] • **angular** displacement² / deformity / stress

(Teil)verrenkung, (Sub)luxation
Verschiebung, Dislokation, Fehlstellung¹ Achsenknickung, -fehlstellung² verrenken, luxieren³ verschieben, dislozieren⁴ subluxiert⁵ neuerliche Verschiebung⁶ einen Winkel bilden⁷ Winkel-, Achse betreffend⁸ Hebel⁹ heraushebeln¹⁰ Luxationsfraktur¹¹ Teilverrenkung¹² habituelle L.¹³ Spontanluxation¹⁴ angeborene (Hüftgelenk)subluxation¹⁵ S. des Facettengelenks¹⁶ dislozierte Fraktur¹⁷ (nicht) tolerierbare Achsenknickung¹⁸ (ad axim) verschobene Radiushalsfraktur¹⁹   4

avulsion [əvʌlʃᵊn] **(chip fracture)** n term → U44-3
　　　　　　　　　　　　sim **disruption¹** [ʌ] n term → U3-18

fracture that occurs when soft tissue (joint capsule, ligament, muscle insertion or origin) is pulled away from the bone; fragments of the bone may come away with it

avulse² v term • avulsed³ adj • disrupted⁴ adj

» Avulsion of the ulnar [ʌ] styloid [aɪ] may accompany the distal radius [eɪ] fracture. X-rays [eks] may show a bit of bone avulsed from the fibular head.

Use traumatic / cortex / tooth / minor [aɪ] **avulsion** • **avulsion** (flap) injury⁵ • **avulsed** teeth⁶ / (bone) fragment⁷ • traumatic / bone⁸ / articular / wound⁹ [uː] **disruption** • ligamentous / (soft) tissue¹⁰ / pelvic / intimal¹¹ **disruption** • **disrupted** muscle¹² [mʌsl]/ disk¹³ / operative wound

Ab-, Ausrissfraktur, knöcherner Ausriss
Ruptur, Riss¹ ab-, ausreißen² ab-, ausgerissen³ zer-, (auf)gerissen⁴ Ausrissverletzung⁵ ausgeschlagene / luxierte Zähne⁶ Knochenabsprengung⁷ Knochenbruch⁸ Klaffen d. Wunde, Wunddehiszenz⁹ Weichteilzerreißung¹⁰ Intimaruptur¹¹ Muskelriss¹² rupturierte Bandscheibe¹³
　　　　　　　　　　　　5

impacted fracture n term → U44-3　　sim **compression fracture¹** n term

fracture with one of the fragments driven into the cancellous tissue² of the other fragment

impaction³ [ɪmpækʃᵊn] n term • impact⁴ n

» Impacted and minimally angulated fractures can be treated by means of a shoulder immobilizer. Most surgeons prefer to use internal fixation for impacted fractures. Closed manipulation is justifiable [aɪ], but if possible impaction or locking of the fragments is desirable [aɪ].

Use **impacted** tooth⁵ / foreign [fɒːrɪn] bodies / gallstone [ɔː]/ cerumen⁶ [sɪruːmᵊn] • lateral / multiple / stable⁷ [eɪ] **compression fractures** • dorsal / food⁸ **impaction**

Stauchungsbruch
Kompressionsfraktur¹ Spongiosa² Impaktion, Einkeilung³ Auswirkung, Einfluss⁴ impaktierter Zahn⁵ Zeruminalpfropf, Cerumen obturans⁶ stabile Kompressionsfrakturen⁷ Retention / Impaktion v. Speiseresten⁸
　　　　　　　　　　　　6

comminuted fracture n term　　sim **splinter(ed) fracture¹** n term

fracture in which the bone is crushed [ʌʃ] or broken into several fragments

comminution² n term • non/uncomminuted adj • splinter³ v & n

» Comminuted fractures of the clavicle with displacement can usually be managed successfully by closed reduction. First the severity⁴ [e] of comminution and magnitude⁴ of the displacement were determined by x-rays. Often the fracture line⁵ will splinter to reach the medial [iː] wall of the inner ear.

Use to check for **comminution** • **comminuted** bone fragments • minor [aɪ]/ extensive / severe⁶ [ɪə] **comminution** • spiral / butterfly⁷ **fracture** • **splintered** to pieces / fragments

> Note: Butterfly fracture is not equivalent with the German term Schmetterlingsfraktur (= bilateral fracture of the pubic rami).

Trümmerbruch
Splitterbruch¹ Zertrümmerung, -splitterung² zersplittern; Splitter³ Ausmaß⁴ Frakturlinie⁵ starke Zertrümmerung⁶ (Schaft)fraktur m. beidseitigen Biegungskeilen⁷
　　　　　　　　　　　　7

skull [ʌ] **fracture** n clin　　syn **cranial** [eɪ] **fracture** n term

break of the cranium [eɪ] resulting from trauma [ɒː] which may be associated with injury to underlying brain

» These skull fractures may also injure [ɪndʒɚ] cranial nerves that course [ɔː] through the skull base. Basal skull fractures may be recognized by the presence of CSF rhinorrhea¹ [raɪnəriːə] or otorrhea.

Use simple / closed / open / compound / comminuted / stellate² [eɪ] / basal [eɪ] or basilar³ / depressed⁴ / expressed⁵ **skull fracture** • **fracture of the** skull vault⁶ [vɔːlt]/ base [eɪ] of the skull³ • temporal bone⁷ / blow-out⁸ **fracture**

Schädelbruch, -fraktur
nasale Liquorrhoe¹ Sternfraktur, sternförmige F.² Schädelbasisbruch³ Impressionsfraktur⁴ Berstungsfraktur⁵ Schädeldach-, Kalottenfraktur⁶ Schläfenbeinfraktur⁷ Blow-out F.⁸
　　　　　　　　　　　　8

fracture by contrecoup [kɒːtrəkuː] n term

fracture of the skull at a point opposite to where the blow¹ [oʊ] was received

» Deceleration [s] of the brain against the inner skull causes contusions [tʲuː], either under a point of impact² (coup lesion) or in the antipolar area (contrecoup lesion).

Use **contrecoup** lesion [liːʒᵊn] / injury [ɪndʒɚ] contusion³

Gegenstoß-, Contrecoup-Fraktur
Schlag, Stoß¹ Stoßherd² Contrecoup-Hirnprellung³
　　　　　　　　　　　　9

Colles' [kɒlɪs] **fracture** n term　　sim **silver-fork fracture** or **deformity¹** n term

fracture of the lower end of the radius with displacement of the distal fragment dorsally

» Colles' fracture is typically caused by falls on the outstretched [tʃ] hand, the wrist [rɪst] in dorsi-flexion, and the forearm in pronation so that the force is applied to the palm [pɑːm] of the hand².

Use Smith's or reversed³ **Colles' fracture** • Pott's⁴ **fracture** • bony / gross [oʊ]/ buttonhole⁵ [ʌ]/ cloverleaf skull⁶ / ulnar [ʌ] drift⁷ / Volkmann's compression-type⁸ **deformity**

Radiusfraktur an typischer Stelle, Fractura radii loco classico
F. radii loco classico m. Bajonettfehlstellung¹ Handfläche² Smith-, Radiusflexionsfraktur³ Pott-, Bimalleolarfraktur⁴ Knopflochdeformität⁵ Kleeblattschädel⁶ Ulnadeviation⁷ Volkmann-Sprunggelenkdeformität⁸
　　　　　　　　　　　　10

Fractures GENERAL CLINICAL TERMS 67

fissure(d) [fɪʃɚ] *or* **hairline** *or* **linear fracture** *n term*   *sim* **crack¹, cleft²** *n clin*   **Fissur, Haarbruch**
  fracture in which there is a crack in the cortex but not through the entire [aɪ] bone   Riss, Fissur¹ Spalt² gespalten, rissig³
  fissure¹ *n term* • fissured³ [fɪʃɚd] *adj*   Os lunatum, Mondbein⁴ Fraktur-
  » A fissure fracture can be treated by immobilization [aɪz] in plaster for 3 weeks.   ausläufer⁵ Gesichtsspalte⁶
  Fracture of the lunate⁴ [luːneɪt] may be manifested by a crack, by comminution, or   Gaumenspalte⁷
  by impaction. Linear fractures usually extend from the point of impact toward the
  base of the skull.
  Use multiple [ʌ] **fissure fractures** • **linear** skull fracture • direction / obliteration /
  extension⁵ / configuration **of the fracture cleft** • widened [aɪ]/ oblique [-iːk]/
  facial⁶ [feɪʃəl]/ palatal⁷ **cleft** • **crack** fracture¹   11

greenstick fracture *n term*   *sim* **bending fracture¹** *n term*   **Grünholzfraktur**
  bending of a bone with incomplete fracture involving the cortex on the convex side (typically   Biegungsfraktur¹
  seen in children)
  » If angulation of a greenstick fracture exceeds [iː] 15 degrees, reduction should be
  carried out. An undisplaced valgus greenstick fracture of the proximal tibia had
  caused the deformity.
  Use bent¹ *fracture*   12

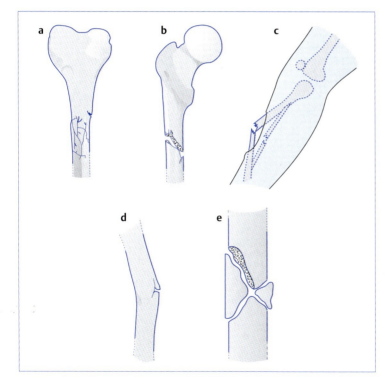

Types of Fractures
a comminuted fracture
b spiral fracture
c compound fracture
d greenstick fracture
e butterfly fracture

68 GENERAL CLINICAL TERMS — Therapeutic Intervention

fatigue [fəti:g] **fracture** n term   syn **stress fracture** n,
sim **march** [mɑːrtʃ] **fracture**[1] n clin
mostly transverse crack in bones that are subjected to excessive or unusual endogenous [ɒːdʒ] stress
» Fatigue fracture of the shafts of the metatarsals has been given various names (e.g. march, stress, strain and insufficiency fracture). Patients with march fractures typically have pain and point tenderness[2] but do not always have a history of dramatically increased activity.

Ermüdungsbruch
Marschfraktur[1] punktuelle Druckschmerzhaftigkeit[2]

[13]

crepitation n term   syn **crepitus, crepitance** n term
(i) crackling sound or sensation produced by the grating[1] [eɪ] of the fragments at a fracture site[2]
(ii) sound heard on auscultation [ɒː] over areas of consolidation in lung inflammation
» Fracture is suggested [dʒe] by crepitance or palpably mobile bony segments. Did you note any tenderness, crepitation, or movement of the fractured bones on palpation?
Use leathery[3] [e] **crepitation** • subcutaneous [eɪ]/ soft tissue / joint[4] [dʒ]/ marked[5] / bony[6] **crepitus**

(i) Krepitation, Crepitatio, Reibegeräusch
(ii) Knisterrasseln
Reiben[1] Bruchstelle[2] lederartiges Reibegeräusch[3] Gelenkreiben[4] deutl. Reibegeräusch[5] ossäre Krepitation[6]

[14]

bone or **bony union** n clin   rel **callus** [kæləs] **formation**[1] n term
growing together of the ends of fractured bone as fibrous [aɪ] callus[2] forms between the fragments
(un/mal)united[3] adj term • callous[4] [kæləs] adj • callosity[5] n
» A persisting fibrous callus forming between fractured bone is termed fibrous union. The callus holding the break [eɪ] firm until new bone is remodeled eventually turns into bone. Callus bridging a fracture may deform plastically and angulate if the fracture is loaded too early.
Use to be in (direct)[6] **union** • **bone** formation / healing[7] [iː] • postfracture bone[7] / fibrous / faulty[8] [ɒː]/ delayed[9] [eɪ]/ stable [eɪ] **union** • cartilaginous [ædʒ]/ advancing [æ]/ mal[8]/ non[10]-**union** • exuberant [uː] **callus** formation[11] • provisional[12] / definitive[13] **callus** • **malunited** fracture[8] • to avoid/treat/repair [eɚ] **nonunion** • complete / partial [ʃəl]/ tibial / infected[14] **nonunion** • **nonunion** site [aɪ]/ of bone / of the fracture[10]

Knochen-, Frakturheilung
Kallusbildung[1] bindegewebiger Kallus[2] vereinigt[3] kallös; schwielig[4] Callositas, Schwiele[5] Knochen ist verheilt[6] Frakturheilung[7] Frakturheilung in Fehlstellung[8] verzögerte Heilung[9] Pseudarthrose[10] überschießende Kallusbildung, Callus luxurians[11] provisor. K., Intermediärkallus[12] knöcherner K., Sekundärkallus[13] Infektpseudarthrose, infizierte P.[14]

[15]

Unit 18   Therapeutic Intervention
Related Units: 19 Pharmacologic Treatment, 20 Surgical Treatment, 28 Wound Healing, 29 Fracture Management, Dentistry

treatment [iː] n clin, abbr **T**ₓ   syn **therapy** [θerəpi] n term, **management** n jar
care for the sick or injured [ɪndʒɚd] by conservative measures [eʒ], medical treatment, surgical intervention, etc.
treat[1] v • manage[1] v • manageable[2] adj • treatable[2] adj
» Patients with positive tests are treated as having syphilis. Microbial infections are best treated early. Many of these patients will gradually improve without treatment. Treatment consists of administering magnesium. This does not require further treatment. The patient was managed symptomatically[3]. The patient refused to submit to treatment[4].
Use to be under[5]/start/initiate [ɪʃ]/discontinue[6]/interrupt [ʌ]/undergo[4] **treatment** for a disease • preferred[7] / primary [aɪ] or first-line[8] / definitive / long-term **treatment** • life-long / operative / gold standard / multimodality / drug[9] **treatment** • a course [ɔː] of[10] / emergency[11] [ɝː]/ post/ self-/ over**treatment** • **treatment** of choice[7] / of sepsis / failure[12] [eɪ]/ center / room • to treat on an outpatient basis[13] / at an early stage / in hospital[14] • **treated** for 2 weeks / for gastritis[15] [aɪ]/ acutely / topically[16] • **treated** conservatively or medically / surgically / adequately • **treated** with 0.45% saline [eɪ]/ with cold compresses / by fixation / by a physician / as indicated[17] • insulin-/ placebo-**treated** • vigorously[18] [ɪg]/ promptly / successfully / previously[19] **treated** • prehospital[20] / patient / dietetic / home[21] **management**

Behandlung, Therapie
behandeln[1] behandelbar[2] symptomatisch behandelt[3] sich einer Behandlung unterziehen[4] in B. sein[5] B. absetzen[6] B. der Wahl[7] Primärbehandlung[8] medikamentöse B.[9] Kur, Behandlungszyklus[10] Notfallversorgung[11] Therapieversagen[12] ambulant behandeln[13] stationär b.[14] auf Gastritis b.[15] lokal b.[16] laut Indikation b.[17] intensiv b.[18] vorbehandelt[19] präklinische Versorgung[20] häusliche Pflege[21]

[1]

Therapeutic Intervention GENERAL CLINICAL TERMS 69

cure [kjʊɚ] v & n sim **heal**[1] [hiːl] v → U28-4

(v) to restore health by treating successfully
(n) a promising drug or course of treatment[2] (also at a spa[3])

curative[4] adj term • (in)curable[5] adj clin • curability[6] n • healing[7] adj & n

» *Physicians should attempt to achieve a cure at least in some patients, relieve symptoms as often as possible and always comfort[8] the patient. This is a promising new drug which may cure 60-80% of patients in first remission. The only cure for eclampsia is termination of pregnancy[9]. The outlook for cure[10] remains poor for children with high-grade gliomas* [aɪ]. *Hysterectomy alone is usually curative.*

Use to effect a[11]/be treated with intent to/have a chance of **cure** • water / clinical / complete / permanent **cure** • **cure** rate[12] • **curative** approach [oʊtʃ]/ intent[13] / resection / treatment[14] • **curable** cancer[15] / by surgery

heilen; Behandlung, Heilung, Kur, Heilmittel
(ab-, ver)heilen[1] Kur[2] Kurort[3] kurativ, heilend[4] (un)heilbar[5] Heilbarkeit[6] heilsam, -end; Heilung[7] beruhigen[8] Schwangerschaftsabbruch[9] Heilungsaussichten[10] Heilung bewirken[11] Heilungsrate[12] Heilungsabsicht[13] kurative Behandlung[14] heilbarer Krebs[15]

2

treatment or **therapeutic**[juː] **modality** n term sim **tool**[1] [uː],
rel **option**[2] [ɒːpʃən] n clin & jar

the drug(s), operation, or approach chosen to treat a patient

» *Lithotripsy combined with salt therapy is a valuable treatment modality for single gallstones* [ɒː]. *No therapeutic modality has been shown to be superior[3]* [ɪɚ].

Use preferred treatment[4] / chemotherapeutic [iː] **modality** • combined **modality** therapy[5] • treatment[6] **options**

Behandlungsmethode, -modalität
(Hilfs)mittel, Instrument[1] Wahl, Möglichkeit[2] besser, überlegen[3] Methode der Wahl[4] Kombinationstherapie[5] Behandlungsmöglichkeiten[6]

3

therapy [θerəpi] n term

any of the various treatment modalities, e.g. immunotherapy, genetic, operative therapy, etc.

therapeutic [juː] adj term • therapist[1] n • -therapy comb

» *In elderly patients digitalis* [dʒ] *has a narrow therapeutic window[2].*

Use physical[3] [ɪ]/ antiviral [aɪ]/ laser / electroshock / speech **therapy** • adjuvant[4] [ædʒɚ]/ occupational[5] [eɪʃ]/ standby[6] / high-dose[7] **therapy** • to institute[8]/discontinue[9] **therapy** • **therapeutic** approach[10] / strategy • behavior[11] / rehabilitation nurse[12] / home / speech[13] [spiːtʃ] **therapist** • physio/ chemo[14] [iː]/ radio**therapy**

Therapie, Behandlung
Therapeut(in)[1] therapeutisches Fenster[2] Physiotherapie, physikal. Th.[3] medikam. Zusatztherapie, adjuvante Th.[4] Beschäftigungstherapie[5] Therapiereserve[6] hochdosierte Th.[7] Th. einleiten[8] B. absetzen[9] therap. Ansatz[10] Verhaltenstherapeut(in)[11] Krankengymnast(in)[12] Logopäde/in[13] Chemotherapie[14]

4

regimen [redʒɪmən] n term sim **course**[1] [kɔːrs] clin, **protocol**[2] n term

systematic course of treatment (esp prescribed medication, diet, exercise, change in life-style)

» *Progress in drug therapy has resulted in the development of curative chemotherapy regimens for several tumors. A protocol or treatment plan is an outline of care.*

Use treatment / split course[3] / prescribed[4] /(multi)drug **regimen** • combination / dosage[5] [ɪdʒ] / initial / curative[6] / preparative[7] / recommended **regimen** • 2-dose / low-dose / 5-day / 3-drug / alternate [ɔː] day **regimen** • **regimen** of drugs / for herpes • a **course** of estrogens[8] [e‖iː]

Note: Sometimes incorrectly referred to as *regime*.

therapeut. Maßnahme(n), Diät, Behandlung(sschema)
Kur, Behandlung(szyklus)[1] Behandlungsplan, -protokoll[2] Sequenztherapie[3] verordnete Behandlung[4] Dosierungsschema[5] kurative Behandlung[6] Vorbehandlung, vorbereitende Maßnahmen[7] Östrogenbehandlung, -kur[8]

5

prophylactic [pɒːfəlæktɪk] adj & n term & clin syn **preventive** adj clin

(adj) preventing the onset or spread [e] of disease (preventive medicine[1]) or pregnancy

prophylaxis[2] n term • prevention[3] [prɪvenʃən] n

» *Broad-spectrum antibiotics[3] should never be given for prophylaxis. Routine or prophylactic use of penicillins is not required. Prophylactic therapy consists of increasing renal* [iː] *output[4].*

Use to require/receive **prophylaxis** • **prophylactic** administration[5] / measures[6] [eʒ]/ agent / antibiotics / use • effective for / used as / postexposure[7] [oʊʒ]/ antibiotic[8] / long-term **prophylaxis** • oral / stress ulcer[9] [ʌlsɚ]/ chemo[10] [iː]/ single-dose **prophylaxis** • **prophylaxis** against or for malaria / with antacids

prophylaktisch, vorbeugend, präventiv; vorbeugende Maßnahme; Kondom
Präventivmedizin[1] Prophylaxe, Prävention, Vorbeugung[2] Breitbandantibiotika[3] Harnproduktion[4] prophyl. Verabreichung[5] vorbeugende Maßnahmen[6] postexpositionelle Prophylaxe[7] Antibiotikaprophylaxe[8] Stressulkusprophylaxe[9] Chemoprophylaxe[10]

6

18

Therapeutic Intervention

surveillance [sɚˈveɪləns] *n term* *syn* **watchful waiting, expectant therapy** *n term*

active observation and ongoing monitoring of a patient without actual treatment; a wait-and-see strategy[1]

» Close contacts of patients with diphtheria [ɪɚ] must be kept under surveillance for one week. Continuous surveillance for long-term complications is neccessary. The postoperative management options include either surveillance or 2 cycles of adjuvant chemotherapy.

Use close[2] / ongoing[3] / immune[4] / endoscopic / wound[5] [uː] **surveillance**

Beobachtungsstrategie, Surveillance, Überwachung

abwartende Strategie[1] strenge Überwachung[2] ständige Ü.[3] immunologische Ü.[4] Wundkontrolle[5]

[7]

adjuvant [ˈædʒəvᵊnt] *n & adj term* *syn* **adjunct** [ˈædʒʌŋkt] *n & adj clin & inf*

(n) additional treatment to increase the efficiency of primary therapy, e.g. chemotherapy following surgery

neoadjuvant[1] *n & adj term* • adjunctive[2] *adj*

» We generally use radiation treatment as an adjunct to surgery for these patients. Cytokine [aɪ] immunotherapy has shown promise as an adjunctive measure. Regimens that are not effective against bulky[3] [ʌ] tumors may be curative when used in an adjuvant setting.

Use **adjuvant** regimen / chemotherapy / irradiation[4] • pharmacologic[5] **adjunct** • **adjunctive** nephrectomy / medication[5] / measure[6] / management

Zusatztherapie, Adjuvans; adjuvant

Neoadjuvans, neoadjuvant[1] unterstützend[2] groß, raumfordernd[3] adjuvante Strahlentherapie[4] medikamentöse Zusatztherapie[5] unterstützende Maßnahme[6]

[8]

palliative [æ] *adj & n term* *opposite* **curative**[1] [kjʊɚˈətɪv] *adj clin & term*

(adj) supportive treatment alleviating[2] [iː] or relieving[2] [iː] symptoms without curing the underlying [aɪ] disease[3]

palliate[2] *v term* • palliation[4] *n*

» Strictures at the hilum [aɪ] may be difficult to palliate endoscopically. Surgery may be used for palliation in patients for whom cure is not possible. A smooth [uː] transition[5] in treatment goals[6] [oʊ] from curative to palliative is difficult to achieve in all cases.

Use **palliative** (home) care[7] / needs / procedure / drugs / surgery[8] • to provide / pain / effective / long-term **palliation** • **curative** measure / dose[9] / intent[10] / approach[10]

palliativ, lindernd; Palliativum

kurativ[1] lindern, erleichtern[2] Grundkrankheit, zugrundeliegendes Leiden[3] Linderung[4] fließender Übergang[5] Behandlungsziele[6] palliative (häusliche) Pflege[7] Palliativoperation[8] kurative Dosis[9] kurativer Ansatz[10]

[9]

indication [eɪ] *n term* *opposite* **contra-indication**[1] *n term*

(i) diagnostic basis for initiation[2] of a therapeutic course or for performing a clinical investigation (ii) sign

indicate[3] *v* • indicative (of)[4] *phr* • (contra-)indicated[5] *adj* • indicator[6] *n*

» Breast [e] feeding[7] [iː] is not a contraindication for vaccination[8] [ks]. Heart-lung transplants have been performed for a variety [aɪ] of indications. The ECG changes are indicative of an infarct.

Use clear[9] / clinical / vital[10] [aɪ] / excellent / principal[11] / emergency **indication** • major / compelling or absolute[12] / relative **contraindication** • **to be (contra)indicated** in patients / in pregnancy • diagnostic / prognostic **indicator**

(i) Indikation (ii) (An)zeichen

Kontraindikation, Gegenanzeige[1] Einleitung, Beginn[2] anzeigen, indizieren[3] hinweisen(d) auf[4] (kontra)indiziert[5] Indikator[6] Stillen[7] Impfung[8] eindeutige Indikation[9] vitale I., Vitalind.[10] Hauptindikation[11] absolute Kontraindikation[12]

[10]

response *n term*

(i) reaction of the patient's body to therapy (ii) reaction to stimuli [aɪ], viruses [aɪ], questions, etc.

respond (to)[1] *v term* • (non)responder[2] *n* • (un)responsive(ness)[3] *adj/n*

» Fifty percent of patients failed to respond to[4] this regimen. The tumor was found to shrink in response to tamoxifen withdrawal[5] [-ɔːl]. His diarrhea [iː] was unresponsive to fasting[6].

Use clinical / (durable) complete / poor / partial[7] [ʃ]/ immune[8] **response** • **response** rate • **to respond** well[9] / poorly / inadequately / partially • placebo[10] [siː] **responder** • to be **responsive** to treatment

Ansprechen, Reaktion

ansprechen (auf), reagieren[1] Responder[2] ansprechend; Ansprechen[3] sprachen nicht an auf[4] Absetzen von T.[5] persistierte trotz Nahrungskarenz[6] Teilreaktion[7] Immunantwort, -reaktion[8] gut ansprechen[9] Plazeboresponder[10]

[11]

morbidity *n term* → U13-2, U14-9

undesirable[1] [aɪ] consequences and complications resulting from treatment

» Morbidity is lower if transplantation is performed before the patient is critically ill. This technique is associated with considerable morbidity[2], above all in bilateral procedures.

Use high / low / increased / minimal / long-term[3] / late[4] / septic[5] / infective **morbidity**

Morbidität

unerwünschte[1] beträchtliche M.[2] Langzeitmorbidität[3] Spätmorb.[4] sepsisbedingte M.[5]

[12]

refractory *adj term* **syn intractable, resistant, recalcitrant** [kælsɪ] *adj term*
showing little or no response to treatment
intractability[1] *n term* • refractoriness[1] *n* • resistance[1] *n*
» Hypotension can progress to refractory shock. Notable features[2] [fiːtʃɚz] of this tumor include refractoriness to cytotoxic agents. Abdominal pain and vomiting may become intractable.
Use **refractory** cases / symptoms / period[3] / anemia [iː]/ heart failure • **intractable** pain[4] / ascites [əsaɪtiːz]/ insomnia[5] / to treatment[6] • drug[7] **resistance** • **recalcitrant** disease / case / lesion [iːʒ]

refraktär, (therapie)resistent, hartnäckig
(Therapie)resistenz[1] auffällige Merkmale[2] Refraktärzeit[3] therapieresistente(r) Schmerz(en)[4] therapieresistente Schlaflosigkeit[5] therapieresistent[6] Arzneimittelresistenz[7]
13

aftercare [æftɚkeɚ] *n term* *sim* **followup**[1] [fɒːlouʌp] *n term*
management (treatment, help, supervision[2] [13]) of a patient in the postoperative or convalescent [es] period[3]
» Aftercare following psychiatric [saɪkɪætrɪk] hospitalization involves a continuing program of rehabilitation to reinforce[4] [riːɪn-] the effects of the therapy by partial [ʃ] hospitalization[5], outpatient treatment[6], etc.
Use **aftercare** treatment / plan[7] • long-term[8] **aftercare** • **followup** period[9] / examination[10] • **followup** at 6 months postoperatively[11]

Nachsorge, -behandlung
Nachuntersuchung, Verlaufskontrolle[1] Überwachung[2] Rekonvaleszenz, Genesungszeit[3] unterstützen[4] teilstationäre Behandlung[5] ambulante Beh.[6] Nachbehandlungsplan[7] Langzeitnachbetreuung[8] Nachuntersuchungszeitraum[9] Kontroll-, Nachuntersuchung[10] postop. Verlaufskontrolle nach 6 Monaten[11] 14

(patient) compliance [kəmplaɪəns] *n term* *sim* **adherence**[1] [ɪɚ] *n clin*
consistency[2] and accuracy[3] with which a patient follows the prescribed[4] treatment regimen
(non)compliant[5] *adj term* • noncompliance *n* • (un)cooperative[5] *adj*
» The importance of adherence to the recommended regimens for diet, exercise and glucose monitoring should be stressed. Patient compliance is essential if surveillance is to work.
Use to ensure[6] [ʃʊɚ]/monitor[7] **compliance** • poor[8] / strict[9] / patient **compliance** • **adherence** to treatment[10] • **compliance** with therapy[10] / rate

(Patienten-)Compliance
Befolgung, Einhaltung[1] Konsequenz, Beständigkeit[2] Genauigkeit[3] verordnet[4] (nicht) kooperativ[5] Compliance sicherstellen[6] C. überwachen[7] mangelnde Einhaltung / Compliance[8] genaue Befolgung[9] Therapietreue[10]
15

Unit 19 Pharmacologic Treatment
Related Units: 5 Drugs & Remedies, 20 Pharmacologic Agents, 48 Types of Anesthesia & Anesthetics

prescribe [aɪ] *v term* *sim* **order**[1], **schedule**[2] [skedjuːl‖ʃed-] *v clin*
ordering (in writing) the preparation, dispensing[3] and/or administration[4] of medication or treatment for a particular patient; some medications are available only on prescription[5] others without (over-the-counter[6] [aʊ])
prescription[7] *n term, abbr* R_x • nonprescription[6] *adj*
» Prescriptions include the sign R_x (i.e. take), the names and quantities of the drugs ordered, directions[8] for compounding[9] [aʊ] the ingredients[10] [iː] and designation of the form (pill, powder, solution, etc.) in which the drug is to be made, directions for the patient regarding the dose, route [uː‖aʊ] of administration and times of taking the drug. Drugs are effective only if the patient takes them as prescribed[11].
Use to **prescribe** drugs / baths[12] / a diet [daɪət]/ exercises • **prescribed** dose / regimen [edʒ] *or* course [ɔː] of therapy[13] • to write out a[14] **prescription** • vitamin / dietary[15] / eyeglass[16] **prescription** • **prescription** drugs or medications[17] / preparation / error

> Note: Common *abbr* for the dosage and administration of drugs include: b.i.d. [biːaɪdiː] (twice a day), q.d. (every day), t.i.d. (3 times/day), q.i.d. (4 times/day), q.h. *or* o.h. (every hour), p.r.n. *or* qrs. *or* q.l. *or* q.p. (at will, as needed), a.c. (before meals [iː]), o.n. *or* h.s. (every night), alt.noct. (every other night) and q4 (every 4 hs). These may also be written in upper case letters, e.g. PRN.

verschreiben, verordnen
ver-, anordnen[1] planen, ansetzen[2] Zubereitung, Abgabe[3] Verabreichung[4] auf Rezept, rezeptpflichtig[5] rezeptfrei[6] Verordnung, Rezept[7] Anleitungen[8] (ver)mischen[9] Bestandteile[10] nach Vorschrift, vorschriftsmäßig[11] Bäder verordnen[12] verordnete(s) Therapie(schema)[13] Rezept ausstellen[14] Diätvorschrift[15] Brillenverordnung[16] rezeptpflichtige Medikamente[17]

1

GENERAL CLINICAL TERMS

Pharmacologic Treatment

proprietary [prəpraɪəterɪ] *adj term*   opposite **non-proprietary¹**, **generic¹** [dʒənerɪk] *adj term*

proprietary drug names are protected trade names or trademarks² (e.g. Zovirax®) while generic drug names³ (e.g. acyclovir) are those recognized by official organizations and recommended for general use

» Many proprietary antacids⁴ contain both magnesium and aluminum hydroxides [aɪ].

patentrechtlich geschützt
generisch, allgemein¹ geschützte Handelsnamen / Warenzeichen² Freinamen³ Antazida, säurebindende Mittel⁴

2

---

administration *n term*   sim **application¹** *n term*

the act of giving a patient medication

administer² *v term* • apply³ [əplaɪ] *v* • applicator⁴ *n*

» These preparations can be swallowed whole⁵ [hoʊl] or chewed [tʃuːd] or administered as a patch⁶ or paste [eɪ] via the transdermal route⁷. Heparin is administered to patients with acute thrombosis. This drug must be administered under close supervision [ʒ] of a physician.

Use **to administer** an enema⁸ / a local anesthetic • **administered by** infusion / the parenteral route⁹ / inhalation / jet [dʒet] nebulizer¹⁰ • **administered** at full dose / in doses of • acute / chronic / continuous¹¹ / lifelong¹¹ / long-term / simultaneous [eɪ] **administration** • oral / intravaginal [dʒ]/ systemic / oxygen / once-daily / self-/ patient-**administration** • for ease¹² [iːz]/ safest route¹³ / preferred method¹⁴ / frequency / timing **of administration**

> Note: Common *abbr* for the route of administration include: p.o.¹⁵ (by mouth), i.m. (intramuscular), i.v. (intravenous), i.a. (intra-arterial) and sub-q or s.c. (subcutaneous). These *abbr* may also be written in upper case letters, e.g. IV.

Verabreichung, Gabe
Anwendung, Applikation¹ verabreichen² applizieren, anwenden, auftragen³ Applikator⁴ unzerkaut geschluckt⁵ Pflaster⁶ per-, transkutan⁷ Einlauf machen⁸ parenteral verabreicht⁹ mit Düsenaerosolgerät verabr.¹⁰ Dauermedikation¹¹ zur leichteren Anwendung¹² sicherste Applikationsart¹³ bevorzugte Applikationsart¹⁴ peroral¹⁵

3

---

drug delivery *n term*   sim **drug targeting¹** [g], *rel* **drug release²** [iː] *n term*

(i) route of supplying or providing therapeutic agents (ii) transport of substances to the target tissue³

deliver⁴ *v term* • target⁵ *v* • release⁶ *v*

» Drugs for transdermal delivery⁷ must have suitable [uː] skin penetration characteristics and high potency⁸. Clonidine diffusion through a membrane provides controlled drug delivery over a period of 1 wk.

Use **drug delivery** system⁹ / device [aɪ] • slow-**release** drug¹⁰

Applikation(sart)
Drug targeting (gezielte Konzentr. e. Arzneistoffes am Wirkort)¹ Arzneistoff-, Wirkstofffreisetzung² Wirkort, Zielgewebe³ zuführen, applizieren⁴ abzielen auf⁵ freisetzen⁶ transdermale Applikation⁷ Wirkungsstärke⁸ therapeut. System⁹ Depot-, Retardpräparat¹⁰

4

---

topical *adj term*   opposite **systemic¹** *adj term*

applied or restricted to a specific area (usually the skin)

» Newer, very potent² topical corticosteroids [ɪɚ] may be applied less often.

Use **topical** application³ / agents [eɪ]/ anesthetic⁴ / stimulant / steroids / ointments⁵

> Note: Topical creams [iː], ointments, etc. are *applied* to the skin, while oral, IV drugs, etc. are *administered*.

topisch, lokal
systemisch, generalisiert¹ stark, (hoch)wirksam² topische / lokale Anwendung³ Lokalanästhetikum⁴ Salben z. lokalen Anwendung⁵

5

---

discontinue *v term*   sim **withdraw¹** [wɪθdrɔː]-drew [uː]-drawn *v irr term*

discontinuation or discontinuance² *n term*

» First nonessential medication should be discontinued. Whether to discontinue or switch [ɪtʃ] a drug³ depends on the severity [e] of the skin eruption [ʌ]. The dose is gradually tapered⁴ [eɪ] and discontinued over several days.

Use **to discontinue** drug therapy⁵ / all oral intake⁶ / application of heat • **discontinuation of** therapy / life support⁷

absetzen, -brechen
entziehen, absetzen¹ Abbruch, Unterbrechung² Medikament wechseln³ allmählich reduziert⁴ medikamentöse Behandlung absetzen⁵ Nahrungsaufnahme einstellen⁶ Intensivtherapie absetzen, lebenserh. Maßnahmen einstellen⁷

6

Pharmacologic Treatment | **GENERAL CLINICAL TERMS 73**

dose [doʊs] *n & v term*   *syn* **dosage** [doʊsɪdʒ] *n clin*

n (i) quantity [ɒ:] of medication to be taken at a time (ii) radiation administered or absorbed
overdose[1] *n & v term, abbr* OD • **dose-dependent**[2] *adj* • **dosimeter** *n*

» The **dose-effect curve**[3] of a drug results from its potency (*location of curve along the dose axis*), **peak** [i:] **efficacy** or **ceiling** [i:] **effect**[4] (*greatest attainable response*), **slope**[5] (*change in response per* **equivalent dose**[6]), *and biologic variation of response among tested individuals.*

Use to adjust [ʌ] the[7] **dosage** • oral / missed[8] / minimal effective / **tolerance**[9] **dose** • curative [kju:] *or* therapeutic[10] [u:]/ recommended **dose** • single[11] / initial[12] [ɪʃ]/ maintenance[13] / lethal[14] [i:] (*abbr* LD) **dose** • **dose** fractionation / calculation / distribution /-response curve[3] • **high dose** therapy[15] • liberal / in divided[16] **doses**

Dosis, Dosierung, Gabe; dosieren
Überdosis; überdosieren[1] dosisabhängig[2] Dosis-Wirkungs-Kurve[3] Wirkungsmaximum[4] Steilheit d. Dosis-Wirkungs-K.[5] Dosisäquivalent[6] D. anpassen[7] vergessene Einnahme[8] Toleranzdosis (radiolog.)[9] kurative D., D cur[10] Einzelgabe, -dosis[11] Anfangs-, Initialdosis[12] Erhaltungsd.[13] letale D.[14] hochdosierte Therapie[15] in Teildosen[16]   7

action [ækʃ³n] *n term*   *sim* **activity**[1], **effect**[2] *n term*

» It is important to better understand the mechanism [k] *of* **action**[3] *of these new drugs. These* cephalosporins [s] *have good activity against most gram-positive cocci* [kaɪ‖ksaɪ]. *These drugs reach their* **peak action**[4] *in 4 h. Each agent possesses a* distinct[5] *pharmacodynamic profile of* **action**[6].

Use bactericidal [saɪ]/ broad spectrum of[7] / gram-positive / in vitro **activity** • onset of[8] / pharmacologic / selective / cytoprotective [saɪtoʊ-]/ hypotensive[9] **action**

Wirkung
Wirksamkeit, Wirkung[1] Effekt, (Aus)wirkung[2] Wirkungsmechanismus[3] maximale Wirkung[4] charakteristisches[5] pharmakodynam. Wirkprofil[6] breites Wirkungsspektrum[7] Wirkungseintritt[8] blutdrucksenkende W.[9]   8

potency [poʊtənsi] *n term*   *sim* **efficacy**[1] [efɪkəsi] *n term*

(i) pharmacological effectiveness of a drug (ii) opposite of sexual impotence
potent[2] *adj term* • low-/ high-**potency**[3] *adj*

» Unfortunately the potency of inhaled steroids is not measurable [eʒ] by improvements in asthma [æzmə] activity. Levorphanol has good oral potency. This patient must not be placed on high potency agents. Nitroglycerin [aɪ] loses potency unless stored in a tightly [aɪt] sealed[4] [i:] light-resistant[5] container.

Use clinical / carcinogenic [dʒen]/ antiarrhythmic [ɪ] **potency** • highly / moderately[6] **potent drugs**

(i) Wirksamkeit, Wirkungsstärke (ii)sexuelle Potenz
Effektivität, Wirksamkeit[1] stark, wirksam[2] hochwirksam, -potent[3] (luft)dicht verschlossen[4] lichtundurchlässig[5] Medikamente mittlerer Wirkungsstärke[6]   9

bioavailability [baɪoʊ-] *n term*   *sim* **rate of absorption**[1] *n term*

extent and rate at which a given amount of a drug is absorbed and made available to the target tissue
bioavailable[2] *adj term*

» The concept of bioavailability relates to the efficiency [ɪfɪʃənsi] of the dosage formulation as an extravascular drug delivery system and permits comparison of drug products for relative availability or **bioequivalence**[3]. Although bioavailability generally refers to the extent of input only, it includes consideration of both the amount and rate of absorption into the systemic circulation[4] [sɜːr] following extravascular administration.

Use level of **bioavailability** • low[5] / high / reduced / decreased / poor[5] **bioavailability**

Bioverfügbarkeit, biolog. Verfügbarkeit
Resorptionsgeschwindigkeit[1] biologisch verfügbar[2] Bioäquivalenz[3] Körper- / großer Kreislauf[4] geringe Bioverfügbarkeit[5]   10

drug interactions *n term usu pl*   *sim* **cross-reaction**[1] *n term*

harmful[2] or desirable[3] [aɪ] pharmacological effects of drugs interacting with other drugs or themselves, (non)physiologic chemical agents, components of the diet[4] [daɪət], etc.
interact with[5] *v* • cross-react *v term* • cross-reactivity *n*

» Unwanted interactions can cause adverse [ɜː] drug reactions[6] or therapeutic failure[7] [eɪ]. Pharmacokinetic interactions are mainly due to alteration of absorption, distribution, metabolism, or excretion [iːʃ], which changes the amount and duration of a drug's availability at receptor sites[8]. If a formulation[9] has the potential to interact with food the drug should be administered apart from meals[10].

Use drug-drug / drug-food / nutrient-drug[11] / pharmacokinetic[12] / pharmacodynamic **interactions** • adverse **drug interaction** • **cross**-reaction /-reactive antigen

(Arzneimittel)wechselwirkungen, -interaktionen
Kreuzreaktion[1] schädliche[2] erwünschte[3] Nahrungsstoffe[4] s. gegenseitig beeinflussen[5] Nebenwirkung(en)[6] Therapieversagen[7] Rezeptorstellen[8] Arzneiform[9] nicht mit Mahlzeiten eingenommen werden[10] Wechselwirkung zw. Nahrungsmitteln u. Medikamenten[11] pharmakokinet. Interaktionen[12]   11

74 GENERAL CLINICAL TERMS — Pharmacologic Treatment

tolerate v term & clin

able to endure or resist the action of a drug, poison[1], radiation [eɪ] or food without untoward [ʌntˤwɔːrd] effects[2]

(in)tolerance[3] n term • cross-tolerance[4] n • (in)tolerable[5] adj

» Parenteral quinidine[6] [kwɪn] is generally well tolerated by most patients. The patient developed unacceptable symptoms despite medical therapy to its tolerable limits[7]. The initial dosage of 2 mg tid is increased as tolerated[8].

Use well[9] / better / poorly / not[10] **tolerated** • short-term[11] / acquired[12] [əkwaɪɚd] **tolerance** • drug[13] / food / exercise / cold **intolerance** • minimal / organ[14] / tissue **tolerance dose** • **tolerance** test[15] / to opioids • **intolerable** pain / side effects

vertragen

Gift[1] schädliche Auswirkungen[2] (Un)verträglichkeit, (In)toleranz[3] Kreuztoleranz[4] (un)verträglich[5] Chinidin[6] max. verträgliche Dosis[7] nach Verträglichkeit[8] gut vertragen, verträglich[9] nicht vertragen, unverträglich[10] kurzfristige Verträglichkeit[11] Toleranzentwicklung[12] Arzneimittelunverträglichkeit[13] Organtoleranzdosis (radiol.)[14] Toleranztest[15]

12

---

toxic level or **range** [reɪndʒ] n term   opposite **therapeutic** [uː] **range**[1] n term

dosage of any substance that is beyond[2] the maximal therapeutic dose and produces overdosage[3] toxicity

nontoxic[4] adj term • toxicity[5] [tɒːksɪsɪti] n • toxicology n

» This dosage produces a toxic response on chronic administration. Overdosage toxicity is the predictable toxic effect that occurs with dosages in excess of[2] the therapeutic range for a particular patient. Equivalent mg/kg doses well tolerated by adults can result in serious [ɪɚ] toxicity in neonates[6] [iː]. These drugs are particularly toxic to the organ of Corti.

Use drug / side-effect[7] / digitalis[8] [dʒ] / local / systemic / hepatic[9] / long-term **toxicity** • **toxic** reaction / manifestations[10] / shock / agent / effect • **toxicity** test[11] / study

toxischer Wirkungsbereich

therapeutische Breite[1] (liegt) über[2] Überdosierung[3] ohne toxische Wirkung, ungiftig[4] Toxizität, Giftigkeit[5] Neugeborene[6] toxische Nebenwirkungen[7] Toxizität v. Digitalis[8] Lebertoxizität[9] Intoxikationszeichen[10] toxikologischer Test[11]

13

---

adverse [ɜː] **drug reaction** n term, abbr **ADR**

syn **side** or **untoward effect** n clin

secondary effects of a drug not normally seen in the therapeutic range that may cause minor[1] [aɪ], significant and even life-threatening[2] [e] morbidity

» Serious[3] [ɪɚ] adverse reactions are uncommon. Adverse effects should be discussed with patients to encourage [ɜː] them to mention them to the physician [fɪzɪʃˤn] prior [aɪ] to stopping medication[4].

Use to cause or provoke[5] [oʊ] / minimize **adverse effects** • **adverse** response to[6] / effect on

unerwünschte Arzneimittelwirkung, Nebenwirkung

gering(fügig)[1] lebensbedrohlich[2] ernsthaft, schwer(wiegend)[3] vor dem Absetzen d. Medikamente[4] N. auslösen[5] unerwünschte Reaktion auf[6]

14

---

drug-induced [uːs] adj clin   sim **iatrogenic**[1] [aɪə-] adj → U13-9,
                                   rel **nosocomial**[2] [koʊ] adj term

resulting from the administration of a drug, e.g. a drug rash, psychosis, or liver disease

» Predisposing[3] iatrogenic factors include cancer chemotherapy [kiː], genitourinary instrumentation or catheterization, recent surgery, steroid therapy, and antibiotic administration.

Use **drug-induced** disease / hepatitis / gingivitis • **drug**-fast or -resistant /-related fever /-associated /-free • **iatrogenic** illness[4] / fracture / factors / injury[5] / infection[6]

arzneimittelinduziert, -bedingt

iatrogen, durch d. Arzt verursacht[1] nosokomial, Krankenhaus-[2] prädisponierend[3] iatrogene Erkrankung[4] i. Verletzung / Schädigung[5] infektion[6]

15

Pharmacologic Agents   GENERAL CLINICAL TERMS **75**

Unit 20 Pharmacologic Agents
Related Units: **5** Drugs & Remedies, **19** Pharmacologic Treatment, **48** Types of Anesthesia & Anesthetics

pharmacology [fɑːrməkɒːlədʒi] *n term*
  sim **pharmaceutics**[1] [-suːtɪks] *n term*
  science of natural and synthetic medicinal substances, including pharmacognosy[2], pharmacokinetics[3], pharmacodynamics[4] [aɪ], pharmacogenetics[5] [dʒ], pharmacotherapy and toxicology
  pharma(co)- *comb* • pharmacologic *adj* • pharmacopeia[6] [piːə] *n*, BE -poeia
  » Pharmacokinetics is the study of the activity of drugs within the body, particularly their rates of absorption, distribution[7], binding [aɪ], biotransformation and elimination[8].
Use clinical / biochemical **pharmacology** • **pharmacologic** effect / action / properties[9] / treatment / agent • **pharma**ceutical chemistry[10] /cologist[11] • US / British / International[12] / European **pharmacopeia**

Pharmakologie, Arzneimittellehre
Pharmazie, -zeutik[1] Pharmakognosie[2] Pharmakokinetik[3] Pharmakodynamik[4] Pharmakogenetik[5] Arzneibuch, Pharmakopoe[6] Verteilung[7] Elimination, Ausscheidung[8] pharmakologische Eigenschaften[9] pharmazeutische Chemie[10] Pharmakologe/in[11] internat. Arzneibuch[12]   1

agent [eɪdʒənt] *n term*
  broad term for any substance capable [eɪ] of triggering[1] a chemical, physical [fɪ] or biological [aɪ] effect (e.g. drugs, bacteria, chemical substances, contrast media[2] [iː] etc.)
  » Not all preparations and agents are approved[3] [uː] for this indication. Treatment consists of adding bulk [ʌ] agents[4]. Proteus species [spiːʃiːz] are common causative [ɒː] agents[5].
Use rapidly/long acting / oral / sunscreen[6] **agent** • antipsychotic[7] [saɪkɒː]/ antiulcer [ʌls]/ antiangina [dʒaɪ]/ cholinergic[8] [kɒːlɪnɜːrdʒɪk]/ germicidal[9] [saɪdᵊl] **agent** • alkylating[10] / embedding / foamy [oʊ] antifoaming[11] / retrovirus-like / sclerosing / nephrotoxic / mucolytic[12] [ɪ]/ contrast[2] / infectious[13] [ɪnfekʃəs] **agent**

Mittel, Wirkstoff, Agens, Erreger
auslösen, hervorrufen[1] Kontrastmittel[2] zugelassen[3] Ballaststoffe[4] (Krankheits)erreger[5] Sonnenschutzmittel[6] Antipsychotikum, Neuroleptikum[7] Cholinergikum[8] Desinfektionsmittel, keimtötendes M.[9] Alkylans[10] Entschäumer, Antischaummittel[11] schleimlösendes M.[12] Infektionserreger[13]   2

pharmacologic activity *n term*   *syn* **bioactivity, action, effect** *n term*
  activate[1] *v term* • activator[2] *n* • activation[3] *n* • activating *adj* • active *adj*
  » The balance between cholinergic and dopaminergic activity[4] in the basal ganglia is improved.
Use synergistic [dʒɪ]/ specific / in vitro / peak[5] [iː]/ serotonergic[6] **activity** • **activated** charcoal[7] [tʃ] • antibacterial / site of[8] **action** • extension of[9] **effect**

Arzneimittelwirkung, biologische Aktivität / Wirkung
aktivieren, anregen[1] Aktivator[2] Aktivierung, Anregung[3] dopaminerge Wirkung[4] maximale W.[5] Serotoninaktivität[6] Aktivkohle, Carbo medicinalis[7] Wirkort[8] Wirkungsverlängerung[9]   3

biotransformation [aɪ] *n term*   *sim* **biodegradation**[1] *n clin & inf*
  successive[2] biochemical changes a substance undergoes as it is metabolized[3] in the body
  biodegradable[4] [eɪ] *adj term*
  » The precise kinetics of metallic substances depend on their diffusibility[5], rate of biotransformation[6], availability of intracellular ligands[7] [aɪ‖ɪ], etc.

Biotransformation
biologischer Abbau[1] aufeinanderfolgende[2] abgebaut, umgewandelt, metabolisiert[3] biologisch abbaubar[4] Diffusionsvermögen[5] Biotransformationsrate[6] Liganden[7]   4

pharmacologic half-life [hæf laɪf] *n term*   *sim* **biologic half-life**[1] *n term*
  time required for half the administered dose of a drug or radioactive substance to be eliminated by normal metabolic processes[2]
  » Multiple daily doses are required because of the drug's short half-life.
Use elimination[3] / cellular / serum [ɪə]/ functional **half-life** • **half-life** range[4] [reɪndʒ]

pharmkolog. Halbwertzeit
biologische Halbwertszeit[1] Stoffwechselprozesse[2] Eliminationshalbwertzeit[3] Halbwertbreite[4]   5

antagonist *n term*   *opposite* **agonist**[1], **synergist**[2] [sɪnɚdʒɪst] *n term*
  agent (also physiologic structure or process) neutralizing [uː] or impeding[3] [iː] the action or effect of other agents
  (ant)agonistic *adj term* • antagonism *n* • synergistic *adj* • synergism[4] *n*
  » Some opioid antagonists have mixed[5] agonist/antagonist activity.
Use calcium / competitive[6] / enzyme [zaɪ]/ folic acid[7] / insulin / narcotic / H₂ receptor **antagonist** • potent[8] / partial / moderate **antagonists**

Antagonist
Agonist[1] Synergist[2] hemmen[3] Synergismus[4] sowohl ... als auch[5] kompetitiver A.[6] Folsäureantagonist[7] hochwirksamer A.[8]   6

GENERAL CLINICAL TERMS — Pharmacologic Agents

blocking agent or **blocker** n term   syn **inhibitor** n term
(i) agent that interferes with[1] [ɪɚ] or retards[2] chemical, physiologic, or enzymatic [enzɪmætɪk] activity (ii) nerve which on stimulation represses activity
» Patients with beta-blocker[3] [eɪ‖iː] or ACE inhibitor[4] intolerance should be considered for surgery.
Use angiotensin converting enzyme (abbr ACE)[4] / monoamine oxidase [eɪz] (abbr MAO) **inhibitor** • alpha / ganglionic[5] / calcium channel[6] [tʃænəl] **blocker**

Hemmstoff, Hemmer, Blocker, Inhibitor
hemmen, stören[1] verzögern[2] Beta-(Rezeptoren)blocker[3] ACE-Hemmer[4] Ganglienblocker, Gangliople-gikum[5] Kalziumantagonist, -blocker[6]   7

cholinergic [kɒːlənɜːrdʒɪk] adj & n term   opposite **anticholinergic** or **parasym-patholytic**[1] [ɪ] adj & n term
(n) agent affecting[2] the regulation of the autonomous nervous system[3]
» Unlike[4] phenothiazines [fiːnoʊθaɪəziːnz] (anticholinergic) the drug has powerful peripheral cholinergic effects.
Use **cholinergic** stimulation / blocking agent / fibers[5] [aɪ]/ receptor • **anticholinergic** potency[6] [oʊ]/ preparations

cholinerg; Cholinergikum
anticholinerg, Anticholinergikum, Parasympatholytikum, -lytisch[1] beeinflussen[2] autonomes Nervensystem[3] im Gegensatz zu[4] cholinerge (Nerven)fasern[5] anticholinerge Wirkung[6]   8

antibiotic [æntɪbaɪɒːtɪk] n & adj term   syn **antimicrobial/-bacterial agent** n, sim **antiviral** [aɪ] **agent**[1] n term
(n) drug produced from a mold[2] [oʊ] or similar bacterium which inhibits the proliferation[3] of other micro-organisms
» Broad spectrum antibiotics[4] have a wide range of activity against both Gram-positive and Gram-negative organisms.
Use broad-spectrum / bactericidal[5] [-saɪdəl]/ oral / IV / acquired [kwaɪ] resistance to[6] **antibiotics** • **antibiotic-associated** diarrhea [daɪəriːə] • **antibiotic** use / cover[7] / sensitivity test[8]

Antibiotikum; antibiotisch
Virostatikum, antivirales Mittel[1] Schimmelpilz[2] Wachstum, Proliferation[3] Breitbandantibiotika[4] bakterizide A.[5] erworbene Antibiotikaresistenz[6] antibiot. Abschirmung[7] Antibiogramm[8]   9

penicillin [penɪsɪlɪn] n term
(i) antibiotic substance obtained from cultures of molds
(ii) natural or synthetic variants of penicillic acid
penicillamine[1] [iː] n term • penicillinase[2] n • penicillin-allergic adj
» Penicillins are mainly bactericidal in action (especially active against Gram-positive organisms). Erythromycin [aɪs] may be used in penicillin-allergic individuals.
Use oral / systemic / aqueous[3] [eɪkwɪəs] **penicillin** • **penicillin** B / G / O / G / N / V /-sensitive /-fast[4] / derivative[5]

Penizillin, Penicillin
Penicillamin[1] Penizillinase, Beta-Laktamase[2] wasserlösliches P.[3] penizillinresistent[4] Penicillinderivat[5]   10

anti-inflammatory drugs n term
drugs such as glucocorticoids or aspirin capable of indirectly reducing inflammation[1] by metabolic activity[2]
» All NSAIDs are analgesic [dʒiː], antipyretic[3] [aɪ] and anti-inflammatory in a dose-dependent fashion.
Use non-steroidal[4] **anti-inflammatory drugs** (abbr NSAIDs) • **anti-inflammatory** effect

Antiphlogistika, entzündungshemmende Mittel
Entzündung[1] Stoffwechsel(prozesse)[2] fiebersenkend[3] nichtsteroidale Antiphlogistika, NSA[4]   11

emetic n & adj term   opposite **antiemetic**[1] n & adj term, **antivomiting drug**[1] n clin
(n) agent such as ipecac syrup[2] that induces vomiting; used mainly after ingestion[3] [dʒe] of noxious [kʃ] substances[4]
» The antiemetic can be delivered[5] IM or by rectal suppository[6]. Administration of emetics proved unsuccessful.
Use ectopic / effective / weak[7] **antiemetic** • **antiemetic** medication / effect / therapy / properties

Emetikum; emetisch
Antiemetikum; Übelkeit u. Erbrechen verhindernd[1] Brechwurzelsirup[2] Einnahme[3] schädliche Substanzen[4] appliziert[5] Zäpfchen, Suppositorium[6] leichtes A.[7]   12

laxative [æks] n & adj term   syn **stool** [uː] **softener** n clin, opposite **antidiarrheal**[1] [aɪ] n & adj term
(n) drug stimulating bowel [aʊ] movement[2] and/or softer or bulkier [ʌ] stools[3] (ranging from mild aperients[4] [ɪɚ] to strong purgatives [pɜːrg] or cathartics[5] such as Castor oil[6]
» Epsom salt[7] is used in constipation[8] for its purgative properties[9].
Use chronic / osmotic / rapid-acting / oily / saline [eɪ] / oral / mild[4] **laxatives** • **laxative** abuse[10]

Abführmittel, Laxans, Laxativum; abführend, laxierend
Antidiarrhoikum, stopfendes Mittel[1] Stuhlentleerung[2] voluminösere Stühle[3] schwache Abführmittel, Aperitiva[4] Purganzien, Kathartika[5] Rizinusöl[6] Bittersalz[7] Verstopfung, Obstipation[8] abführende Wirkung[9] Laxanzienabusus[10]   13

Pharmacologic Agents GENERAL CLINICAL TERMS **77**

inhalant [eɪ] n term syn **aerosol** [eəˈɒsɒːl] n term

(i) aerosolized (combinations of) medication taken by inhalation with nebulizers[1] or metered [iː] dose inhalers[2] (ii) generally, any substance that is inhaled, esp. allergens, narcotics, and irritants[3]

inhalation[4] [eɪ] n term • inhale[5] [eɪ] v • inhaler[6] n

» In adults sympathomimetic bronchodilators[7] [k] should be given in aerosol form.
Use water / particulate[8] **aerosol** • **aerosol** inhalation / generator[1] [dʒe] / therapy • broncho**aerosol**

Aerosol, Inhalat(ionsmittel)
Handzerstäuber, Nebulisator[1] Dosierinhalator[2] Irritanzien, Reizmittel[3] Inhalation, Einatmung[4] einatmen, inhalieren[5] Inhalator[6] Broncholytika, -dilatatoren[7] Trocken-, Staubaerosol[8] 14

---

expectorant n & adj term   syn **phlegm** [flem] **loosener** [uː] n clin, **mucolytic** [ɪ] n & adj term

agent promoting bronchial [k] secretion [iː] and expulsion[1] [ʌ] of mucus[2] from the respiratory tract

expectorate[3] v term • expectoration[4] n

» Treatment for mucoviscidosis [s] includes expectorants, and bronchodilators.

Expektorans, Sekretolytikum; schleimlösend
Auswerfen[1] Schleim[2] aushusten, expektorieren[3] Aushusten, Expektoration[4] 15

---

anticoagulants n term   syn **antihrombotic (agents)** n, rel **thrombolytic (agents)**[1] n term

anticlotting[2] drugs that can suppress or delay[3] [eɪ] coagulation

coagulate[4] [koʊægjəleɪt] v term • coagulation[5] n

» The patient is on anticoagulants for coronary thrombosis. Streptokinase [aɪ] and urokinase are thrombolytics capable of disintegrating[6] thrombi [aɪ].

Antithrombotika, Antikoagulanzien, Gerinnungshemmer
Fibrino-, Thrombolytika[1] gerinnungshemmend[2] verzögern[3] koagulieren, gerinnen[4] Koagulation, (Blut)gerinnung[5] auflösen[6] 16

---

vasodilators [veɪzoʊdaɪleɪtɚz] n term
opposite **vasoconstrictors** or **-pressors**[1] n term

agents causing dilation[2] of the blood vessels; often used for their antihypertensive[3] effect

vasodilat(at)ion[4] n term • vasoconstriction[5] n • vasoconstrictive adj

» Alpha-adrenergic agonists are used as nasal decongestants[6] [dʒe] orally and as vasodilators conjunctivally[7] [kəndʒʌŋktaɪ-]. Captopril, an ACE inhibitor, acts as an arteriolar and venous [iː] vasodilator.
Use arterial / pulmonary [ʊ‖ʌ]/ coronary[8] **vasodilator** • topical / intranasal **vasoconstrictor**

Vasodilatanzien, -dilatatoren, gefäßerweiternde Mittel
Vasokonstringenzien, gefäßverengende Mittel[1] Erweiterung[2] blutdrucksenkend[3] Vasodilatation, Gefäßerweiterung[4] Vasokonstriktion, Gefäßverengung[5] abschwellende Mittel[6] bei konjunktivaler Applikation[7] Mittel m. koronardilatator. Wirkung[8] 17

---

antiarrhythmic [æntɪeɪrɪθmɪk] n & adj term   syn **antiarrhythmic agent** n term

medication that can prevent or alleviate[1] [iː] cardiac arrhythmias[2]

» In patients with heart failure[3] quinidine[4] [kwɪnɪdiːn] and other antiarrhythmics had a proarrhythmic effect.

Antiarrhythmikum
lindern, vermindern[1] Rhythmusstörungen, Arrhythmien[2] Herzversagen[3] Chinidin[4] 18

---

antispasmodic n & adj term   syn **spasmolytic** [ɪ] n & adj term

agent that prevents or relieves spasms, esp. of smooth [uː] muscles[1] in the arteries, bronchi, bile ducts[2] [baɪl dʌkts], intestines or sphincters

» It exerts[3] a direct antispasmodic effect on smooth muscle[1].
Use biliary[4] [bɪlɪəri]/ urinary / bronchial / systemic **antispasmodics** • **antispasmodic** action

Spasmolytikum; spasmolytisch, krampflösend
glatte Muskulatur[1] Gallengänge[2] haben, ausüben[3] Spasmolytikum bei Gallenkolik[4] 19

---

anticonvulsive or **-ant** [ʌ] n & adj term   syn **antiepileptic** n & adj term

agent reducing the severity[1] [e] of convulsions[2] and epileptic seizures[3] [siːʒɚz]

» Patients on[4] anticonvulsants such as phenobarbital [iː] and phenytoin may develop osteomalacia [eɪʃ]. Phenytoin prevents the spread [e] of excessive discharges[5] in cerebral motor areas. The anticonvulsant properties of hydantoin [aɪ] derivatives are attributed to[6] their stabilizing effect on the cell membrane.
Use tricyclic / long-term **anticonvulsants**

Antikonvulsivum, -epileptikum; krampflösend, antiepileptisch
Schwere(grad)[1] Krampfanfälle[2] epileptische Anfälle[3] behandelt mit[4] Depolarisationen[5] zugeschrieben[6] 20

20

Pharmacologic Agents

diuretics [daɪjəretɪks] n term   syn **water pills** n inf & clin,
opposite **antidiuretics**[1] n term

agents that increase urinary excretion[2] [iːʃ] (by increasing cardiac output[3], renal perfusion[4] or decreasing reabsorption)

diuresis[2] [iː] n term • diuretic[5] [e] adj

» *Hypokalemia[6] [iː] may occur in hypertensives taking potassium-wasting diuretics[7].*

Use to administer **diuretics** • cardiac / (in)direct / rapidly acting / loop[8] [uː] / injectable / thiazide[9] [θaɪəzaɪd] / K+ sparing[10] [eə] **diuretics** • **antidiuretic** hormone[11] (abbr ADH) / response / therapy

Diuretika, wassertreibende Mittel

Antidiuretika[1] Harnausscheidung, Diurese[2] Herzminutenvolumen[3] Nierendurchblutung[4] diureseförderud, harntreibend[5] Hypokaliämie[6] Saluretika[7] Schleifendiuretika[8] Thiaziddiuretika[9] kaliumsparende D.[10] antidiuret. Hormon, Adiuretin, Vasopressin[11]   21

---

antihistamines n term

drugs used in the treatment of allergic reactions for their antagonistic action on histamine

» *Use a symptom-sign-directed approach including an H_1 antihistamine[1] for the pruritus[2] [aɪ].*

Use nonsedating[3] / IV / oral / OTC[4] / topical **antihistamines**

Antihistaminika, Histamin-antagonisten

H_1-Rezeptorenblocker, H_1-Antihistaminika[1] Hautjucken, Pruritus[2] nicht sedierende A.[3] rezeptfreie A.[4]   22

---

psychoactive [saɪkoʊ-] **substances** n term   syn **psychotropic agents** n term

agents that act on the mind or behavior and are used to treat emotional disorders; these include antidepressants, lithium carbonate (for manic [eɪ] episodes[1]), neuroleptics[2], antianxiety [ængzaɪə] agents[3], stimulants[4], sedatives[5], tranquilizers[6] [aɪz], and hypnotics [ɪ] or sleeping aids[7]

» *Discontinuation[8] of psychotropic or anti-Parkinson drugs[9] should be considered[10].*

Psychopharmaka, psychotrope Substanzen

manische Phasen[1] Neuroleptika[2] Anxiolytika, angstlösende Mittel[3] Stimulanzien[4] Sedativa, Beruhigungsmittel[5] Tranquilizer[6] Hypnotika, Schlafmittel[7] Absetzen[8] Antiparkinsonmittel[9] in Betracht ziehen[10]   23

---

antidepressants n term   opposite **barbiturates**[1] n term,
downers[2] [aʊ] n jar & inf

agents relieving symptoms of depression (e.g. tricyclic [traɪsaɪklɪk] antidepressants[3] and MAO inhibitors[4])

» *Women have a higher frequency of ADRs[5] to antidepressants and anticonvulsants. Benzodiazepine [aɪæ] overdosage potentiates[6] the respiratory depressive effects of barbiturates.*

Antidepressiva

Barbiturate[1] Beruhigungsmittel[2] trizyklische A.[3] Monoaminooxidasehemmer, -inhibitoren[4] Nebenwirkungen[5] verstärken, potenzieren[6]   24

---

anthelmintic n & adj term   syn **anthelminthic (agent)** n term

drug that expels[1] or eradicates[2] parasitic worms (esp. intestinal tapeworms[3] [eɪ], roundworms[4], etc.)

» *Many anthelmintic drugs are toxic and must be given with care. If a tapeworm is the cause of vitamin deficiency[5] [ɪʃ], an anthelmintic agent is indicated.*

Anthelminthikum, Wurmmittel; anthelminthisch

abtreiben[1] abtöten[2] Bandwürmer[3] Rund-, Fadenwürmer, Nematoden[4] Vitaminmangel[5]   25

---

antifungal [fʌŋgəl] n & adj term   syn **antimycotic** [aɪ] n & adj,
sim **fungicide**[1] [-saɪd] n term

agent that destroys fungi[2] [fʌŋgaɪ] and suppresses their growth and reproduction

fungal adj term • fungicidal[3] adj • fungistatic[4] adj

» *The use of powders [aʊ] containing antifungals or chronic use of antifungal creams may prevent recurrences of athlete's foot (tinea pedis [iː])[5]. Cutaneous [eɪ] candidiasis[6] [aɪə] responds well to topical application of an antifungal agent.*

Use systemic / topical[7] / oral / broad-spectrum **antifungal** • **antifungal** drugs / lotion / mouthwash / antibiotics / activity / prophylaxis / therapy

Antimykotikum; antimykotisch

fungizides Mittel, Fungizid (Schädlingsbekämpfungsmittel)[1] Pilze, Fungi[2] fungizid[3] fungistatisch[4] Fußpilzerkrankung, Tinea pedis[5] kutane Candidose[6] lokal wirkendes Antimykotikum[7]   26

---

sympatho- [sɪmpəθoʊ] or **adrenomimetics** n term
opposite **sympatholytic (agents)**[1] n term

agents that mimic[2] the action of the sympathetic nervous system, esp epinephrine[3] and norepinephrine[4]

» *Asthmatics[5] [z] with infrequent symptoms should be given an inhaled sympathomimetic PRN[6]. Some of these patients benefit from[7] sympatholytic drugs such as methyldopa.*

Sympathomimetika

Sympatholytika[1] nachahmen, imitieren[2] Adrenalin[3] Noradrenalin[4] Asthmatiker[5] bei Bedarf[6] profitieren von[7]   27

Pharmacologic Agents **GENERAL CLINICAL TERMS 79**

uricosuric drugs n term syn **urinary acidifiers** [əsɪdɪfaɪɚz], **uric acid reducers** n term

agents reducing serum levels of uric acid[1], e.g. to combat[2] the symptoms of gout[3] [aʊ]
» Serum uric acid is used as an indirect measure [eʒ] of the therapeutic [juː] effect of uricosurics. In quinine [kwɪn-] overdose urinary elimination can be enhanced[4] with an acidifying agent. Because contrast agents are uricosuric, tubule obstruction by crystals of uric acid has been proposed as the pathogenic [dʒe] mechanism [k].

Urikosurika
Harnsäure[1] bekämpfen[2] Gicht[3] gesteigert[4]

28

antacid [æntæsɪd] n & adj term

agent reducing or neutralizing [uː] acidity[1], e.g. of the gastric juice[2] [dʒuːs] in peptic ulcer[3] [ʌlsɚ]
» Treatment of the underlying reflux [iː] with antacids was curative.
Use effervescent[4] / fast-acting / high-dose / liquid / contact[5] / magnesium-containing [iː] **antacid** • **antacid** tablet / action / combinations / preparation

Antazidum; antazid, säurebindend
Azidität, Säuregrad[1] Magensaft[2] Ulcus pepticum[3] brauseförmiges A.[4] schleimhautprotektives A.[5]

29

emollient [ɪmɒːljənt] n & adj term sim **demulcent**[1] [dɪmʌlsənt] n & adj term

agent (e.g. mucilage[2] [mjuːsəlɪdʒ], oil) used to soothe[3] [suːð] and relieve irritation, esp of the mucous [mjuːkəs] layer[4]
» White petrolatum[5] [eɪ] and other topical emollients may be used if the itching[6] [tʃ] skin is dry.
Use **emollient** paste [eɪ]/ dressing[7] / laxative[8] • **demulcent** expectorant

erweichendes Mittel, Emollienzium; lindernd, beruhigend
Demulzenzium, einhüllendes / milderndes Mittel; lindernd[1] Schleim, Mucilago[2] lindern[3] Schleimhaut[4] weiße(s) Vaselin(e), Vaselinum album[5] juckend[6] feuchtwarmer Umschlag[7] Gleitmittel[8]

30

antineoplastic [iː] or **cytostatic agents** n term
  sim **antitumor antibiotics**[1] n term

various groups of agents (e.g. antimetabolites[2], alkaloids, or antihormones[3]) used in chemotherapy [kɪ] for their inhibiting effect on the maturation and proliferation[4] of cancerous cells[5]
» Although little is known about distribution of antineoplastic agents into breast-milk, breast-feeding[6] [e] is not recommended during chemotherapy.

Zytostatika, antineoplastische Substanzen
zytostatische Antibiotika[1] Antimetaboliten[2] Antihormone, Hormonantagonisten[3] Wucherung[4] Krebszellen[5] Stillen[6]

31

cytotoxic [saɪtoʊtɒːksɪk] adj term sim **cytostatic**[1] adj & n term

harmful or destructive to cells; used esp to refer to antitumor drugs that selectively destroy dividing cells
cytotoxicity[2] n term • cytotoxin[3] n • -toxic adj & comb
» Antimetabolites induce cytotoxicity by serving as false [ɔː] substrates[4] [ʌ] in biochemical pathways[5] [æ].
Use **cytotoxic** drug[6] / antitumor agents / therapy • direct / cellular[7] / antibody-mediated[8] [iː] **cytotoxicity** • cardio/ hepato/ nephro[9]/ thyro [θaɪroʊ]/ myelo[10] [aɪ]/ oto**toxic**

zytotoxisch, zellschädigend
zytostatisch; Zytostatikum[1] Zytotoxizität[2] Zytotoxin, Zellgift[3] Substrate[4] biochem. Abläufe[5] zytotox. Substanz[6] Zelltoxizität[7] antikörpervermittelte Zytotoxizität[8] nephrotoxisch, nierenschädigend[9] myelotoxisch[10]

32

teratogenic [-dʒenɪk] adj term sim **embryotoxic**[1] adj term

capable of inducing disturbed fetal [iː] growth, malformations[2] and deformities
teratogenicity[3] n term • teratogen[4] n • teratogenesis[5] n
» Because of its teratogenicity thalidomide is contraindicated in women of childbearing age[6] [eɚ].
Use **teratogenic** potential / effect / drug

teratogen
embryotoxisch[1] Missbildungen[2] Teratogenität[3] Teratogen[4] Teratogenese[5] im gebärfähigen Alter[6]

33

biologic response modifiers [mɒːdɪfaɪɚz] n term
  syn **immunomodulators** n term

chemical agents capable of modifying the response of the immune system, e.g. by stimulating antibody formation or inhibiting WBC[1] activity
» Biologic response modifiers such as interleukin-2 [uː] have received much attention recently.

Immunmodulatoren
Leukozyten, weiße Blutkörperchen[1]

34

20

Unit 21 Surgical Treatment

Related Units: 22 Basic Operative Techniques, 23 The Surgical Suite, 24 Surgical Instruments, 25 Perioperative Care, 26 Sutures & Suture Material, 27 Medical & Surgical Asepsis, 28 Wound Healing, 29 Fracture Management, 44 Oral Surgery, 43 Dental Implantology, 45 Maxillofacial Surgery, Plastic & Reconstructive Surgery

---

operate on *v term*

performing surgery in a patient [eɪʃ] with the help of instruments in order to remove or repair damaged tissue

operation[1] *n term & clin* • (in)operable[2] *adj* • preoperated *adj*

» The patient should be operated on immediately following chest x-ray[3]. Resuscitation[4] [SAS] is continued as the patient is being operated on. Complications occur in approximately 2% of all people operated on for biliary tract disease[5]. The prognosis is good if the patient is operated on in the early stages of the illness.

Use **to operate on** the heart [ɑː]/ leg • to undergo[6]/be subjected to/perform[7]/postpone[8]/schedule[9] [skˈʃedjuː]/ **an operation** • chest-wall / hip / gynecologic [gaɪnəˈdʒɪnɪ-] / major[10] [eɪdʒ] **operation** • open[11] / high-risk / repeat[12] [iː]/ second-look[13] / prolonged **operation** • preoperated abdomen[14] • **(in)operable** tumor / lesion • newly **operated** patient[15]

> Note: Mark the difference between *to operate*[16] (e.g. a machine) and *to operate* on (e.g. a patient). The preposition must not be dropped, also in the passive.

operieren
Operation, chir. Eingriff[1] (nicht)operierbar, (in)operabel[2] Thorax-Röntgen[3] Reanimation[4] Gallenerkrankung[5] s. einer Op. unterziehen[6] Op. durchführen[7] Op. verschieben[8] Op. ansetzen[9] großer Eingriff[10] offenchir. Eingriff[11] Reoperation[12] (diagnost.) Zweiteingriff, Second-look-Operation[13] voroperiertes Abdomen[14] frischoperierte(r) Patient(in)[15] bedienen[16]

1

---

operative *adj term*   *syn* **operating, surgical** [sɜːrdʒɪkəl] *adj term*

pre/ postoperative *adj term* • intra/ perioperative *adj*

» When fever [iː] appears after the second postoperative day, we ought [ɒːt] to reconsider[1] the diagnosis. This kind of hematoma [iː] requires operative intervention[2].

Use **operative** field[3] / site[4] / time / approach[5] [-oʊtʃ]/ risk / scar[6] / management or treatment / mortality rate / permit[7] / wound [uː] • **operating** room[8] (*abbr* OR) or BE theatre[8] (*abbr* OT)/ (micro)scope / table[9] / team • **preoperative** evaluation / history[10] / hospital stay / fasting[11] • **preoperative** diagnosis / management[12] / workup[13] / counseling [aʊ]/ cessation [s] of smoking • **postoperative** pain / course[14] [ɔː]/ period / day 2 / care[15] / followup[16] • **intraoperative** findings[17] [aɪ]/ evaluation / monitoring[18]

operativ, Operations-, chirurgisch
sollten überdenken[1] chir. Eingriff[2] Operationsfeld[3] Operationssitus[4] operativer Zugang[5] Operationsnarbe[6] Operationseinwilligung[7] Operationssaal, OP[8] OP-Tisch[9] präop. Anamnese[10] präop. Nahrungskarenz[11] Operationsvorbereitung[12] präop. Anamnese u. Diagnostik[13] postop. Verlauf[14] p. Nachsorge[15] p. Nachuntersuchung[16] intraop. Befund[17] intraop. Überwachung[18]

2

---

surgery [sɜːrdʒəri] *n term & clin*

(i) operative treatment (ii) in BE the room where a doctor or dentist sees and treats patients

surgeon[1] *n* • surgical *adj* • electro-/ micro-/ cryosurgery[2] [kraɪoʊ-] *n term*

» In the hands of an experienced surgeon the operative mortality rate should approach zero[3] [zɪəroʊ]. This problem demands immediate surgical attention[4].

Use minor[5] / major / elective[6] / emergency[7] [ɜːrdʒ]/ radical / exploratory[8] **surgery** • corrective / abdominal / hand / day[9] / plastic / palliative **surgery** • general / vascular[10] /assistant **surgeon** • **surgical** treatment / candidate / margin[11] [dʒ]/ center / ward[12] [ɔː]/ case / condition / correction / excision[13] / outcome[14]

**(i) Chirurgie, chir. Eingriff
(ii) Ordination, Praxis**
Chirurg(in), Operateur(in)[1] Kryochirurgie[2] bei Null liegen[3] chir. Behandlung[4] kleiner chir. Eingriff[5] Wahl-, Elektiveingriff[6] Not(fall)op.[7] explorative Op.[8] op. Eingriff i. einer Tagesklinik[9] Gefäßchirurg(in)[10] chir. Schnittrand[11] chir. Station[12] op. Entfernung[13] Operationsergebnis[14]

3

(surgical *or* **operative) procedure** [prəsiːdʒər] *n term*
syn **technique** [tekniːk] *n term*

specific type of surgery the steps and maneuvers [uː] of which are more or less standardized

technical [k] *adj* • technically *adv*

» The awake patient may experience cough[1] [kɒːf] during the procedure. The key factor for achieving optimal healing [iː] after operation is good surgical technique. Many cases of healing failure[2] [feɪljər] are due to technical errors.

Use adjunctive[3] [dʒʌ] / invasive [eɪ] / dental / termination / staged [eɪdʒ] / two-stage[4] / salvage[5] [sælvɪdʒ]/ V-Y[6] / staging[7] **procedure** • laser [eɪ] / closed[8] / irrigation / childbirth[9] **technique** • technically feasible[10] [iː]

Operation(stechnik), operative(s) Verfahren / Methode
Husten[1] schlechte (Ver)heilung[2] unterstützende Maßnahme[3] zweizeitige Op.[4] organ-, lebensrettender Eingriff[5] V-Y Plastik[6] Staging-Operation[7] nicht invasives Verfahren[8] Entbindungstechnik[9] technisch durchführbar[10]

4

Surgical Treatment · **GENERAL CLINICAL TERMS** 81

elective adj term   opposite **emergency** [ɜːrdʒ], **urgent**[1] [ɜːrdʒᵊnt] adj
   an elective procedure is one that can be scheduled without any pressure of time
   » Elective surgical repair is indicated to prevent complications. There is no need for an urgent or emergency operation.
Use **elective** procedure[2] / treatment / case / resection / left colectomy / abortion [-ɔːrʃᵊn]/ dental surgery • **emergency** situation[3] / consultation / measures[4] [eʒ]/ room[5] (abbr ER) / ward / department[5] / physician[6] [fɪzɪʃᵊn]/ treatment / surgical care / amputation[7] • in (case of) an[8] / medical **emergency** • on an **emergency** basis • **urgent** attention / admission[9] / evaluation[10] / referral[11] / intervention / transfusion / laparotomy

elektiv, zum Zeitpunkt d. Wahl
Not(falls)-[1] Wahl-, Elektiveingriff[2] Notfall[3] Notmaßnahmen[4] Notaufnahme(zimmer, -station)[5] Notarzt[6] Notamputation[7] im Notfall[8] Notfallaufnahme[9] dringende Abklärung[10] dringende Überweisung[11]

5

(surgical) approach [əproʊtʃ] n term   sim **access**[1] [ækses], **route**[2] [uː‖aʊ] n term
   specific anatomic dissection by which access is gained[3] [eɪ] to the operative field
   approach[4] v • (in)accessible[5] adj • accessibility n
   » The left chest approach affords[6] limited access to the esophagus [ɪsɒːf-]. The laparoscopic approach provides good access with low morbidity. Submandibular abscesses are best approached through an incision 2 cm below the inferior [ɪɚ] border of the mandible. An extraperitoneal approach via the flank is preferred for upper retroperitoneal and perirenal [iː] lesions [iːʒ].
Use combined / lateral / transpalatal **approach** • to gain[3]/allow (for) or provide[7]/have/ limit[8] **access to** • operative / vascular / intravenous[9] [iː]/ limited / easy / good / wide[10] **access** • **access** route[1] • surgically **(in)accessible** areas • easily **accessible**

  Note: Access (the right, privilege or possibility to enter or make contact) and approach (the way or route of entering or doing something) are clearly different in usage and meaning. Also do not confuse accessible and accessory[11].

Operationsweg, operativer Zugang
Zugang(sweg)[1] Zugangsweg, -art[2] Zugang erlangen[3] s. nähern, herangehen an[4] (un)zugänglich[5] ermöglicht[6] Zugang ermöglichen[7] Z. beschränken[8] venöser Z.[9] breiter Z.[10] zusätzlich, Hilfs-[11]

6

(surgical) exposure [ɪkspoʊʒɚ] n term   → U46-7
   the extent to which the operative field is visualized[1] [ʒ], accessible and provides sufficient [ɪʃ] working space[2]
   expose[3] v term • (un)exposed[4] adj
   » The hepatic flexure [kʃ] may have to be mobilized to expose the duodenum. The tissue must be either retracted upward[5] or divided to allow for adequate exposure of the trachea [treɪkɪə].
Use to achieve[6]/allow for or permit[7] **adequate exposure** • good / wide **exposure**

Freipräparierung, Freilegung, Darstellung
dargestellt[1] genügend Arbeitsraum[2] freilegen, -präparieren[3] (nicht)freiliegend[4] n. oben gezogen[5] ausreichend darstellen[6] ausreichende Darst. ermöglichen[7]

7

landmark n term
   a distinctive site[1] or anatomic feature[2] [fiːtʃɚ] used by surgeons to facilitate[3] orientation in the operative field
   » Use the brachial [eɪk] artery as a landmark. All landmarks were obliterated[4] by the swelling.
Use anatomic **landmark** • to locate[5]/find/identify/visualize[6] [ʒ]/lose **landmarks**

Orientierungs-, Bezugspunkt
markante Stelle[1] anatomische Struktur[2] erleichtern[3] verdeckt[4] O. lokalisieren[5] O. darstellen[6]

8

21

incise [ɪnsaɪz] v term   sim **circumcise**[1] v term, **cut**[2] v jar, opposite **excise**[3] v term
   cutting the skin or a tissue layer with a scalpel to open up the operative field
   incision[4] [ɪnsɪʒᵊn] n term • incisional adj • incised adj
   » The lung is incised over the cyst [sɪst]. A transverse incision[5] overlying the upper trachea is developed by separating[6] the muscles of the neck in the midline.
Use to make[7]/deepen **an incision** (into) • the **incision** is carried/developed/continued[8] along the ... • **incise** and drain[9] • flank[10] / skin[11] (crease) [iː] / Pfannenstiel / stab[12] **incision** • circular[13] / midline[14] / muscle-splitting[15] / relaxing[16] / inadvertent[17] / Z-shaped **incision** • **incisional** biopsy[18] [aɪ]/ hernia[19] / drainage [ɪdʒ]

inzidieren, ein-, aufschneiden
um-, beschneiden[1] (ein-, durch-, ab)schneiden[2] exzidieren, (her)ausschneiden[3] Eröffnung, (Ein)schnitt, Inzision[4] Querinzision[5] (Durch)trennen, Spalten[6] inzidieren, einschneiden[7] Schnitt w. geführt[8] inzidieren u. (durch Drain) ableiten[9] Flankenschnitt[10] Hautschnitt[11] Stichinzision[12] kreisförm. / zirkulärer Schnitt[13] Medianschnitt[14] Wechselschnitt[15] Entlastungsschnitt[16] unbeabsichtigter Einschnitt[17] Probeexzision[18] Narbenbruch[19]

9

section [sɛkʃən] *v & n term*   *syn* **sectio** *n term*, **sectiones** *pl*

(i) making an incision (ii) a cut surface¹ (iii) segmentation of an anatomic structure

cross-section² *n term* • cross-sectional *adj*

» The transverse carpal ligament had to be sectioned to liberate³ the median [iː] nerve. The vessel was doubly [ʌ] ligated [aɪ] and sectioned⁴.

Use histologic / frozen⁵ / serial⁶ [ɪɚ]/ cesarean⁷ [sɪzɛrɪən] **section** • **cross-sectional** area⁸ / plane [eɪ]/ view / image / study • nerve **sectioning**

inzidieren, durchtrennen; Schnitt(fläche), Abschnitt
Schnittfläche¹ Querschnitt² freilegen³ zwischen zwei Ligaturen abgesetzt⁴ Gefrierschnitt⁵ Serienschnitt⁶ Kaiserschnitt, Sectio caesarea⁷ Querschnittfläche⁸   10

---

exploration *n term*   *sim* **inspection¹** *n term*

(i) surgical or clinical examination for diagnostic purposes (ii) initial step in some surgical procedures performed either for gaining orientation or strategy planning

(re)explore *v term* • inspect *v* • exploratory² *adj term*

» Arteriography or surgical exploration of the neck is recommended for penetrating injuries. Exploratory laparotomy³ or laparoscopy is advisable [aɪz] if all investigations prove inconclusive⁴.

Use vaginal [dʒ]/ manual⁵ / visual [ʒ] **exploration** • **exploratory** incision / biopsy / puncture⁶ [pʌŋktʃɚ]/ surgery • **to explore** the depth of the wound⁷

Exploration, Untersuchung, Austastung
Inspektion, Prüfung, Kontrolle¹ explorativ, Probe-² Explorativ-, Probelaparotomie³ ergebnislos⁴ Austastung⁵ Probepunktion⁶ Tiefe einer Wunde feststellen⁷   11

---

dissect *v term*   *sim* **free¹, liberate¹** *v jar*

to cut and separate body tissues in surgery, autopsy [ɒ], or for anatomic study

dissection² *n term* • dissect free¹ *v phr* • dissector³ *n*

» The surrounding tissue is carefully dissected away from⁴ the tumor. The dissection was carried upward to the axilla. The ureter was freed and wrapped [r] in omentum.

Use **dissected** bluntly⁵ [ʌ]/ off or free from⁶ • extensive / meticulous⁷ / gentle [dʒ]/ sharp⁸ / blunt / finger / (lymph) node⁹ / subintimal **dissection** • **dissecting** microscope¹⁰ [aɪ]/ aneurysm¹¹ [jɚ]

präparieren, sezieren
freilegen, -präparieren¹ Präparation, (Dis)sektion, Obduktion² Prosektor; Dissektor³ abpräpariert⁴ stumpf präpariert⁵ frei-, abpräpariert⁶ exakte Präparation⁷ scharfe P.⁸ Lymphadenektomie, -knotendissektion⁹ Präpariermikroskop¹⁰ Aneurysma dissecans¹¹   12

---

preserve *v term*   *syn* **spare** [spɛɚ] *v*, **leave** [iː] **intact** *v phr*

(i) to maintain in normal, healthy or unchanged condition (ii) not affected by dissection or disease

preservation¹ *n* • (life-)preserving² *adj* • organ-sparing³ *adj*

» Every effort must be made to preserve antegrade ejaculation [ɪdʒæk-]. The technique spares⁴ the patient a second anesthetic [e].

Use **to preserve** viable [aɪə] tissue / normal weight-bearing [weɪt]/ full range of motion⁵ / the duodenum • functional⁶ **preservation** • **preservation of** length / health⁷ / position sense⁸ / arterial [ɪɚ] blood flow • nerve-**sparing** procedure⁹

erhalten, schonen
Erhaltung, Konservierung¹ (lebens)erhaltend² organerhaltend³ erspart⁴ volle Beweglichkeit erhalten⁵ Funktionserhaltung⁶ Gesunderh.⁷ E. der Lageempfindung⁸ nerv(en)schonender Eingriff⁹   13

---

transect *v term*   *sim* **bisect¹** [aɪ], **divide²**, **split²** *v term*

to incise and separate transversely, esp. vessels and tubes; sever³ is also used for traumatic amputations

transection⁴ *n term* • division⁵ [dɪvɪʒən] *n*

» Take care not to transect the vein or puncture its outer wall. Stapled [eɪ] transection⁶ has replaced the older technique of direct suture [suːtʃɚ] ligation⁷ of varices [vɛəːɪsːz].

Use partial [ʃ]/ gastric⁸ / ureteral / line of **transection** • **split**-thickness graft⁹ / tongue¹⁰ [tʌŋ]/ rectus muscle [mʌsl] • transverse / longitudinal¹¹ / cell **division**

(quer) durchtrennen, -schneiden
(zwei)teilen¹ trennen, spalten² abtrennen³ Querschnitt; Durchtrennung⁴ Durchtrennung⁵ Absetzen zw. Klammerreihen⁶ Umstechungsligatur⁷ Absetzen d. Magens⁸ Spalthauttransplantat⁹ Spaltzunge¹⁰ Längsteilung¹¹   14

---

resection *n term*   *syn* **excision, extirpation** *n term* → U22-1

surgical removal of an organ or part of an organ

resect¹ *v term* • resectable *adj* • excise² [aɪz] *v* • extirpate³ *v*

» Obstructing lesions of the left colon are best managed by resection. Nonsurgical modalities should be reserved for patients who are poor candidates for resection.

Use rib / wedge⁴ [dʒ]/ segmental / transurethral⁵ / (en) bloc(k)⁶ / complete / curative [kju] **resection** • **resectable** lesion [liːʒən] or tumor⁷ • **resected** tissue / tonsil / aneurysm • **resecto**scope⁸

Resektion, Exzision, Entfernung
resezieren, entfernen¹ exidieren² exstirpieren³ Keilresektion⁴ transurethrale R.⁵ En-Bloc R.⁶ resezierbarer Tumor⁷ Resektoskop⁸   15

Unit 22 Basic Operative Techniques

Related Units: 21 Surgical Treatment, 26 Sutures & Suture Materials, 24 Surgical Instruments, 44 Oral Surgery, 43 Dental Implantology, 45 Maxillofacial Surgery, Plastic & Reconstructive Surgery

-ectomy comb → U21-15

word ending for terms referring to surgical removal or excision [eksɪɜ⁻n]

gastr<u>e</u>ctomy[1] n term • gingiv<u>e</u>ctomy [dʒɪndʒ-] n • append<u>e</u>ctomy[2] n

-ektomie, -exzision, -entfernung
Gastrektomie, totale op. Magenentfernung[1] Appendektomie[2]   1

-(o)tomy comb → U21-9f

word ending for terms denoting surgical incision

lapar<u>o</u>tomy[1] n term • oste<u>o</u>tomy n • cyst<u>o</u>tomy[2] n • episi<u>o</u>tomy[3] n

-tomie, -schnitt, -eröffnung
Laparotomie, Bauchschnitt, -höhleneröffnung[1] Zystotomie, Blasenschnitt[2] Episiotomie, (Scheiden)dammschnitt[3]   2

-stomy comb

word ending denoting surgical creation of an opening into a h<u>o</u>llow v<u>i</u>scus[1] [sk] or the artif<u>i</u>cial [ɪʃ] communication[2] (also termed st<u>o</u>ma[3]) between two spaces

col<u>o</u>stomy[4] n term • antr<u>o</u>stomy[5] n • trache<u>o</u>stomy[6] n

-stomie, -stoma, op. angelegte Öffnung
Hohlorgan[1] künstl. Verbindung[2] Stoma[3] Kolostomie[4] Kieferhöhlenfensterung[5] Tracheostoma[6]   3

-plasty comb → U49-3

word ending denoting surgical repair or restoration of form and/or function of organs or structures

angi<u>o</u>plasty[1] [dʒ] n term • arthr<u>o</u>plasty[2] n • rhin<u>o</u>plasty [aɪ] n • geni<u>o</u>plasty[3] n

-plastik, -ersatz, op. Korrektur
Angioplastie, Gefäßplastik[1] Arthroplastik, Gelenkersatz[2] Genio-, Kinnplastik, Kinnkorrektur[3]

Note: Many (in BE practically all) terms with the above endings carry the main stress on the vowel that comes before the ending, e.g. an<u>a</u>tomy, ...<u>o</u>stomy, ...<u>o</u>plasty.

4

m<u>i</u>crosurgery [aɪ] n term sim **micron<u>eu</u>rosurgery** [ʊɚ] n term

dissection of t<u>i</u>ny[1] [aɪ] structures using a micromanip<u>u</u>lator[2] or laser b<u>ea</u>m [iː] and m<u>a</u>gnifying lenses

micros<u>u</u>rgical(ly) adj term • micros<u>u</u>rgeon[3] n • microdiss<u>e</u>ct [ɪ‖aɪ] v

» A laser micr<u>o</u>probe[4] was used to v<u>a</u>porize[5] [eɪ] a min<u>u</u>te[1] [maɪnuːt] area of tissue.
Use laser / pit<u>ui</u>tary[6] / transsphen<u>oi</u>dal **microsurgery** • **microsurgical** techn<u>i</u>que / excision / coniz<u>a</u>tion[7]

Mikrochirurgie
winzig[1] Mikromanipulator[2] Mikrochirurg(in)[3] Mikrosonde[4] verdampfen, vaporisieren[5] mikrochirurg. Eingriff a. d. Hypophyse[6] mikrochir. Konisation[7]   5

<u>o</u>perating m<u>i</u>croscope n term sim **m<u>a</u>gnifying loupe** [luːp] or **lens**[1] n term

specially designed loupe for surgery on d<u>e</u>licate[2] structures not visible to the naked [neɪkɪd] eye[3]

magnific<u>a</u>tion[4] n term • m<u>a</u>gnify v

» An operating microscope with two viewing bin<u>o</u>cular [baɪ-] lenses[5] and swaged-on needles[6] [swedʒd] of 60 μm are required.
Use 3-fold / 8 times / with × 100[7] **magnification**

Operationsmikroskop
Lupe(nbrille)[1] zarte [2] mit bloßem Auge[3] Vergrößerung[4] Binokularmikroskop[5] atraumatische Nadeln[6] bei 100facher Vergrößerung[7]   6

laser [l<u>eɪ</u>zɚ] n term

acronym for light amplific<u>a</u>tion by st<u>i</u>mulated em<u>i</u>ssion of radi<u>a</u>tion; a high-energy narrow beam of nondiv<u>e</u>rgent[1] [-daɪvɜːrdʒənt] electromagnetic radiation highly useful in microsurgery (eye, spine [aɪ], brain surgery)

lase[2] [leɪz] v term • laser-assisted adj

» Carcin<u>o</u>ma in situ can be er<u>a</u>dicated[3] by cauterization, cryotherapy, laser vaporiz<u>a</u>tion[4], cone b<u>i</u>opsy [aɪə], or electrosurgical loop [uː] excision[5].
Use **laser** surgery / ablation / excision / photocoagulation / iridotomy • **laser** pr<u>o</u>be[6] [oʊ]/ tip / b<u>ea</u>m[7] [iː]/ <u>e</u>nergy / argon / krypton [ɪ]/ Nd:YAG[8] / helium-n<u>eo</u>n [iː]/ carbon di<u>o</u>xide [aɪ]/ dye[9] [daɪ]/ thermal / endosc<u>o</u>pic **laser**

Laser
nicht divergierend[1] lasern[2] völlig beseitigt[3] Laservaporisation[4] Abtragung mittels Diathermieschlinge[5] Lasersonde[6] Laserstrahl[7] Neodym-YAG-Laser[8] Farbstofflaser[9]

7

GENERAL CLINICAL TERMS — Basic Operative Techniques

cryosurgery [kraɪoʊ-] n term

operating on tissue subjected to extreme cold, e.g. by application of carbon dioxide

cryoprobe[1] n term • cryocautery[2] [ɔː] n • cryothalamotomy n

» The hemorrhoids [e] were necrosed by freezing with a cryoprobe of liquid nitrogen[3] [naɪtrədʒən].

Use **cryosurgery** technique • **cryosurgical** destruction • **cryo**therapy[4]

Kryochirurgie

Kryo-, Kältesonde[1] Kryokauter[2] flüssiger Stickstoff[3] Kryotherapie, Kältebehandlung[4]

[8]

---

electrosurgery n term   sim **diathermy**[1] [daɪəθɜːrmi], **electrocautery**[2] [ɔː] n term

searing[3] [ɪɚ] and coagulating tissue using high-voltage current[4] [ɜː] from an electrosurgical unit

electrosurgical adj term • cauterize[5] v • cautery[6] n • cauterization n

» The bleeding site was cauterized. Mild degrees of cervicitis [sɜːrvɪsaɪtɪs] can be treated by office cauterization[7], either chemically with 20% silver nitrate [aɪ] solution on cotton-tipped applicators, by light radial cauterization with nasal-tipped thermal cautery or electrocautery.

Use **electrosurgical** pencil[8] • monopolar / bipolar [aɪ] shortwave[9] **diathermy** • **diathermy** tips • snare[10] [eɚ]/ cold[11] / wet field / steam [iː]/ gas **cautery** • **cautery** knife [naɪf]/ probe • **electro**resection /desiccation

> Note: The terms cauterization, cautery, cauterize, and cauter also include the application of heat and caustic[12] [ɔː] substances to destroy tissue.

Elektrochirurgie

Diathermie[1] Elektrokauterisation[2] verschorfen[3] Strom[4] kauterisieren[5] Kauter; Kauterisation[6] ambulante Kauterisation[7] Diathermiestift[8] Kurzwellendiathermie[9] Schlingenelektrode[10] Kryokauter(isation)[11] ätzend, kaustisch[12]

[9]

---

hemostasis [hiːmoʊsteɪsɪs] n term, BE **haemostasis**   sim **coagulation**[1] n term

stopping a bleeding either by surgical means or physiologically by blood clotting[1]

coagulate[2] v term • coagulator[3] n • electrocoagulation n • hemostatic[4] [iː] adj & n • hemostat[5] n

» In this patient who has a coagulation disorder[6] adequate hemostasis was achieved with fibrin [faɪbrɪn] glue[7] [gluː].

Use to secure[8]/accomplish[9]/maintain **hemostasis** • bipolar **coagulation** • **coagulated** bleeding points / tissue • **hemostatic** clamp[5] / material

Hämostase, Blutstillung

Koagulation, Blutgerinnung[1] koagulieren; gerinnen[2] Koagulator[3] blutstillend; Hämostyptikum, -statikum[4] Gefäßklemme[5] Koagulopathie, Gerinnungsstörung[6] Fibrinkleber[7] H. sicherstellen[8] H. erreichen[9]

[10]

---

snare [sneɚ] n term

wire [aɪ] loop[1] [uː] used for removing small pedunculated[2] [ʌ] growths, e.g. polyps [ɪ]

(en)snare[3] v term • (electro)cautery snare[4] n

» Small polyps can be snared during endoscopy.

Use polypectomy[5] **snare** • **snare** technique

Schlinge

Drahtschlinge[1] gestielte[2] anschlingen[3] elektr. Schlinge, Diathermieschlinge[4] Polypenschlinge[5]

[11]

---

conization [kɒːn-‖koʊnɪzeɪʃən] n term   sim **electroconization**[1], **cone biopsy**[2] [aɪ] n term

electrosurgical or cold knife [naɪf] resection of a cone[3] of tissue, e.g from the uterine [aɪ‖ɪ] cervix

» Cervical cone biopsy[4] alone is therapeutic [pjuː] in many cases.

Use cold[5] / laser / excisional[6] / cervical[4] **conization** • **cone biopsy** specimen[2]

Konisation

Elektrokonisation[1] Konusbiopsie[2] Konus, Kegel[3] Zervix-, Portiokonisation[4] Schnittkonisation[5] Exzisionskonisation[6]

[12]

---

ablation [æbleɪʃən] n term   sim **extirpation**[1], **resection**[2] n term

surgical detachment[3] [tʃ], removal[4] or destruction of tissue

cryoablation[5] n term • ablate[6] [eɪ] v • ablative adj • resect v

» Many supraventricular arrhythmias [ɪ] can be definitely treated by catheter ablation[7] procedures.

Use laser[8] / tissue / catheter-induced[7] / radio frequency **ablation** • **ablative** techniques / surgery

> Note: The term ablation is also used for hormone withdrawal therapy[9] but not for the pathologic detachment[3] of tissue layers (e.g. ablatio placentae or retinae).

Ablatio, Abtragung

op. Entfernung, Exstirpation[1] Resektion[2] Ablösung[3] Entfernung[4] Kryo-, Kälteablation[5] abtragen, amputieren[6] Katheterablation[7] Laserablation[8] Hormonentzugstherapie[9]

[13]

Basic Operative Techniques   **GENERAL CLINICAL TERMS**   **85**

fulguration [fʌlgjəˈeɪʃən] *n term*   *syn* **electrodessication** *n term*
destruction of tissue with sparks[1] from a high-frequency current applied with needle electrodes
fulgurate[2] *v term* • fulgurating[3] *adj*
» Patients who are poor surgical risks may be palliated[4] with laser fulguration of the tumor mass.
Use direct / indirect / endoscopic / intraurethral [iː] *fulguration*

Elektrodesikkation, Fulguration
Funken[1] elektrochir. zerstören[2] blitzartig[3] Erleichterung verschaffen[4]
    14

vaporize [ˈveɪpəˌraɪz] *vt term*   *sim* **evaporate**[1] [æ] *vt/i term*
converting a solid or liquid into vapor[2] [eɪ]; in surgery it mostly refers to tissue ablation by laser
vaporization[3] [eɪ] *n term* • evaporation[4] [æ] *n*
» Using the endoscopic laser part of the tumor was vaporized to relieve her symptoms.

(Gewebe) verdampfen, vaporisieren
verdampfen; sich verflüchtigen[1] Dampf[2] Vaporisation[3] Verdampfung, -dunstung[4]
    15

suction [sʌkʃən] *n & v term*   *syn* **aspiration, suctioning** *n*,
                      sim **tap(ping)**[1] [æ] *n term*
(n) in surgery, a procedure to aspirate fluids or material from the body through a tube or needle
aspirate[2] [-eɪt] *v term* • aspirator[3] *n* • aspirate[4] *n* [-ət] • tap[5] *v*
» Suction evacuates[6] blood or serum [ɪə] accumulating[7] in the wound [uː] bed. The aspirate was heavily [e] contaminated. The diagnosis may be established[8] by fine-needle aspiration[9] and a cytologic [saɪ-] study of abnormal nodes. The material was aspirated for culture. The suction tube was plugged[10] [ʌ] with secretions.
Use to apply[2] **suction** • **suction** device[3] [dɪvaɪs]/ drainage[11] [-ɪdʒ]/ curettage[12] / (naso)gastric / low intermittent / continuous[11] **suction** • blood / bronchial [k]/ foreign body[13] (*abbr* FB) / synovial [aɪ] fluid **aspiration** • **aspiration** biopsy[14] • gastric **aspirate** • suprapubic (bladder) / lumbar [ʌ] *or* spinal[15] [aɪ]/ (non)traumatic / bloody / dry **tap**

Aspiration, Saug-; aspirieren, absaugen
Punktion[1] ab-, ansaugen, aspirieren[2] Saugvorrichtung, Aspirator[3] Punktionsflüssigkeit, Aspirat[4] punktieren; perkutieren[5] entfernen[6] ansammeln[7] gesichert[8] Feinnadelbiopsie[9] verlegt[10] Saugdrainage[11] Saugkürettage[12] Fremdkörperaspiration[13] Saug- Aspirationsbiopsie[14] Lumbalpunktion[15]

Note: *Aspiration* and *aspirate* can refer to the withdrawal of fluids or tissue specimens as well as to accidental inhalation of fluids or FBs into the respiratory tract.
    16

irrigation *n term*
to flush[1] [ʌ] and wash out a cavity or wound [uː] with fluid
irrigate[2] *v term* • irrigator[3] *n* • irrigating *adj*
» Irrigate the eyes gently[4] with sterile [sterɪl‖aɪl] saline [eɪ] solution. Then the wound was debrided[5] [aɪ] and irrigated again. In this case the use of jet irrigators[6] for cleaning teeth is not advisable.
Use daily / throat [oʊ]/ mouth / copious[7] [oʊ]/ whole gut[8] [ʌ] **irrigation** • bladder[9] / pressure[10] / (non)sterile / local antibiotic **irrigation** • **irrigating** solution[11]

Irrigation, (Aus-, Durch)spülung
(durch)spülen[1] (aus-, durch)spülen[2] Irrigator[3] vorsichtig[4] Wundränder w. angefrischt[5] Munddusche[6] gründliche Spülung[7] Darmspülung[8] Blasenspülung[9] Druckspülung[10] Spülflüssigkeit[11]   17

22

(venous) [iː] **cutdown** *n term*   *sim* **vene-** *or* **venipuncture**[1] [e‖iː] *n term*
small incision to gain access to[2] a subcutaneous vein [eɪ] for insertion of a needle or cannula
» Three IV lines are necessary for severe shock, two of them being large-bore catheters[3] placed by cutdown. An intraluminal device was implanted via a jugular [dʒʌgjələ] venous cutdown[4]. Allow enough time for the first venipuncture to clot, or leave the catheter in place to occlude the venipuncture site.
Use saphenous [iː] vein / antecubital fossa **cutdown** • emergency / jugular[4] **venous cutdown** • **cutdown** site / procedure / approach / tray • routine / subclavian[5] [eɪ] **venipuncture** • **venipuncture** technique

Venae sectio, Venenschnitt, Phlebotomie
Venenpunktion[1] Zugang schaffen[2] großlumige Katheter[3] Jugulariseröffnung[4] Subklaviapunktion[5]

    18

catheter [ˈkæθɪtə] *n term*   *syn* **line** [aɪ] *n clin & jar*
tube used for insertion into blood vessels, urinary passages or body cavities to inject or withdraw[1] [ɔː] fluids, keep the passage patent[2] [eɪ], etc.
catheterization[3] *n term* • catheterize[4] *v*
» The stricture [strɪktʃə] may be dilated[5] [aɪ] with a transhepatic balloon-tipped [uː] catheter[6]. Change the arterial [ɪə] line sites every 3-4 days. This requires insertion of a radial or femoral [e] arterial line.
Use to insert[7]/introduce[7]/place[7]/remove *a catheter* • ureteral[8] / cardiac[9] / suction / central venous[10] / subclavian / balloon[6] **catheter** • pigtail[11] / olive tip / indwelling[12] / Swan-Ganz / Foley / angio**catheter** • **catheter** tip[13] / site / dilatation / fever[14] [iː] • intermittent[15] / self-**catheterization**

Katheter
absaugen, aspirieren[1] offen, durchgängig[2] Katheterisierung[3] katheterisieren[4] (auf)gedehnt[5] Ballonkatheter[6] K. legen / einführen[7] Harnleiter-, Ureterkatheter[8] Herzk.[9] zentraler Venenk.[10] Doppel-J-K.[11] Dauer-, Verweilkatheter[12] Katheterspitze[13] Katheterfieber[14] intermittierende Katheterisierung[15]
    19

stent n & v term

thin, mostly catheter-like metal or resin tube[1] for supporting healing vessels or ducts and ensure [-ʃʊɚ] patency[2] or for holding surgical grafts[3] in place
stenting n term
» A stent of minimally reactive foreign material, (e.g. Silastic) that fills the lumen above and below the intubated area should be placed.
Use to insert/place **a stent** • urethral[4] [iː]/ bile [aɪ] duct [ʌ]/ intraoral / percutaneous[5] [eɪ]/ self-expandable[6] (metal) / occluded[7] **stent** • **stent** tube / placement / plugging[7] [ʌ]

Stent, Splint, Endoprothese; Stent plazieren, schienen
Kunststoffschlauch[1] offenhalten[2] Transplantate[3] Harnröhrenstent[4] perkutaner Stent[5] selbstexpandierender Stent[6] Stentverlegung[7]

20

Unit 23 The Surgical Suite
Related Units: 21 Surgical Treatment, 25 Perioperative Care, 27 Medical & Surgical Asepsis, Anesthesiology

operating room BE **theatre** [θɪətəʳ] n term   abbr **OR**, BE **OT**

hospital room equipped and used for performing surgical procedures
» The OR may only be entered by persons wearing [eɚ] clean operating attire[1] [ətaɪɚ] not worn elsewhere. Traffic[2] and talking in the OR should be minimized. A patient with shock or unexplained hemorrhage [-ɪdʒ] should be taken to the OR for emergency exploration.
Use to be rushed[3] [ʌ]/taken/brought/transferred **to the OR** • **OR** facilities[4] [sɪ]/ personnel / procedure [-iːdʒɚ]/ temperature

Operationssaal, OP
OP-Kleidung[1] Aus- u. Eingehen[2] schnell in den OP gebracht werden[3] OP-Einrichtung[4]

1

presurgical suite [swiːt] n term   sim **operating** or
   surgical [sɜːrdʒɪkəl] **suite**[1] n term

holding or catchment area[2] on the operating floor[1] where the ward [ɔː] nurse[3] hands the patient and the chart[4] [tʃ] over to the anesthesiologist; also includes rooms with facilities for scrubbing[5] [ʌ], gowning[6] [aʊ] and gloving [ʌ]
» Even though the patient appears to be safely dozing[7] [oʊ] with a strap in place[8], he should not be left alone in the presurgical suite.

Vorräume zum OP-Saal
Operationstrakt[1] Wartebereich (vor OP-Schleuse)[2] Stationsschwester, -pfleger[3] Krankenblatt[4] chir. Händereinigung[5] Anlegen d. OP-Kleidung[6] (vor sich hin)dösen[7] angegurtet[8]

2

induction room [ʌ] n term   sim **prep room**[1] n jar

a quiet room adjoining[2] the OR where the anesthesiologist administers[3] the preoperative anesthetic [e]
» In the induction room undesirable [aɪ] noise and conversations should be avoided as the patient may be acutely aware[4] of everything he hears.

Narkose(prämedikations)-raum
Vorbereitungsraum[1] neben[2] verabreicht[3] (bewusst) wahrnehmen[4]

3

operating or **surgical team** n term

includes the surgeon [dʒ], the surgeon's assistant[1], the anesthesiologist, the circulating and scrub nurses
» Nonsterile ORs and the operating team remain a source [ɔː] of infection[2]. Members of the surgical team should not operate if they have viral [aɪ] infections that may cause coughing [kɒfɪŋ] or sneezing[3] [iː].

Operationsteam
Operationsassistent(in)[1] Infektionsquelle[2] Niesen[3]

4

surgeon [sɜːrdʒ³n] n term   syn **operator** n term

physician who specializes in surgery; in the UK they are traditionally addressed[1] as Mr X rather than Dr X.
operator-dependent[2] adj term
» Given an accomplished[3] surgeon and good preoperative preparation this nerve can be preserved[4] in more than 98% of cases. In this technique skillful operators make only minimal use of sutures [tʃ].
Use attending[5] / general / plastic / house[6] (BE) / assistant / experienced **surgeon** • **the surgeon's** technical [k] skills / judgement[7] [dʒʌdʒ-]/ responsibility / experience

  Note: Do not be confused by the fact that the *operator* is commonly the person who works on a telephone switchboard or operates any other apparatus or machine.

Chirurg(in), Operateur(in)
angesprochen[1] abhängig v. Chirurg(in)[2] gut, fähig[3] erhalten[4] behandelnde(r) Chirurg(in)[5] Arzt od. Ärztin i. Praktikum / Turnusarzt od. -ärztin a.d. chir. Abteilung[6] Ermessen d. Chirurgen/-in[7]

5

The Surgical Suite **GENERAL CLINICAL TERMS 87**

anesthesiologist [ænəsθiːzɪɒːlədʒɪst] *n term*
    syn **anaesthetist** [əniːsθətɪst] *n term BE* → U47-2
physician who administers the anesthetic [e] and monitors[1] the patient while under anesthesia [-iːʒə]
» *The anesthesiologist continuously assesses[2] the depth of anesthesia[3].*
Use **anesthesiologist-on-call[4]**

> **Note:** Unlike in the U.K., the *anesthetist* in the U.S. is a nurse [ɜː] *anesthetist[5]* [e], a registered nurse[6] with extra qualifications working under the supervision of an *anesthesiologist*.

anesthesia screen [ænəsθiːʒə skriːn] *n term*
protective screen attached above the patient's chest to preclude airborne contamination[1] from the anesthesiologist or the patient him/herself

surgical nurse [nɜːrs] *n term* *syn* **scrub** [ʌ] **nurse** *n jar*
(s)he is responsible for the scrub-up procedures, lays [leɪz] out[1] sterile instruments and equipment, assists by providing the required sutures, drains, etc. and checks to ensure that all sponges[2] [ʌ], etc. are accounted for[3]
» *Have the scrub nurse label[4] [eɪ] the specimen[5] and send it to the lab.*

circulating nurse *n jar* *sim* **OR tech(nician)[1]** [teknɪʃᵊn] *n term*
(s)he manages the OR (proper temperature, lighting[2], availability of supplies[3], etc.) coordinates activities of lab or x-ray staff, and monitors aseptic practices to avoid breakdowns in technique[4]
» *The circulating nurse must observe the patient to ensure that his needs are provided for[5].*

operating table *n term*
special table on which the patient is positioned during the surgical procedure; sandbags, straps[1] and braces[2] [eɪs] may be used to keep the patient stable [eɪ] and comfortable
» *Proper positioning[3] of the patient on the operating table is crucial[4] [kruːʃᵊl].*
Use **to flex or break[5] [eɪ]/incline [aɪ] or tilt[6]/elevate[7] the operating table**

position *n & v term* *sim* **positioning[1]** *n term*, **place[2]** *v*
(n) depending on the procedure scheduled[3] [skǁʃedjuːld] the patient is brought into a position on the table which is as comfortable as possible (e.g. no undue[4] [ʌnduː] pressure on nerves), does not interfere [ɪɚ] with[5] respiration or circulation, and provides adequate exposure[6] [oʊʒ] of the operative field
reposition[7] *v term* • **repositioning** *n*
» *Improper positioning of the patient can result in immediate and long-term complications. The legs were positioned in stirrups[8] [ɜː].*
Use **to be in/bring into/place in/remain in /assume[9] [suː]/adopt[9] a position • satisfactory / patient positioning • change of[10] / left lateral[11] / supine[12] [aɪ]/ with the patient/foot (placed) in a ... position**

dorsal recumbent [ʌ] **position** *n term*
the standard position with the patient flat on the back, legs slightly flexed[1] and straddled[2]; one arm is placed palm[3] [pɑːm] down alongside the trunk[4] [ʌ] while the other is positioned on an armboard[5] for IV infusion
» *Laparoscopy is usually performed with the patient in the dorsal recumbent position.*

Trendelenburg('s) position *n term* *opposite* **reverse** [ɜː] **Trendelenburg position[1]** *n term*
supine position[2] on the operating table, which is inclined[3] [aɪ] so that the pelvis is higher than the head; the patient is supported by padded shoulder braces[4] [eɪ] and thigh [θaɪ] straps[5]
» *The Trendelenburg position is employed for procedures on the pelvis and lower abdomen to obtain good exposure by displacing[6] the intestines somewhat more cephalad[7] [sefəlæd].*

Anästhesist(in), Narkosearzt/ärztin
überwacht[1] überprüft[2] Narkosetiefe[3] diensthabende(r) Anästhesist(in)[4] Narkoseschwester /-pfleger[5] Diplom-, staatl. geprüfte(r) Krankenschwester /-pfleger[6]
 6

Abgrenzung d. Sterilbereichs, Sichtschutz z. Anästhesiebereich
Kontamination über die Atemluft verhindern[1] 7

Instrumentier-, OP-Schwester
auflegen[1] Tupfer[2] abgezählt[3] etikettieren[4] (Gewebe)probe[5]
 8

unsterile Hilfe
OP-(Ge)hilfe[1] Beleuchtung[2] Verfügbarkeit von OP-Bedarf[3] Verstöße gegen aseptische Kautelen / Vorsichtsmaßregeln[4] dass er entsprechend versorgt ist[5] 9

Operationstisch
Gurte[1] Stützen, Schienen[2] richtige Lagerung[3] sehr wichtig[4] O. knicken[5] O. neigen / kippen[6] O. anheben[7] 10

Lage, Position, Stellung; legen, positionieren
Lagerung[1] lagern[2] geplant[3] übermäßig[4] beeinträchtigen[5] Darstellung[6] umlagern[7] Fußstützen, -halter[8] Stellung einnehmen[9] Positionswechsel, Umlagerung[10] linke Seitenlage[11] Rückenlage[12]
 11

Rückenlage m. angewinkelten, gespreizten Beinen
angewinkelt[1] gespreizt[2] Handfläche[3] Rumpf[4] Armstütze[5]
 12

Kopftief-, Trendelenburglage
Anti-Trendelenburg-, Fußtieflage[1] Rückenlage[2] geneigt[3] gepolsterte Schulterstützen[4] Oberschenkelgurte[5] verlagern[6] nach kranial[7]
 13

lithotomy position n term   syn **dorsosacral** [eɪ] **position** n term
a supine position with the buttocks [ʌ] extending over the table[1], the hips and knees [iː z] are flexed at 90° and the feet held in position by strapping them to stirrups
» For nearly all rectal and vaginal [dʒ] operations the patient is brought into the lithotomy position.

Steinschnittlage
Gesäß bis an den Rand der Unterlage hervorgezogen[1]

14

semiprone [oʊ] or **English position** n term   syn **Sims'** or **lateral (recumbent) position** n term
the patient lies on the side with the under arm behind the body; the upper leg[1] is flexed more than the lower one; this is the position of choice for vaginal and rectal procedures (exams, enemas[2], etc)
» Delivery[3] may be accomplished[4] in either the lithotomy or the Sims' position.

Sims-Lage
Oberschenkel[1] Einläufe[2] Entbindung[3] erfolgreich durchgeführt[4]

15

lateral decubitus [uː] **position** n term   syn **flank** [æ] **position** n term
lateral recumbent position, but with the lower leg flexed, the upper leg extended, and the table broken at the patient's waistline[1] [eɪ]
» The flank position is used for nephrectomy. The patient is placed on his well side[2]. An intra-operative x-ray in the lateral decubitus position is usually the best way to assess[3] the problem.
Use left/right lateral / dorsal[4] / ventral[5] **decubitus position**

Seitenlage(rung)
Taille[1] gesunde Seite[2] abklären[3] Rückenlage[4] Bauchlage[5]

16

recovery [ʌ] **room** n clin, abbr **RR**   syn **postanesthesia** [-iːʒə] **recovery area** n term, abbr **PAR**
unit or room adjoining the ORs staffed and equipped with facilities[1] to provide optimal care during the recovery period[2] until the patient can be safely transferred[3] back to the surgical ward[4] [ɔː]
» While en route[5] from the OR to the recovery area the patient is accompanied by a physician. In the recovery room the anesthesiologist generally exercises primary responsibility[6].
Use **recovery** area / room nurse[7] / room staff • **recovery** system / score card[8]

Aufwachraum
Einrichtungen[1] Aufwachperiode[2] verlegt[3] chir. Station[4] auf dem Weg[5] hat die Hauptverantwortung[6] Aufwachschwester /-pfleger[7] Beurteilungsschema im Aufwachprotokoll[8]

17

recovery (room) bed n clin
special bed for patients in the immediate postoperative period; it is supplied with side rails[1] [eɪ] which can be raised[2] [eɪ], receptacles[3] for IV poles[4] [oʊ], and often has a chart [tʃ] storage rack[5]
» If the patient is unattended[6], the side rails of the recovery bed are placed in position[2].

Aufwachbett
seitl. Gitter[1] hochgezogen[2] Haltevorrichtung[3] Infusionsständer[4] Ablage f. Fieberkurve / Aufwachprotokoll[5] unbeaufsichtigt[6]

18

instrument cart [kɑːrt] n clin
small table on wheels on which the scrub nurse lays [leɪz] out the set of sterilized instruments; many other mobile[1] carts supplied with various special equipment are used in hospitals (e.g. the crash cart[2] for emergencies)
» Hospital ERs[3] usually have several crash carts equipped with analgesics, antiseptics, sponges[4] [ʌndʒ], swabs[5] [ɒː], hemostats[6] [iː], etc.

Instrumentenwagen
fahrbar[1] Notfallwagen[2] Notaufnahmen[3] chir. Tupfer[4] Tupfer (z. Desinfektion)[5] Gefäßklemmen[6]

19

Unit 24   Surgical Instruments
Related Units: 32 Dental Instruments, 22 Basic Operative Techniques

instrument n & v term   sim **instrumentation**[1], **instrumentarium**[2] n term
equipment[3], tools[4] or appliances[5] [aɪ] or any means [iː] used to perform surgical procedures
instrumental[6] adj genE & term
» The mobility of the tumor can be determined by manipulation with the tip of the instrument.
Use to sterilize/hand-wash/lay [eɪ] out[7]/sharpen/pass or insert[8]/scald[9] [ɒː] **instruments** • soiling[10] / successful passage / set[11] / stock[12] **of instruments** • dissecting[13] / gas sterilized [aɪ] / microsurgical / lensed[14] **instruments** • endoscopy / urethral [iː] **instrumentation** • **instrumental** birth[15] / perforation / malfunction • by **instrumental** means[16] • **instrument** tray[17]

Instrument; instrumentieren
Instrumentieren, -ation[1] Instrumentarium[2] Ausrüstung[3] Werkzeuge, Geräte[4] Vorrichtungen, Geräte[5] förderlich, behilflich; instrumentell[6] I. auflegen[7] I. einführen[8] I. thermisch desinfizieren[9] Kontamination von I.[10] Instrumentensatz, chir. Besteck[11] Instrumentenbestand[12] Präparierbesteck[13] optische Geräte[14] operative Entbindung[15] instrumentell[16] Instrumentenschale, -tray[17]

1

sharps n jar

instruments for cutting and transfixing[1] tissue that are razor [reɪzɚ] sharp[2] and therefore require special [eʃ] safeguards[3] for handling (often marked by a red stripe [aɪ] on the handle[4] and disposed of[5] in a sharps container)

Use **sharp** blade[6] [eɪ] / curette[7] / tip / dissection[8] / -edged[9] / -pointed

scharfe bzw. spitze Instrumente

durchstoßen, -stechen[1] messerscharf[2] Sicherung, Schutz[3] Griff[4] entsorgt[5] scharfe Klinge[6] scharfe Kürette[7] scharfes Präparieren[8] scharfkantig[9] 2

scalpel n term   syn knife [naɪf] n inf & jar

surgical knife usually with an interchangeable blade[1] and a straight handle or blade [eɪ] holder[2]

» A No. 15 blade is used to scrape[3] [eɪ] the lesion [iːʒ] until it is flat.

Use to cut/incise/excise/probe[4] **with a scalpel** • disposable[5] / dissecting[6] / micro/ cold / heated / laser-assisted **scalpel** • **knife** blade / point[7] / handle / edge[8] / needle • crescent[9] [s] / slit **blade** • needlepoint / spoon[10] [uː] / hook [ʊ] / gum[11] **knife**

Skalpell, chir. Messer

Wechselklinge[1] Klingenhalter[2] ausschaben[3] m. e. Skalpell sondieren[4] Einmalskalpell[5] Seziermesser[6] Messerspitze[7] Messerschneide[8] sichelförm. Klinge[9] scharfer Löffel[10] Zahnfleischmesser[11] 3

scissors [sɪzɚz] n pl   sim shears[1] [ɪɚ] n pl term

a cutting instrument with two crossed shearing blades which may have a sharp or blunt [ʌ] nose[2]

microscissors[3] [aɪ] n term • shear[4] v irr

» Do you want the scissors with dissecting or plain [eɪ] blades[5]?

Use a pair of long / short / curved[6] [ɜː]/ straight[7] **scissors** • medium-sized / heavy[1] [e]/ double-action / pointed / delicate or fine **scissors** • dissecting[8] / suture[9] [suːtʃɚ]/ ligature[10] [-tʃʊɚ] / wire cutting[11] / Metzenbaum **scissors** • bone[12] / rib / sternum [ɜː] / plaster[13] **shears**

Schere

(große / stabile) Schere[1] stumpfe Spitze[2] Mikroschere[3] scheren, schneiden[4] ungezahnte / glatte Schneidblätter[5] gebogene S.[6] gerade S.[7] Präparierschere[8] Naht-, Fadenschere[9] Ligaturschere[10] Draht(schneide)schere[11] Knochenschere[12] Gipsschere[13] 4

(surgical) needle [iː] n term → U26-1 ff   sim awl[1] [ɒːl] n term

sharp instrument used for puncturing [ʌ] and/or suturing; the shaft may be cutting or round-bodied; at the tip there is usually a tapered[2] [eɪ] point and the suture is threaded[3] [e] at the eye[4] or it is already swaged[5] [eɪdʒ] to the needle for atraumatic sewing[6] [oʊ] (so-called armed sutures[7])

needle-shaped adj term • needle-like adj • needling[8] n

» Precautions[9] [ɒː] must be taken against leaving needles, clamps, sponges, etc. inside the patient.

Use to pass/push/pull/rotate/withdraw[10] [ɒː] **the needle** • straight / curved / suture[11] / arterial [ɪɚ] suture[12] / intestinal or abdominal suture[13] / Reverdin / punch[14] [ʌ]/ swaged-on[15] **needle** • hollow / hypodermic[16] [aɪ]/ fine / large-bore[17] **needle** • **needle** count / point / shaft / site[18] [aɪ]/ holder

(chirurgische) Nadel

Ahle[1] spitz zulaufend[2] eingefädelt[3] Öhr[4] übergangslos verbunden[5] (Ver)nähen[6] armierte / atraumatische Nähte[7] Ritzen (m. N.), Punktion[8] (Sicherheits)vorkehrungen[9] N. zurückziehen / entfernen[10] Nähnadel[11] Gefäßnadel[12] Darmnadel[13] stanzende Biopsienadel[14] Nadel-Faden-Kombination, öhrlose Nadel[15] Injektionsnadel[16] großlumige Hohlnadel[17] Punktions-, Einstichstelle[18] 5

24

Curved atraumatic needle

cannula n term

tube introduced into a vessel, duct or body cavity

cannulate[1] v term • cannular adj • cannul(iz)ation n

» The cannula may be left in place for two weeks. Inability to cannulate the subclavian [eɪ] vein [eɪ] is among the most common technical [k] complications.

Use to insert or introduce[1]/place[2] **a cannula** • IV / central venous[3] [iː]/ (intra-)arterial / plastic / flexible / small-bore / 18-gauge[4] [geɪdʒ] / infusion[5] / needle-tipped **cannula** • suction[6] [sʌkʃən]/ nasal / wash or irrigating[7] / ointment[8] **cannula** • **cannula** insertion / removal • percutaneous [eɪ] **cannulation**

Kanüle, Hohlnadel

K. einführen[1] K. legen[2] zentraler Venenkatheter[3] Kanüle, Größe 18[4] Infusionskanüle[5] Saugkanüle[6] Spülkanüle[7] Salbenkanüle[8]

 6

Surgical Instruments

trocar [oʊ] *n term*   *sim* **stylet** or **stilet(te)**[1] [ˈstaɪlət] *n term*

metal tube (cannula) with a sharp-tipped, three-cornered obturator[2] (trocar) inside which is withdrawn after insertion; strictly speaking the complete instrument is termed trocar and cannula

» Seeds[3] [iː] are placed into the residual tumor[4] with a trocar.
Use to place/insert/introduce **a trocar** • working[5] **trocar** • **trocar** sheath[6] [iː] • floppy or flexible / introducing / lighted [aɪ]/ needle **stylet**

Trokar
Mandrin[1] Trokardorn m. Dreikantspitze[2] radioaktive Implantate[3] Resttumor[4] Arbeitstrokar[5] Trokarhülse[6]

7

probe [proʊb] *v & n term*   *syn* **sound** [aʊ] *n*, *sim* **director**[1] *n term* → U32-9

(v) to explore a wound [uː], duct [ʌ] or cavity (n) slender[2] instrument inserted for exploration[3] cryoprobe[4] *n term* • probing[5] *adj & n*

» Introduction of the probe is tricky[6] and care must be exercised to avoid perforation.
Use ultrasonic[7] / suction [ʌ]/ antrum[8] / rectal **probe** • blind[9] / gentle **probing** • uterine[10] [aɪ‖ɪ] **sound** • (rectal) grooved[11] [uː]/ hernia [ɜː] **director**

sondieren; Sonde
Führungs(hohl)sonde[1] fein[2] Austastung, Exploration[3] Kryo-, Kältesonde[4] sondierend; Sondierung[5] schwierig[6] Schallsonde[7] Kieferhöhlensonde[8] Sondieren ohne Sichtkontrolle[9] Uterussonde[10] Rektal-Hohlsonde[11]

8

hook [hʊk] *n & v*   *sim* **loop**[1] [luːp] *n*

(n) instrument with a curved[2] tip for elevating[3] or trapping[4] and ensnaring[5] [eɚ] tissues

» Foreign [ˈfɒrɪn] bodies[6] may be removed with a loop or a hook without irrigation.
Use wire[7] / suture[8] / tape / cautery[9] [ɒː]/ cord **loop** • right-angled [æŋgld]/ electrosurgical **hook** or **hook** electrode[9] • to place or ensnare in a **loop**[5]

Haken; festhaken
Schlinge[1] (auf)gebogen[2] anheben[3] fassen[4] anschlingen[5] Fremdkörper[6] Drahtschlinge[7] Nahtschlinge[8] Diathermieschlinge[9]

9

curet(te) [kjʊɚˈet] *v & n term*   *sim* **spoon** [uː] or **scoop**[1] [uː] *n jar*

(v) remove layers of tissue from a surface such as the uterus [juː]
(n) a long and thin spoon-shaped instrument
curettage [kjʊɚˈetɪdʒ] or curettment *n term* • scoop or scrape[2] [eɪ] *v jar & inf*

» Necrotic nodes should be curetted out. The curettings[3] were suggestive [dʒe] of[4] ectopic pregnancy.
Use skin / metal / blunt or dull[5] [ʌ]/ sharp / plastic **curette** • sharp / subgingival [-dʒɪndʒ-]/ cervical / root[6] / suction[7] **curettage** • dilatation and[8] **curettage** (abbr D & C)

kürettieren, auskratzen; Kürette
Löffel[1] auskratzen, -schaben[2] kürettiertes Gewebe[3] hindeuten auf[4] stumpfe K.[5] Wurzelglätten[6] Saugkürettage[7] Uterusdilatation u. -kürettage[8]

10

rongeur (forceps) [rɒːndʒɚ] *n term*   *sim* **bone chisel** [tʃɪzᵊl] or **osteotome**[1], **gouge**[2] [gaʊdʒ] *n term*

heavy-duty forceps for cutting bone, enamel[3], or other tough [tʌf] tissue;
an osteotome is a wedge-like[4] [dʒ] tool with a cutting edge at the tip of the blade

» A gouge is a hollow chisel for cutting away bone chips. Osteotome tips are not beveled[5]. Rongeurs were used to procure[6] [-kjʊɚ] small bone chips from bony protuberances.
Use bone[7] / intervertebral disk[8] / laminectomy[9] **rongeur** • rounded[2] / straight[10] **osteotome** • sternum / hemostatic[11] **chisel**

Knochen(fass-), Luer-Zange
Knochenmeißel, Osteotom[1] Hohlmeißel[2] (Zahn)schmelz[3] keilförmig[4] abgeschrägt[5] entnehmen[6] Hohlmeißel-, Luer-Knochenzange[7] Bandscheiben-Rongeur[8] Laminektomie-Stanze[9] Flachmeißel[10] Blutstillungsmeißel[11]

11

raspatory *n term*   *syn* **bone scraper, rasp, rugine** [ruːʒiːn] *n jar*, *sim* **file**[1] [faɪl] *n & v* → U32-12

hardened steel tool with cutting ridges used to lift or scrape away[2] periosteum;
files serve to smoothen[3] [uː] surfaces, e.g. of a tooth or root canal

» After lifting the periosteum with a raspatory, the implant bed was prepared. Alveoloplasty was performed using bone-cutting burs, rongeurs, and bone files.
Use bone / rib[4] / nasal[5] / antrum[6] **raspatory** • bone[7] / nail **file**

Raspatorium, Raspel, Schabeisen
Feile; feilen[1] abschieben, -präparieren[2] glätten[3] Rippenraspatorium[4] Nasenraspel[5] Antrumraspel[6] Knochenfeile[7]

12

grasper [æ] *n term & jar*   *syn* **grasping forceps** *n term*, *sim* **clamp**[1] *n term*, **tweezers**[2] [iː] *n clin pl*

instruments with two tongs[3] [ʌ] that can be clamped to lift, seize[4] [iː] or compress tissue
grasp[4] *v* • clamp[5] *v term* • cross-clamping[6] *n*

» The mucosa above the hemorrhoid is grasped with forceps. Gently [dʒ] spread [e] the clamp to dilate the vein. The duct proximal to the stone must be temporarily clamped. The appendix was serially clamped[7] and cut.
Use three-prong(ed)[8] [ɒː] **grasper** • to apply/place/release [iː] **clamps** • aortic cross-**clamping** • doubly[9] **clamped** • vascular[10] / right-angle / Kocher's / crushing[11] [ʌ]/ noncrushing[12] / towel[13] [aʊ]/ bulldog[14] **clamp**

Fasszange
Klemmzange, Klemme[1] Pinzette[2] Branchen[3] fassen[4] (ab)klemmen[5] vollständiges Abklemmen[6] mehrfach abgeklemmt[7] F. mit 3 Maulteilen[8] zweifach abgeklemmt[9] Gefäßklemme[10] scharfe K., Gewebe(fass)kl.[11] atraumatische K.[12] Tuchklemme[13] Bulldog-, Gefäßklemme[14]

13

Perioperative Care   GENERAL CLINICAL TERMS **91**

forceps [fɔːrseps] n pl term   sim **tweezers**[1] n clin, **applicator**[2] n term
  instruments with two blades to grasp or compress tissue or dressings[3] in surgery
  » It was done with a mosquito [k] forceps[4]. Tweezers are small forceps that can be held between the thumb [θʌm] and forefinger.
  Use to apply/place/release **forceps** • delivery[5] / high[6] / low / hemostatic[7] [iː]/ splinter[8] / dressing[9] / ear[10] / clip removing **forceps** • ring / cup / biopsy[11] [aɪ]/ nasal / polyp / tissue[12] **forceps** • smooth[13] [uː]/ toothed or hooked[14] / four-prong[15] / thread[16] [e]/ sterile [aɪ] **forceps** • cotton(-tipped)[17] / sonic / sealed [iː]/ laryngeal [dʒ] **applicator** • a pair of / fine tipped **tweezers**

Zange, Klemme, Pinzette
kleine Zange, Pinzette[1] Applikator[2] Wundauflagen[3] Moskitoklemme[4] Geburtszange[5] hohe Z.[6] Gefäßklemme[7] Splitterzange, -pinzette[8] Tupferzange[9] Ohrpinzette[10] Biopsiezange[11] Gewebefassz.[12] anatomische P., Gefäßp.[13] chirurgische P.[14] Vierkrallen-Fasspinzette[15] Fadenpinzette[16] Watteträger[17]   14

needle holder n term   syn **suture** [suːtʃɚ] **forceps** n
  forceps used to grasp the needle and pass it through the tissue

Nadelhalter
                                                                                         15

retractor n term   syn **tenaculum** n term
  pointed or hooked instrument used for holding the wound [uː] edges[1] apart[2] or vessels and other tissues out of the operative field; may have one or several claws [ɒː] or teeth[3] at either end
  retract[4] v term • retraction n
  » Retractors out! The vein was retracted medially. The injury was due to a misplaced retractor.
  Use sharp or toothed[5] / blunt[6] / (non-)malleable[7] / self-retaining[8] **retractor** • lip / cheek[9] /vaginal [dʒ]/ abdominal[10] **retractor** • **retracting** clamp

Wundhaken, -sperrer, -spreizer
Wundränder[1] auseinander[2] Zinken, Zähne[3] zurückziehen, auseinanderspreizen[4] scharfer / gezahnter Wundhaken[5] stumpfer W.[6] (nicht) federnder W.[7] selbsthaltender Wundspreizer[8] Wangen(ab)halter[9] Bauchdeckenhalter[10]   16

dila(ta)tor [daɪl(ət)eɪtɚ] n term   sim **bougie (boule)**[1] [buːʒɪ] n term
  instrument to expand and enlarge the diameter[2] [daɪæmətɚ] of a tube or passage [-ɪdʒ], e.g. a narrowed[3] duct
  dila(ta)te[4] v term • dila(ta)tion n • bougi(e)nage[5] [-ɑːʒ] n
  » How much dilatation is desirable? A 32F dilator was passed orally.
  Use anal[6] [eɪ]/ antegrade / retrograde / tent / Hegar's[7] **dilator** • dilating[1] / olive-tipped / medicated **bougie** • catheter / balloon[8] [uː] **dilation** • **dilation** and evacuation / of stricture [-ktʃɚ]

  Note: The F in 32F dilator stands for French, a measure to indicate the diameter or thickness of dilators, catheters, bougies and similar instruments.

Dilatator, Erweiterer, Dehner
(Dilatations)bougie, Dehnsonde[1] Durchmesser[2] verengt[3] dilatieren, aufdehnen, (sich) erweitern[4] Bougierung[5] Analdehner[6] HegarStift, -Uterusdilatator[7] Ballondilatation[8]

                                                                                         17

25

(surgical) sponge [spʌndʒ] n term & jar
  sterile, absorbent material used to control bleeding sites, mostly a compressed pad of aseptic gauze[1] [ɡɔːz] that swells[2] when moistened[3]
  » Dry sponges are used and weighed [weɪd] to estimate intraoperative blood loss. Sponge and needle count are correct.
  Use alcohol[4] / (sterile) gauze[5] **sponge** • **sponge** biopsy[6] [aɪə]/ count / forceps[7] / stick[8]

Tupfer
Verbandsmull, Gaze[1] (auf)quellen[2] befeuchtet[3] Alkoholtupfer[4] Gazekissen[5] Abstrich, Tupfpräparat[6] Tupferzange[7] Tupferträger[8]
                                                                                         18

Unit 25 Perioperative Care
Related Units: 21 Surgical Treatment, 23 The Surgical Suite, 27 Medical & Surgical Asepsis, 28 Wound Healing, Anesthesiology

preoperative assessment n term   syn **preoperative workup** n jar
  patient evaluation[1] including a detailed history[2], PE[3], and specific diagnostic investigations[4]
  » The nutritional [ɪʃ] status[5] [eɪ] of the patient is an essential factor in the preoperative workup. Additional workup including skin testing and a biopsy [aɪ] is required. The preoperative evaluation should be completed before hospitalization.
  Use to undergo or have[6] **a workup** • (non)emergency / initial / outpatient[7] / diagnostic[4] / routine / extensive / laboratory / complete urologic / prebiopsy **workup**

Anamnese u. präop. Diagnostik
Abklärung[1] Anamnese[2] körperl. Untersuchung, Status(erhebung)[3] diagnost. Untersuchungen[4] Ernährungsstatus[5] s. einer Durchuntersuchung unterziehen[6] ambulante Untersuchungen[7]   1

GENERAL CLINICAL TERMS — Perioperative Care

patient selection [sɪlɛkʃən] n term

select[1] v & adj • selective adj • unselectively adv

» Specific indications for the selection of patients for curative radiotherapy are listed below.

Use **in selected** patients[2] / cases • donor-recipient[3] [sɪ]/ drug **selection** • **selection** criteria[4] [aɪ] • **selective** angiography[5]

Patientenselektion
auswählen; -gewählt[1] bei ausgewählten Patienten[2] Spender-Empfänger-Auswahl[3] Selektions-, Auswahlkriterien[4] selektive Angiographie[5] 2

informed consent n term   sim **operative permit**[1] n term

agreement (usually in writing[2]) by a patient, guardian[3] [gɑːrdiən] or next of kin[4] to treatment suggested [dʒ] by the physician or surgeon

informed waiver[5] [eɪ] n term

» Informed consent must be based on a full discussion of the potential benefits[6], risks, and complications of the treatment proposed as well as a discussion of alternative options.

Use to obtain[7]/be (in)capable of giving / full / written / voluntary / presumed[8] **informed consent** • **informed consent** form[9] / for removal of tissue for grafting[10]

Einwilligung(serklärung) nach Aufklärung
Operationseinwilligung[1] schriftlich[2] gesetzliche(r) Vertreter(in), Vormund[3] Angehörige(r)[4] aufgeklärte Verzicht(s)erklärung[5] mögliche Vorteile[6] E. einholen[7] angenommene E.[8] Einwilligungsformular[9] E. zur Gewebeentnahme für e. Transplantation[10] 3

presurgical anxiety [æŋzaɪəti] n term

commonly includes emotional strain[1] [eɪ] created by the prospect[2] of surgery, worries about losing job, friends, etc.

» Anxiety and fear [fɪɚ] are normal in patients undergoing surgery[3]. Patients facing surgery[4] may be beset by[5] fears of anesthesia [-iːʒə], death, or cancer. Relieving anxiety[6] and restlessness[7] is one of the principal goals[8] [oʊ] of preoperative medication[9].

Operationsangst
emotionelle Belastung[1] Aussicht[2] s. einer Op. unterziehen[3] denen eine Op. bevorsteht[4] befallen von[5] Angstabbau[6] Unruhe[7] Hauptziele[8] Prämedikation[9] 4

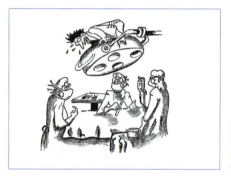

Proper psychological preparation for the operative stress includes permitting the patient some degree of anxiety, as it will eventually help him to develop effective ways of coping with the situation.

(operative) risk n & v term   sim **hazard**[1] n term

at-risk[2] adj term • high-/good-/poor-/low-risk[3] adj • risk-benefit ratio[4] [reɪʃioʊ] phr

» Their risk of acquiring [kwaɪ] cancer is two times that of age-matched controls[5]. Patients who have sustained[6] [eɪ] head injuries are at risk for/of spinal injury. This patient is a good operative risk[7]. The risks associated with the procedure are too high.

Use to face/run or take[8]/have/expose to/carry or involve[9]/avoid/lessen/reduce/minimize/eliminate **a risk** • (peri)operative / increased / long-term / overall[10] / potential / low **risk** • **high-risk** patient[11] • **risk** factor / group • life-threatening[12] [e] **hazard**

(Operations)risiko; Risiko eingehen
Risiko, Gefahr[1] Risiko-[2] risikoarm, m. geringem R.[3] Risiko-Nutzen-Verhältnis[4] Kontrollpersonen[5] erlitten[6] hat ein sehr geringes Operationsrisiko[7] R. eingehen[8] mit R. verbunden sein[9] Gesamtrisiko[10] Risikopatient(in)[11] lebensbedrohliche Gefahr[12] 5

preoperative bowel [baʊəl] **preparation** n term   syn **bowel prep** n jar

in elective procedures[1] most patients are put on a light diet[2] or fasted[3] overnight and may be given a cleansing [e] enema[4] the evening before; esp. for intestinal surgery mechanical [k] cleansing of the bowels[5], laxatives[6], or whole-gut [ʌ] lavage[7] [ləvɑːʒ] and systemic antibiotics may be required

» Measures taken to eliminate the fecal mass[8] [iː] and reduce the number of bacteria [ɪɚ] as much as possible prior [aɪ] to surgery[9] are known as the "bowel prep".

präop. Darmentleerung
elektive Eingriffe[1] auf leichte Kost gesetzt[2] nüchtern bleiben müssen[3] Klistier, Einlauf[4] Darmreinigung[5] Abführmittel[6] Darmspülung[7] Stuhl[8] präoperativ[9] 6

Perioperative Care　　　　　　　　　　　　　　　　　　　　　　　　　　　GENERAL CLINICAL TERMS 93

postoperative course [kɔːrs] *n term*

progress[1] the patients makes after the operation (surgical outcome, convalescence[2] [-esəns], complications)

» *The appearance of a* pleural [ʊɚ] *effusion[3] late in the postoperative course suggested[4] the presence of a subdiaphragmatic* [aɪə] *inflammation. At this time the surgeon should explain the operation and the expected postoperative course to the patient.*

Use smooth [uː] or uneventful or uncomplicated[5] **course** • preoperative **course**

postanesthetic observation *n term*　　*syn* **monitoring** *n,*
　　　　　　　　　　　　　　　　　　sim **surveillance**[1] [sɚveɪləns] *n term*

as the patient recovers from the effects of the anesthetic[2] the vital [aɪ] signs[3] [aɪ] are closely watched; in some patients invasive [eɪ] monitoring, cardiopulmonary [ʊ‖ʌ] support and critical care management[4] are required

observe[5] *v* • observer *n* • monitor[6] *v & n term*

» *Appearance of a mass while the patient is under observation may be a sign of local perforation. Pulse* [ʌ] *oximetry is increasingly becoming a standard of care in patient monitoring during general anesthesia.*

Use period of / close[7] / continuous[8] / frequent **observation** • cardiac[9] / Holter **monitor** • hourly[10] [aʊɚli]/ hemodynamic [iː]/ intraoperative **monitoring**

complication *n term*
　　　　　　　　sim **sequel** [siːkwəl] *or* **sequela**[1] [sɪkwelə] *n term* -ae [iː] *pl*

(i) generally the occurrence [ɜ] of concomitant disorders[2] in a patient (ii) in surgery, any intra- or postoperative event, injury or disorder that sets back[3] or delays the patient's convalescence

(un)complicated[4] *adj* • uneventful[5] *adj*

» *Complications are most common on the 2nd to 5th postoperative days. Major bleeding is the most worrisome[6] complication. Vitreous* [ɪ] *hemorrhage is a common sequela. The postoperative course was uneventful.*

Use to avoid[7]/prevent/preclude[8]/suspect/develop/lead to/contribute to[9]/be due to[10] **complications** • rare / minor [aɪ] / serious [ɪɚ]/ life-threatening[11] [e]/ anesthetic-related / late[12] / wound [uː] **complication** • **complication** rate[13] [eɪ] • **(un)complicated** postoperative course / delivery[14] / fracture • long-term[15] **sequelae**

adhesion [ædhiːʒ³n] *n term*　　*sim* **adherence**[1] [ɪɚ] *n term*

two surfaces which are normally separate adhere to each other[2] due to scar formation[3], e.g. after abdominal surgery; adhesions which produce intestinal obstruction [ʌ] have to be released[4] [iː] on repeat [iː] surgery[5]

adhesiolysis[6] [-pːlɪsiːz] *n term* • adherent[7] *adj* • adhesio- *comb*

» *Formation of adhesions acquired from abdominal operations is more commonly seen in adults.*

Use to form/produce/cause/develop/prevent/free[8]/lyse[8] [aɪs‖z] **adhesions** • fibrous [aɪ]/ bowel[9] [baʊəl]/ inflammatory **adhesions** • **adhesio**tomy[6]

postoperative hospitalization *or* **hospital stay** [steɪ] *n term*

time of required postop inpatient care[1] (observation and treatment) until discharge[2] [dɪstʃɑːrdʒ]

» *Early surgery can reduce the length of postoperative hospitalization by[3] 5-7 days. In the event of[4] complications the hospital stay will be longer. The laparoscopic technique reportedly achieves similar results with a shorter hospital stay and convalescence.*

Use short / prolonged[5] / reduced **hospital stay**

postoperative oral intake *n term*

most patients are first put on TPN[1] or a clear liquid diet[2] [daɪət] and only gradually resume regular oral intake[3]

» *These patients do not benefit from[4] total parenteral nutrition[1] and can resume an oral diet.*

Use (un)restricted[5] / permissible[6] **oral intake** • fluid[7] / protein / nutrient[8] / salt **intake**

postoperativer Verlauf
Fortschritte[1] Rekonvaleszenz[2] Pleuraerguss[3] deutete hin auf[4] komplikationsfreier Verlauf[5]

7

postop. Überwachung
Beobachtung[1] Anästhetikum[2] Vitalfunktionen[3] Intensivtherapie[4] beobachten[5] überwachen; Monitor, Überwachungsgerät[6] intensive Ü.[7] ständige Ü.[8] Herzmonitor[9] stündliche Überprüfung[10]

8

Komplikation
Folge(erscheinung)[1] Begleiterkrankungen[2] zurückwerfen[3] komplikationslos, -frei[4] unauffällig[5] beunruhigend[6] Komplikationen vermeiden[7] K. ausschließen[8] zu K. beitragen[9] auf K. zurückzuführen sein[10] lebensbedrohliche K.[11] Spätkomplikation[12] Komplikationsrate[13] schwierige/komplikationslose Entbindung[14] Langzeitfolgen[15]

9

Verwachsung, -klebung, Adhäsion
Anhaftung, Adhärenz[1] miteinander verkleben[2] Narbenbildung[3] gelöst[4] Reoperation[5] Adhäsiolyse, Lösen v. Adh.[6] adhärent, verklebt, -wachsen[7] Verwachsungen lösen[8] Darmadhäsionen[9]

10

postop. Krankenhausaufenthalt
stationäre Behandlung[1] Entlassung[2] um[3] bei (Auftreten von)[4] längerer Krankenhausaufenthalt[5]

11

postop. Nahrungsaufnahme
künstl. Ernährung[1] flüssige Nahrung (ohne Einlage)[2] zur normalen Kost zurückkehren[3] profitieren von[4] eingeschränkte N.[5] erlaubte N.[6] Flüssigkeitszufuhr[7] Nährstoffzufuhr[8]

12

25

94 GENERAL CLINICAL TERMS — Perioperative Care

ambulation *n term sing* *sim* **mobilization**[1] *n term* | **Umhergehen, Mobilisation**
Mobilisation, -sierung[1] umhergehen[2] bettlägrig[3] mobilisieren[4] gehfähig, mobil; ambulant[5] Bettruhe[6] Gehen m. Krücken[7] ausgelöst durch[8] Frühmobilisation[9] vorsichtige Belastung[10] übermäßige Mobilis.[11] gehfähige(r) Patient(in)[12] ambulante Behandlung[13]

walking about[2] and not confined [aɪ] to bed[3] (e.g as a result of surgery or disease)
ambulate[2] *v term* • mobilize[4] *v* • ambulatory[5] *adj*

» Initial treatment consists of bed rest[6] for a few days followed by ambulation on crutches[7] [ʌtʃ]. Vomiting was precipitated[8] by ambulation. The catheter can be removed if the patient is expected to ambulate. Dietary measures [eʒ], early mobilization[9] and active rehabilitation are essential in all cases. Gradual mobilization with protected weight [weɪt] bearing[10] [eɚ] follows.

Use early[9] / crutch[7] / indoor / progressive / limited / prolonged **ambulation** • controlled / exaggerated[11] [ædʒ]/ passive **mobilization** • **ambulatory** patient[12] / care[13] / therapy / monitoring

13

return to normal activity *phr term* *sim* **recovery**[1] [ʌ], **recuperation**[1] [uː], **convalescence**[1] *n clin*

Wiederaufnahme d. Aktivitäten d. tägl. Lebens
Genesung, Rekonvaleszenz[1] fortschreitende Besserung[2] genesen, sich erholen; etw.wiedererlangen[3] genesend; Rekonvaleszent(in)[4] minimal invasive Chirurgie[5] Amputierte[6] Genesungszeit[7] Sehkraft wiedererlangen[8] Genesung beschleunigen[9] G. verzögern[10] Spontanheilung[11] Erholungsheim[12]

progressive improvement[2] as the symptoms disappear and body functions return to normal
convalesce[3] [-les] *v* • convalescent[4] *adj & n* • recuperate[3] *v* • recover[3] *v i/t*

» Recuperation and return to normal activity are usually faster in minimal access surgery[5]. Most patients improve sufficiently [ɪʃ] to return to full activity. In these young amputees[6] anything but return to full function is not acceptable.

Use **time to** recovery[7] / disease progression / recurrence • **to recover** from an illness / one's eyesight[8] [-saɪt] • to resume **normal activities** • to accelerate[9] [kse]/promote/delay[10] [eɪ]/prolong **recovery** • partial / (in)complete / prompt / quick or rapid • spontaneous[11] [eɪ] / functional **recovery** • hope / chance / period[7] [ɪɚ] extent **of recovery** • **convalescent** stage / period[7] / home[12]

14

postoperative follow-up *n term* *syn* **followup**, *abbr* **f/u** *or* **F/U**

Nachuntersuchung, -sorge, Verlaufskontrolle
nachuntersuchen, Verlaufsk. durchführen[1] terminisiert[2] zur Nachsorge kommen[3] prakt. Arzt, Hausarzt[4] Verlaufskontrollstudie[5] zur Nachsorge überweisen[6] zur Nachsorge entlassen werden[7] Nachuntersuchungstermin[8] intensive Nachsorge[9] ambulante N.[10] bei der / zum Zeitpunkt der Nachunters.[11]

examining, monitoring or observing the progress made by the patient in the postoperative course
follow[1] *v term*

» Follow-up visits should be scheduled[2] [sk‖ʃ] at 4- to 6-week intervals. The patient was advised to seek followup consultation[3] with his primary-care physician[4]. This is a 10-year follow-up study[5].

Use to require/receive/arrange/refer for[6]/be discharged [-tʃɑːrdʒd] to[7] **follow-up** • **follow-up** examination / care / appointment[8] / instructions / period / evaluation / testing • long-term / 5-year / telephone / periodic / close[9] / daily / outpatient[10] **followup** • at[11] **followup**

15

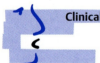

Clinical Phrases

Are you on any medication? Nehmen Sie irgendwelche Medikamente? • Nurse, please prepare Mr. Smith for a colectomy on Monday. Schwester, bereiten Sie bitte Herrn S. für die am Montag geplante Kolektomie vor. • The patient was put on a clear liquid diet. Der Patient bekam nur flüssige Nahrung. • Early ambulation should be encouraged. Der Patient sollte möglichst früh mobilisiert werden. • Mrs. Moore has made a complete recovery. Frau M. ist vollkommen wiederhergestellt. • Ten out of 154 patients were lost to followup. Zehn von 154 Patienten erschienen nicht mehr zur Nachuntersuchung. • Followups were performed at 6 and 12 months postoperatively. Verlaufskontrollen wurden 6 und 12 Monate nach dem chirurgischen Eingriff durchgeführt.

GENERAL CLINICAL TERMS 95

Unit 26 Sutures & Suture Material
Related Units: 22 Basic Operative Techniques, 28 Wound Healing, 24 Surgical Instruments

suture [suːtʃɚ] *n & v term*   *syn* **stitch** [stɪtʃ] *n & v clin & jar*

(n, i) the seam[1] [iː] formed by surgical sewing[2] [oʊ] (ii) material used to approximate[3] wound [uː] edges (iii) a suture joint, e.g. in bones of the skull (v) closing a wound or surgical incision with surgical stitches

suturing *n term* • sutureless *adj* • resuture *v*

» The subcutaneous tissue should always be sutured, care being taken to "bury" [e] the knot[4] [nɒːt]. Facial [eɪʃ] skin sutures should be removed no later than on the 4th day. The suture is placed so that it does not break[5] or pull free[6].

Use to apply or place[7]/tie [aɪ]/secure[8]/remove or take out[9] **sutures** • **to suture** into place • approximation[10] / subcutaneous / fine[11] / buried[12] [e] **suture** • vascular / layered[13] [eɪ]/ relaxation[14] / fixation[15] **suture** • inverting[16] / primary[17] / delayed[18] [eɪ]/ (double) armed[19] **suture** • **suture** closure / material / line • to place or take[7] **stitches** • **stitch** abscess • **suturing** instruments / in layers[20]

(i,ii) Naht(material) (iii) Sutura; Naht legen, (an)nähen
Naht[1] chir. Nähen[2] adaptieren[3] Knoten versenken[4] reißen[5] aufgehen[6] Nähte legen[7] N. sichern[8] N. entfernen[9] Situations-, Adaptationsnaht[10] feines Nahtmaterial[11] versenkte Naht[12] Schicht-, Etagennaht[13] Entlastungsnaht[14] Haltenaht[15] invertierende N.[16] Primärnaht[17] aufgeschobene Primärnaht[18] armierte Naht[19] schichtweiser Wundverschluss[20]   1

-rrhaphy [rəfi] *comb*

word ending denoting surgical suturing, e.g. neurorrhaphy[1] [ʊɚ] is a nerve suture or neurosuture[1]

herniorrhaphy [ɜː] *n term* • tenorrhaphy[2] • colporrhaphy

» The duration of immobilization after tenorrhaphy is generally for no more than 3-4 weeks.

-naht, -rrhaphie
Nervennaht[1] Sehnennaht[2]

2

ligate [laɪɡeɪt] *v term*   *rel* **tie** [taɪ] **off** *v phr jar*

(i) tying a blood vessel, pedicle[1], etc. with a suture or wire to constrict it
(ii) in dentistry, using a wire [aɪ] to secure[2] an orthodontic attachment to an archwire[3]

clip[4]-/suture[5]-ligate *v term* • ligature[6] [ɪ] *n & v* • ligation[7] [aɪ] *n*

» The common hepatic artery can be safely ligated. Venous injuries are best managed by ligation. Now the umbilical [ʌ] cord[8] can be ligated.

Use to do/place/apply/anchor[9] [k] **a ligature** • **ligature** loop[10] [uː]/ needle / wire[11] [aɪ] • tubal[12] / varix / caval[13] [eɪ]/ high / suture[14] / rubber band[15] / occluding **ligature** • suture / proximal **ligation** • doubly / clamped and[16] **ligated**

ab-, unterbinden, Ligatur legen, ligieren
Gefäßstiel[1] befestigen[2] Drahtbogen[3] clippen, m. Clip ligieren[4] umstechen, Umstechungsnaht setzen[5] Ligatur (legen)[6] Unterbindung[7] Nabelschnur[8] L. sichern[9] Ligaturschlinge[10] Ligaturendraht[11] Tubenunterbindung[12] Vena cava-Ligatur[13] Umstechung[14] elast. Ligatur[15] abgeklemmt und ligiert[16]   3

secure [sɪkjʊɚ] *v & adj term*   *rel* **tack**[1] *v jar*

(v) to fix or attach firmly (adj) safe

» Use staples[2] [eɪ] to secure a patch of mesh[3] over the internal inguinal ring. Take care to repair the fascial [ʃ] defect securely. Bleeding points were secured. The flap[4] is tacked into position.

Use secured in place[5] / with tape • secure closure[6] [ʒ] • securely knotted[7] [nɒːt] • tacking suture[8]

sichern; sicher
anheften, klammern[1] Klammern[2] Meshtransplantat[3] Lappen[4] fixiert[5] sicherer (Wund)verschluss[6] fest verknotet[7] Heftnaht[8]

4

26

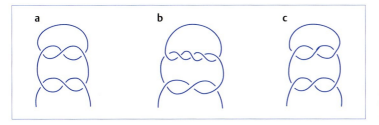

a square knot
b surgical knot
c false knot

GENERAL CLINICAL TERMS — Sutures & Suture Material

coapt [kouæpt] *v term*   *sim* **(re)approximate¹, appose¹** *v term*

to join or fit together two surfaces or stumps² [ʌ], e.g. a severed³ nerve or wound margins⁴ [dʒ]

coaptation⁵ *n term* • (re)approximation *n* • apposition⁶ *n* • apposing *adj*

» The skin edges can be approximated with tapes. Sutures should accurately appose skin edges without undue⁷ tension. Meticulous⁸ nerve coaptation is essential.

Use proper / incomplete **coaptation** • **coaptation** suture⁹ / splint¹⁰ • to achieve *or* obtain *or* bring into¹¹ / close / accurate **approximation** *or* **apposition**

adaptieren

(wieder) annähern, adaptieren¹ Stümpfe² durchtrennt³ Wundränder⁴ Koaptation, (Nerven)adaptation⁵ Apposition, Anlagerung⁶ übermäßig⁷ exakt⁸ Stoß-auf-Stoß-Naht⁹ Führungsschiene¹⁰ (wieder) vereinigen, aneinanderlegen¹¹   5

---

knot [nɒːt] *v & n term*   *syn* **tie** *v jar*

(v) to tie and fix suture ends (n) the result of knot-tying

knot-tying¹ *n term* • knotting¹ *n* • slipknot² *n*

» Synthetic sutures must be knotted at least four times. To tie a surgical knot³ the thread [e] is passed twice through the first loop⁴ [uː] and then once through the second. The suture knots should be placed on the outside.

Use to tie/tighten⁵ [aɪt]/secure/cinch⁵ [sɪntʃ] *a knot* • to pull a *knot* taut⁵ [ɒː]/tight⁵ • surgeon's³ / double / square⁶ [eɚ]/ microsurgical [aɪ]/ false⁷ [ɔː] *knot*

(ver)knoten -knüpfen; Knoten

Knoten(technik)¹ Schiebeknoten² chir. Knoten³ Schlinge⁴ K. zuziehen⁵ Schifferknoten⁶ Weiberknoten⁷   6

---

suture material *n*   *sim* **thread¹** [e], **strand¹** [æ], **filament¹** *n term*

monofilament² *adj term* • multifilament *or* braided³ [eɪ] *adj*

» Monofilament plastic will not harbor⁴ bacteria. Sutures are available in various diameters⁵ (e.g fine 8-0 sutures) and tensile [ɪ] strengths⁶. Even buried nylon sutures are better tolerated than braided or absorbable sutures. Wait a few minutes to allow the suture material to swell⁷.

Note: The caliber of suture lines⁵ ranges from fine 10-0 to coarse⁸ [ɔː] 2-0 and 0 to 4 (the largest) sutures.

Nahtmaterial

Faden¹ monofil² multifil, geflochten³ enthalten, beherbergen⁴ Fadenstärke, -durchmesser⁵ Zugfestigkeit⁶ quellen lassen⁷ dick⁸   7

---

absorbable *adj term*   *opposite* **non-absorbable¹** *adj term*

type of suture material that can be digested² [daɪdʒestɪd] by the body and need not be removed

resorb³ *v term* • resorption *n*, *espBE* absorption

» The urethra [iː] is closed with a single layer of 4-0 absorbable suture. Extra precautions⁴ [ɒːʃ] include using nonabsorbable suture materials for fascial [æʃ] closure. Catgut⁵ will eventually⁶ resorb but the resorption time⁷ is highly variable.

resorbierbar

nicht resorbierbar¹ abgebaut² resorbieren³ Vorsichtsmaßnahmen⁴ Katgut⁵ schließlich⁶ Resorptionszeit⁷   8

---

catgut [kætgʌt] *n term*

traditional absorbable suture material; catgut is a misnomer¹ as it is usually made from the intestines of sheep or cattle²

» There is little use for catgut sutures in modern surgery. I generally use interrupted 4-0 chromic catgut sutures³ to close the mucosal edges of the renal pelvis. Modern synthetic suture materials are clearly superior [ɪɚ] to⁴ catgut for fascial closure.

Use plain⁵ [eɪ]/ hardened / chromic³ **catgut** • **catgut** suture / thread

Katgut, Catgut

irreführende Bezeichnung¹ Rinder² Chromkatgut(nähte)³ besser als, überlegen⁴ reines K.⁵   9

---

synthetic [sɪnθetɪk] *adj term*   *opposite* **organic¹** *adj term*

common synthetic suture materials are prolene, nylon and Surgilon (nonabsorbable) and Vicryl, PDS, and Dexon (absorbable); types of organic suture materials include silk², cotton³ and catgut

» Synthetic nonabsorbable materials are mostly inert⁴ [ɜː] and retain⁵ [eɪ] tensile strength longer.

Use Monocryl / GORE-TEX / Teflon-coated⁶ [oʊ] polyester⁶ / black silk (*abbr* BSS) *suture*

synthetisch

organisch¹ Seide² Baumwolle³ biologisch inaktiv / reaktionslos⁴ behalten⁵ teflonbeschichtete Polyesternaht⁶   10

---

seal [siːl] *v & n term*   *syn* **seal over** *v phr jar & inf* → U34-16

(v) to achieve a tight closure (n) tight closure

sealant¹ [siːlənt] *n term*

» Fibrin [aɪ] glue² [gluː] is a useful operative sealant to achieve hemostasis³ [iː] in a variety [aɪ] of procedures. Perforations may be sealed by omentum. The leak⁴ [iː] in the ureter was effectively sealed.

Use to produce a **seal** • water-⁵/air-tight⁶ [taɪt] / hermetic *seal*

abdichten, (dicht) verschließen; Verschluss, -siegelung

(Ab)dichtungsmittel, Versiegler¹ Fibrinkleber² zur Blutstillung³ Leck, undichte Stelle⁴ wasserdichter Verschluss⁵ luftdichter V.⁶   11

Sutures & Suture Material   GENERAL CLINICAL TERMS **97**

staple [steɪəl] *n & v term*

(n) U-shaped metal (mostly stainless steel[1]) applied in rows[2] [oʊ] or circles with a stapling device[3] [aɪs] to approximate wounds or cut edges[4]

stapler[3] *n term* • stapling *n* • (double-)stapled *adj*

» Then the graft can be stapled into place and dressed with pressure. Use staples to secure the patch of mesh. Now you can fire[5] the staples. Two 10-cm rows[2] of staples are placed adjacent [dʒeɪs] to each other[6].

Use to place or apply[7]/remove **staples** • absorbable **staples** • **staple** line / disruption[8] [ʌ] • **stapled** closure / anastomosis • GIA (gastrointestinal anastomosis) / TA (tissue autosuture) / end-to-end **stapler**

Klammer; klammern, Klammernaht anlegen
rostfreier Stahl[1] Reihen[2] Klammernahtgerät[3] Schnittränder[4] einschießen[5] nebeneinander[6] Klammern setzen[7] Aufgehen von Klammern[8]

12

clip *n & v term*

(n) mostly metal clasp-like surgical device used for hemostasis or approximation of cut edges
(v, i) to place clips (ii) in genE to trim or shorten hair, fingernails, etc.

clip-ligate *v term* • clip applier[1] *n*

» Control the leak by application of stainless steel clips directly to the bleeding vessels.

Use to fire or place or apply[2]/transect between[3] **clips** • a rack of[4] **clips** • wound / occlusive[5] / towel[6] [taʊəl]/ metal / absorbable / titanium **clip** • **clip** forceps [s] or holder[7] • multi-load[8] **clip applier**

Clip, Klammer, Klemme;
(i) Clip setzen, (ab)klemmen
(ii) (zurück)schneiden
Clip-Applikator[1] Clips setzen[2] zwischen Clips absetzen[3] Clip-Magazin[4] Gefäß-, Ligaturclip[5] Tuchklemme[6] Clipzange[7] Mehrfachapplikator[8]

13

fibrin [faɪbrɪn] **glue** [gluː] *n term*

blood product rich in[1] fibrinogen [faɪbrɪnədʒən] and admixed[2] with thrombin [θ] used to coagulate surgical wounds

» Fibrin glue can be made from the patient's own blood donated[3] at least three days before surgery. Instillation of fibrin glue directly into the fistula is still a matter of controversy.

Use **fibrin** spray gun / foam[4] [oʊ]

Fibrinkleber
reich an[1] durchmischt[2] gespendet[3] Fibrinschaum[4]

14

interrupted [ʌ] **suture** *n term*   *sim* **over-and-over suture**[1] *n term*

single sutures each of which is tied separately with a surgical knot

» Small wounds are ideally closed with fine interrupted sutures placed loosely[2] and conveniently [iː] close[3] to the wound edges. We prefer a running 2-0 Prolene fascial closure [-ɜɚ] reinforced[4] with interrupted polyglycolate [aɪ] suture to ensure [-ʃʊɚ] a dry wound.

Einzelknopfnaht
Knopfnaht[1] lose[2] entsprechend nahe[3] verstärkt[4]

15

running [ʌ] or **continuous suture** *n term*
                          rel **(inter)locking** or **lock-stitch suture**[1] *n term*

uninterrupted series of stitches with a single suture the ends of which are fastened [fæsnd] by a knot[2]

» A running permanent suture can also be used and pulled out after healing has progressed. The pouch[3] [paʊtʃ] is then closed with two layers of 3-0 PGA running sutures to ensure water-tightness of the closure.

Use **running** lock-stitch suture[4] • plain or simple[5] **continuous suture** • **locking** running suture[4]

fortlaufende Naht
eingewendelte Naht[1] verknotet[2] Tasche[3] eingewendelte Fortlaufnaht[4] einfache fortlaufende N.[5]

16

mattress suture *n term*   *syn* **quilt(ed)** [kwɪlt] **suture** *n jar*

double stitch that forms a loop[1] [uː] about the tissue on both sides of a wound

» A horizontal running mattress suture is useful to produce eversion [ɜː] of the skin edges[2]. Buried [e] half-mattress (flap) sutures are recommended for tacking skin flaps into position.

Use interrupted / continuous / vertical / horizontal **mattress suture**

Matratzennaht
Schlinge[1] Ausstülpung der Wundränder[2]

17

purse-string [ɜː] **suture** *n term*

circular [sɜː] continuous suture used for closure of openings, e.g. in hernias[1] [ɜː] or appendectomy

» Create [krɪeɪt] a purse-string type of stitch around the cervix[2] [sɜːr]. High ligation of the hernia sac was performed with a purse-string suture of 3-0 silk.

Raff-, Tabakbeutelnaht
Hernien, Brüche[1] Gebärmutterhals, Zervix[2]

18

26

figure-of-eight suture n term

a stitch in which the thread begins at the deepest layer on each side of a wound and crosses over to the superficial layers on the opposite side following the contours of the figure 8; used, e.g. to close muscle and fascial layers of an abdominal incision

» *Definite hemostasis can be achieved* [tʃiː] *with figure-of-eight sutures or hemostatic clips. Repair by wire cerclage¹* [sɜːrklɑːʒ] *or figure-of-eight wire is preferred.*

Achternaht
Drahtcerclage¹

19

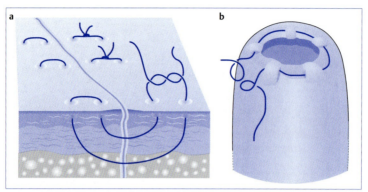

a interrupted mattress suture
b purse-string suture

Unit 27 Medical & Surgical Asepsis
Related Units: 25 Perioperative Care, 23 The Surgical Suite, 28 Wound Healing

aseptic [eɪ‖əseptɪk] adj term   opposite septic¹ adj term

aseptic surgical techniques involve precautions² [ɒː] against the introduction of infectious [-fekʃəs] agents [eɪ]

asepsis³ n term • sepsis⁴ n • antisepsis⁵ n • antiseptic⁶ adj & n

» *Strict aseptic technique is of critical importance in catheterization. The wound* [uː] *was aseptically dressed⁷. In these critically septic patients the mortality rate is 30%.*
Use to render⁸ **aseptic** • to adhere [ɪɚ] to **aseptic** techniques⁹ • **aseptic** surgery / wound / fever [iː] • surgical / medical **asepsis** • to observe⁹/maintain/relax **aseptic precautions** • **septic** complications / patient / process / shock¹⁰ / wound • localized / generalized / abdominal / late / deep¹¹ / lethal [iː] **sepsis** • bowel [aʊ] **antisepsis** • **antiseptic** solution / gauze¹² [ɒː]/ cleansing [e]/ dressing¹³ • skin¹⁴ / topical / urinary [jʊ] **antiseptic**

keimfrei, aseptisch, steril
septisch, verunreinigt, nicht keimfrei¹ Sicherheitsmaßnahmen² Asepsis, Keimfreiheit³ Sepsis, Blutvergiftung⁴ Antisepsis⁵ keimtötend, antiseptisch; Antiseptikum⁶ verbunden⁷ keimfrei machen, sterilisieren⁸ s. an die asept. Kautelen / Vorsichtsmaßregeln halten⁹ septischer Schock¹⁰ schwere Sepsis¹¹ antiseptische Gaze¹² a. (Wund)verband¹³ Hautdesinfektionsmittel¹⁴

1

sterile [sterəl‖aɪl] adj term   opposite non-sterile, contaminated¹ adj term

(i) free from micro-organisms and their spores²; aseptic (ii) infertile [-əl‖aɪl]
(re)sterilize³ [-laɪz] v term • sterilization⁴ n • sterility⁵ n • sterilizer⁶ n

» *Although much of the OR environment* [aɪ] *is sterile, the operative field itself is not. This must be done under sterile conditions. Total sterilization by this method requires 10 hours.*
Use **sterile** field⁷ / dressing / fluid • **sterilized** equipment / syringe⁸ [sɪrɪndʒ]/ enema set⁹ / catheter • to (with)stand¹⁰ **sterilization** • dry heat or hot air¹¹ / saturated steam¹² [iː]/ safe **sterilization** • (in)adequately **sterilized** • **sterilizing** chamber¹³ [tʃeɪ-]

(i) steril, keimfrei
(ii) steril, unfruchtbar
kontaminiert, verunreinigt¹ Sporen² sterilisieren, entkeimen³ Sterilisation, -sierung⁴ Sterilität, Keimfreiheit⁵ Sterilisator⁶ steriler Bereich⁷ st. Spritze⁸ st. Einlaufgerät / Irrigator⁹ sterilisierbar sein¹⁰ Heißluftsterilisation¹¹ Dampfsterilisation¹² Sterilisierbehälter, -trommel¹³

2

autoclave [ɒːtəkleɪv] n & v term

(n) apparatus [æ‖eɪ] for sterilizing instruments with superheated¹ steam [iː] under pressure; the articles are inserted in a wire [aɪ] basket and wrapped² [ræ] if necessary
autoclaving n term • autoclavable³ adj

» *Gas sterilization of materials that cannot withstand autoclaving⁴ has largely replaced soaking* [oʊ] *in antiseptics⁵.*
Use high-pressure⁶ / high-vacuum / gas **autoclave**

Autoklav; autoklavieren
sehr heiß¹ eingehüllt, verpackt² autoklavierbar³ nicht autoklavierbar sein⁴ in keimtötende Flüssigkeiten legen⁵ Hochdrucksterilisator⁶

3

Medical & Surgical Asepsis — GENERAL CLINICAL TERMS

disposable *adj term*   opposite **reusable**[1] [riːjuːzəbl] *adj term*

materials and instruments that cannot withstand sterilization and must be discarded[2] after single use

dispose of[3] *v* • disposal[4] *n* • discard *v*

» New guidelines [aɪ] for disposal of materials contaminated by bacteria have been established[5].

Use **disposable** equipment / drapes[6] [eɪ]/ gloves[7] [ʌ]/ cannula • **reusable** appliances [aɪ] • sewage[8] [suːɪdʒ] / waste[9] **disposal**

Einmal-, Einweg-
wiederverwendbar[1] weggeworfen[2] entsorgen[3] Entsorgung, Beseitigung[4] festgelegt[5] Einmal-Abdecktücher[6] Einmalhandschuhe[7] Abwasserentsorgung[8] Müllentsorgung[9]
4

disinfect *v term*   *sim* **cleanse**[1][e], **rinse**[2] *v clin*

to destroy harmful microorganisms or inhibit[3] their growth [grouθ] or pathogenic [dʒe] activity

disinfection[4] *n term* • disinfectant[5] *n & adj* • detergent[6] [ɜːrdʒ] *n*

» Painting[7] with mild disinfectants may be helpful. Disinfection of clothing, bedclothes[8] and the patient's living quarters[9] is necessary.

Use chemical / skin / wet / terminal[10] / antisepsis, sterilization and **disinfection** • **disinfectant** solution[11]

desinfizieren
reinigen[1] (ab-, aus)spülen[2] hemmen[3] Desinfektion, Entkeimung, Entseuchung[4] Desinfektionsmittel; desinfizierend[5] Reinigungsmittel[6] (ein)pinseln[7] Bettwäsche[8] Wohnung[9] Schlussdesinfektion[10] Desinfektionsmittel[11]
5

scrub(-up) [ʌ] *n & v jar*

(v) to rub[1] [ʌ], disinfect and rinse before surgery, esp. the hands and forearms[2] of the operative team

scrubbing[3] *n jar* • scrub suit[4] [suːt] *n*

» For preoperative preparation hands should be scrubbed for 5-10 min. Shorter scrubs are acceptable between operations.

Use hand / chlorhexidine / surgical **scrub** • scrub routine / nurse[5] [nɜːrs]/ room[6] • **(un)scrubbed** personnel[7] / team members

chir. (Hände)desinfektion; Hände desinfizieren
(ab)reiben[1] Unterarme[2] präoperative Desinfektion[3] Operationskleidung[4] OP-Schwester[5] Wasch-, Händedesinfektionsraum[6] (nicht) steriles Personal[7]
6

drape [dreɪp] *v & n usu pl term*

(v) to cover body parts other than the operative field with sterile materials

» The skin is prepared with an antiseptic solution and then the area is draped.

Use skin / patient / operative field or area **is draped** • scrubbed, sterilely prepped[1] and **draped** • adherent[2] [ɪɚ] **drape** • sterile[3] **draping**

(m. sterilen Tüchern) abdecken; (steriles) Abdecktuch
steril gemacht[1] Abdeckfolie[2] sterile Abdeckung[3]
7

ventilation [ventᵊleɪʃᵊn] **system** [ɪ] *n term*

conditioner which provides clean air for the sterile zone[1] [zoʊn], eliminates airborne bacteria[2] [ɪɚ] and avoids microbial [aɪ] dissemination[3] by controlled air flow patterns[4]

» This ventilation system avoids microbial emission[3] between the air source and the clean zone[1] by downstream[5] turbulence [ɜː] and even works without restrictive side panels[6].

Use laminar flow[7] / outward or exflow **ventilation**

Belüftungsanlage
Sterilzone, sterile Z.[1] Keime i. d. Luft[2] Verbreitung von Mikroorganismen[3] Luftströmung[4] nach unten gerichtet[5] seitliche Begrenzung[6] Laminar-Flow-System[7]
8

contamination *n term*   *rel* **infection**[1] *n term*

soiling[2] or making impure [-pjʊɚ] or unhealthy [e] by contact with bacteria or other harmful[3] agents

(de)contaminate[4] *v term* • contaminant[5] *n* • contaminated *adj* • decontamination *n*

» Additional intraincisional antibiotics [aɪǁɪ] failed to reduce wound infection rates in contaminated abdominal surgery. They are nonpathogenic [dʒe] surface contaminants but may be opportunistic invaders[6] in immunosuppressed[7] patients.

Use **contaminated** wound / procedure • **contamination from** instruments / ambient hospital air[8] / linens[9] • cross-[10]**contamination** • airborne[11] / surgical / bacterial / fecal[12] [iː]/ radioactive[13] **contamination** • heavily [e] **contaminated**

Kontamination, Verunreinigung, Keimverschleppung
Infektion[1] Verunreinigung, Verschmutzung[2] schädlich[3] kontaminieren, verunreinigen[4] Schadstoff, Kontaminant[5] opportunistische Erreger[6] immunsupprimiert[7] Kontamination durch d. Raumluft i. Krankenhaus[8] K. durch Bettwäsche[9] Übertragung(sinfektion)[10] durch Luft verursachte Kont.[11] fäkale Kont.[12] radioakt. Kont. / Verseuchung[13]
9

colony forming unit *n term*   *abbr* **cfu**

» It is prudent[1] to prevent cfu from infecting the wound rather than rely [aɪ] on[2] prophylactic antibiotics[3].

koloniebildende Einheit
sinnvoll, klüger[1] sich verlassen auf[2] Antibiotikaprophylaxe[3]
10

GENERAL CLINICAL TERMS — Medical & Surgical Asepsis

cross infection n term

infection transmitted between patients or from hospital staff[1] to patients or vice versa[2] [vaɪsə vɜːrsə]

» Surgical patients must be protected from cross-infection with virulent [ɪ] strains [eɪ] of bacteria[3].

Use **cross infection** control policies[4]

Kreuzinfektion
Krankenhauspersonal[1] umgekehrt[2] virulente Bakterienstämme[3] Vorschriften zur Vermeidung v. Kreuzinfektionen[4]

11

---

hospital-acquired [əkwaɪəd] adj term   syn **nosocomial** adj term

a new disorder (esp. an infection) a patient develops while hospitalized[1]

» It led to a significant increase in hospital-acquired wound infections and septicemia [siː], particularly among the aged[2] [eɪdʒd] and debilitated[3].

nosokomial, Krankenhaus-
in stationärer Behandlung[1] Betagte[2] Geschwächte[3]

12

---

prophylactic antibiotic coverage [kʌvərɪdʒ] n term
    syn **antibiotic prophylaxis** [prɒːfɪlæksɪs] n term

preoperative administration of a broad [ɒː] spectrum antibiotic[1] to patients at risk of[2] infectious [ekʃ] complications

» In the case of open injuries prophylactic antibiotics should be given.

Antibiotikaprophylaxe
Breitbandantibiotikum[1] Gefahr besteht[2]

13

---

preoperative skin preparation n term   syn **prep** n jar

includes bathing [eɪ], shaving[1] [eɪ] and disinfecting the operative area to render the skin as free of microorganisms[2] as possible without causing irritation

» A 1-minute skin prep was applied followed by an adherent drape[3]. In uncooperative patients a depilatory cream[4] [iː] can be used instead of skin shaving.

Use abdominal / knee **prep**

präop. Hautdesinfektion
Rasur[1] die Haut keimfrei machen[2] Abdeckfolie[3] Enthaarungscreme[4]

14

---

scrub [ʌ] **suit** [suːt] n term   syn **OR attire** [aɪ], **gown** [aʊ] n term

close-fitting dresses, pants, suits, etc. worn with surgeon's aprons[1] [eɪ], shoes or shoe coverings [ʌ] and other protective gear[2] [ɡɪə] to keep the clean zone as aseptic as possible

gowning[3] n term

» Scrub suits should only be worn in the OR. When the gown is donned[4] [ɒː] the glove[5] [ʌ] is grasped with the fingers still inside the sleeve[6] [iː]. Fresh OR attire is put on each time a person enters the OR.

Use to don/secure/fasten sterile[7] **gowns** • **gown** cuffs[8] [ʌ]

OP-Kleidung, -anzug, -mantel
OP-Schürzen[1] Schutzvorrichtungen[2] Ankleiden[3] angezogen wird[4] (OP-)Handschuh[5] Ärmel[6] sterile OP-Kleidung zuschnüren[7] Abschlussbund am OP-Mantel[8]

15

---

total body exhaust [ɪɡzɒːst] **gown** n term

system to capture[1] [-tʃɚ], contain[2], and remove the continuous infective body emissions[3] from the operating team

» This garment[4] is supplied with a negative pressure necklace [nekləs] exhaust[5].

OP-Anzug mit Absaugvorrichtung
einfangen[1] einschließen[2] Körperabsonderungen[3] Anzug[4] Absaugvorrichtung (unterhalb d. Visiers)[5]

16

---

surgical gloves [ʌ] n term

gloving n term • gloved adj • glove-wearing [eɚ] adj & n

» Palpate gently [dʒ] with the gloved hand. Surgical gloves should be wiped [aɪ] clean[1] of lubricants[2] [uː] before handling abdominal viscera[3] [vɪsɚə]. If a glove is torn it should be replaced as promptly as patient safety permits.

Use to wear/handle with **gloves** • double[4] [ʌ] **gloving** • latex [eɪ]/ disposable[5] / protective[6] / punctured[7] [ʌ] **gloves** • **glove** cuff / lubricant / (dusting [ʌ]) powder[8] [aʊ]

Operationshandschuhe
sauber abgewischt[1] Gleitmittel[2] Eingeweide[3] Doppelhandschuhe[4] Einmalhandschuhe[5] Schutzhandschuhe[6] perforierte H.[7] Handschuh(gleit)puder[8]

17

(face) mask n & v term   sim **face shield**[1] n, rel **surgical cap**[2] n term

(n) worn at all times in the OR to minimize airborne contamination

» When the moistened[3] [mɔɪsᵊnd] mask is changed during operations only the strings[4] must be handled.

Use full[1]-**face mask**

Mundschutz; M. anlegen
Visier[1] OP-Haube[2] feucht gewordene[3] Bänder[4]

18

Unit 28 Wound Healing

Related Units: 3 Injuries, 17 Fractures, 27 Medical & Surgical Asepsis, 26 Sutures & Suture Material, 29 Fracture Management

wound [uː] **care** *or* **management** *n clin*   *sim* **wound repair**[1] [rɪpeɚ] *n term*
includes cleansing[2] [e], closing and dressing[3] the wounded area, irrigation[4], infection control, drainage [eɪ], etc.
» She requires a visiting nurse[5] to assist with wound care at home. A carefully applied dressing assures the patient that good wound care has been provided. This is how the wound should be cared for.
Use to provide/assist with **wound care** • appropriate / negligent[6] [-dʒənt]/ postoperative / local / deep[7] **wound care**

> Note: The term *wound repair* may refer to surgical wound care as well as the body's healing process following an injury (→ U28-5).

Wundversorgung, -behandlung
chir. Wundversorgung[1] Reinigen[2] Verbinden[3] Spülung[4] Hauskrankenpfleger(in)[5] nachlässige Wundversorgung[6] Versorgung einer tiefen Wunde[7]

1

approximate *v term*   *sim* **align**[1] [əlaɪn] *v term* → U29-1, 26-5
bringing two surfaces (e.g. wound edges[2]) or stumps[3] [ʌ] (fractured bone, vessels, nerves) close together
reapproximate *v term* • approximation[4] *n* • alignment[5] *n* • approximator *n*
» The wound edges can be approximated with tapes. Simple approximation of the freshened edges[6] is sufficient. Precise alignment facilitates[7] rapid healing, return of function and a good cosmetic result.
Use loosely **approximated** • to provide/allow for/permit/(re)check **approximation** • primary [aɪ]/ simple / loose[8] / skin / tissue / end-to-end / close or exact[9] **approximation** • rib **approximator** • **approximator** clamp

adaptieren, annähern, wiedervereinigen
reponieren, einrichten[1] Wundränder[2] Stümpfe, Bruchenden[3] Adaptation[4] Einrichtung, Reposition[5] angefrischte Wundränder[6] ermöglicht[7] lockere Adaptation[8] gute / exakte A.[9]

2

wound closure [klouʒɚ] *n term*
approximation of the wound edges over the wound cavity[1] by means of tapes[2], sutures or dressings[3]
» Tapes are the skin closure of choice[4] for clean wounds. The ideal type of wound closure is primary approximation of the wound edges[5].
Use to achieve/delay [eɪ] **wound closure** • early / primary[5] / adequate / precise / burn / abdominal / layered[6] [eɪ] **wound closure** • type / safety **of wound closure** • to close[7] **a wound**

Wundverschluss, -naht
Wundhöhle[1] Klebebänder, (Heft)pflaster[2] Wundauflagen, Verbände[3] der Wahl[4] primärer Wundverschluss, Primärnaht[5] schichtweiser W.[6] Wunde schließen[7]

3

heal [hiːl] *v i/t* → U18-2
(i) to recover and become healthy [e] again (ii) to provide therapy to support this process
healing[1] [iː] *n & adj* • heal up[2] *v* • healed *adj* • healer[3]
» A fractured leg cannot be healed, it has to be set[4]. The ulcer failed to heal with local care. He has a poorly healing burn on his hip. These donor sites are slower to heal.
Use **to heal** spontaneously [eɪ] • **healing** process[5] / rate / by first intention[6] [-ʃən] / earth[7] [ɜː] • spontaneous[8] / wound / bone / ulcer[9] [ʌlsɚ] **healing** • faith[10] [eɪ] **healer** • **heal**-all[11]

> Note: While *heal* is mainly used to describe the recovery the body makes (esp. self-healing) and less commonly for restoring sb.'s health with the help of medication or therapy, *cure* is used exclusively in the second meaning.

(ver)heilen
Heilung; (ab)heilend, heilsam[1] ver-, zuheilen[2] Heiler(in)[3] reponiert, eingerichtet[4] Heilungsprozess[5] Primärheilung[6] Heilerde[7] Spontanheilung[8] Geschwür-, Ulkusabheilung[9] Gesundbeter(in)[10] Allheilmittel[11]

4

wound healing *n*   *syn* **wound repair** *n term*
natural process including blood clotting[1], tissue regeneration, and scar formation[2]
» Wound healing is faster if the state of nutrition[3] is normal. In healing by first intention or primary union[4] wound repair occurs directly without granulation.
Use to support/accelerate[5]/delay or interfere with[6] / moist[7] / poor **wound healing** • **wound healing by** first[4]/second[8]/third **intention**

Wundheilung
Blutgerinnung[1] Narbenbildung[2] Ernährungszustand[3] primäre Wundheilung[4] W. beschleunigen[5] W. beeinträchtigen / verzögern[6] Wundversorgung mittels Okklusionsverband, feuchte Kammer[7] sekundäre Wundheilung[8]

5

GENERAL CLINICAL TERMS — Wound Healing

epithel(ial)ization n term

growth [oʊ] of new tissue in the healing process that forms an epithelial [iː] bridge[1] in the wound cavity

» A scab[2] [æ] forms and peels [iː] off[3] from the edges as epithelialization is completed underneath.

Use to heal by / to produce / squamous[4] [ɒː‖eɪ] *epithelialization*

Epithelisierung, -isation
Epithelbrücke[1] Kruste, Schorf[2] sich ablösen[3] Schuppen-, Plattenepithelbildung[4]   6

granulation tissue [tɪʃuː‖tɪsjuː] n term

red granular tissue containing newly formed vessels and collagen [kɒːlədʒən] formed in open wounds

granulate[1] v term • granulating adj • granular[2] adj

» Exuberant [uː] granulation tissue[3] on the wound surface is termed proud [aʊ] flesh[4].

Use healthy / infected **granulation tissue** • *granulating* wound / ulcer[5]

Granulationsgewebe
granulieren[1] körnig, granulär[2] überschießendes Granulationsgewebe[3] wildes Fleisch, Caro luxurians[4] granulierendes Ulkus[5]   7

wound contraction n term   rel **contracture**[1] [kɒːntræktʃɚ] n term

as the wound heals the defect shrinks[2] and closes spontaneously; contracture, by contrast, is a pathologic process resulting from processes like excessive scar formation[3]

» Although [-ðoʊ] a normal event during healing, wound contraction may give rise to[4] contracture.

Narbenretrakion, -schrumpfung
Kontraktur[1] schrumpft[2] übermäßige Narbenbildung[3] führen zu[4]   8

scab [skæb] n&v   sim **eschar**[1] [eskɑːr] n term

thick crust or slough[2] [slʌf] formed by coagulation of blood, pus[3] [ʌ], and/or serum [ɪɚ] on the surface of a wound; the sloughy[4] tissue typically seen in thermal [ɜː] burns[5] or cauterization [ɒː] are called eschars

» The pustules[6] [pʌstjuːlz] become crusted and scab over[7] but they leave no scar.

Use dry[8] **scab** • **scabs** form[9] / fall off • burn / necrotic[10] **eschar**

Kruste, Schorf; verschorfen
Verbrennungs-, Ätzschorf[1] Schorf[2] Eiter[3] verschorft[4] Verbrennungen[5] Pusteln[6] verschorfen[7] trockener Schorf[8] Krusten bilden sich[9] nekrotische Verschorfung[10]   9

scar [skɑːr] n&v   syn **cicatrix** [sɪkətrɪks] pl **-ces** n term

mark left on the skin by a wound that has healed; excessive scar formation is termed keloid[1] [iː] (un)scarred[2] [ɑː] adj • scarring[3] n • cicatricial [-trɪʃəl] adj term

» The ulcers disappeared without leaving a scar. The scar may fade[4] [eɪ] to a varying degree. These superficial linear fissures may leave scars on healing.

Use wide[5] [aɪ] / fine(-line) / hypertrophic[6] / depressed / unsightly[7] [saɪt] / pliable[8] [aɪ] **scar** • acne [ækni]/ burn / facial [eɪʃ] **scar** • scar formation[3] / tissue / marks[9] /-like / revision • to produce/promote/minimize scarring • progressive / permanent / severe / renal scarring • scarred face[10] • cicatricial stenosis[11]

Narbe, Cicatrix; vernarben, Narbe bilden
Wulstnarbe, Keloid[1] narbig, vernarbt[2] Narbenbildung[3] blass werden[4] breite Narbe[5] hypertrophe N.[6] unschöne / hässliche N.[7] geschmeidige N.[8] Narben[9] narbiges Gesicht[10] narbenbedingte Stenose[11]   10

wound irrigation n term   sim **lavage**[1] [ləvɑːʒ] n term → U22-17

cleansing [e] a wound with a medicated irrigating solution[2] to remove secretions[3] and promote healing

» After irrigation the site is dried with sterile sponges[4] [ʌ] working from the wound out. The wound bed[5] should be irrigated with a wound cleanser, e.g. saline[6] [seɪliːn‖laɪn].

Use copious[7] [oʊ] **irrigation** • to rinse or flush[8] [ʌ]/wash out *a wound* • *irrigating* catheter / solution

Auswaschen d. Wunde; Wundspülung
Lavage, Spülung[1] medizinische Spülflüssigkeit[2] Wundsekret[3] Tupfer[4] Wundbett[5] physiolog. Kochsalzlösung[6] gründliche Spülung[7] Wunde (aus)spülen[8]   11

debridement [dɪbriːdmənt‖mɔː] n term   sim **freshening**[1] n jar

surgical resection of devitalized[2] [aɪ] and/or contaminated[3] tissue from a wound together with cellular debris[4] [dəbriː], foreign bodies[5], etc. to expose the adjacent [dʒeɪs] healthy tissue

debride[6] [iː] v term

» In this case it is better to explore and debride the wound. Now the freshened edges can be approximated. Hospitalize the patient for debridement and closure in the OR.

Use **to debride** devitalized tissue / and close a wound • surgical[7] / radical **debridement**

Wundrandexzision, -ausschneidung, Debridement
Wundanfrischung[1] abgestorben, nekrotisch[2] verunreinigt, kontaminiert[3] Zelltrümmer[4] Fremdkörper[5] ausschneiden[6] Wundtoilette, -exzision[7]   12

Wound Healing GENERAL CLINICAL TERMS 103

exudate [ˈeksjʊdeɪt] n term   rel **weep**[1] [iː] v clin, sim **transudate**[2] n term

fluid discharged[3] from an injury (e.g the exudate that forms a scab over a skin abrasion[4] [eɪʒ]) or inflammation (peritoneal pus in peritonitis [aɪ])

exude [ɪɡˈzuːd] v term • exudative[5] adj • trans-/exudation[6] n • transudative adj

» Viral [aɪ] conjunctivitis is typically marked by a watery discharge[7] with very scanty[8] exudate. Compresses or soaks[9] [oʊ] help to soothe[10] [uː] weeping lesions[11]. A thin[12] hemorrhagic [-ˈrædʒɪk] exudate may be seen.

Use hemorrhagic [e]/ inflammatory / seropurulent[13] **exudate** • **exudative** lesion [iːʒ]/ inflammation • clear / low-viscosity / serous [ɪə] / pleural [ʊ] **transudate** • fluid / perivascular / serosanguineous[14] **transudation**

suppurate [ˈsʌpjʊəreɪt] v term   syn **fester** v inf

forming and/or discharging [tʃ] pus[1] [ʌ] from infected wounds or inflamed[2] [eɪ] tissues

suppuration[3] n term • suppurative[4] adj • purulent[4] [ˈpjʊərələnt] adj

» The furuncle was associated with gross [oʊ] suppuration[5]. Peritonitis is an inflammatory [æ] or suppurative response of the peritoneal lining[6] to direct irritation.

Use acute / prolonged / chronic / pleural[7] **suppuration** • **suppurative** lymphadenitis [aɪ]/ otitis media[8] [iː] / complications

drain [dreɪn] n & v t/i term

(n) patent[1] [eɪ] tube placed into wounds, infected sites etc. to prevent an accumulation[2] of fluids, blood or pus

drainage[3] [ˈdreɪnɪdʒ] n term

» Incise and drain the involved area. Penrose drains[4] should not be left in place for more than about two weeks. Sump [ʌ] drains[5] are attached to a suction [ʌ] device[6] [aɪs]. Drains were left in place to evacuate[7] small amounts of blood.

Use to place[8]/remove **drains** • wound **drain** • (closed) suction[9] / surgical / closed[10] (tube) / open / percutaneous / continuous[11] / abscess **drainage** • bladder / lymphatic[12] / postural[13] / water-sealed [iː]/ catheter / vacuum[9] / endoscopic / irrigation-aspiration[14] **drainage** • **drainage** bag / bottle / tube[15] / system

(wound) dehiscence [dɪˈhɪsəns] n term

disruption[1] [ʌ] of some or all layers of a sutured wound; when associated with extrusion[2] [uːʒ] of abdominal viscera it is termed evisceration[3] [vɪs]

dehiscent adj term • dehisce[4] [dɪˈhɪs] v

» The patient's unruly[5] [uː] behavior precipitated[6] dehiscence of a fresh laparotomy incision. Most wounds dehisce because the sutures cut through the fascia [ˈfæʃ(ɪ)ə].

Use partial / total **dehiscence** • **dehiscence** without evisceration / of a wound

dressing n

(i) a protective, sterile covering of a wound or sore[1] (ii) the application of a dressing

dress[2] v • redress[3] v

» When you remove a dressing be sure to wrap[4] [ræp] it for disposal. Nonadherent [ɪ] dressings[5] should be favored because they do not disturb sutures or coated [oʊ] wound edges[6] when removed.

Use to **dress** a wound[2] • to apply or put on[7]/change or replace[3]/reinforce[8]/discard[9] **a dressing** • surgical[10] / sterile / wet / moist[11] / dry / pressure[12] **dressing** • (non)absorbent / transparent [eə] film[13] / hydrocolloid [aɪ] / (semi)occlusive[14] / soiled[15] / antiseptic **dressing** • **dressing** room[16] / and stockinette[17] applied

(surgical) gauze [ɡɒːz] n

loosely woven[1] [oʊ] cotton[2] dressing for covering wounds

» Open fractures should be covered with saline-soaked [oʊ] gauze[3].

Use paraffin-coated[4] / fine-mesh[5] / ribbon / wrap-around roller[6] **gauze** • **gauze** bandage / dressing / pad[7] / squares[7] / sponge[8] [ʌ]/ cut / mesh • **gauze** fluff[9] [ʌ]/ wick[10] / strip[9] • expanded **gauze** roll • **gauze**-covered cotton

---

Exsudat
nässen, sezernieren[1] Transsudat[2] abgesondert[3] Hautabschürfung[4] exsudativ[5] Exsudation[6] wässrige(s) Absonderung / Sekret[7] wenig[8] Bäder, feuchte Umschläge[9] beruhigen[10] nässende Wunden[11] wässrig[12] eitrig-seröses E.[13] blutig-seröses Transsudat[14]

13

eitern
Eiter[1] entzündet[2] Eiter(bild)ung, Suppuration[3] eitrig, eiternd, purulent[4] starke Eiterbildung[5] Bauchfell, Peritoneum[6] Pleuraempyem[7] eitrige Mittelohrentzündung[8]

14

Drain; ableiten, -fließen
offen, durchgängig[1] Ansammlung[2] Drainage[3] Penrose-Drains[4] doppellumige D.[5] Saugvorrichtung[6] ableiten[7] D. legen[8] Saugdrainage[9] geschlossene Drainage[10] Dauerdrainage[11] Lymphdrainage[12] Lagedrainage[13] Spül-Saug-D.[14] Drainagerohr[15]

15

Wunddehiszenz
Auseinanderweichen, -klaffen[1] Hervortreten[2] Eingeweidevorfall[3] aufplatzen, klaffen[4] ungestüm, wild[5] verursachte[6]

16

(i) Verband(smaterial), Wundauflage (ii) Verbinden
Läsion[1] (Wunde) verbinden[2] Verband wechseln[3] einschlagen, -wickeln[4] nicht adhärente Wundauflagen[5] bedeckte Wundränder[6] V. anlegen[7] V. verstärken[8] V. entsorgen[9] Wundauflage[10] feuchter V.[11] Druckverband[12] Sprüh-, Filmverband[13] Okklusivverb.[14] schmutziger V.[15] Verband(s)raum[16] Wundauflage u. Trikotschlauch[17]

17

Gaze, Verband(s)mull
weitmaschig[1] Baumwolle[2] kochsalzimprägnierte G.[3] paraffingetränkte Gaze[4] feinmaschiger V.[5] Mullbinde[6] Gazekissen, Mullkompresse[7] Gazetupfer[8] Gazestreifen[9] Gazetampon[10]

18

28

GENERAL CLINICAL TERMS — Wound Healing

pad [pæd] n & v   sim **padding**[1] n

(n) soft cushion-like [ʊ] material, e.g for relieving pressure[2] from a dressing, absorbing fluids, etc.

» A padded dressing was applied. Thick foam [oʊ] pads[3] can help prevent pressure sores[4].

Use foam[3] / gauze / warming[5] / protective / sanitary or perineal[6] [iː]/ corn[7] / eye[8] **pad**
• well / lightly[9] / loosely **padded** • **padded** splint[10] • cast[11] **padding**

Kissen, Kompresse; polstern
Polsterwatte, Polsterung[1] Druck mindern[2] Schaumpolster[3] Wundliegen, Dekubitus[4] Heizkissen[5] Vorlage, Damen-, Monatsbinde[6] Hühneraugenpflaster[7] Augenkompresse[8] leicht gepolstert[9] gepolsterte Schiene[10] Polsterung (im Gipsverband)[11]   19

---

bandage [bændɪdʒ] n & v   sim **binder**[1] [aɪ] n, **wrap**[2] [ræp] n & v

roll or patch [pætʃ] of gauze[3] or other material applied to an injury to absorb secretions, prevent motion, achieve compression, or keep surgical dressings in place

» This lesion may be bandaged with wet dressings. A triangular [aɪ] or scarf bandage[4] was used as a sling[5]. In wound dehiscence the abdomen must be wrapped with a binder or corset[6].

Use to apply/put on/remove[7] **a bandage** • roller[8] / four-tailed[9] / spiral / protective / spica[10] [aɪ] **bandage** • plaster[11] / triangular / Esmarch('s)[12] [k]/ Ace® **bandage** • elastic[13] / compression[14] **bandage** • absorbable mesh / protective **wrap** • abdominal[15] / breast [e]/ T-**binder**

Bandage, Binde, Verband; bandagieren, verbinden
Binde[1] Umschlag, Wickel; einwickeln[2] Mullkompresse[3] Dreieckstuch[4] (Arm)schlinge[5] Korsett[6] V. abnehmen[7] Rollbinde[8] Schleuderverband, Funda[9] Kornährenverb., Spica[10] Gipsverband[11] Staubinde, Esmarch-Binde[12] elastische B.[13] Kompressionsverband[14] Leibbinde[15]   20

(sterile) adhesive [iː] **tape** [eɪ] or **plaster** n   syn **Steri-strip**® n jar → U29-11

» Unless there is bleeding from the wound the skin is preferrably closed with adhesive strips.

Use cloth[1] [ɒː]/ water-repellent[2] **adhesive tape** • **adhesive** strapping[3] / plaster • hypoallergenic [dʒe]/ restraining[4] [eɪ] **tape**

(Heft)pflaster, Klebeband
Textilpflaster[1] wasserabweisendes Pflaster[2] Heftpflaster-, Tape-Verband; Tapen[3] Stützklebeband[4]   21

Band-Aid® n

small adhesive strip with a gauze pad in the middle for covering minor [aɪ] skin lesions[1] [iː]

Heftpflaster
kleine Hautverletzungen[1]   22

---

pledget [pledʒɪt] n term   syn **cotton ball**, **swab** [ɒː] n term & clin

a tuft[1] [ʌ] or small compress of gauze, absorbent cotton, or lint[2] placed over a wound or into a cavity, e.g. to apply medication or absorb the wound discharge[3]

swab[4] v term

» Nosebleeds[5] can be stopped by placing long pledgets into the nasal [eɪ] cavity.
Use cotton[6] / prethreaded [e] Teflon **pledget** • to **swab** a wound[7]

(Watte)bausch, Tupfer
Bausch[1] Verband(s)mull[2] Wundsekret[3] (ab-, be)tupfen[4] Nasenbluten[5] Wattebausch[6] Wunde abtupfen[7]   23

---

pack n & v   syn **packing** n, sim **tampon**[1] n & v

(n, i) dressing used to check bleedings (ii) wrapping a limb or the entire body in towels[2] [aʊ], etc. (iii) absorbent material used to plug[3] [ʌ] cavities or apply medication

» Early application of ice packs[4] to reduce swelling is indicated.
Use to apply a **pack** • moist[5] / cold / ice[4] / mud[6] [ʌ]/ hot / hot wet[7] **pack** • tracheal [eɪk]/ nasal[8] **tampon** • vaginal [dʒ]/ gauze / nasal[8] **packing**

Packung, Wickel; einwickeln, W. machen, tamponieren
Tampon; tamponieren[1] (Hand)tücher[2] zustopfen, tamponieren[3] Eispackungen[4] feuchter Wickel[5] Moor-, Schlammpackung[6] feuchtwarme Packung[7] Nasentampon(ade)[8]   24

---

compress n term   sim **poultice** [poʊltɪs] or **fomentation**[1] [oʊ] n clin

cloth [ɒː] pad[2] or dressing (with or without medication) applied firmly to a lesion

» Apply cold compresses and a sterile eye patch[3]. Prescribe warm compresses 3-4 times daily.

Use to prescribe/apply/cover with/treat with **compresses** • cold / cool / tap-water[4] / hot[5] / dry / moist / vinegar[6] [ɪ] **compress** • mustard[7] [ʌ]/ paraffin / linseed[8] **poultice**

Kompresse, Umschlag
Breiumschlag, Kataplasma[1] Stoffauflage[2] Augenklappe[3] U. m. Leitungswasser[4] warme Kompresse[5] Essigumschlag[6] Senfpackung[7] Leinsamenkataplasma[8]   25

28

Fracture Management GENERAL CLINICAL TERMS 105

truss [trʌs] n & v sim **corset**[1], **brace**[2] [breɪs] n → U29-7

padded belt[3] around the abdomen kept in place by straps[4] to retain[5] a reduced hernia[6] [ɜː]

» The patient's herniated bowel needs to be supported by a truss or binder. A corset or back brace provides external support and allows patients with lower back pain to return to activity earlier. Lumbosacral [eɪ] corsets with steel stays[7] provide mechanical [k] support for the spine [aɪ] by compressing and reinforcing the flaccid[8] [æks] abdominal wall.

Use to wear/prescribe/fit/support by *a truss* • elastic *corset* • extension-type[9] *brace*

Bruchband; mit B. stützen

(Stütz)korsett[1] Schiene[2] Gürtel[3] Riemen[4] stützen[5] reponierte(r) Hernie / Bruch[6] Stahleinlagen[7] schlaff[8] Extensionsschiene[9]

26

Unit 29 Fracture Management
Related Units: 3 Injuries, 17 Fractures, 28 Wound Healing, 21 Surgical Treatment, 45 Maxillofacial Surgery

alignment [əlaɪnmənt] n term sim **apposition**[1] n term

(i) longitudinal position of a bone or limb [lɪm] (ii) bringing sth into line, e.g. fractured ends of a bone or teeth relative to supporting, adjacent [dʒeɪs] or opposing structures

align[2] v clin • malalignment[3] [æ] n • appose[4] [oʊ] v • appositional[5] [ɪʃ] adj

» The elbow was placed in marked flexion to preserve fracture alignment. Primary repair[6] can occur only when the fracture is stable [eɪ] and aligned and its surfaces closely apposed. Healing of the fracture in malalignment may cause limitation of shoulder motion [oʊʃ].

Use to bring into[7]/obtain[7]/improve/restore/maintain *alignment* • gross[8] [oʊ]/ correct / accurate / unstable / *fracture*[9] / femoral [e] *alignment* • joint / anatomical (position and) / longitudinal / rotational[10] [eɪʃ] *alignment* • to achieve/be in *apposition* • side-by-side or bayonet[11] [eɪ]/ adequate / mal[3]/ non*apposition* • direct / close / level[12] *bone apposition* • *to be apposed* to sth.[13] / by sth. • *appositional bone* formation[14] / fixation • gross / significant / patellar *malalignment*

(i) Achsenstellung
(ii) Ausrichtung, Herstellung normaler Bissverhältnisse

Apposition, An-, Auflagerung, Adaptation[1] aus-, einrichten[2] Fehlstellung[3] aneinanderlegen, adaptieren[4] angelagert, Appositions-[5] Primärheilung[6] adaptieren, einrichten[7] makroskop. korrekte Stellung[8] Frakturrichtung[9] Rotationsstellung[10] Bajonettstellung[11] höhengleiche Knochenapposition[12] anliegen[13] Knochenanbau[14]

1

reduction [ʌ] n term syn **setting** n, sim **realignment**[1] n, rel **manipulation**[2] n clin

repositioning broken bones to their anatomical relationships by surgical or manipulative procedures

reduce[3] [uː] v term • realign[4] v • set[3] v clin • unset[4] adj • manipulate[5] v

» If reduction by closed manipulation is anatomic, transverse fractures tend to be stable. When the fracture has been properly set, a splint[6] should be applied.

Use to obtain[2]/confirm/prevent/undergo *reduction* • open[7] / closed or manual or manipulative[8] / (non)operative[7] / failure of *reduction* • anatomic / (in)complete / end-on-end / fracture / joint *reduction* • *reduction* under anesthesia [iː] • closed[8] *manipulation* • *to set* a fracture[9]

Reposition, Einrichtung

Wiederherstellung d. Achsenausrichtung[1] Handgriff, Manipulation[2] reponieren, einrichten[3] nicht reponiert[4] manipulieren, handhaben[5] Schiene[6] offene Reposition[7] geschlossene R.[8] Fraktur / Bruchfragmente reponieren[9]

2

skeletal [skelətəl] **traction** [trækʃən] n term rel **extension**[1], **suspension**[2] n term

(i) pulling or dragging force exerted on a broken limb in a distal direction (ii) the act of pulling

re/dis/protraction[3] n term • distract[4] v • suspend[5] v • extend[6] vi/t

» Reduce gross deformity by applying traction to the tibia and manipulating it as needed to align it with the femur [iː]. Finger extension splints[7] can potentiate grip.

Use to apply[8]/exert/maintain *traction* • to place[8]/be held[9] *in traction* • sustained [eɪ] skeletal / axial / lateral / counter-[10] [aʊ]/ cranial [eɪ] / cervical [ɜː] / arm extension / head halter [ɔː] or halo[11] [eɪ] *traction* • skin / manual / gentle [dʒ] / weight[12] [weɪt]/ continuous[13] / intermittent / elastic *traction* • *traction* splint[7] / device [-aɪs]/ suture[14] • balanced[15] / frontomaxillary wire [aɪ] *suspension* • *suspension* sling / wire[16] • *extension* wire

Traktion, Zug, Extension

Streckung, Extension, Verlängerung, (Aus)dehnung[1] Suspension, Aufhängung[2] Re/Dis/Protraktion[3] distrahieren[4] aufhängen, suspendieren[5] (aus)strecken, reichen bis[6] Extensionsschienen[7] Zug anwenden, Streckverband anlegen[8] in Extension behandeln[9] Gegenzug[10] Ext. m. Kopfhalter (Glisson-Schlinge)[11] Gewichtszug[12] Dauerzug[13] Entlastungsnaht[14] Aufhängung in d. Schwebe[15] Suspensionsdraht[16]

3

29

GENERAL CLINICAL TERMS — Fracture Management

fracture fixation [eɪ] n term   syn **stabilization** n,
    rel **osteosynthesis**[1] [-sɪnθəsɪs] n term

fastening [fæsnɪŋ] a broken bone in a firmly attached or stable position by internal or external fixation devices

transfix[2] v term • fixator[3] n • (in)stability[4] n • (un)stable [5] adj

» Good results are most readily[6] [e] obtained by rigid [dʒ] internal fixation of the fractured ulna with plate and screws and complete reduction of the dislocated radial head. Pins and wires [aɪ] were incorporated into the cast to transfix the major bone fragments.

Use (prompt/temporary/failed) external[7] / (immediate/prophylactic/rigid [dʒ]) internal[8] **fixation** • / two-point / percutaneous [eɪ] / intermaxillary[9] (abbr IMF) **fixation** • mini-plate / intramedullary[10] / (axial / lateral) pin[11] **fixation** • **fixation screw**[12] [skruː]/ device • external[13] / internal **fixator** • bony / emergency / surgical **stabilization** • **stabilization** bar[14] • **(un)stable** joint / spinal [aɪ] fracture[15] • midcarpal / patellar / spinal / recurrent [ɜː] / shoulder[16] **instability** • fracture / mechanical [k] **stability**

Fixation, Stabilisierung
Osteosynthese[1] transfixieren[2] Fixateur[3] (In)stabilität[4] (in)stabil[5] am besten[6] sofortige externe Fixation[7] starre innere F.[8] mandibulomaxilläre F.[9] Marknagelung[10] Stiftfixation, Spickung[11] Fixierschraube[12] Fixateur externe[13] Stabilisierungstab[14] instabile Wirbelfraktur[15] rezidivierende Schulterinstabilität, -gelenkluxation[16]

4

---

immobilization n term   opposite **mobilization**[1] n term

rendering a person or a body part incapable [eɪ] of moving

(im)mobilize[2] [oː] v term • (im)mobile[3] [moʊbəl‖aɪl] adj • (im)mobility[4] n

» Immobilization is obtained by incorporation of the traction pin or wire in a full extremity plaster with the knee [niː] flexed 30 degrees and the foot in plantar flexion.

Use to provide excellent/treat by **immobilization** • wound [uː]/ shoulder / spine [aɪ]/ spica[5] [aɪ] **immobilization** • duration or length[6] / time / position / preferred [ɜː] method **of immobilization** • complete / prolonged[7] **immobility** • restricted[8] **mobility** • gradual / progressive / early[9] **mobilization**

Immobilisation, -sierung, Ruhigstellung
Mobilisation, Mobilisierung[1] ruhigstellen, immobilisieren[2] immobil, unbeweglich[3] Mobilität, Beweglichkeit[4] Immobilisierung durch Kornährenverband[5] Immobilisationsdauer[6] Langzeitimmobilität[7] eingeschränkte Mobilität / Beweglichkeit[8] Frühmobilisation[9]

5

(plaster) [plæstɚ] **cast** [kæst] n term   syn **plaster (of Paris cast)** n term, abbr **P.O.P.**

firm covering made of plaster of Paris to immobilize broken bones while they heal

casting[1] [æ] n term

» A well-molded[2] [oʊ] plaster cast is applied to maintain this position. At potential pressure sites[3] a window should be cut out of the cast. Recurrent angular displacement can be corrected by cast wedging[4] [dʒ], which involves dividing the plaster circumferentially [enʃ] and inserting wedges in the appropriate direction. Today we can apply a walker[5] [wɒːkɚ] to the cast.

Use to apply[6]/encase [eɪ] in[7]/place in[7]/immobilize in/split/spread [e]/remove **a cast** • (below-knee) walking[8] / hanging / (short/long) leg[9] **cast** • arm / forearm / boxing glove[10] [ʌ]/ (hip/shoulder) spica[11] [aɪk]/ body[12] **cast** • tubular or circumferential[13] / articulated / weight-bearing [eɚ]/ snugly [ʌ] fitting[14] / (excessively) tight [taɪt]/ well-padded[15] **cast** • **cast** treatment / immobilization / removal / (re)application • corrective[16] **casting** • **plaster** dressing or bandage[17] / boot[18] [uː]/ gauntlet[19] [ɒː] • **plaster of Paris** (abbr P.O.P.) jacket[12] [dʒæ]

Gipsverband
(Ein)gipsen[1] gut anmodelliert[2] Druckstellen[3] Keilen[4] Gehstollen, Sohlenplatte[5] Gips(verband) anlegen[6] eingipsen[7] Gehgips[8] Unterschenkelgips[9] Gipsverband m. Fingereinschluss[10] Spica humeri[11] Gipsmieder/-korsett[12] Gipstutor, -hülse, zirkulärer G.[13] gut sitzender G.[14] gepolsterter G.[15] Redressionsgips[16] Gipsverband[17] Gipsstiefel[18] Gipshandschuh[19]

6

---

splint [splɪnt] n clin & term   sim **brace**[1] [eɪ], **jacket**[2], **corset**[2] n clin

orthopedic [iː] device [aɪ] used to immobilize, align, support, or protect fractured or traumatized [ɒː] sites

splint[3] v term • splinting[4] n • brace[3] v

» The elbow should be splinted in sufficient [ɪʃ] extension to avoid interfering[5] [ɪɚ] with perfusion [uː]. Splints are most commonly used to immobilize broken bones or dislocated joints. Loosen[6] the splint if the extremity becomes cold, discolored or dusky[7] [ʌ]. Braces allow motion of the braced part, in contrast to a splint, which prevents motion.

Use external / internal / active or functional or dynamic[8] / (inflatable [eɪ]) air[9] / anchor[10] [k]/ coaptation[11] / contact **splint** • intraoral / wrist [rɪst] / knee / tenodesis [iː]/ wire [aɪ] or ladder[12] **splint** • plaster[13] / jacket[14] / surgical / pillow[15] **splint** • neck / back / ischial [sk] weight-bearing / long leg / Milwaukee[16] / forearm / removable / cast[17]-**brace** • emergency [ɜː]/ abduction **splinting** • plastic **jacket** • to wear or use[18] **a corset** • lumbosacral [ʌ]/ elastic / surgical **corset**

Schiene
(Gelenk)schiene, Stützkorsett, Brace, Manschette[1] Mieder, Korsett[2] stützen, schienen[3] Schienung[4] Beeinträchtigung[5] lockern[6] bläulich verfärbt[7] Bewegungsschiene[8] aufblasbare Sch.[9] Kieferbruchschiene[10] Adaptationsschiene[11] Draht(leiter)schiene[12] Gipsschiene, -schale, -longuette[13] Rumpforthese[14] gepolsterte Schiene[15] Milwaukee-, Extensionskorsett[16] Funktions-, Bewegungsgips[17] ein Korsett tragen[18]

7

Fracture Management — GENERAL CLINICAL TERMS

sling [slɪŋ] *n term*   *sim* **harness**[1], **cuff**[2] [ʌ] *n*, **swathe**[3] [sweɪð] *n & v clin*

supporting or suspensory bandage used to fix or immobilize body parts, esp the arm

» *Treatment of bicipital* [aɪs] *tendinitis* [aɪ] *includes* cessation[4] [s] *of offending activities and short-term immobilization of the shoulder in a sling. Splint the extremity in a sling for comfort.*

Use to apply/treat in/support in[5]/wear *a sling* • suspension / triangular [aɪ] bandage[6] / arm **sling** • **sling** traction / and swathe • Pavlic[7] / head **harness**

Schlinge
Gurt, Zügel, Bandage[1] Manschette[2] Binde, Umschlag; um-, einwickeln[3] Einstellen[4] durch eine Schlinge stützen[5] Mitella, Dreieckstuch[6] Pavlik-Bandage[7]

8

---

cervical [sɜːrvɪkəl] **collar** [ɒː] or **orthosis** [ɔːrθoʊsɪs] *n term*
rel **head halter**[1] [ɒː] *n term*

orthopedic appliance [aɪ] worn around the neck to support the head (used in cervical spine [aɪ] injuries)

orthotics[2] [ɒː] *n term* • orthotic[3] *adj* • orthotist[4] *n*

» *In stable injuries of the cervical spine, cervical collars or* cervical thoracic [s] *braces*[5] *(4-poster) are adequate. A hard cervical spine collar is then applied, and the head is taped to a backboard, surrounded by some means of* cushioning[6] [ʊ] *(e.g.* rolled blankets[7] [æ]*).*

Use rigid[8] [dʒ]/ light **cervical collar** • firm plastic / tight / loose / soft foam[9] [oʊ]/ inelastic **collar** • halo-type[10] [heɪloʊ]/ four-poster[10] / dynamic / flexion [kʃ] **orthosis** • cervical **halter** • **halter** traction[11]

Halskrause, Schanz-Krawatte
Kopfhalterung[1] Orthese-, Stützapparate[2] gerade, aufrecht, gestreckt[3] Orthetiker[4] Kopf-Brust-Gipsverband, Minerva-Gips[5] Polsterung[6] zusammengerollte Decken[7] starre Halskrawatte[8] Schaumstoff-Halskrawatte[9] Halo-Fixateur[10] Haloextension[11]

9

---

stockinet(te) *n clin*   *sim* **elastic** or **compression stockings**[1] *n clin*

tube of elastic material applied underneath casts or splints to protect the skin, prevent thrombosis, etc.

» *The palmar splint is padded with a thin* foam pad[2] *and held in place with a loosely* wrapped [r] *roll of plaster of Paris*[3], *stockinet or elastic* bandage[4]. *Conservative measures* [eɪ] *such as leg* elevation[5], *or elastic stockings may be helpful.*

Use **stockinette** dressing[6] / amputation bandage[7] • heavy-duty[8] [e]/ knee-length / full-length / waist-high [eɪ]/ custom [ʌ] fitted[9] **elastic stockings** • support[10] / body[11] **stocking**

Baumwoll-, Trikotschlauch
Kompressions-, Antithrombosestrümpfe[1] Schaumstoffpolster[2] Gipsbinde[3] elastische Binde[4] Hochlagerung[5] Schlauchverband[6] Amputationsstrumpf[7] starke Gummistrümpfe[8] maßgefertigte Gummistrümpfe[9] Stützstrumpf[10] Rumpftrikotschlauch[11]

10

---

strapping [æ] *n clin*   *syn* **taping** [eɪ] *n clin*

application of overlapping strips of adhesive [iː] tape[1] [eɪ] to exert pressure or increase stability

strap[2] *n & v term* • tape[3] *n & v* • (un)strapped[4] *adj* • (un)taped[5] *adj*

» *A* supple[6] [ʌ] *foot that is easily corrected by strapping and casting has a more favorable prognosis. Splint the injury by taping the injured toe to its neighbor.*

Use knee / shoulder / rib / metatarsal / figure-of-eight[7] / eversion [ɜːrʒ] tape[8] / imbricated[9] **strapping** • chin [tʃ]/ head / cuff [ʌ] suspension[10] **strap** • **strap** sling • buddy[11] [ʌ]/ (medial [iː]) patellar / adhesive[12] **taping** • occlusive [uː]/ sterile / strips of[13] **tape** • **tape** dressing[14] / closure of wounds

Tape-, Pflasterverband
Pflaster, Klebeband[1] Riemen, Gurt; fest-, anschnallen[2] Band, elast. Pflasterbinde, (Heft)pflaster; (m. Heftpflaster) verkleben[3] bandagiert; festgeschnallt[4] getapet[5] beweglich[6] Achtertourenpflasterverband[7] Eversions-Tapeverband[8] Dachziegelverband[9] (Schulter)gurtverband[10] Fixation durch Nachbarfinger, -zehe[11] Anlegen e. Pflasterverbandes[12] Klebestreifen[13] Tape-Verband[14]

11

---

osteosynthesis [ɒstɪoʊsɪnθəsɪs] *n term*   *sim* **osteorrhaphy** [-rəfi] or **osteosuture**[1] *n term*

surgical fixation of bone fragments by mechanical [k] means (e.g. wires, sutures)

» *A flexible multistrand cable system was used in posterior spinal osteosynthesis for cervical fracture-dislocation.*

Use stable / orthodontic[2] **osteosynthesis** • **osteosynthesis** screw [skruː]

Osteosynthese
Knochennaht[1] kieferorthopäd. Osteosynthese[2]

12

---

spinal [aɪ] or **vertebral fusion** [fjuːʒən] *n term*   *rel* **arthrodesis**[1] [iː] *n term*

joint stiffening surgery to achieve bone ankylosis[2] [oʊ] between two or more vertebrae[3] [eɪ‖iː]

» *Management of spine instability may include spinal fusion with metal plates and screws in combination with bone fusion. Fusion of the joint may be necessary due to irreparable instability or persistent infection. Surgical fusion of the* talonavicular [eɪ], talocalcaneal [eɪ], *and* calcaneocuboid [kjuː] *joints is known as triple arthrodesis.*

Use bony / joint[2] / cervical / atlanto-occipital [ksɪ] **fusion** • **fusion** procedure • thumb [θʌm]/ shoulder **arthrodesis**

op. Wirbelsäulenversteifung, Spondylodese
operative Gelenkversteifung, Arthrodese[1] Gelenkversteifung, Ankylose[2] Wirbel, Vertebrae[3]

13

108 GENERAL CLINICAL TERMS — Fracture Management

circumferential wiring [waɪɚɪŋ] n term sim **figure-of-eight wire**[1] n term

passing a slender pliable[2] [aɪ] stainless steel wire around a fractured bone for internal fixation
wire[3] n & v term • wired[4] adj • wiring[5] n

» Temporary percutaneous wire fixation[6] was advocated. The best method of fracture fixation and restoration of the articular surface is compression by figure-of-eight wires. Significant displacement requires overhead skeletal traction[7] by means of a Kirschner wire[8] inserted through the proximal ulna [ʌ].

Use to insert[9] **a wire** • stiff / pull-out[10] / stainless steel / Kirschner or K-[8] / guide[11] / pinning[12] / hook[13] [ʊ]/ gold plated [eɪ] metal[14] wire • No. 22 / biodegradable [aɪ]/ coated[15] / supporting / suspension **wire** • **wire** fixation[5] / loop[16] [uː]/ coil[17] / cerclage[18] [sɚklɑːʒ]/ stump [ʌ]/ saw[19] [ɒː]/ extension / sutures[20] • circummandibular / interosseous / transosseous / tension band[21] **wiring** • orthodontic arch[22] [ɑːrtʃ] **wire**

> Note: The expression wire is traditionally applied to pliable as well stiff wires or pins (e.g. K-wires). This is why wiring and pinning are often used synonymously.

Drahtumschlingung
Achterdraht(schlinge), Achterligatur[1] biegsam, verformbar[2] (Bohr)draht; (ver)drahten[3] gedrahtet, gespickt[4] Drahtung, Drahtosteosynthese, Spickung[5] perkutane Spickung[6] Overheadextension[7] Kirschner-(Bohr)draht, -Bohrstift[8] Draht einbringen[9] Ausziehdraht[10] Führungsdraht[11] Spickdraht, Stift[12] Hakendraht[13] vergoldeter Metalldraht[14] beschichteter D.[15] Drahtschlinge[16] Drahtspirale[17] Drahtumschlingung, -cerclage[18] Drahtsäge[19] Drahtnähte[20] Zuggurtung(sosteosynthese)[21] kieferorthopäd. Drahtbogen[22] 14

pin [pɪn] n clin & term →U40-14

(i) flexible but not pliable stainless steel spike[1] [aɪ] used for internal fixation (ii) pointed metal rod[2] [ɒː] used to immobilize fractures (iii) thin metal peg[3] or dowel[3] [aʊ] for attaching things
pinning[4] n term • pin[5] v • micropin n • pinprick[6] n clin

» These fractures tend to be very unstable and frequently require percutaneous fixation with pins or open reduction. Most surgeons prefer to use internal fixation by multiple screw or pin fixation for impacted fractures to allow maintenance of reduction, earlier crutch [krʌtʃ] ambulation, and earlier weight bearing.

Use to insert or place[7]/secure with/pull out **a pin** • fixation / straight / lateral / crossed / Steinmann[8] / olecranon / (skeletal) traction **pin** • metal / dental[9] / external fixation / safety[10] **pin** • **pin** fixation[4] / fixator / tract (infection)[11] / site / placement / implant • cross- or crossed / double [ʌ]/ percutaneous / K-wire[12] **pinning**

(i) Bohrstift, Spick-, Bohrdraht
(ii) (Knochen)nagel
(iii) Stift, (Steck)nadel
Stift, Dorn[1] Stift[2] Stift, Dübel[3] Stiftfixation, Nagelung, Stift-, Spickdrahtosteosynthese, Spickung[4] fixieren, spicken, (an)heften[5] Nadelstich[6] Spickdraht/Nagel (in d. Knochen) einbringen/-bohren[7] Steinmann-Nagel[8] Wurzelstift[9] Sicherheitsnadel[10] Bohrlochosteitis[11] Kirschnerdraht-Fixation[12] 15

(medullary) nail [neɪl] n term rel **screw**[1] [skruː], **bolt**[2] [oʊ] n clin & term

solid tubular and often flanged [dʒ] rod[3] inserted into the marrow [mæroʊ] cavity[4] for fixation of fractured long bones
nailing[5] n term • screw[6] v • bolt v • bolting[7] n

» The functional outcome in closed interlocking nailing of femoral [e] shaft fractures was excellent. The cut bones are then reshaped, repositioned, and fixed with a combination of wires or miniplates and screws.

Use to drive a **nail** into the bone[8] • intramedullary[9] / flanged[10] [dʒ]/ interlocking or locked or locking[11] / (un)reamed[12] [iː] **nail** • **nail** extension • closed[13] / open / intramedullary[14] **nailing** • bone[15] / transverse / (non)sliding [aɪ] or lag[16] [æ]/ titanium[17] [eɪ]/ transarticular / dynamic condylar[18] / bi-/unicortical[19] **screw** • **screw** fixation /-plate system • **bolt**head / shank

Marknagel
Schraube[1] (Schrauben)bolzen[2] Stift, Stab[3] Markhöhle[4] (Mark)nagelung, Stiftfixation[5] (ver)schrauben[6] Bolzung[7] Nagel in d. Knochen hineintreiben[8] intramedullär plazierter Nagel, Marknagel[9] geflanschter Nagel[10] Verriegelungsnagel[11] (un)aufgebohrter (Mark)nagel[12] gedeckte Nagelung[13] Marknagelung[14] Knochenschraube[15] Gleitlochschr.[16] Titanschr.[17] dyn. Kondylenschr.[18] monokortikale Schr.[19] 16

(bone) plate [pleɪt] n term sim **mini-plate**[1] n term

strip of metal applied to a fractured bone in order to keep its ends in apposition
plating[2] [eɪ] n term

» A clinical and radiographic comparison of tension band wiring and plate fixation[2] was performed. At operation excellent stability was achieved with bone plates.

Use fracture / metal[3] / stainless steel / side / U-shaped / nail **plate** • (sliding[4] [aɪ]/ locking[5]) screw / slotted[6] [ɒː] **plate** • compression[7] / ancillary[8] [sə] **plating** • affixed **mini-plate**

(Knochen)platte
Miniplatte[1] Plattenosteosynthese[2] Metallplatte[3] dynamische Kompressionsplatte[4] Rundlochplatte[5] Langlochplatte[6] Kompressions-osteosynthese[7] zusätzl. Plattenosteosynthese[8] 17

Unit 30 Basic Dental Materials
Related Units: 7 Basic Dental Equipment, 31 Dental Lab Procedures & Equipment

(dental) amalgam [əmælgəm] *n term*

silver colored alloy[1] of metals including mercury (Hg)[2] and silver, tin[3], copper or zinc that is used to fill cavities

amalgamator[4] *n term* • amalgamate[5] *v* • amalgamation *n*

» The first premolar was a virgin [vɜːrdʒɪn] tooth[6] and the 1st and 2nd molars had been restored with Class I amalgam 50 years ago. This agent also bonds to set amalgam[7].

Use to pack[8]/carve[9]/polish **amalgam** • **amalgam** restoration or filling[10] / allergy / poisoning[11] • **amalgam** condensation / gun[12] / finisher / alloy / core[13] / lathe-cut[14] [leɪð-] • zinc-containing / high-copper **amalgam** • sterile **amalgam** carrier[15] • pin(-retained) / multisurface / large / cusp-overlay / leaking[16] [iː]/ fast-setting[17] **amalgam** • HG spillage[18] [-ɪdʒ] • **amalgamation** process

(Dental)amalgam
Legierung[1] Quecksilber[2] Zinn[3] Amalgammischgerät, Amalgamator[4] amalgamieren[5] unversehrter Zahn[6] erhärtetes Amalgam[7] A. stopfen[8] A. schnitzen[9] Amalgamfüllung[10] Amalgamintoxikation[11] Amalgampistole[12] Amalgamkern[13] Amalgamfeilung[14] steriler Amalgamträger[15] undichtes A.[16] rasch härtendes A.[17] Quecksilberaustritt[18] 1

dental acrylic [əkrɪlɪk] *n term*   *syn* **acrylic resin** [rezɪn] *n term*

general term for resinous materials[1] of the esters [iː] of acrylic acid[2] used for denture bases[3], trays[4], etc.

» The patient is satisfied with acrylic-resin restorations and does not want to change these prostheses to porcelain[5] [pɔːrsᵊlɪn] or gold.

Use heat-cured[6] [kjuːrd] **acrylic resin** • **acrylic-resin** filling / veneer [-ɪɚ]/ prosthesis [iː]/ plate / bite [aɪ] blocks[7] • **acrylic** trimmer[8] / polishing rubber / acid[2]

Akrylat, Dentalkunststoff
Kunststoffe[1] Akrylsäure[2] Prothesenbasen[3] Abformlöffel, Schienen[4] Keramik[5] heißpolymerisiertes Akrylat[6] Bissschablonen aus Kunststoff[7] Kunststofftrimmer[8] 2

composite resin *n term*

plastic tooth-colored filling material; a mixture of plastic resin and finely ground[1] [aʊ] glass

» Wear [weɚ] resistance[2] of posterior composite resins is being examined.

Use **composite resin** biomaterial [aɪ]/ veneer[3] / crown • self-curing[4] / light-curing[5] **resin** • **composite** adhesive[6] [iː]/ core /-dentine strength[7] / etched bridge[8] [tʃ]/ inlay • **resin** curing agent[9] /-bonded /-bound [aʊ]/ core • luting[10] [uː] **composites**

Komposit
fein gemahlen[1] Abrasions-, Verschleißfestigkeit[2] Kompositverblendschale, -veneer[3] autopolymerisierender / selbsthärtender Kunststoff[4] lichthärt. K.[5] Kompositkleber[6] Komposit-Dentin-Verbundfestigkeit[7] Kompositadhäsivbrücke[8] Kunststoffhärter[9] Befestigungskomposite[10] 3

porcelain [pɔːrsᵊlɪn] *n term*   *sim* **ceramic**[1] [sɪræmɪk] *adj & n term*

fine, tooth-colored ceramic material consisting mainly of feldspar[2], kaolin [eɪ] and quartz [kwɔːrts] which fuse[3] [fjuːz] at high temperature to form a hard, enamel-like substance

» Porcelain has a high resistance to wear. All-ceramic, metal-ceramic and porcelain crowns were evaluated.

Use **porcelain** jacket crown / inlay[4] / tip / coverage[5] [-ɪdʒ]/ powder / firing [aɪ]/ polishing wheel • **porcelain**-fused-to-metal restoration[6] /-veneered gold fixed prostheses[7] • **ceramic** alloy /-coated / facing (crown)[8] / glaze[9] [eɪ]/ veneering[10]

Porzellan, Keramik
keramisch; Keramik[1] Feldspat[2] verschmelzen[3] Keramikinlay[4] Keramikmantel, -überzug[5] Metallkeramik[6] Goldknopfzähne[7] Keramikfacette(nkrone)[8] Keramikglasur[9] Keramikverblendung[10] 4

kaolin [keɪəlɪn] *n term*   *syn* **aluminum silicate** *n term*, **China clay** [kleɪ] *n clin*

fine whitish clay[1] used in dentistry as a filler or extender for ceramics

» Kaolin is used to add toughness[2] [ʌf] and opacity [æs] to porcelain teeth.

Porzellanerde, Kaolin
Ton[1] Härte, Festigkeit[2] 5

cement [sɪment] *n & v term*

(n) material used for luting[1], sealing[2] [iː] and filling[3] purposes, made by mixing components into a mass which sets[4], or as an adherent[5] [ɪɚ] in attaching [ætʃ] various dental restorations in or on the tooth

cementation[6] *n term* • cementable *adj* • cementless *adj*

» The cement bond[7] could fail when stressed. Temporary cementing material was used for crown retention. The restoration must be secured[8] [kju] before the cement sets.

Use luting / restorative / lining [aɪ]/ dual affinity[9] / zinc oxide-eugenol [juːdʒ]/ composite[10] / temporary[11] **cement** • **cement** line[12] / film / leakage / plugger[13] [ʌ] • **cement**-retained prosthesis • **cemented** retention pin

(Befestigungs-, Klebe)zement; (ein)zementieren
Befestigung[1] Abdichtung, Versiegelung[2] Füllung[3] abbinden[4] Kleber[5] (An/Auf)zementieren[6] Zementverbindung, -haftung[7] fixiert, verankert[8] dualhärtender Zement[9] Kompositkleber[10] provisorischer Zement[11] Zementfuge[12] Zementstopfer[13] 6

30

DENTISTRY | Basic Dental Materials

alloy [ælɔɪ] *n & v term*

(n) mixture of two or more metals or metalloids used to obtain special properties¹ for constructing denture bases, frameworks², etc. that are not found in the pure components

» *Prefabricated³ gold-alloy bars were soldered⁴* [sɒːdəd] *to the mesial* [iː] *aspects.*

Use to cast⁵ **alloys** • chrome-cobalt / silver-palladium / wrought [rɒːt] gold⁶ / wire **alloy** • binary / castable magnetic / high-noble⁷ / semi-precious⁸ [eʃ] **alloy** • **alloy**-ceramic interface / base⁹ / gold¹⁰ / plastic bonding / wire

Legierung; legieren

Eigenschaften¹ Gerüstkonstruktionen² konfektionierte, vorgefertigte³ gelötet⁴ Legierungen gießen⁵ gehämmerte Goldlegierung⁶ Edelmetalleg.⁷ edelmetallreduzierte L.⁸ Legierungsbasis⁹ legiertes Gold¹⁰   7

---

cohesive [iː] **gold** *n term*   *rel* **gold foil**¹ [ɔɪ] *n term*

nearly pure gold free of adsorbed surface gases and impurities; used as a restorative material placed directly into a prepared cavity and welded² by pressure

» *Filling small dental cavities with cohesive gold is still one of the most durable means of restoring a tooth. The most common fillings used for the occlusal surfaces of posterior teeth are amalgam and gold inlays, while gold foil is less common.*

Use **cohesive gold** restorations • class I / II / III / IV dental **gold** alloy • (crystalline) sponge³ / platinized **gold** • **gold** framework⁴ / coping / inlay⁵ / collar⁶ / clasp⁷ /-platinum foil • **gold** annealing⁸ [iː]/ cast /-plated or gilded⁹ / plating bath¹⁰ / frit / filings¹¹ [aɪ] / content / finishing • low¹² / non¹³-**gold alloy**

Stopfgold

Goldfolie, Blattgold¹ verschweißt² Schwammgold³ Goldgerüst⁴ Goldinlay, -gussfüllung⁵ sichtbarer Goldrand⁶ Goldklammer⁷ Goldvergütung⁸ vergoldet⁹ Vergoldungsbad¹⁰ Goldspäne¹¹ goldarme Legierung¹² goldfreie L.¹³

8

---

platinum foil [plætᵊnəm fɔɪl] *n term*

pure platinum (abbr Pl) rolled into extremely thin sheets [iː]; used as a matrix [eɪ] for various soldering procedures¹ and for providing internal form to porcelain restorations during their fabrication²

» *There are several ways to fabricate veneers, but I use the platinum foil technique for most of my cases. Use an intermediate layer of tin oxide between the dental porcelain and the platinum foil.*

Use **platinum foil** technique / crown / matrix / impression³ • porcelain bonded to **platinum foil** • scrap⁴ / irido⁵**platinum** • **platinum** metal (bath) / gold (foil) / rivet⁶ /-bonded porcelain crown / shoulder • **platinum**-palladium /-rhodium⁷ /-silver **alloy**

Platinfolie

Lötverfahren¹ Fertigung, Herstellung² Platinfolienabdruck³ platinhaltiges Gekrätz⁴ Platin-Iridium Legierung⁵ Platinstift, -krampon⁶ Platinrhodiumlegierung⁷

9

---

titanium [taɪteɪniəm‖tɪtæ-] *n term*   *abbr* **Ti** *(chemical symbol)*

silvery gray, very light but strong metallic element used mostly in alloys for dental implants and coatings¹ [oʊ]

» *The reaction of soft tissue cells to titanium surfaces with differing degrees of surface roughness* [rʌf-] *was analyzed. We have developed a system of tissue-integrated (osseointegrated) titanium implants, suitable for use in edentulous jaws.*

Use **titanium** white or dioxide² [daɪɒːksaɪd]/ polishing kit /-sprayed surface / coating / porcelain bond³ / implant⁴

Titan(ium)

Beschichtungen¹ Titanoxid, $TiO_2$² Titan-Keramikverbund³ Titanimplantat⁴

10

---

tungsten carbide [tʌŋstən kɑːrbaɪd] *n term*   *abbr* **TC**

one of the hardest known materials used as an abrasive [eɪ] for coating cutting instruments

» *After sandblasting¹ 0.5 mm was ground off²* [aʊ] *with tungsten carbide burs³* [ɜː].

Use **tungsten carbide** fissure [fɪʃɚ] drill / excavating bur / bone cutter⁴ • **tungsten** vanadium [eɪ] steel bur

Wolframkarbid

Sandstrahlen¹ abgetragen² Hartmetallbohrer³ Hartmetallknochenfräse⁴

11

---

gypsum [dʒɪpsəm] *n term*   *sim* **plaster** [æ] **(of Paris)**¹ *n clin & jar, abbr* **POP**

the natural hydrated [aɪ] form of calcium sulfate [ʌ]; a component of stones, plasters, and investments²

» *The accuracy of casts produced from three impression materials and the effect of a gypsum hardening agent were evaluated. Impression material shrinkage³ [-ɪdʒ] and gypsum expansion⁴ need to be considered. A fast-setting⁵ plaster mix was used.*

Use to imbed⁶ (*espBE* embed) in plaster • fibrous⁷ [aɪ] / dried⁸ **gypsum** • **gypsum** powder / spar⁹ / cast die¹⁰ / rock • **gypsum** edentulous master cast • type I (dental) or impression¹¹ / type II (dental)¹² plaster • plaster matrix / key¹³ / cast / wash¹⁴ / model¹⁰ / impression¹⁵ / hardener / accelerator¹⁶ / retarder / chisel¹⁷ [tʃ]

(Natur)gips

(Alabaster)gips, β-Halbhydrat¹ Einbettungen² Schrumpfung, Schwindung³ Gipsausdehnung, -expansion⁴ schnellabbindend⁵ in Gips einbetten⁶ Fasergips⁷ gebrannter G.⁸ Gipsspat, Marienglas⁹ Gipsmodell¹⁰ Abformgips¹¹ Alabastergips¹² Gipsvorwall, –schlüssel¹³ erste dünne Gipsbeschichtung d. Abdrucks¹⁴ Gipsabformung, -abdruck¹⁵ Gipsabbindebeschleuniger¹⁶ Gips-, Ausbettmeißel¹⁷   12

Basic Dental Materials DENTISTRY 111

(dental) stone *n term* *syn* **artificial** [ɪʃ] **stone** *n term*
  special nonporous gypsum derivative stronger than plaster used for making dental casts[1]
  » The impressions were filled with die stone[2]. The existing stone cast[3] was no longer accurate. A preliminary cast was poured[4] [ɔː] in dental stone before fabrication of a final impression.
  Use class I[5] / class II[6] **(dental) stone** • **(dental) stone** die / powder[7] [aʊ]/ surface sealer / hardness

(Spezial)hartgips, α-Halbhydrat
Modelle[1] Modellgips[2] Hartgipsmodell[3] gegossen[4] Hartgips Typ III[5] H.Typ IV, Superhartgips[6] Hartgipspulver[7]
13

guttapercha [ʌ] *or* **gutta-percha** [pɜːrtʃə] **point** *n term*
  pins of a coagulated, purified, dried, milky juice of trees used as a root filling material
  » If all screws [uː] were stable, the access holes[1] were sealed with guttapercha and composite resin. The softened gutta percha cone was tamped[2] [æ] into the canal. Excess gutta percha is seared off[3] [ɪɚ] with a heated plugger.
  Use **gutta-percha** marker / (master) cone[4] [koʊn]/ spreader[5] [e]/ cement / (root) filling / seal / carrier system • chloro**percha**

Wurzelkanal-, Guttaperchastift
Zugangsöffnungen[1] gestopft[2] heiß abgetragen[3] Guttapercha-(Haupt)stift[4] G.-Spreizer, -Spreader[5]
14

alginate [ældʒɪneɪt] *n term*
  salt of alginic acid[1]; a colloidal substance used in dental impression materials in the form of calcium, ammonium[2] or sodium alginate[3]
  » After the diagnostic wax-up a full arch alginate impression[4] is made and poured[5].
  Use **alginate** impression[6] / impression tray[7] / foam [oʊ] gel [dʒel]/ varnish[8] / stabilizer / gauze [gɒz] • to pour/make **an alginate impression**

  Note: Mark the difference between ammonia[9] (NH₃) and ammonium (NH₄).

Alginat
Alginsäure[1] Ammonium[2] Na-Alginat[3] Alginatabformung d. Kiefers[4] ausgegossen[5] Alginatabformung[6] Alginatabformlöffel[7] A.-Isoliermittel, -lack[8] Ammoniak[9]
15

eugenol [juːdʒənɒl] *n term* *syn* **eugenic acid** *n term*, *rel* **clove** [oʊ] **oil**[1] *n clin*
  aromatic liquid used with zinc oxide [aɪ] as a base for impression materials and for analgesic [dʒiː] purposes
  » A topical analgesic (gauze saturated in eugenol[2]) was placed in the socket[3] and changed daily. Topical covering with zinc-eugenol cement[4] is used if the pulp is not exposed[5].
  Use **eugenol** impression paste[6] [eɪ]/ foam / filling / dressing[7] • **zinc oxide eugenol cement type** II[8] / III[9] • non**eugenol** paste[10]

Eugenol
Nelkenöl[1] mit E. getränkte Gaze[2] Extraktionswunde[3] Zinkoxid-Eugenol-Zement[4] freigelegt, eröffnet[5] Eugenol-(Abform)paste[6] E.-Verband[7] Zinkoxid-Eugenol-Befestigungszement[8] Zinkoxid-Eugenol-Füllungszement[9] eugenolfreie Paste[10]
16

casting wax [kæstɪŋ wæks] *n term* *sim* **inlay wax**[1] *n term*
  paraffin-based wax used for a variety [aɪə] of dental techniques [k], esp. for casting dental alloys
  wax (up[2]/to[3]) *v* • wax-up[4] *n term* • waxing(-up)[4] *n*
  » The hard and soft tissue was contoured with wax. A framework waxup was completed and cast in gold alloy. Then the wax is boiled out[5].
  Use **casting wax** pattern[6] / sheets[7] • **wax** check bite[8] / try-in[9] / melter /-coated / paper / residue[10] [resᵊduː]/ trimmer / smoother [uː] / final **wax** trial [aɪ] prosthesis • diagnostic *or* pretreatment[11] **wax-up** • **wax-up** material / technique[12] / die / instruments • **waxed-up** crown[13] • **waxing** sleeve • occlusal detection[14] / impression[15] **wax**

Guss-, Modellierwachs
Inlay-, Gusswachs[1] aufwachsen[2] anwachsen[3] Wachsaufstellung[4] ausgebrüht[5] Wachsformling[6] Wachsplatten[7] Wachsbiss[8] Wachseinprobe[9] Wachsrückstand[10] diagnostisches Aufwachsen[11] Aufwachstechnik[12] wachsmodellierte Krone[13] Bisswachs[14] Abformwachs[15]
17

(flour [flaʊɚ] **of) pumice** [pʌmɪs] *n term*
  volcanic cinders[1] [sɪn] ground [aʊ] to particles of varying sizes; used for polishing restorations or teeth
  » The rubber [ʌ] cup with flour of pumice left a smoother[2] surface than the interdental brush [ʌ].
  Use **pumice** grinder[3] [aɪ]/-containing wheel[4] [iː]/ polishing paste [eɪ]/ pan[5] • (tooth) cleanser [e] **pumice**

Bimsstein(pulver), Pumex
erstarrte Lavamasse[1] glattere[2] Bimssteinmühle[3] bimssteinhaltiges Polierrad[4] Bimssteinbehälter[5]
18

etching [etʃɪŋ] **liquid** *or* **solution** *n term* *syn* **etchant** [etʃənt] *n term*
  material used in various cementing and bonding techniques
  etch[1] *v & n term* • (acid [æsɪd]) etching[2] *n* → U39-21
  » The problem was caused by inadequate rinsing[3] after a hydrofluoric [aɪ] acid[4] etch.
  Use **acid etch** (composite) technique[2] / cemented splint • hot **acid etch** • **etch(ing)** acid / paste[5] / time / depth / pattern[6] • to be (acid) **etched** • **etched** surfaces / bridge[7] • resin[5] **etchant**

Ätzflüssigkeit, -mittel
ätzen; Ätzverfahren[1] Säureätzverfahren[2] Spülen[3] Flusssäure, HF[4] Ätzgel[5] Ätzmuster[6] Ätz-, Adhäsivbrücke[7]
19

30

sprue pin or **former** [spruː] n term   rel **sprue**[1] n & v term

wax or metal used to form the opening for molten metal to flow into a mold[2] [oʊ] when making a casting

» The sprues are removed and the taper[3] [eɪ] of the wall refined by mechanical milling techniques[4]. The complete framework is sprued, invested[5], and cast.
Use **sprue** reservoir[6] / hole[1] / button[7]

Gussstift
Gusskanal; m. Gussstiften versehen[1] Gussform[2] Verjüngung[3] Schleifverfahren[4] eingebettet[5] Gussreservoir[6] Gusskegel[7]
20

frit [frɪt] n & v term   rel **fritting**[1] n term

(n, i) mass of fused porcelain obtained by firing and subsequent immersion[2] [ɜːrʃ] in water
(ii) material from which the glaze[3] [gleɪz] for artificial [ɪʃ] teeth is made
(v) to heat ceramics to cause them to fuse and/or increase their transparency

» Then the frit is ground to make porcelain powders[4].

Fritte; fritten
Fritten[1] anschließendes Eintauchen[2] Glasur[3] pulverförm. Keramikmassen[4]
21

varnish [vɑːrnɪʃ] n & v term   sim **cavity liner**[1] [aɪ] n term

(n) liquid preparation painted[2] onto surfaces of teeth, restorations, etc. to form a protective coating[3]

» Fluoride gels and varnish had no corrosive effect on the titanium abutments[4] [ʌ].
Use fluoride[5] [aɪ]/ waterproof **varnish**

Lack; Lack auftragen
Kavitätenlack, Liner[1] aufgetragen[2] Schutzschicht[3] Titanpfeiler[4] Fluoridlack[5]
22

retarder [rɪtɑːrdɚ] n term   opposite **accelerator**[1] [əkselɚeɪtɚ] n term

agent used to slow the chemical hardening of gypsum, resins, or impression materials

Verzögerer
Beschleuniger[1]
23

desensitizing [diːsensɪtaɪzɪŋ] **paste** [eɪ] n term
                syn **dental (protective) paste** n term

caustic[1] [kɔːstɪk], coagulating or cytotoxic ointment[2] applied to the cervix of a tooth to obtund[3] [ʌ] pain from sensitive, exposed cementum or dentin
desensitize[4] v term • desensitizer[5] n • desensitization[6] n

» Application of an emollient[7] dental paste (e.g. Orabase®) reduces discomfort and promotes healing.

Desensibilisierungspaste
kaustisch, ätzend[1] Salbe[2] dämpfen, lindern[3] desensibilisieren, unempfindlich machen[4] Desensibilisierungsmittel[5] Desensibilisierung[6] schmerzlindernd[7]
24

Unit 31   Dental Lab Procedures & Equipment
Related Units: 30 Basic Dental Materials, 32 Dental Instruments

articulator [ɑːrtɪkjʊleɪtɚ] n term   sim **cast relator**[1] n term

device[2] [dɪvaɪs] representing the TMJ[3] and the jaws [dʒɔːz] and on which casts[4] may be mounted[5] [oʊ]

» Our aim was to measure [eʒ] the steepness of the occlusal plane produced by three different semi-adjustable articulators. We studied casts on articulators that are used to plan orthognathic surgery. Students will be able to perform laboratory exercises on dental articulators, e.g. mounting casts onto an articulator and fabrication of removable partial dentures.
Use (fully) adjustable [dʒʌ] (gnathologic) or class IV[5] / semi-adjustable or class III[7] / non-adjustable or class I[1] **articulator** • **articulator** joint / mounting[8]

Artikulator
Okkludator[1] Gerät, Vorrichtung[2] Kiefergelenk[3] Modelle[4] montiert, einartikuliert[5] (voll)justierbarer A.[6] teil-, halbjustierbarer A.[7] Modellmontage[8]
1

(dental) impression n term   rel **cast**[1] [kæst] n & v term

imprint[2] of teeth made by placing a tray of soft material (alginate) into the mouth; when it has hardened plaster[3] [æ] is poured [ɔː] into the impression to make a model of the teeth

» To secure impressions for the fabrication of master cast replicas[4], custom [ʌ] trays[5] were made from autopolymerizing acrylic resin[6].
Use to make[7]/obtain[7]/secure[7] **an impression** • alginate [dʒ]/ master / preliminary[8] / (altered cast partial) denture / sectional (facial moulage [ɑːʒ]) / tube **impression** • square / tapered[9] [eɪ] **impression coping** • **impression** appointment / post[10] [oʊ]/ fabrication[10] / compound / wax / area / jig[11] [dʒɪg]/ form • master / preliminary / working[12] / stone[13] / soft-tissue[14] **cast**

Abdruck, -formung
Modell, Guss(stück); gießen, abformen[1] Abdruck[2] Gips[3] Nachbildungen v. Meistermodellen[4] individuelle Abformlöffel[5] Akrylat, Kunststoff[6] Abdruck nehmen[7] Erstabformung[8] konische Abform- u. Übertragungskappe[9] Abdruckpfosten[10] Positionierungshilfe (z. Kieferrelationsbestimmung)[11] Arbeitsmodell[12] Spezialhartgipsmodell[13] Weichgewebemodell[14]   2

Dental Lab Procedures & Equipment — DENTISTRY

impression tray [treɪ] *n term*   *rel* **mold**[1] [oʊ] *n term, BE* **mould**

receptacle[2] used for pressing the alginate against the gums when making impressions for dentures

» After polymerization the tray was removed and allowed to bench cure[3] [benʃ kjʊɚ] for 24 hours.

Use custom / foil[4] [fɔɪl]/ resin[5] / mesh[6] **tray** • custom **tray** waxup • **impression tray** holder[7] / outline form / compound[8] • embedding[9] **mold**

mold [moʊld] *v term, BE* **mould**   *syn* **cast-cast-cast** [kæst] *v irr term*

to form a negative copy of an object in wax or any other material

castable[1] *adj term* • castability[2] *n* • molding *n*

» An alginate impression of the model with the tapered impression copings in place was made, and a cast fabricated with type IV dental stone. The hydroxylapatite [ɪ] particles are introduced with a sterile amalgam carrier[3] and molded into shape.

Use **molded** onto • firmly **molded** • **molding** time / stability[4] / process • injection[5] **molding** • **casting** mold[6] / muffle[7] [ʌ]/ stress[8] / material / properties[9] / unit[10] / flux[11] [ʌ]/ wax[12] / temperature[13]

die [daɪ] *n term*   *rel* **counterdie** [aʊ] *or* **female die**[1] *n term*

positive reproduction of teeth in hard substances, e.g. metal or special dental stone

» All dies fit into their predetermined positions. The impressions were filled with die stone[2].

Use **die** method[3] / system / pin[4] / spacer[5] / hardener • master[6] / gypsum [dʒɪpsəm] cast[7] **die**

setting expansion [æ] *n term*   *opposite* **shrinkage**[1] [ʃrɪŋkɪdʒ], **contraction**[1] *n term*

increase in size and volume occurring in the hardening of some materials, e.g. plaster of Paris[2]

expand[3] *v term* • shrink[4]-shrank-shrunk(en) *v irr* • contract[4] *v*

» Expanding wax patterns are used to compensate for the shrinkage of gold during the casting process. The resin is allowed to set[5] fully so that polymerization shrinkage[6] takes place. A thicker casting has a greater degree of shrinkage. The inaccuracies[7] related to the setting expansion of the stone base can be eliminated.

Use material / casting / curing[6] / low[8]-**shrinkage** • stone[9] / thermal[10] **expansion** • **shrinkage** compensation[11]

mounting [aʊ] *n term*   *sim* **mount**[1] *n & v term*

laboratory procedure of attaching the maxillary and/or mandibular cast to an articulator

» The master casts are mounted on a semi-adjustable articulator.

Use **mounting** device[2] [aɪs]/ medium [iː]/ resin / plate [eɪ] *or* ring[3] / plaster[4] • **mounted** diagnostic cast

invest *v term*   *syn* **imbed** *or espBE* **embed** *v*

covering or enveloping a denture, tooth, wax form, or crown, etc. wholly or in part with a refractory investment material[1] before curing, soldering, or casting

investment[2] *n term* • investing machine[3] *n*

» The two wax segments were invested and cast with Type III gold. The framework is recovered[4] from the investment to verify the fit on the master cast.

Use **investment** material[5] / liquid / cast[6] / casting mold[7] [oʊ]/ soldering[8] • **investing** dough[9] [doʊ]/ aids[10] / plaster / binder / tissue[11] • prosthesis-fixture-**investing** bone system

---

Abform-, Abdrucklöffel

Gussform, Gussstück[1] Träger[2] nachpolymerisieren[3] Metall-Abformlöffel[4] Kunststoff-Abformlöffel[5] perforierter Abformlöffel[6] Abformlöffelhalter[7] Löffel-, Abformmasse[8] Küvette[9]   3

(aus)gießen, formen, modellieren

gießfähig, Guss-[1] Gießfähigkeit[2] Amalgamträger[3] Formbeständigkeit[4] Spritzgussverfahren[5] Guss(hohl)form[6] (Guss)muffel, (Gieß)küvette[7] Gussspannung[8] Gusseigenschaften[9] Gussgerät[10] Flussmittel[11] Gusswachs[12] Gießtemperatur[13]   4

Modell(stumpf), Stumpfmodell

Konter, Gegenguss[1] Modellgips[2] Modellherstellungsverfahren[3] Modellstift[4] Stumpflack[5] Meistermodell[6] Gipsmodell[7]   5

Abbindeexpansion

Abbinde-, Erstarrungskontraktion, Schwindung, Schrumpfung[1] (Alabaster)gips, ß-Halbhydrat[2] ausdehnen, expandieren[3] kontrahieren, schwinden[4] polymerisieren, aushärten[5] Polymerisationsschrumpfung[6] Ungenauigkeiten[7] schrumpfarm[8] Abbindeexpansion v. Spezialhartgips[9] Wäremausdehnung, thermische Expansion[10] Schrumpfausgleich[11]   6

Modellmontage; Einartikulieren

Montage, montieren, einartikulieren[1] Montagehilfe[2] Montageplatte[3] Montagegips[4]   7

einbetten

feuerfeste Einbettmasse[1] Einbettung[2] Einbettgerät[3] ausgebettet[4] Einbettmasse[5] Einbettmassemodell[6] Gussmuffel, Gießküvette[7] Löten auf Einbettmasse[8] angerührte Einbettmasse[9] Einbetthilfen[10] umgebendes Gewebe[11]   8

114 DENTISTRY — Dental Lab Procedures & Equipment

(casting or **denture) flask** n & v term   rel **deflasking**[1] n term

(n) metal tube in which a refractory mold is made for casting dental restorations

» *To standardize the fabrication of the tray, a mold was fabricated using a denture flask. The cast and custom tray waxup were then flasked and boiled out[2] for 10 minutes. Separating medium was placed on both halves of the flask.*

Use to place or invest[3] **in a flask** • processing / tissue **flask** • **(denture) flask** holder / cross bar[4] / press[5] / basket / polymerization[6] / opener / removal[1] / cleanser [e] • trial[7] [aɪ]/ final **flask closure**

Küvette; einbetten, küvettieren
Ausbettung, -en[1] ausgebrüht[2] küvettieren[3] Küvettenbügel[4] Küvettenpresse[5] Küvettenpolymerisation[6] provisorischer Küvettenschluss[7]   9

waxup or **wax-up** n term & jar   syn **waxing** n jar

(i) technique of shaping the contours of a trial denture or crown in wax before metal casting (ii) the product of this procedure

» *A fully contoured waxing is completed on the preoperative casts.*

Use diagnostic[1] / framework[2] **waxup** • **waxing** technique[3] / pattern / sleeve • **wax-up** material / brush[4] [ʌ]/ die[5]

(i) Aufwachsen (ii) aufgewachstes Modell
diagnostisches Aufwachsen[1] Aufwachsen d. Gerüsts[2] Aufwachstechnik[3] Aufwachspinsel[4] Modellstumpf[5]   10

transfer coping [koʊpɪŋ] n term

cap-like covering of acrylic resin[1] or metal used to position dies in impressions

» *You may experience problems in seating the transfer copings. Impressions were made with transfer copings connected with acrylic resin[1].*

Use direct / indirect / one-piece / square [skweɚ]/ tapered[2] [eɪ] **transfer coping** • **transfer coping** technique

Übertragungs-, Transferkappe
Akrylat, Kunststoff[1] konische Übertragungskappe[2]   11

dowel [daʊəl] **(pin)** n term   syn **die pin** n, sim **impression post**[1] [oʊ] n term

metal pin placed in stone casts to be able to remove die sections[2] and replace them in their positions

» *The position of the dowel pin must be determined after the impression is cast. Care must be exercised not to allow the impression post to move from its positive seat in the impression material when the impression is vibrated [aɪ] and poured [ɔː] with stone[3].*

Use to cement/cast/cut back[4]/draw out/vibrate [aɪ] **dowels** • parallel / two-sided / notched[6] [tʃ]/ tapered [eɪ]/ stainless steel **dowel** • **dowel** length / space

Modellstift, Dowel pin
Abdruckpfosten[1] Modellstümpfe[2] m. Spezialhartgips ausgegossen[3] Stifte kürzen[5] gekerbter Modellstift[6]   12

(surgical) template [templɪt] n term

(i) a pattern, gauge[1] [geɪdʒ] or mold[2] used as a guide for duplicating[2] anatomic relationships
(ii) curved or flat surface pattern used as an aid[4] in fitting in[5] restorations
(iii) a guide used to assist in proper placement of dental implants

» *The acrylic template is separated from the cast, and its borders are smoothed [uː] and polished. Surgical guide templates[6] approximating the mandibular arch form were used.*

Use **template** fabrication / setting[7] • measuring / matching / guiding / reference / (transparent) overlay[8] [eɪ] **template** • well-fitting / flat[9] / positively seated / clear acrylic resin[10] / surgical implant **template**

Schablone, (Aufstell)kalotte
Messlehre[1] Gussform[2] D(o)ublieren[3] Hilfsmittel[4] Aufstellen[5] chir. Führungsschablonen[6] Kalottenartikulation, -aufstellung[7] (transparente) Röntgenschablone[8] flache Aufstellungshilfe[9] transparente Kunststoffschablone[10]   13

trituration n term   syn **amalgamation** n term → U30-1

breaking[1] and mixing substances such as amalgam in a mortar[2] with a pestle[3] [pesl] or a mechanical [k] device [aɪs]

triturate[4] v & n term • triturator[5] n • amalgamator[5] n

» *Triturate the tablets in a clean raised center mortar with a close fitting pestle using a light load. Sources of mercury vapor[6] in the dental office[7] include the trituration, handling, and placement of amalgam, the polishing of amalgam restorations, and the removal of old amalgam with a dental handpiece. Once amalgamation occurs, practically no free mercury is associated with the amalgam restoration.*

Use mortar and pestle **trituration** • **trituration** ratio[8] [reɪʃ(ɪ)oʊ] • mechanical **amalgamator**

Anmischen, Trituration
Verreiben[1] Mörser[2] Mörserkolben, Pistill[3] amalgamieren, verreiben; Amalgam[4] Amalgammischgerät, -vibrator[5] Quecksilberdampf[6] Zahnarztpraxis[7] Amalgamierungsverhältnis[8]   14

Dental Lab Procedures & Equipment — DENTISTRY 115

annealing [iː] n term   rel **annealing furnace**[1] [fɜːrnɪs] n term

heating materials followed by controlled cooling to remove internal stresses or brittleness[2], to achieve a desired degree of toughness[3] [tʌf-] or temper[3], or to volatilize impurities[4] from their surface and increase their cohesive properties[5]

anneal v term • annealing adj • annealer[1] n

» Then the material was transferred to an annealing furnace. Its structure was refined[6] [aɪ] by annealing at 800°C for 1 hour. An alcohol lamp with a soot-free[7] [uː] flame used e.g. to drive off the protective NH3 gas coating from the surface of cohesive [iː] gold foil[8] is called annealing lamp[9].

Jse **annealing** treatment / temperature / lamp[9] / cycle [saɪkl]/ tray • **(non)annealed** joints • **annealed** metal-ceramic [sɪr–] transition regions

Vergüten, Tempern, Anlassen
Vergütungsofen[1] Sprödigkeit[2] Härte(grad)[3] Verunreinigungen[4] Kohäsionskraft[5] vergütet[6] rußfrei[7] Stopfgoldfolie[8] Lötlampe, Gasbrenner[9]

15

---

solder [sɒːdɚ] n & v term   sim **brazing**[1] [breɪzɪŋ] n term

(n) fusible [fjuːz-] alloy[2] used to unite metals of a higher melting point[3] (v) joining two pieces of metal with such an alloy

soldering[4] n & adj term • braze v

» The framework is cast, tried in to confirm the fit and soldered after application of porcelain. Vacuum brazing[5], which offers one of the strongest bonding methods for metal joining, results in minimal distortion, leak-tight joint areas and clean and bright assemblies.

Jse to **solder** together / to / into / off • **hard**[6] / **main**[7] / **repair**[8] / **gold-based**[9] **solder** • **soldering** iron[10] [aɪɚn]/ technique / dish / furnace[11] / procedure / agent[12] / aid[13] / gap[14] / index • **solder** joint[15] • partially **soldered** framework • postceramic **soldering** • **brazing** temperature[16] / alloy / paste / investment material[17] • infrared / torch[18] [tʃ] / furnace / dip[19] / high-temperature **brazing** • **brazed** seam[20] [iː]

(Weich)lot; (weich)löten
Hartlöten[1] schmelzbare Legierung[2] Schmelzpunkt[3] Löten; löt-[4] Vakuumlöten[5] Hartlot[6] Erstlot[7] Nach-, Reparaturlot[8] Goldlot[9] Lötkolben[10] Lötofen[11] Löt-, Flussmittel[12] Löthilfe[13] Lötspalt, -fuge[14] Lötstelle[15] Löttemperatur[16] Löteinbettmasse[17] Flammenlötung[18] Tauchlöten[19] Hartlötnaht[20]

16

---

luting agent [luːtɪŋ eɪdʒənt] n term

fastening material or cement; e.g. plaster or wax to hold casts to an articulator, crowns to teeth, etc.

lute v term

» The restoration was fitted with a soft luting agent to ensure [ɪnʃʊɚ] that it can be removed. The coping on the master cast was luted with autocure resin[1].

Jse **to be luted** to / into place[2] / in position[2] / together • **luted** framework[3]

Kleber, Klebstoff, Haftvermittler
autopolymerisierender Kunststoff[1] fixiert werden[2] geklebtes Gerüst[3]

17

---

fire [faɪɚ] v term   syn **bake** [beɪk], **frit** v term

fusing[1] [fjuːzɪŋ] water and a powder containing kaolin, feldspar[2], etc. to produce porcelain for restorations etc.

refire[3] v term • rebake[3] v

» Firing was carried out in a furnace with platinum winding. Porcelain was fired onto the prefabricated copings. During the bisque-bake[4] [bɪsk] trial, the contour of the restoration was adjusted [dʒʌ] to a favorable emergence profile[5].

Jse **fired** porcelain[6] • **fire**-polished[7] • **firing** chamber[8] / temperature / cycle or regimen[9] [redʒ-]/ time / crack[10] • **baking** shrinkage[11] / in[12] / (on)to[13] (metal)

brennen
verbacken[1] Feldspat[2] nachbrennen[3] Bisquitbrand[4] Austritts-, Emergenzprofil[5] gebranntes Porzellan[6] glanzgebrannt[7] Brennkammer[8] Brandführung[9] Hitzeriss[10] Brennschwund[11] Einbrennen[12] Aufbrennen[13]

18

---

curing [kjʊɚɪŋ] n term → U32-23

polymerization process of resinous materials[1] causing them to become rigid[2] [dʒ] to form denture bases[3], fillings, impression trays[4], etc.

» The resin is then cured under pressure and carefully removed from the cast to avoid stone breakage[5] [breɪkɪdʒ].

Jse **chemically** / **room-temperature** / **poorly**[6] / **light**[7]-/ **heat**[8]-**cured** • **denture**[9] [-tʃɚ]/ **extended curing** / **curing** technique / agent[10] / cycle / lamp or light[11] / unit[12] • **self-curing**[13] • depth of[14] **cure** • dual-**cure** material[15]

Härten, Polymerisation
Kunststoffe[1] hart[2] Prothesenbasen[3] Abformlöffel[4] Hartgipsbruch[5] schlecht ausgehärtet[6] lichtpolymerisiert, -gehärtet[7] hitzegehärtet, heißpolymerisiert[8] Prothesenhärtung[9] Härter[10] Polymerisationsleuchte[11] Lichtofen[12] Autopolymerisation[13] Durchhärtungstiefe[14] dualhärtendes Material[15]

19

---

glaze [gleɪz] v & n term

(v) coating[1] ceramics [s] and other materials (esp. porcelain) to give them a glossy [ɒː] finish[2]

» Highly glazed porcelain was shown to promote a favorable soft-tissue response.

Jse **glazing** and soldering / furnace[3] [ɜː] / (ceramic) material[4] / liquid / brush[5] [ʌ]/ varnish[6] • **glaze** baking or firing[7] • **glazed** appearance

glasieren, emaillieren; glänzen; Glasur
Beschichten[1] glänzende Oberfläche[2] Keramikofen[3] Glasurmasse[4] Glanzlackpinsel[5] Glanzlack[6] Glanzbrand[7]

20

31

burnish [bɜːrnɪʃ] *v term*   *sim* **polish¹** [pɒːlɪʃ] *v & n term*

(i) to adapt margins [dʒ] of restorations by rubbing with an instrument (ii) to make dental surfaces smooth² [smuːð] and glossy

burnisher³ *n term* • burnishability *n* • polishing⁴ *adj & n* • polishable⁵ *adj*

» Condense and burnish the amalgam or place the selfcure⁶ composite in the usual way. A small double-ended ball burnisher may be used to burnish contacts⁷ and post-carve burnish amalgam restorations⁸.

Use **to burnish** restorations / margins [dʒ]/ necks / away a seamline⁹ [iː]/ out tool marks • hot / cold / light¹⁰ / citric [sɪ] acid **burnishing** • **burnishing** agent / machine³ / instruments / technique • **polishing** kit¹¹ / file / unit¹² / heat / lathe¹³ [eɪð]/ paste or gel¹⁴ [dʒel]/ dolly¹⁵

(i) (an)brünieren (ii) glätten
(glanz)polieren; Politur¹ glatt² Brünierer³ Polier-; Polieren⁴ polierbar⁵ selbsthärtend⁶ Kontaktflächen⁷ Glätten v. geschnitzten Amalgamfüllungen⁸ Nahtlinie glätten⁹ leichtes Anbrünieren¹⁰ Poliersatz¹¹ Poliergerät¹² Poliermaschine¹³ Polierpaste¹⁴ Schwabbel¹⁵

21

Unit 32   Dental Instruments
Related Units: 24 Surgical Instruments, 31 Dental Lab Procedures & Equipment, 37 Orthodontic Appliances

armamentarium [eɚ] *n term*   *sim* **instrumentarium¹**, **instrument(ation)²** *n term* → U7-1 ff

general term for dental chairs, ambient lights³, casting machines⁴ and other devices⁵ [aɪ] and equipment

» There is a need to improvise with a growing armamentarium to satisfy⁶ the atypical [eɪ] clinical situation. During surgery the lingual aspect of the mandible should be investigated with a probing instrument⁷.

Use compatible / implant **armamentarium** • dental / sharp / cutting / blunt⁸ [ʌ] **instruments** • inhalation / ingestion [dʒe] of⁹ **instruments** • **instrument** stroke¹⁰ / sterilization / tray

Ausrüstung, Einrichtung, Armamentarium
Instrumentarium¹ Instrument; Instrumentation² Praxisleuchten³ Gussmaschinen⁴ Vorrichtungen, Apparate⁵ gerecht werden⁶ Sonde⁷ stumpfe / atraumatische Instr.⁸ Verschlucken v. Instr.⁹ Instrumentbewegung¹⁰

1

lip *and/or* **cheek** [tʃiːk] **retractor** *n term*   → U24-16

small plastic pieces used to draw back¹ lips and cheeks

retract¹ *v term* • retraction *n* • retractability² *n*

» The use of multiple, single lip, wound [uː], or cheek retractors requires too many assisting hands. Soft tissues were incised [saɪz] and retracted to expose³ the alveolar [ɪə] crest⁴.

Use plastic / broad **retractor** • protraction and **retraction** forces • forceful⁵ /soft tissue **retraction** • **retraction** suture⁶ [suːtʃɚ] • tissue **retractability** • self-**retracting** flap

Lippen- bzw. Wangen(ab)halter
abhalten, zurückziehen, retrahieren¹ Retraktionsfähigkeit² freilegen, zugänglich machen³ Alveolarkamm⁴ starke / übermäßige Retraktion⁵ Haltenaht⁶

2

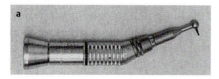

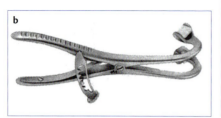

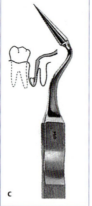

a handpiece
b mouth gag
c elevator

Dental Instruments | DENTISTRY 117

mouth gag [maʊθ gæg] n term, **gagger** n jar → U10-16
 sim **tongue** [tʌŋ] **depressor¹** n term
instrument used for opening the mouth, depressing the tongue to facilitate² examination, maintaining the airway³, and transmitting volatile anesthetics⁴ [e] during oropharyngeal [-ɪndʒɪəl] surgery
Use Davis-Crowe / Whitehead's **mouth gag** • **gag** reflex⁵

Mundsperrer
Zungenspatel¹ ermöglichen² Atemwege freihalten³ (volatile) Inhalationsanästhetika⁴ Würgreflex⁵   3

mouth mirror n clin   syn **dental mirror** n term
small mirror on a handle to facilitate visualization¹ [ʒ] in the examination of the teeth
» *Implant mobility was examined manually by tapping² with a dental mirror.*
Use plane³ [eɪ]/ magnifying⁴ [aɪ]/ fogging of the⁵ **mirror** • **mirror** handle⁶ / image⁷

Mund-, Zahnspiegel
Darstellung, Sichtbarmachung¹ Perkussion, Beklopfen² planer Spiegel³ Vergrößerungsspiegel⁴ Beschlagen d. Spiegels⁵ Spiegelgriff⁶ Spiegelbild⁷   4

(dental) handpiece n term   syn **dental drill** n jar
rotary power-driven dental instrument supplied with a mandrel¹ to hold cutting, polishing or grinding [aɪ] tools² [uː]
» *The embedded blocks were trimmed³ using a dental handpiece with a separating disk⁴.*
Use air-driven / low-speed / contra-angle⁵ [æŋgl]/ high-torque⁶ [k]/ torque-reduction **handpiece** • **handpiece** angulation

Handstück
Scheibenträger, Mandrel¹ Schleifkörper, -instrumente² zurechtschneiden³ Trennscheibe⁴ Winkelstück⁵ Handstück m. hohem Drehmoment⁶   5

bur [ɜː] n term or **burr** rare   syn **(bur) drill** n term, sim **diamond¹** [aɪ] n clin & jar
drilling tool with a small metal shaft and a head designed in various shapes; used at various rotational velocities for excavating decay [eɪ], shaping cavity forms, etc.
drill² v term • drilling n • drill bit³ n
» *The neck is reduced with a diamond bur and water-cooled. A bur mark is placed on the apex.*
Use (medium-grit [iː]) diamond⁴ / aqueous [eɪkwɪəs] dental⁵ / cross-cut⁶ / end-cutting⁷ **bur** • bud [ʌ] or rose-head⁸ / finishing⁹ / fissure [ɪʃ]/ no.6 round / tap / conical or inverted cone¹⁰ / microhead **bur** • long-shafted cylindrical / high-speed diamond¹¹ **bur** • hollow contouring / no. 8 carbide¹² [aɪ]/ 3.3-mm cannon **bur** • **bur** tip / hole / mark • through-the-**bur** internal irrigation¹³ • **drilling** technique / device / site • low rotatory **drill(ing)** speed • guide or pilot¹⁴ [aɪ]/ twist / spiral [aɪ]/ trephine¹⁵ [triːfaɪn]/ countersink¹⁶ **drill** • single-patient-use¹⁷ **diamond**

(Zahn)bohrer
Diamantschleifer, -schleifkörper¹ bohren² Bohrstück³ mittelkörniger Diamant⁴ wassergekühlter Bohrer⁵ Querhiebbohrer⁶ Stirnfräse⁷ Rosenbohrer⁸ Finierer⁹ Kegelbohrer¹⁰ hochtouriger Diamant¹¹ Hartmetallbohrer¹² intern gekühlter B.¹³ Pilotbohrer¹⁴ Trepanb.¹⁵ Versenkbohrer¹⁶ Einmaldiamantschleifkörper¹⁷   6

Note: In communication among dentists *drills* are quite commonly referred to as the *diamond*¹ since most burs, disks, and other cutting instruments are hardened with numerous small diamond pyramids [ɪ].

polishing brush [ʌ] n term
brush usually mounted¹ [aʊ] on a mandrel used to polish teeth or artificial [ɪʃ] replacements²

Polierbürste
befestigt¹ Zahnersatz²   7

emery disk n term, BE **disc**
disk coated¹ [oʊ] with emery powder² used to abrade³ [eɪ] or smooth⁴ [uː] the surface of teeth or fillings
Use rotating / diamond / end-cutting separating⁵ **disk** • snap on⁶ / water-cooled / sandpaper⁷ **disk**

Schleifscheibe
belegt¹ Schmirgel² be-, abschleifen³ glätten⁴ Trennscheibe⁵ aufsteckbare Scheibe⁶ Polierscheibe⁷   8

explorer n term   syn **probe** [oʊ], **sound** [aʊ] n term → U24-8
hook-like instrument with a fine pointed end (the tine¹ [aɪ]) used for examining the teeth
probe² v term • explore² v • sound² v
» *Anesthesia [-θiːʒə] of the tissues was confirmed by probing with an explorer.*
Use micro/ hook / thin / endodontic **explorer** • long tapered³ [eɪ] **tines** • double-ended / bulb-headed or bulbous⁴ [ʌ]/ antrum⁵ **probe** • hollow⁶ **sound**

(Zahn)sonde
Sonde(nspitze)¹ sondieren² lange, spitze Sonden³ Knopfsonde⁴ Kieferhöhlensonde⁵ Hohlsonde⁶   9

surveyor [səveɪɚ] n term
instrument for delineating¹ the contour of abutment [ʌ] teeth² and associated structures, e.g. before designing a removable partial denture³
» *The pins⁴ can be inserted into a surveyor to coordinate precision [sɪʒ] attachment⁵.*

Parallelisierungshilfe, -spiegel
erheben¹ Pfeiler-, Ankerzähne² abnehmbare Teilprothese³ Stifte⁴ Präzisionsverankerung⁵   10

32

DENTISTRY — Dental Instruments

reamer [iː] *n term*   *syn* **broach** [broʊtʃ] *n term*

rotating drilling tool for removing the pulp [ʌ], exploring, widening and cleaning the canal

ream[1] *v term* • reaming *n*

» *Preparation of the site included four-stage hand reaming to the final diameter of 6 mm.*

Use endodontic / hand(held) / engine[2] [endʒɪn] **reamer** • smooth [uː] / barbed[3] **broach**

Reamer, (Wurzel)kanalerweiterer
Wurzelk. ausräumen[1] maschineller R.[2] Exstirpationsnadel, Pulpaextraktor[3]

11

---

file [aɪ] *n term*   *sim* **rasp(atory)**[1] [æ] *n term* → U24-12

instrument with pointed ridges [dʒ] for grinding [aɪ] and smoothing[2] [uːð] surfaces; coarse[3] [ɔː] files are called rasps[1]

file *v term* • filed *adj* • rasp[4] *v*

» *Use of bone-cutting burs[5], rongeurs[6] [rɒˈndʒɚz], and bone files[7] was limited to patients with knife-edged [naɪf] ridge contours. A root canal file[8] is a pointed, flexible, steel tool used for rasping canal walls.*

Use bone[7] / flexible / endodontic or root canal[8] **file**

Feile
Raspatorium, Schabeisen, Grobfeile[1] glätten[2] grob[3] (ab)raspeln[4] Knochenfräsen[5] Luer-Knochenzangen[6] Knochenfeile(n)[7] Wurzelkanalfeile[8]

12

---

scaler [skeɪlɚ] *n term*   *sim* **interproximal stripper**[1] *n term*

tool with a curved hook used to remove tartar[2] or excess cement, check for cavities, etc.

scaling[3] *n term*

» *Presently, titanium rather than stainless steel scalers are recommended for instrumentation procedures involving the transmucosal abutments.*

Use metal / ultrasonic / air sonic / piezo-ceramic[4] [pieɪzoʊ] / stainless [eɪ] steel[5] / hoe[6] [hoʊ] **scaler** • root or deep[7] **scaling**

Scaler, Zahnsteinentferner
diamantierte(s) Feile / Band[1] Zahnstein[2] Scaling, Zahnstein- u. Konkrementenfernung[3] Zahnsteinentfernungsgerät[4] Edelstahlscaler[5] Hakenscaler[6] subgingivale Konkrementenfernung, deep scaling[7]

13

---

excavator *n term*   *sim* **curet(te)**[1] *n term* → U24-10

small spoon [uː] for cleaning out and shaping a carious cavity to prepare it for filling

excavation *n term* • excavate[2] *v*

» *The socket[3] was curetted[4] with a spoon excavator[5].*

Use hatchet[6] [hætʃɪt] / hoe[7] **excavator**

Exkavator
Kürette[1] exkavieren[2] Zahnfach, Alveole[3] kürettiert[4] Löffelexkavator[5] beilförm. Exk.[6] hauenförm. Exkavator[7]

14

---

elevator *n term*   *sim* **dental** or **extracting forceps**[1] [s] *n clin pl*

dental lever [eːǁiː *BE*] used to luxate [ʌ] and remove teeth and roots that cannot be engaged[2] by the beaks[3] [iː] of a forceps

elevate[4] *v term* • exolever[5] *n* • leverage[6] *n*

» *Extraction forceps or a dental elevator cannot be applied to the root without damaging the alveolar bone. Now the root fragment can be elevated gently up the socket.*

Use surgical / dental / small-tip / tissue / root[7] / periosteal[8] / sharp paddle[9] **elevator** • **elevator** edge

Hebel, Elevatorium
Zahn-, Extraktionszange[1] gefasst[2] Branchen, Maul[3] ab-, anheben, herausheben[4] Krallenhebel[5] Hebel(wirkung)[6] Wurzelheber[7] Periostelevatorium[8] scharfes flaches Elevatorium[9]

15

---

pliers [plaɪɚz] *n term pl*

grasping [æ] instrument[1] with two hinged[2] [dʒ] arms and (usually) serrated [eɪ] jaws[3] [dʒɔːz]

» *Enough of the material was trimmed[4] to allow it to be seized[5] [iː] with pliers.*

Use (telescope) crown / matrix [eɪ] / straight [streɪt] / curved [ɜː] contouring[6] **pliers** • sterile cotton / locking / clasp-adjusting[7] [dʒʌ] **pliers** • bird beak[8] [iː] / wire [aɪ] cutting[9] / torquing[10] [k] / three-prong[11] / flat nose[12] **pliers**

(Draht)zange
Fassinstrument[1] mit Scharnier[2] gezahntes Maul[3] entfernt[4] gefasst[5] gebogene Konturzange[6] Klammerjustierz.[7] Vogelschnabelz.[8] Drahtschneidezange[9] Torque-Z.[10] Aderer Z.[11] Flachzange[12]

16

---

plugger [ʌ] *n term*   *syn* **condenser** *n*, *sim* **spreader**[1] [e] *n term*

manual or powered instrument used for packing[2] unset[3] restorative material into a cavity of a tooth with a smooth [uː] or serrated nib[4] at the end

condense[2] *v term* • plug[2] *v* • plugging *n* • condensation *n*

» *Pluggers are instruments designed for vertical condensation, while spreaders are used for lateral condensation of gutta [ʌ] percha [tʃ] in the root canal.*

Use (fine) finger[5] / serrated / amalgam[6] / ball-shaped[7] / drop-shaped[8] / finishing[9] **plugger** • **plugger** nib • finger / hand[10] **spreader**

(Wurzelkanal)stopfer, Plugger
Spreizer, Spreader[1] verdichten, kondensieren[2] (noch) nicht ausgehärtet[3] glattes oder gezahntes Arbeitsende[4] Fingerstopfer, -plugger[5] Amalgamstopfer[6] Kugelst.[7] tropfenförm. St.[8] Planstopfer[9] Handspreader[10]

17

32

enamel cleaver [iː] *n term*   *sim* **hoe**[1] [hoʊ] *n term*

instrument with a heavy [e] shank[2] and a very short blade[3] [eɪ] at about 90° to the axis of the handle[4]; used with a hoeing motion to strip[5] enamel from the axial surfaces of a tooth in preparation for a crown

Schmelzmesser, -meißel, Gingiva(l)randschräger
Haue[1] breiter Schaft[2] Schneide[3] Griff[4] absprengen[5]   18

rubber [ʌ] **dam** [æ] *n term*

thin piece of rubber that can isolate teeth to control moisture[1] [mɔɪstʃɚ] during treatment
» In some instances[2] the application of a dam or clamp is physically not possible. The rubber dam prevented the water coolant spray[3] from draining into the abutment [ʌ].
Use **rubber dam** clamp[4] / clamp forceps[5] / punch[6] / frame

Kofferdam, Spanngummi
Feuchtigkeit[1] Fällen[2] Spraywasser (f. Kühlung)[3] Kofferdamklammer[4] Kofferdam-Klammerzange[5] Kofferdam-Lochzange[6]   19

pulp [ʌ] **tester** *n term*   *syn* **vitalometer** [aɪ] *n term*

electrical device for determining[1] the vitality [aɪ] of the tooth pulp
» X-rays, pulp testers, and percussion aid[2] in the diagnosis. A tooth may have a negative response to a pulp test[3] and still be sensitive to[4] percussion.
Use electric / thermal **pulp tester**

Pulpaprüfer, -tester
feststellen[1] helfen[2] Sensibilitäts-, Vitalitätsprüfung[3] empfindlich reagieren (auf)[4]   20

matrix [eɪ] **retainer** [eɪ] *n term*

mechanical [k] device to hold a matrix[1] around a tooth during restorative procedures by drawing the matrix band tight[2] [taɪt]

Matrizenhalter, -spanner
Matrize[1] Matrizenband spannen[2]   21

wedge [wedʒ] *n & v term*   *sim* **space maintainer**[1] [eɪ] *n term* → U37-12

(n) device for separating the teeth, maintaining[2] the separation obtained[3], or holding a matrix in place
» Both the treated and untreated implants were firmly wedged into the sockets.
Use interproximal[4] / interocclusal reference **wedge** • (aluminum) reference (step) **wedge** • **wedge**-shaped[5]

Keil, Separator; verkeilen
Lücken-, Platzhalter[1] Aufrechterhalten[2] erreicht[3] Interdentalkeil[4] keilförmig[5]

22

curing [kjʊɚɪŋ] **light** *n term*   *syn* **blue light (source)** *n term* → U31-19

special UV or halogen [-dʒən] light used to help plastic materials become rigid[1] [dʒ] to form a denture base[2], filling, etc.
» Composites can be cured[3] by any blue light source. Blue light sources may cause eye damage.

Aushärtelicht, Polymerisationsleuchte
fest, hart[1] Prothesenbasis[2] (aus)gehärtet, polymerisiert[3]   23

abrasive [eɪ] **paper** *n term*   *syn* **abrasive strip** *n term*

a ribbon[1] bonded with abrasive particles[2] on one side for contouring and polishing proximal surfaces
» The surfaces were polished to 600 grit[3] with silicon carbide[4] [aɪ] abrasive paper.

Polierstreifen
Streifen, Band[1] m. Abrasivpartikeln besetzt[2] Grit (Maß f. Körnung)[3] Siliciumcarbid[4]   24

articulating paper *n term*   *syn* **disclosing** or **occlusal paper** or **foil** [fɔɪl] *n term*

inked paper or ribbon[1] placed between the mandibular and maxillary teeth to check for[2] tooth contacts
» The occlusal contacts were checked directly with disclosing paper.

Okklusionsfolie, -papier, Artikulationspapier
m. Farbstoff beschichteter Papierstreifen[1] überprüfen[2]   25

Unit 33   Dental Imaging Techniques
Related Units: 46 Basic Radiologic Terms, Dentistry

x-ray tube [eksreɪ tʲuːb] *n term*

housed in the tube head[1] (together with the transformer[2]) of the dental x-ray machine[3]
» When children have their first x-rays taken it is wise to explain the procedure and equipment such as the tube head, camera, etc. to them in easy-to-understand language.
Use fogged[4] **x-ray tube**

Röntgenröhre
Röhrenschutzhaube, -gehäuse[1] Transformator[2] Röntgenstrahler[3] beschlagene Röntgenröhre[4]

1

Dental Imaging Techniques

(radiographic or x-ray) film n term

(i) x-ray-sensitive substance used in taking radiographs (ii) jargon for radiograph

» The *two-film procedure (stereoroentgenography[1])* is helpful for assessing marginal [dʒ] *bone height* [haɪt]. *The films were exposed at right angles* [ŋg] *to the field with the fixtures[2] parallel to the film.*

Use underexposed[3] / fogged[4] / sequential / gridded[5] / self-developing / scout[6] [aʊ] **film** • **film**-holding forceps or holder[7] / cassette[8] / packet / placement /-tooth relationship / density • occlusal / double emulsion[9] [ɪmʌlʃən]/ nonscreen[10] / blackness of the[11] **film** • **film** contrast / bending[12] / development / badge[13] [bædʒ]

Röntgenfilm, -aufnahme, -bild
Röntgenstereographie[1] Implantate[2] unterbelichteter Film[3] F. mit Grauschleier[4] gerasterter F.[5] Screeningaufnahme[6] Filmhalter[7] Filmkassette[8] beidseitig beschichteter F.[9] folienloser Film[10] Filmschwärzung[11] Knicken d. Films[12] Strahlenschutzplakette[13] 2

lead [e] **shield** [ʃiːld] n term

guard[1] [gɑːrd] or screen of lead and rubber protecting the patient, radiologic technician[2] [-knɪʃən] or radiologist from x-rays[3]

» *Modern dental x-ray equipment, fast film[4], collimated beams[5]* [iː] *and lead shields have significantly reduced the patient's risk of gonadal* [eɪ] *exposure[6]* [-oʊʒɚ].

Use gonad[7] / portable **shield** • **lead** or protective apron[8] [eɪ] • proper **shielding**

Bleigummiabdeckung
Schutz[1] Röntgenassistent(in)[2] Röntgenstrahlen[3] Film für Schnellaufnahmen[4] gebündelte / kollimierte Strahlen[5] Gonadenbelastung[6] Gonadenschutz[7] Bleischürze[8] 3

intraoral views [vjuːz] n term *opposite* **extraoral views[1]** n term

x-rays obtained[2] with the film package placed inside the oral cavity

» *Frequently employed extraoral radiographs* [eɪ] *include panoramic and lateral jaw* [dʒɔː] *radiographs[3].*

Use **intraoral** radiograph / bitewing film / x-ray film viewer[4] • long-cone[5] / conventional **intraoral radiograph** • axial / lateral / occipitomental [ks]/ occlusal[6] / submentovertex **view**

intraorale (Röntgen)-aufnahmen
extraorale (Röntgen)aufnahmen[1] angefertigt[2] laterale Kieferaufnahme[3] Röntgenbildbetrachter f. intraorale Aufnahmen[4] io. Aufnahme mit Langtubus[5] Aufbiss-, Okklusalaufnahme[6] 4

panoramic radiograph n term *syn* **pan** n jar

x-ray taken by a machine that rotates around the head and produces a view of the entire maxillary and mandibular arch [tʃ] including the TMJ[1]; sometimes also termed dental panoramic tomograph[2]

» *The major drawback[3] of panoramic radiographs, which are commonly used to visualize* [ʒ] *the canal, is image distortion[4]* [-ʃən] *(lingual objects appear higher than the buccal* [ʌ] *ones).*

Use **panoramic** radiographic evaluation / survey[5] / view[6] / CT[2] / rotating machine[7]

Panorama(röntgen)aufnahme
Kiefergelenk[1] Panorama-Schichtaufnahme[2] Nachteil[3] Verwischung[4] Panorama-Vergrößerungsaufnahme[5] Panoramaaufnahme[6] Panorama-Röntgengerät[7] 5

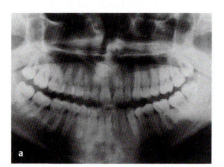
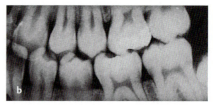

a Panoramic radiograph
b Bitewing radiograph

bitewing [baɪtwɪŋ] **film** or **radiograph** n term *syn* **interproximal film** n term

x-ray (taken with a film package held between the occlusal surfaces) that shows the coronal portion and cervical third of the root of the teeth in near occlusion

» *Bitewing films are useful in detecting interproximal caries[1] and determining alveolar* [ɪə] *septal height. In children with low caries potential a bitewing exam every 18-24 months is sufficient* [ɪʃ].

Use reverse[2] / posterior **bitewing**

Bissflügelaufnahme
Approximalkaries[1] umgekehrter Bissflügel[2] 6

Dental Imaging Techniques DENTISTRY 121

periapical [eɪ] **radiograph** n term

radiograph demonstrating tooth apices[1] [eɪpɪsiːz] and surrounding structures of a selected area
» *Ultraspeed film[2] was used for all periapical images. On inspection of the periapical radiographs small radiolucent [uːs] zones[3] [z] were visible around the failed[4] implants.*
Use **periapical** (dental) film / view / image / (intraoral) x-rays

periapikale Aufnahme
Wurzelspitzen[1] hochempfindlicher Film[2] strahlendurchlässige / radioluzente Bereiche[3] gelockert[4]

7

T-Scan n term

computerized sensing system[1] for assessing occlusal forces[2]
» *The T Scan can provide analysis of the bilateral [aɪ] similarity[3] of occlusal contacts[4].*
Use **T-Scan** occlusal analysis system[5] / sensor

T-Scan
Erfassungssystem[1] okklusale Kräfte[2] beidseitige Übereinstimmung[3] okklusale Kontakte[4] T-Scan-System[5]

8

cephalometry [sefəl-] or **-metrics** n term
                                                sim **cephalometric radiograph**[1] n term

scientific assessment[2] of the cranial [eɪ] bones, head and face (including soft tissue profile) with relation to specific reference points[3] using a fixed, reproducible position for lateral radiographic exposure
» *Longitudinal cephalometric studies revealed growth-related problems in two dental implants.*
Use **cephalometric** tracing[4] [eɪs]/ analysis[5] / landmarks[3] / view / film / head positioner[6] (cephalostat[6]) / relationship • lateral / serial **cephalogram**

Kephalometrie
kephalometrische Röntgenaufnahme[1] wissensch. Untersuchung[2] kephalom. Bezugs-, Referenzpunkte[3] kephalom. Befund-(erheb)ung[4] kephalom. Analyse[5] Kephalostat[6]

9

skull x-ray or **radiograph** n term   syn **skull film** n jar

» *The lateral skull radiograph showed a wide alveolar [ɪə] crest[1] down to the base of the mandible.*

Schädelröntgen(aufnahme)
breiter Alveolarkamm[1]

10

(ultra)sonography n term   syn **ultrasound** [ʌ], abbr **US** n term

visualization, measurement [eɜ], or delineation[1] of deep structures by measuring the reflection or transmission of high frequency or ultrasonic waves
    ultrason(ograph)ic[2] adj term • ultrasonogram[3] n
» *In dentistry ultrasound is used mainly for the analysis of soft-tissue thickness in periodontal diagnosis or preimplantologic evaluation.*
Use **ultrasound** image • gray-scale[4] [eɪ]/ Doppler[5] / real-time[6] / diagnostic / pulsed[7] [ʌ] **ultrasound** • ultrasonographic echo [ekoʊ] • **ultrasonic** waves[8] • A-mode / B scan[9] **ultrasonography**

Ultraschalldiagnostik, Sonographie
Darstellung[1] sonographisch, Ultraschall-[2] Sonogramm[3] Grauwertsonographie[4] Doppler-Sonographie[5] Echtzeitsonographie[6] Impulsechoverfahren[7] Schallwellen[8] B-Mode Darstellung[9]

11

magnetic resonance imaging n term   abbr **MRI**

diagnostic imaging modality using the radiofrequency radiation from hydrogen [aɪ] ions[1] [aɪənz]; depending on H+ concentration the signals vary in strength as the body is placed in a magnetic field
» *MRI is particularly useful for imaging the TMJ and facial [feɪʃəl] soft tissues[2], while the structure of cortical bones yields[3] a signal void[4], so they are black inside while the margins[5] are visualized.*

Magnetresonanz- (MRT), Kernspintomographie
Wasserstoffionen[1] Weichteile, -gewebe[2] stellt sich dar als[3] signalfreier Bereich[4] Ränder, Umrisse[5]

12

sialography [saɪəlɒːgrəfi] n term   syn **ptyalography** [taɪəlɒː-] n term

x-ray examination of the salivary glands[1] and ducts after the introduction of contrast material[2]
» *Interventional sialography[3] can be performed for retrieval[4] of salivary calculi[5] [-laɪ].*

Sialographie
Speicheldrüsen[1] Kontrastmittel[2] Interventionssialographie[3] Extraktion, Entfernung[4] Speichelsteine, Sialolithen[5]

13

arthrography n term   rel **arthrogram**[1] n term

radiography of a joint (e.g. the TMJ) usually following injection of contrast media [iː]
» *In TMJ arthrography both the upper and lower joint spaces can be injected with contrast material under fluoroscopic control[2] and real-time images of meniscus movement can be obtained and recorded on video.*
Use air[3] / opaque [eɪk] **arthrography** • double-contrast[4] **arthrogram**

Arthrographie
Arthrogramm[1] unter fluoroskopischer Sicht[2] Arthropneumo-, Pneumarthrographie[3] Doppelkontrastarthrogramm[4]

14

radioautography or **-gram** *n term*   *rel* **radiovisiography**[1] *n term*

reproduction of the distribution and concentration of radioactivity in a tissue or substance by placing a photographic emulsion on the surface of or in close proximity[2] to the substance

autoradiograph[3] *n term* • radioautographic *adj*

» The radioautographic results were obtained from sections poststained[4] with toluidine [təluːədiːn] blue[5] through the emulsion. Radiovisiography is performed with an x-ray set, an intraoral sensor, a display processing unit and a printer.

Use **radioautographic** evidence / labeling[6] [eɪ]/ study

Autoradiographie
Radiovisiographie[1] Nähe[2] Autoradiogramm[3] nachgefärbt[4] Toluidinblau[5] autoradiographische Markierung[6]

15

digital [dʒ] **subtraction radiography** *n term*   *sim* **videosubtraction**[1] *n term*

computer-assisted imaging modality that allows for[2] visualization of the soft tissues without the overlying bone (e.g. images made before and after contrast injection allow subtraction of unenhanced[3] structures) as well as assessment of changes in radiographs over time

» The digital subtraction image[4] shows areas where remodeling[5] of the peri-implant bone has occurred.

digitale Subtraktionsradiographie
Videosubtraktion[1] ermöglicht[2] ohne Kontrastverstärkung[3] digitale Subtraktionsaufnahme[4] Umbau(vorgänge), Remodellierung[5]

16

dental xerography [zɪɔrɒː-] *n term*   *syn* **dental xeroradiography** *n term*

radiograph produced on a rigid[1] [rɪdʒɪd] aluminum photoreceptor plate instead of a regular film which is developed with a dry powder rather than liquid chemicals

Xeroradiographie
fest[1]

17

computed or **computerized tomography** *n term*   *abbr* **CT** or **CAT (scan)**

gathering of anatomical information from a cross-sectional plane[1] [eɪ] of the body, presented as an image generated [dʒe] by a computer synthesis of x-ray transmission data obtained in many different directions through the given plane[2]

» CT images are invaluable[3] in assessing extensive trauma or pathology and planning surgery.

Use **computed** axial[4] (*abbr* CAT scan) / computerized transaxial (*abbr* CTAT scan) / linear / spiral [aɪ]/ cross-sectional **tomography** • presurgical / high-resolution[5] / 3D[6] / quantitative **computerized tomography**

Computertomographie, CT
Querschnitt, Schicht[1] festgelegte Ebene[2] besonders wertvoll[3] CT[4] hochauflösende Computertomographie (HRCT)[5] 3-dimensionales / 3-D CT[6]

18

multiplanar [-pleɪnəˑ] **reconstruction** *n term*   *sim* **3D imaging**[1] *n term*

three-dimensional image reconstructed from CT cross-sections[2]

» The multiplanar reconstruction and display technique [tekniːk] frequently demonstrated underestimations[3] of the coronal and sagittal [dʒ] slices[4] [slaɪsiːz].

3D-Schichtrekonstruktion
3D-Darstellung[1] CT-Schichtaufnahmen[2] Unterbewertung[3] Sagittalschnitte[4]

19

Unit 34   Oral Hygiene & Prophylactic Dentistry

Related Units: 40 Restorative Dentistry, 35 Periodontics, 42 Prosthodontics, 39 Cosmetic Dentistry

oral hygiene [haɪdʒiːn] *n term*   *syn* **dental care, oral physiotherapy** *n term*

caring for teeth by means of a toothbrush, interdental stimulator[1], dental floss, irrigating device[2], etc.

hygienic [eǁiː] *adj term* • oral hygienist[3] [iːǁe] *n* • dental hygienist[4] *n*

» Without scrupulous oral hygiene[5] and repeated fluoride [aɪ] treatments, tooth decay [-keɪ] will increase.

Use to improve / lack of[6] / adequate **oral hygiene** • **oral hygiene** instructions • **hygienic** measures [eʒ]/ check[7]

Mundhygiene, Zahnpflege
Interdentalstimulator[1] Munddusche[2] Prophylaxehelfer(in), Mundhygieniker(in)[3] Dentalhygieneassistent(in)[4] gründliche M.[5] mangelnde M.[6] Mundhygienekontrolle[7]

1

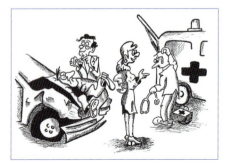

Did you call for a dental hygienist to help with disimpaction?

Oral Hygiene & Prophylactic Dentistry — DENTISTRY

oral or **dental prophylaxis** n term   syn **sanitization** n, **prophy** n jar

removal of accretions[1] [iːʃ], esp. plaque [plæk] from enamel surfaces by scaling and polishing with rubber wheel[2] [iː], etc.

prophylactic[3] adj term

» In addition to providing direct prophylactic treatment, the hygienist also may be responsible for assistance in suture removal, exposure of radiographic films, etc.

Use fluoride **prophylactic** agents[4] • **prophylactic** treatment • caries / periodontal **prophylaxis** • rubber **prophy** point[2]

Zahn-, Kariesprophylaxe
Beläge[1] Gummipolierer[2] prophylaktisch, vorbeugend[3] fluoridhaltige Präparate zur Kariesprophylaxe[4]

2

(tooth)brush [ʌ] n & v   sim **cleanse**[1] [e], **clean**[1] [iː] v

(n) consists of a long handle[2] and bristles[3] [sl] fixed to a small head[4]

» Use of interdental brushes[5] should be encouraged [ɜː] and patients warned against toothpicks[6].

Use **to brush** one's teeth[7] • soft/hard bristled[8] / bent angle [æŋgl]/ end-tufted[9] [ʌ]/ electric / ultrasonic / spiral [aɪ] **(tooth)brush** • **brush** stick[10] • tongue[11] [tʌŋ] • rotary **brushing** • **brushing** strokes[12] / technique[13] • **toothbrush** trauma[14] [ɔː] • to be **brushed** away / off

Zahnbürste; bürsten, putzen
reinigen[1] Griff[2] Borsten[3] (Bürsten)-kopf[4] Zwischenraum-, Interdentalbürstchen[5] Zahnstocher[6] Zähne putzen[7] Zahnbürste m. harten Borsten[8] Büschelbürste[9] Mikro-Zahnbürste[10] Zungenreinigung[11] Putzbewegungen[12] Zahnputztechnik[13] Zahnbürstentrauma, Putzläsionen[14]

3

---

dentifrice [dentɪfrɪs] n term

preparation for cleansing[1] [e] teeth, e.g., toothpaste, tooth powder[2] [aʊ], mouth rinses[3] or mouthwash[3]

» Periodic application of fluoride compounds should be supplemented[4] by daily use of a fluoride-containing dentifrice.

Zahnpflegemittel
Reinigen, Putzen[1] Zahnpulver[2] Mundwasser[3] ergänzt[4]

4

(dental) floss [ɒː] n & v clin   syn **floss silk** n, sim **dental tape**[1] n

untwisted thread[2] [e] made from fine silk[3] fibers [aɪ] used for cleansing interproximal spaces

» Use a regular flossing pattern so that no area is neglected[4]. Tooth loss is less frequent among persons who floss or use stick brushes and visit their dentist regularly.

Use **flossing** cords[1] • **floss** dispenser[5] / threader[6] • implant **flossing** • (un)waxed[7] **floss** • superdental[8] **floss**

Zahnseide; mit Z. reinigen
Zahn(reinigungs)band[1] Faden[2] Seide[3] vernachlässigt[4] Zahnseidenspender[5] Einfädler[6] (un)gewachste Z.[7] Spezialzahnseide[8]

5

---

rinse n & v clin   sim **flush** [ʌ] **(away)**[1] v clin

(n) mouthwash used for rinsing or gargeling[2] (v) cleaning or flushing debris[3] [dəbriː] with fluids

» Try rinsing the mouth by vigorously[4] swishing water back and forth[5] between and around the teeth.

Use **to rinse** off[6] / out[7] / one's mouth[8] / one's hands • to have[8]/give sth. **a rinse** • **rinse** water • daily **rinsing** • **rinsing** time / agent[9] / liquid • mouth[10] **rinses**

Spülung; (aus)spülen
(weg)spülen[1] Gurgeln[2] Speisereste[3] kräftig, tüchtig[4] Wasser durch d. Zähne pressen[5] abspülen[6] ausspülen[7] Mund ausspülen[8] Spülmittel, -flüssigkeit[9] Mundspülungen[10]

6

---

accretion [əkriːʃ°n] n term

foreign [fɔːrɪn] material (plaque or calculus) deposited[1] on the surface of a tooth or in a cavity

» This creates a niche [niːʃ] for plaque accumulation[2] and prevents effective accretion removal.

Use to prevent/remove[3] **accretions** • **accretion** prevention[4] • microglobular **accretions**

Auflagerung, Belag
ab-, an-, aufgelagert[1] Ansammlung[2] Beläge entfernen[3] Plaque-Hemmung[4]

7

(dental) plaque [plæk‖BE plɑːk] n term

thin colorless, sticky film[1] containing saliva[2] [aɪ], acids and bacteria forming on teeth that causes tooth decay

» Air-abrasive [eɪ] polishing is used to remove plaque from hard-to-reach areas[3].

Use **to** disclose[4]/remove **plaque** • **plaque** accumulation / formation[5] / inhibiting agent[6] • calcified[7] [s] **plaque** • adequate **plaque** control[8] • **plaque**-like film /-free /-retaining • **plaque-disclosing** tablet[9] / solution[9] / liquid[9] • **plaque** index or score[10]

(Dental)plaque, Zahnbelag
klebrige Schicht[1] Speichel[2] schwerzugängliche Bereiche, Retentionsstellen[3] Plaque anfärben[4] Plaquebildung[5] Plaquehemmstoff[6] mineralisierte P.[7] Plaquebekämpfung, -beseitigung[8] Plaque-Färbemittel, -Indikator[9] Plaqueindex[10]

8

DENTISTRY — Oral Hygiene & Prophylactic Dentistry

(dental) calculus [æ] n term syn tartar [ɑː], calcified plaque [æ] n term

hardened cement-like deposit[1] consisting of mineral salts[2] and organic matter[3] forming on teeth when plaque is not regularly removed

» The calculus was primarily of the supragingival [dʒ] type and tenaciously [eɪʃ] adherent[4] in nature.

Use calculus formation / deposition / retention[5] / removal by hand[6] • tartar-like /-susceptible[7] [sep]/ inhibitor / inhibitory toothpaste[8] / solvent[9] / scaler[10]

Zahnstein
Ablagerung, Belag[1] Mineralsalze[2] organische Substanzen[3] fest anhaftend[4] Zahnsteinhaftung[5] Zahnsteinentfernung m. Handinstrumenten[6] zahnsteinanfällig[7] zahnsteinhemmende Zahnpasta[8] Zahnsteinlöser[9] Zahnsteinentferner, Scaler[10]   9

acquired [əkwaɪəd] (oral) pellicle n term
syn acquired (enamel) cuticle [kjuː-] n term

thin film forming over the surface of a cleansed tooth crown when exposed to[1] saliva [aɪ]

» The formation of pellicle-like thin layers [eɪ] was observed on all surfaces.

Use pellicle-coated surfaces[2] • salivary / dental pellicle formation

erworbenes / tertiäres Schmelz-, Zahnoberhäutchen, Cuticula dentalis
ausgesetzt[1] m. einem Schmelzoberhäutchen überzogene Flächen[2]   10

stain [steɪn] n & v clin & term syn (colored) spot n inf

deposits produced by chromogenic [dʒen] bacteria, smoking, metal oxides [aɪ], etc. that cause discolorations[1]

» Air-abrasive polishing[2] has proved an effective means for removing tenacious, gross [oʊ] stains[3] and heavy plaques[4].

Use brown / white / green / black[5] stain

> Note: The term staining[6] also refers to coloring materials (dyes[7] [daɪz]) used in diagnostic procedures to visualize structures.

Zahnverfärbung, farbiger Belag; (an)färben
Verfärbungen[1] Polieren m. Pulverstrahlgerät[2] massive, auffällige Z.[3] starker Plaquebefall[4] Melanodontie[5] Anfärbung, Färbetechnik[6] Farbstoffe, Färbemittel[7]   11

plaque-disclosing tablets n term

solutions or tablets selectively staining[1] soft debris, pellicle, and bacterial plaque on teeth

» Plaque-disclosing tablets or liquids may be used to check the efficacy[2] [efɪkəsi] of plaque removal.

Plaquefärbetabletten
anfärben[1] Gründlichkeit, Effektivität[2]   12

stannous [æ] fluoride [flʊəraɪd] n term

prophylactic gel [dʒ] containing stannous tin[1] and fluoride which hardens teeth and prevents tooth decay

» Excessive fluoride ingestion[2] during tooth formation may result in mottled enamel[3], which varies in appearance from small white opacities[4] [æs] to yellow and black stains. Dean's fluorosis index[5] measures [eʒ] the degree of mottled enamel (fluorosis) in teeth.

Use fluoride content[6] / intake[2] / application[7] / poisoning[8] / treatments / varnish[9] / mouthwash / gel • fluoridation of drinking water[10] • fluoridated table salt[11] / water • dental[3] fluorosis

Zinn-Fluorverbindung
Zinn[1] Fluoridaufnahme, -zufuhr[2] Dentalfluorose[3] weiße, opake Stellen[4] Dean-Fluorose-Index[5] Fluoridgehalt[6] Fluoridierung[7] Fluoridintoxikation[8] Fluoridlack[9] Trinkwasserfluoridierung[10] fluoridiertes Kochsalz, Fluoridsalz[11]   13

root [uː] planing [eɪ] n term sim scaling[1] [eɪ], curettage[2] [kjʊəetɪdʒ] n term

using metal scalers to remove and smoothe[3] [uː] hard deposits on the root surface (esp. the subgingival portions) to allow for[4] pocket reduction[5] and reattachment[6] of the gums[7] [ʌ]

» Patients received routine periodontal treatment including scaling and root planing. Implants cannot be scaled or root planed.

Use subgingival [dʒ] or deep[8] scaling • root smoothing[9] • removed by curettage

Wurzelglättung
Zahnsteinentfernung[1] Kürettage[2] glätten[3] ermöglichen[4] (Zahnfleisch)taschenreduktion[5] Wiederanheftung[6] Gingiva, Zahnfleisch[7] subgingivale Konkrementenfernung, deep scaling[8] Wurzelglättung[9]   14

enamel grooves [uː] n usu pl sim enamel pits[1] / porosities[2] / fissures[3] [ɪʃ] n term

depressions, furrows [ɜː] or deep clefts in the enamel favoring deposition of caries-producing agents [eɪdʒ]

» Sealing enamel pits[1] and fissures is highly effective in preventing caries.

Use grooving from brushing[4] • groove wall / edge / width[5] [wɪdθ]/ depth • grooved surfaces

Schmelzfurchen
Schmelzgrübchen[1] Schmelzporositäten[2] Schmelzfissuren[3] Putzrillen, -furchen[4] Grübchenbreite[5]   15

Oral Hygiene & Prophylactic Dentistry — DENTISTRY

sealant [siːlənt] *or* **sealer** *n term*   *rel* **seal**[1] *v & n*   → U26-11

plastic coating material[2] applied e.g. to nonfused [uː], noncarious grooves, pits and fissures of teeth to achieve an airtight [-taɪt] closure[3] [oʊʒ] and prevent decay

Use dental[4] / fissure[5] **sealant** • palatal / peri-implant[6] **seal** • **sealing** material / compound[7] / varnish[4] / wax[8] • **sealed** filling

Versiegler, Versiegelungslack
versiegeln, (ab)dichten; Versiegelung, Abdichtung[1] Beschichtungsmaterial[2] luftdichter Verschluss[3] Versiegelungslack[4] Fissurenversiegler[5] perimplantäre Abdichtung[6] Abdichtungsmasse[7] Siegelwachs[8]   16

(tooth *or* **dental) decay** [dɪkeɪ] *n & v term*

(n) loss of calcified tooth structure[1] due to caries; decalcification begins on the tooth surface and if left unchecked penetrates the enamel and dentin layers and may reach the pulp [ʌ]

» *Are any teeth decayed? Resistance to dental decay was improved.*

Use extensive / deep[2] / subgingival **decay** • deeply **decayed** • **decayed** pulp /-missing-filled teeth surfaces index[3] • **decay** involving the pulp[2] / resistant

Zahnfäule, Karies;
kariös werden, faulen
Zahnhartsubstanz[1] tiefgehende Karies, Caries profunda[2] DMFS-Index[3]
17

(dental) caries [keəriːz] *n term*

microbial destruction of teeth which become discolored and porous[1]

(pre)carious[2] [keəriːəs] *adj term* • caries-prone[3] [oʊ] *adj* • cario- *comb*

» *Caries spreads* [e] *rapidly because of the lower mineral content of dentin and cementum.*

Use **carious** lesion[4] [iː]/ cavity[5] / tooth • (senile [siːnaɪl]) dental / nursing bottle[6] / coronal / cervical[7] [ɜː]/ pit (and fissure) / rampant[8] **caries** • **caries**-resistant /-free /-susceptible[3] /-promoting[9] /-producing / prophylaxis[10] / treatment • active[11] / arrested[12] / buccal [ʌ]/ cemental **caries** • compound / distal / incipient[13] [sɪ]/ interdental / mesial [iː]/ occlusal **caries** • primary / secondary / recurrent[14] [ɜː]/ root / smooth surface[15] **caries** • **cario**static[16] /genesis [dʒen]

(Zahn)karies
porös[1] kariös, kariesbefallen[2] kariesanfällig[3] kariöse(r) Defekt / Läsion[4] Kavität[5] Flaschenkaries[6] Zahnhalskaries[7] floride K., Caries florida[8] kariesfördernd[9] Kariesprophylaxe[10] Caries acuta[11] stationäre / arretierte K.[12] Initialkaries[13] Kariesrezidiv[14] Glattflächenkaries[15] Kariostatikum[16]
18

---

cavity [kævɪti] *n clin & inf*   *sim* **cavitation**[1] *n term*

(i) space in a tooth resulting from dental decay
(ii) hollow space inside the body, e.g the nasal [eɪ]/ oral cavity[2]

» *After removal of tooth decay the fillings are inserted*[3] *in the cavities.*

Use deep / open / closed / compound[4] / buccal **cavity** • to fill / to prepare[5] **cavities** • **cavity** toilet[6] / formation[1] / preparation[7] / wall[8] / margin[9] [dʒ]/ outline[10] / trimmer[11] / varnish[12] / condensation / restoration

(i) Kavität, Loch
(ii) Höhle, Cavum, Cavitas
Kavitation, Defektbildung[1] Mundhöhle[2] Füllungen w. eingebracht[3] mehrflächige Kavität[4] K. präparieren[5] Kavitätenreinigung[6] -präparation[7] Kavitätenwand[8] Kavitätenrand[9] Kavitätenumriss[10] Kavitätenbohrer[11] Kavitätenlack[12]   19

---

breath [breθ] **odor** [oʊdɚ] *n term, BE* **odour**   *syn* **bad breath** *clin*, **halitosis, fetor** [iː] **oris** *n term*

foul[1] [aʊ] offensive[2] odor from the mouth

» *His chief symptoms are acutely painful bleeding gingiva, salivation, and fetid breath*[3]*. Extensive dental caries, periodontal disease, or tonsillitis* [aɪ] *are causes of breath odor often accompanied by a bad taste. GI disorders*[4] *do not generally cause halitosis, and it is a fallacy*[5] *that breath odor reflects the state of digestion* [dʒe] *and bowel* [aʊ] *function. Mouthwashes and chewable* [tʃuː-] *breath fresheners gave him limited improvement.*

Use unpleasant [e]/ fetid[3] [e‖iː]/ fruity / mousy **breath odor** • to have/be aware of one's own **bad breath** • to hold[6]/catch[7] one's **breath** • **breath** freshener[8]

(übler) Mundgeruch, Foetor
ex ore
übel(riechend)[1] widerlich, abstoßend[2] übler Mundgeruch[3] Erkrankungen d. Magen-Darm-Traktes[4] Irrtum[5] Atem anhalten[6] Atem holen, verschnaufen[7] Mundwasser[8]
20

Oral Hygiene Index *n term*   *abbr* **OHI**

index used in field surveys[1] [ɜːrveɪz] for measuring the current oral hygiene status [eɪ] based on the amount of debris and calculus occurring on six representative tooth surfaces in the mouth

Use Simplified[2] **Oral Hygiene Index** (*abbr* OHI-S) • caries **index** • DEF or def / df / dmfs **caries index**[3] (decayed, missing, and filled surfaces of deciduous or permanent teeth) • RDFT (ratio of decayed and filled teeth)

oraler Hygieneindex (OHI)
Reihenuntersuchungen[1] vereinfachter OHI[2] DMF Flächenindex[3]
21

Clinical Phrases

Try to relax as much as you can. Versuchen Sie, sich so gut wie möglich zu entspannen. • I'll now check the efficiency of plaque removal with this disclosing liquid. Ich werde nun mit dieser Farblösung kontrollieren, ob die Plaque gründlich entfernt wurde. • This may hurt a bit. Das tut jetzt vielleicht ein wenig weh. • This way you get access to those hard-to-reach surfaces. Damit erreichen Sie auch die schwer zugänglichen Flächen. • To reduce the amount of oral bacteria I'd recommend using this tongue scraper twice daily. Um die Bakterien im Mund zu reduzieren, würde ich Ihnen empfehlen, die Zunge zweimal täglich mit diesem Zungenschaber zu reinigen. • The patient, who reeked of mouthwash, was obviously being self-conscious about his breath. Der Patient roch stark nach Mundwasser; offensichtlich war ihm sein Mundgeruch peinlich.

Unit 35   Periodontics

Related Units: 34 Oral Hygiene & Prophylactic Dentistry, 40 Restorative Dentistry, 39 Cosmetic Dentistry, 41 Endodontics

periodontal [perɪoʊdɒntᵊl] adj term

related to the periodontium[1] [-ʃ(ɪ)əm], i.e. the gums (gingiva) and bone structures that surround and support the teeth

periodontics or -ology[2] n term • periodontist or -ologist n or perio[3] n jar

» He's a practicing periodontist. The patient had mechanical periodontal prophylaxis for 3 months. Natural teeth are cushioned[4] [ʊ] in their alveoli [aɪ‖i] by periodontal fibers which distribute compression, tension, and rotational forces to all the roots.

Use **periodontal** health / chart[5] [tʃ]/ disease[6] / tissue / ligament [ɪg] (abbr PDL)[7] / bone loss • **periodontal** surgery / wound [uː] healing / pack[8] / probe[9] [oʊ]/ prophylaxis[10] / therapy • **periodontics** research • **periodontally** healthy / involved / compromised[11]

parodontal
Parodont(ium)[1] Parodontologie[2] Parodontologe/-in[3] eingebettet[4] parod. Befundkarte[5] Erkrankung d. Zahnhalteapparats, Parodontopathie[6] Desmodont[7] Parodontalverband[8] Parodontalsonde[9] Parodontalprophylaxe[10] m. schlechtem Parodontalstatus[11]

1

free gingiva [dʒɪndʒɪvə] n term   opposite **attached** [ætʃ] **gingiva**[1] n term

portion of the gums forming the outer wall of the gingival sulcus which is not directly attached to the tooth

supra/subgingival [ʌ] adj term • trans/buccogingival [ʌ] adj

» There was a shortage[2] [-ɪdʒ] of attached gingiva in the edentulous mandible.

Use alveolar [ɪə]/ healthy / interdental / marginal[3] [dʒ] **gingiva** • inflamed[4] [eɪ]/ keratinized / excess **gingiva** • zone / band / width[5] [wɪdθ]/ loss **of attached gingiva** • **attached gingiva** index • **subgingival** plaque [plæk]/ microflora / irrigation / crown margin • **supragingival** deposits / bacteria [ɪɚ] • **mucogingival** junction[6] [dʒʌŋkʃᵊn]

freie (marginale) Gingiva
befestigte G., G. propria[1] zu wenig[2] Gingivarand, Gingivalsaum, marginale G.[3] entzündetes Zahnfleisch[4] Breite d. befest. Gingiva[5] Mukogingivalgrenze[6]

2

gingival margin [mɑːrdʒɪn] n term   syn **gingival crest** [k] n term

(i) edge of the free gingiva (ii) most coronal portion of the gingiva surrounding the tooth

» The gingival margins were thickened and fibrous with a purulent[1] exudate present on probing[2]. The gingival margin was greater than 2 mm and well above the cementoenamel junction[3].

Use free / attached **gingival margin** • height [haɪt] of the **gingival crest** • **gingival** connective tissue / fibers[4] [aɪ]/ contours / epithelium[5] [iː] • **gingival** collar [ɒː]/ changes / color [ʌ]/ tenderness[6] / bleeding[7] • **gingival** hyperplasia[8] [eɪʒ(ɪ)ə]/ analog[9] / margin trimmer[10]

Gingiva(l)rand, -saum, Zahnfleischrand, Margo gingivalis
eitrig[1] beim Sondieren[2] Schmelz-Zement-Grenze[3] Gingivafasern[4] Saumepithel[5] empfindliches Zahnfleisch[6] Zahnfleischbluten[7] Gingiva-, Zahnfleischhyperplasie[8] Zahnfleischmaske[9] Gingiva(l)randschräger[10]

3

gingival crevice [krevɪs] or **sulcus** [sʌlkəs] n term

trough-like[1] [trɒːf] space between the surface of the tooth and the free gingiva

crevicular adj term • sulcular adj

» The probing depth[2] of the gingival crevice was recorded. Explore the gingival crevice for a foreign [fɒːrɪn] object. Then the blade is thrust[3] [ʌ] to the depth of the gingival sulcus and the gingival attachment is severed[4] [e] circumferentially.

Use **gingival** crevicular fluid[5] (abbr GCF) / crevice former[6] / retractor • **sulcus** fluid flow rate[7] (abbr SFFR) / fluid meter [iː]/ depth • buccal [ʌ]/ shallow[8] [æ] **sulcus** • **crevicular** space / probing / sampling • **sulcular** epithelium[9] / incision

Gingivalsulkus, Zahnfleischfurche, Sulcus gingivalis
furchenförmig[1] Sondierungstiefe[2] gestoßen[3] durchtrennt[4] Sulkusflüssigkeit[5] Sulkusformer[6] Sulkusflüssigkeits-Fließrate[7] flacher Sulkus[8] (orales) Sulkusepithel[9]

4

gingival papilla pl -ae [i‖aɪ] n term   syn **interdental papilla** n term

cone-shaped[1] [oʊ] projection of interdental gingiva normally filling the space up to the contact area[2]

papillary[3] adj term

» The partial denture [-tʃɚ] was strangling[4] the gingival papilla underneath. The outstanding signs of simple gingivitis [-aɪtɪs] are a band of red, inflamed gingiva along the necks of teeth and edematous [iː] swelling of the interdental papillae.

Use to preserve[5]/suture [-tʃɚ] **the papilla** • molar **gingival papillae** • atrophied **papillae** • **papillary** gum[6] [ʌ] (zone) / epithelial [iː] hyperplasia[7] [eɪ]

Interdental-, Zahnfleischpapille
kegelförmig[1] Kontaktfläche[2] papillär[3] abschnüren[4] Papille erhalten / schonen[5] interdentale Gingiva[6] Papillenhyperplasie[7]

5

gingival status [eɪ] n term   rel **gingival examination**[1] n term

assessment[2] of color (uniform in color, coral pink, marginal redness, bright red, cyanotic [saɪə-]), contour (bulbous[3] [ʌ], punched [tʃ] out[4], cratered [eɪ]), consistency and pliability [aɪ] of the gums[5] (firm, spongy[6] [spʌndʒi])

» The gingival status was assessed clinically by probing. The gingival status was calculated by means of the sulcus bleeding index (evaluating redness[7], swelling, and bleeding when moving a periodontal probe gently [dʒ] along the inner margin of the gingiva). The surface of the gingiva shows increased stippling[8].

Use **gingival** health / response / parameters / indexes[9] / score

Parodontal-, Gingivastatus
Zahnfleischuntersuchung[1] Beurteilung[2] verdickt[3] ausgestanzt[4] Zahnfleischfestigkeit u. -beweglichkeit[5] schwammig[6] Rötung[7] (Zahnfleisch)tüpfelung, Stippling[8] Gingivaindices[9]

6

gingival index n term, abbr **GI**   syn **periodontal (disease) index** n term, abbr **PDI**

measurement of six representative teeth for gingival inflammation, pocket depth[1] [depθ], calculus and plaque, attrition[2] [ɪʃ], mobility[3], and lack of contact to estimate[4] the degree of periodontal disease

» The patient had a high gingival index score. The PDI was routinely evaluated.

Gingiva-, Parodontalindex
(Zahn)taschentiefe[1] Attrition[2] Beweglichkeit[3] einstufen, -schätzen[4]

7

sulcus bleeding index n term, abbr **SBI**   syn **marginal bleeding index** n term, abbr **MBI**

a percentage score of the number of teeth in which bleeding occurs after running a probe gently[1] [dʒ] around the gingival sulcus; a clinical parameter for the early detection of gingivitis [-aɪtɪs] and periodontitis

» Bleeding on probing the lining[2] [aɪ] of the pocket is due to the inflammation and ulceration [ʌls-] of the gingival mucosa resulting from the deposition of plaque and tartar.

Use mean [iː]/ modified / papillary[3] / periodontal pocket **bleeding index**

Sulkus-Blutungs-Index, SBI
vorsichtig[1] Auskleidung[2] Papillen-Blutungs-Index, PBI[3]

8

attachment [ətætʃmənt] **level** n term

distance (in mm) between the cemento-enamel junction and the point where the PDL[1] attaches[2] to the root surface

» Probing depth, attachment loss[3], and the SBI were used as indicators of periodontal disease. Thirteen patients were evaluated for probing depth, probing attachment levels, gingival index, and plaque index.

Use to probe the / probing / clinical **attachment level** • **attachment level** measurement • creeping[4] **attachment** • clinical **attachment** loss • **attached** gingiva index

Attachment level (Sulkusboden i. Relation z. Schmelz-Zementgrenze)
Desmodont[1] anhaften, angewachsen sein[2] Attachmentverlust, verminderte Anheftung[3] Creeping attachment, Wanderung d. befest. Gingiva n. koronal[4]

9

gingival recession [rɪseʃən] n term   syn **gingival shrinkage** [ʃrɪŋkɪdʒ] or **retraction** n term

migration [aɪ] of the gingival margin in apical [eɪ] direction with increasing exposure[1] [oʊʒ] of tooth surface; clinically commonly referred to as receding [iː] gums

recede[2] [iː] v • receding adj

» Gingivae [iː] may recede and expose more of the crown and even part of the roots. Mean gingival recession from the cementoenamel junction was 1.9 mm.

Zahnfleischschwund, -rückbildung, Gingivarezession, -retraktion
Entblößung, Freilegung[1] s. zurückbilden, schwinden[2]

10

periodontal pocket [pɒːkɪt] n term   sim **pocketing**[1] n term

pathologically deepened[2] gingival sulcus (greater than 3 mm in depth)

» If abnormal gingival contour and pockets go uncorrected[3] surgery will be required. Is this pocket-probing depth clinically tolerable[4]?

Use true / supra-/ infrabony[5] / deep / false[6] or pseudo**pocket** [suː-] • **pocket** depth • (non)surgical **pocket therapy** • soft-tissue[7] **pocketing**

Zahnfleischtasche
Taschenbildung[1] vertiefte[2] nicht behandelt werden[3] klinisch tolerierbar[4] infraalveoläre Knochentasche[5] Pseudotasche[6] Weichteiltaschenbildung[7]

11

35

DENTISTRY

Periodontics

root coverage [kʌvrɪdʒ] n term   opposite **root exposure**[1], **mucogingival** [mjuːkoʊ-] **defect**[2] n term

Lack or absence of attached gingiva as a result of gingival recession or bone loss[3] due to gum disease is termed mucogingival deficiency [fɪʃ] or defect[2].
Use receded / denuded[4] [uː] *roots* • **root coverage** graft [æ]

Wurzel(ab)deckung
Wurzelfreilegung, -denudation, parodontale Rezession[1] Mukogingivaldefekt[2] Knochenabbau[3] freiliegende Wurzeln[4]   12

gingivitis [dʒɪndʒɪvaɪtɪs] n term

inflammation [eɪ] of the gums due to plaque and/or tartar formation which is marked by erythema[1] [iː] and swelling; unless treated gingivitis may progress to periodontitis
» Sites demonstrating gingivitis did not always correspond to sites harboring [ɑː] plaque[2].
Use acute / chronic edematous [iː]/ early onset **gingivitis** • juvenile [dʒuːvənaɪl]/ senile [-aɪl]/ atrophic / desquamative[3] [ɑː] **gingivitis** • hyperplastic / plaque-related / drug-induced / refractory[4] / marginal **gingivitis**

Gingivitis, Zahnfleischentzündung
Rötung, Erythem[1] plaquebehaftete Stellen[2] G. desquamativa[3] refraktäre, rezidivierende G.[4]   13

acute (necrotizing) ulcerative [ʌ] **gingivitis** [aɪ] n term   abbr **ANUG** or **AUG**

condition also known as trench [tʃ] mouth[1], Vincent's gingivitis, and ulceromembranous gingivitis that is characterized by painful papillary white or yellow ulcers which bleed readily[2] [e]
» ANUG patients often complain of a metallic taste and a sensation[3] of their teeth being wedged [dʒ] apart[4]. ANUG is associated with poor oral hygiene [haɪdʒiːn], smoking and stress.

akute nekrotisierende ulzeröse Gingivitis; G. ulcerosa
Plaut-Vincent Angina[1] leicht[2] Gefühl[3] auseinandergekeilt, -gedrängt[3]   14

periodontitis [perɪoʊdɒːntaɪtɪs] n term

advanced inflammation of the periodontium which leads to loosening[1] [uː] and eventual[2] destruction and loss of the tissue anchoring [k] the teeth[3]
» Periodontal disease usually begins as gingivitis and progresses to periodontitis, which affects[4] more than 10% of the world's population and is a common cause of tooth loss.
Use chronic / generalized / localized / marginal[5] / apical[6] [eɪ]/ refractory **periodontitis** • destructive / rapidly progressive[7] / juvenile [dʒuː-]/ advanced[8] / terminal **periodontitis**

Paradontitis
Lockerung[1] schließlich[2] Zahnhalteapparat[3] betrifft[4] Parodontitis marginalis[5] P. apicalis[6] rasch fortschreitende P.[7] P. marginalis profunda[8]   15

stomatitis [stoʊmətaɪtɪs] n term

term for inflammatory diseases of the oral mucosa (e.g. glossitis); may be due to a variety [aɪə] of causes including cheek-biting[1], poorly fitting dentures, allergy [-dʒi], and infection
» There was soreness[2], ulceration and stomatitis of the maxillary mucosa.
Use erosive or ulcerative[3] / aphthous[4] [æfθəs]/ herpetic / gangrenous / epidemic[5] **stomatitis**

Stomatitis
Wangenbeißen[1] Brennen[2] Stomatitis ulcero(membrano)sa[3] St. aphthosa[4] St. epidemica, Maul- u. Klauenseuche[5]   16

aphtha [æfθə], pl **-ae** [iː] n term   sim **canker sore**[1] [kæŋkɚ sɔːr] n clin

(i) small ulcer [ʌlsɚ] of the mucous membrane
(ii) in the plural, it refers to aphthous stomatitis or canker sores
aphthous[2] adj term • aphthosis[3] n
» Aphthous stomatitis is characterized by intermittent episodes of painful ulcers limited to the oral mucosa[4] covered by gray exudate, surrounded by an erythematous [e‖iː] halo[5] [heɪloʊ].
Use minor [aɪ]/ major [eɪdʒ] recurrent[6] [ɜː]/ chronic[6] **aphtha** • **aphthous** lesion [iːʒ]/ ulcer / fever [iː]

Aphthe
Gingivostomatitis herpetica, Stomatitis aphthosa[1] aphthös[2] Aphthose[3] Mundschleimhaut[4] geröteter Randsaum[5] chronisch rezidivierende A.[6]   17

interdental col [kɒl] n term

crater-like depression of the interproximal gingiva connecting the lingual and buccal [ʌ] interdental papillae

Zahnfleischsattel, Col, interdentaler Sattel   18

occlusal trauma [əkluːzəl trɒːmə] n term

loosening[1] [uː] of the teeth due to periodontal infection and bite trauma; may be compounded[2] [aʊ] by inadequate bone support (secondary occlusal trauma)
» Primary occlusal trauma is often due to parafunctional biting habits.

traumatische Okklusion, okklusales Trauma
Lockerung[1] verstärkt[2]   19

combined lesion [liːʒ°n] n clin   syn **endodontic-periodontal abscess** [æbses] n term

a localized collection of pus[1] [ʌ] involving both the pulp [ʌ] and periodontal tissues

Endo-Paro-Läsion
Eiter[1]   20

Periodontics   DENTISTRY 129

(inflammatory) fistula [fɪstʃələ], *pl* **-ae** *or* **-as** *n term*   → U13-25

tract through which pus from an abscessed tooth can escape

fistulation¹ *n term* • fistulous *adj* • fistulotomy *n* • fistulectomy² *n*

» There was no evidence³ of a fistulous tract⁴ in the gingival mucosa.

Use periodontal / gingival / oroantral⁵ **fistula** • **fistula** formation¹

gingival fibromatosis [aɪ] *n term*   *syn* **keloid** [iː] **of the gums** *n term*

localized or generalized fibrous proliferation¹ of gum tissue which becomes firm, pink and leathery² [e] with a pebbled³ surface and in severe cases may completely cover the teeth

» Unsightly⁴ [aɪt] fibrous hyperplasia [eɪ] of the gingiva, which may cover the teeth and interfere [ɪɚ] with⁵ eating, can be due to idiopathic familial gingival fibromatosis.

Use familial **gingival fibromatosis**

furcation [fɜːr-] **defect** *n term*   *syn* **furcal** *or* **furcation involvement** *n term*

condition in which periodontal disease has denuded¹ the furcation of a multirooted tooth of its periodontal ligament² and bone

» GTR procedures were performed in furcation defect sites using expanded polytetrafluoroethylene (ePTFE) membranes, while the other non-furcated molars received only scaling and root planing [eɪ]. Furcation plasty is an open procedure involving a mucoperiosteal flap³ and removal of tooth structure in the furcation area to allow for root planing⁴ and scaling.

Use severe / through-and-through *or* class II⁵ **furcation involvement** • **furcation** site / plasty⁶ • bi/ tri**furcation**⁷ [traɪ-]

pocket elimination *n term*

treatment directed at reduction or elimination of inflamed [eɪ] or infected gum tissue

» The periodontal pocket areas were opened, all irritants¹ removed, and depth was reduced.

crown lengthening *n term*   *rel* **gingivectomy¹** *n term*

operative procedure to increase the size of the clinical crown by means of gingivectomy with or without osteoplasty

» Root length and bone support are a concern² in crown lengthening procedures.

gingival recontouring [uː] *n term*   *syn* **gingivoplasty** *n term*

» Minor surgical procedures, e.g. gingivoplasty can help reestablish¹ natural gingival contours.

Use osseous² **recontouring**

periodontal reattachment [rɪətætʃ-] *n term*

reunion of connective tissue¹ with a root surface on which viable² [aɪə] periodontal tissue is present; reunion with a root surface without its periodontal ligament is called new attachment³

» Cells from the periodontal ligament occupy the site and form new periodontal attachment.

guided [gaɪdɪd] **tissue regeneration** [dʒ] *n term*   *abbr* **GTR** → U44-12

technique which encourages¹ [ɜː] regeneration of lost periodontal structures by selective cell and tissue repopulation of the periodontal wound [uː] using barrier materials² (ePTFE, collagen [-dʒen], polyglactin, etc.) to exclude tissues with little or no regenerative capacity

» The original GTR membrane material was non-resorbable, requiring a second surgery for removal. As use of GTR has progressed, several varieties of resorbable materials have been introduced, obviating the need³ for a second surgery. Non-resorbable material is still used for procedures where long-term membrane retention is desirable.

Use periodontal / bone-supplemented [ʌ] **GTR** • **GTR** technique / site / treatment / barrier material / membrane [membreɪn]

(entzündliche) Fistel / Fistula
Fistelbildung¹ Fistelexzision² Hinweis, Anzeichen³ Fistelgang⁴ oroantrale F., Mund-Antrum-Verbindung⁵
21

gingivale Fibromatosis, F. gingivae
Wucherung¹ lederartig² kieselsteinartig³ unschön⁴ behindern, stören bei⁵
22

Furkationsbefall, -defekt, -beteiligung
freigelegt¹ Desmodont² Mukoperiostlappen³ Wurzelglätten⁴ tunnelierte Furkation⁵ Furkationsplastik⁶ Trifurkation⁷
23

Beseitigung v. Zahnfleischtaschen
irritierende Faktoren¹
24

Kronenverlängerung
Gingivektomie, Zahnfleischabtragung¹ wichtige Faktoren²
25

Zahnfleisch-, Gingivoplastik
wiederherstellen¹ Osteoplastik²
26

Wiederanheftung d. Zahnfleisches, Reattachment
Bindegewebe¹ lebensfähig² bindegewebige Regeneration, Neubildung v. Parodontalgewebe³
27

gesteuerte Geweberegeneration, GTR
fördert¹ Regenerations-, Trennmembran² unnötig machen³
28

35

barrier membrane or **material** n term

thin film-like material placed around the tooth root which keeps the gingiva away and provides a space for the remaining healthy periodontal ligament to regenerate and connect new fibers with the tooth root as well as to allow for bone regrowth

» In this case a non-dissolving barrier which is removed in a minor secondary procedure 4-6 weeks after the GTR procedure is best.

Use nonabsorbable[1] / absorbable / hydrophobic [haɪdrəfoʊbɪk] **barrier material** • membrane / degradable[2] [eɪ]/ polymer / collagen-based **barrier**

Regenerationsmembran
nicht resorbierbare Regenerationsmembran[1] abbaubare R.[2]

29

Unit 36   Orthodontic Dentistry

Related Units: 37 Orthodontic Appliances, 10 Dentition & Mastication, 38 TMJ Disorders, 39 Cosmetic Dentistry

orthodontics n term   syn **orthodontia** [-dɒːnʃə], **corrective dentistry, dental** or **dentofacial** [-feɪʃəl] **orthopedics** [iː] n term

branch of dentistry concerned with the correction and prevention of occlusal abnormalities[1]

orthodontist[2] n term • orthodontic adj

» Function and esthetics are the main indications for orthodontic treatment.

Use conventional / surgical / preventive / corrective / interceptive[3] **orthodontics** • **orthodontic** arch alignment[4] [aɪn]/ appliances[5] [aɪ]/ camouflage[6] [ɑːʒ]/ assessment[7] / correction / tooth movement[8] / forces • Index of Orthodontic Treamtent Need (abbr IOTN)

Kieferorthopädie, Orthodontie; Zahn- u. Kieferregulierung
Bissanomalien[1] Kieferorthopäde/in[2] Interzeptivbeh., kieferorthopädische (kfo.) Frühbehandlung[3] kfo. Zahnbogenkorrektur[4] kfo. Geräte[5] dentoalveoläre Kompensation, Camouflage[6] kfo. Befunderhebung[7] kfo. Zahnbewegung[8]

1

interocclusal [z‖s] **registration** [dʒ] or **record** n term
       syn **maxillomandibular registration** n term → U42-14

record of the positional relationship of the teeth or jaws to each other

» The interocclusal record may be registered in centric or eccentric (i.e. centric jaw position[1] or other than centric relation), lateral, and protrusive[2] positions. An opposing arch impression[3] and interocclusal records were also made.

Kieferrelationsbestimmung, Checkbiss
zentrische Kiefergelenkposition[1] in Protrusionsstellung[2] Abformung, Abdruck[3]

2

articulation n term   rel **vertical dimension**[1] n term

(i) contact relationship of the occlusal surfaces during jaw movement
(ii) joint (iii) verbal expression

articulate v term • articulating adj

» The distance between the maxilla and the mandible when the teeth are in occlusion is termed vertical dimension. Check for optimal occlusion and articulation at the determined vertical and horizontal dimensions.

Use to adjust[2]/equilibrate[2]/compromise[3] **articulation** • **articulation** movement • **articulating** paper[4] / surface

(i & iii) Artikulation
(ii) Gelenk
Vertikaldimension[1] die Artikulation ausgleichen[2] die Artikulation beeinträchtigen[3] Artikulationsfolie[4]

3

arch length [leŋθ] n term   sim **arch** [ɑːrtʃ] **form** or **shape**[1] n term

amount of space required for the permanent teeth; measured from labial surface of the incisors at midline to a line between the mesial [iː] aspects of the first molars

» As the permanent incisors erupt, there is usually little change in mandibular arch length.

Use to increase / shortened **arch length** • **arch length** deficiency[2] / discrepancy[3] • u- or v-shaped / horseshoe[4] **arch form** • **arch** width[5] [wɪdθ]/ dimensions / location / distorsion / reconstruction

Zahnbogenlänge
Zahnbogenform[1] Zahnbogenverkürzung[2] OK/UK Platzdiskrepanz[3] hufeisenförmiger Zahnbogen[4] Zahnbogenbreite[5]

4

curve of Spee n term   syn **Spee('s) curve** [ɜː] n term   → U39-11

anatomic curvature of the mandibular occlusal plane from the tip of the lower cuspid following the buccal [ʌ] cusps[1] of the posterior teeth to the terminal molar

» For treatment planning vertical dimension of occlusion, smile line[2], amount of lip support, arch form, occlusal table, and the curve of Spee were evaluated.

Use reverse[3] **curve of Spee**

Spee Kurve
Höckerspitzen[1] Lachkurve[2] umgekehrte Spee Kurve[3]

5

Orthodontic Dentistry   DENTISTRY 131

leeway [iː] **(space)** *n term*

difference in combined mesiodistal widths of the deciduous cuspids[1] and molars and their successors[2]

» In the permanent dentition[3] the leeway space is used to permit improvement of crowding[4] [aʊ].

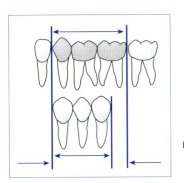

Leeway space in the lower jaw

Leeway Space
Milcheckzähne[1] nachstoßende Zähne[2] bleibende Zähne[3] Zahnengstand[4]

6

occlusion [əkluːʒᵊn] *n term*   *syn* **bite** [baɪt] *n clin & jar*

relationship between the occlusal surfaces of the maxillary and mandibular teeth in contact
(inter)occlusal *adj term* • (dis)occlude[1] v

» Ankylotic teeth in infraocclusion often give rise to malocclusion[2]. Implants were used for orthodontic anchorage [æŋkərɪdʒ] to correct cross-occlusion relationship. If anterior disocclusion is not possible, balanced occlusion[3] is recommended.

Use ideal / normal / distal[4] / lingualized **occlusion** • cross-[5] / mesio[6] / non[7] / infra**occlusion** • **occlusal** discrepancies[2] / contact / scheme [skiːm]/ arrangement [eɪ] • **occlusal** level or plane[8] / stress / stop[9] / interferences[10] / equilibration[11] • **interocclusal** clearance [ɪə] or distance[12] / record / relationship / wedge[13] [dʒ] • **occluding** cusp [ʌ]/ force • **bite** correction

Okklusion, Verzahnung
diskludieren; okkludieren[1] Okklusionsstörung[2] balancierte O.[3] Distalbisslage, -okklusion, Rückverzahnung[4] Kreuzbiss[5] Mesialbiss[6] Nonokklusion[7] Okklusionsebene[8] okklusaler Stopp[9] okkl. Interferenzen[10] Okklusionsausgleich[11] Interokklusalabstand[12] Bisskeil[13]

7

malocclusion *n term*   *sim* **disocclusion**[1] *n term*

malposition of opposing dentitions

» Malocclusion is categorized as class I (crowding or malpositioning[2] of anterior teeth, teeth occlude normally), class II (lower arch retrudes[3]) and class III (lower arch protrudes[4]).

Use to correct / cross-bite / acquired[5] / class I[6] **malocclusion** • severe / unrecognized / persistent / denture [dentʃə]/ iatrogenic [aɪə] **malocclusion**

Malokklusion, Okklusionsstörung
Disklusion, Zahnfehlstellung[1] Fehlstellung[2] mandibuläre Retrusion[3] Progenie, mandibuläre Prognathie[4] erworbene Okklusionsstörung[5] Gebissanomalie d. Angle Klasse I[6]   8

(occlusal) contact point *n term*   *sim* **contact area**[1] *n term*

part of the proximal tooth surface which touches the adjacent [dʒeɪs] tooth[2] mesially or distally

» Placing a restoration slightly out of occlusal contact is no guarantee of light loading.

Use (non)working[3] / excursive [ɜː] / tooth[4] / premature[5] **contacts** • intercuspal[6] / incisal[7] **contact points** • **contact** guidance[8] [aɪ]/ situation

(okklusaler) Kontaktpunkt
Kontaktfläche[1] Nachbarzahn[2] funktionelle Kontakte[3] exzentrische Kontakte[4] Vor-, Frühkontakte[5] Interkuspidationskontaktpunkte[6] inzisale Kontaktpunkte[7] Kontaktführung[8]

9

milled-in paths [æ] *n term*   *syn* **milled-in curves** *n term*

contours developed by masticatory or gliding movements[1] of occlusion rims[2] which are composed of materials including abrasives (so-called scribing studs), e.g. to obtain a functional chew-in record

mill[3] *v & n term*

Use trephine [triːfaɪn]/ bone[4] **mill** • **milling** machine[3]

selbsteingeschliffene Führungsflächen
Kaubewegungen[1] Bisswälle[2] einschleifen; Fräse(r)[3] Knochenfräse[4]

10

36

bruxism [brʌksɪzm] n term
habit of grinding¹, clenching², gnashing¹ [n] or clamping of the teeth, esp. during sleep which may give rise to abnormal wear³ [ɚ] of the chewing surfaces, affect the TMJ, and cause spasms of the muscles [sl] of mastication
brux⁴ v term • **bruxing** n • **bruxer**⁵ n jar
» Joint pain on awakening may indicate bruxism during sleep. The patient was obviously bruxing on the prosthesis [iː]. He denied⁶ [aɪ] bruxing or clenching.
Use **bruxing** habit⁷ • to aggravate⁸ **bruxism**

Bruxismus
Knirschen¹ Pressen² Abnützung³ bruxieren⁴ Knirscher(in)⁵ verneinte⁶ Knirschunart, -habit⁷ B. verstärken⁸

11

anterior open bite n term, abbr **AOB**   opposite **closed** or **deep bite**¹ n term
malocclusion in which the anterior teeth do not close (due to large interarch distance)
» The patient's open bite had to be corrected by orthognathic [θ] surgery.
Use normal / balanced² / faulty³ [ɔː]/ rest⁴ / working⁵ / edge-to-edge or end-to-end⁶ **bite** • lateral⁷ / frontal / class II skeletal⁸ **open bite** • **open bite** tendency / malocclusion

frontal/vorne offener Biss
Tiefbiss¹ balancierte Okklusion² pathologischer B.³ Ruheschwebe⁴ Okkl. d. Arbeitsseite⁵ Kanten-, Kopfbiss⁶ seitlich offener B.⁷ skelettal offener Biss⁸

12

overbite n term, abbr **OB** or **o/b**   syn **vertical overlap** n term
vertical relationship between the maxillary and mandibular incisors when the incisal edges are in maximum intercuspidation¹ and centric occlusion²
» Lingual tipping³ of the lower incisors following extraction increased the overbite.
Use (in)complete / anterior or incisal⁴ / increased⁵ / deep⁶ **overbite** • **overbite** reduction

vertikale(r) Überbiss / Frontzahnstufe, Overbite
maximale Interkuspidation¹ zentrische Okklusion² Lingualkippung³ Frontzahnstufe, -überbiss⁴ vergrößerter Überbiss⁵ Tiefbiss⁶

13

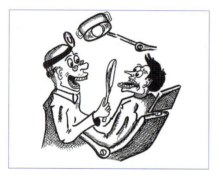

Great job correcting that overbite of yours, isn't it Mr. Wilde!

overjet n term, abbr **OJ** or **o/j**   syn **overjut** n term,
opposite **underbite** or **class III malocclusion**¹ n term
horizontal overlap of the upper incisors over the lower ones
» Unless otherwise specified, the term overjet generally refers to the central incisors. Reverse overjet¹ is most commonly associated with a large mandible and/or a retrusive maxilla (i.e. in class III malocclusion).
Use excess / 6mm / reverse¹ **overjet** • **overjet** discrepancy

sagittale(r) Frontzahnstufe / Überbiss, Overjet
umgekehrter Überbiss, negative Frontzahnstufe¹

14

crossbite n term   syn **Xbite** n jar
abnormal relation of one or more teeth in one arch to the opposing tooth/teeth of the other arch
» The occlusal scheme [skiːm] involved a crossbite situation. The mandible was prognathic with a crossbite preventing contact in centric occlusion.
Use buccal [ʌ]/ lingual / Class III / anterior / posterior / transverse¹ / bi-/ unilateral² **crossbite** • jumping the bite³ • **crossbite** relationship / malocclusion

Kreuzbiss
transversaler Kreuzbiss¹ einseitiger K.² Kreuzbiss überstellen³

15

(dental) crowding [kraʊdɪŋ] n term   opposite **spacing**¹ [speɪsɪŋ] n term
orthodontic problem in which the dental arch provides too little space for the teeth, resulting in altered positions such as bunching² [ʌ], overlapping³, or displacement⁴ in various directions
(un)crowded adj term • **crowd** v • **well-spaced**⁵ adj
» This is a case with sufficient crowding to warrant⁶ [ɔː] premolar extraction in the lower arch. A bulky⁷ [ʌ] prosthesis may crowd the tongue and compromise⁸ speech.
Use moderate / severe / relief [iː] of / tongue / lower labial segment **crowding** • mildly **crowded** • interdental⁹ **spacing** • **well-spaced** teeth

(Zahn)engstand
Zahnlückenstand¹ Gruppenbildung² Überlagerung³ Verschiebung, -lagerung⁴ m. ausreichendem Platzangebot⁵ erfordern⁶ überdimensioniert, zu groß⁷ beeinträchtigen⁸ Vergrößerung d. Interdentalraumes⁹

16

Orthodontic Dentistry

diastema [daɪəstiːmə] *n term, pl* **-mata**

space or gap between two adjacent[1] [eɪ] teeth in the same dental arch

» *If the teeth are of normal width, try and talk the patient into[2] accepting his diastema, as orthodontic space closure[3] [kloʊʒɚ] requires prolonged retention and has a high tendency to relapse[4].*

Use to close a **diastema** • frontal / lateral / midline or median[5] [iː] **diastema**

tooth-size *or* **Bolton discrepancy** *n term*   *abbr* **TSD**

dimensions of the lower or upper teeth are not in proportion with those of their counterparts[1]

» *Malocclusion often reflects a disproportion[2] between jaw and tooth size, e.g. a jaw so small or teeth so large that the jaw cannot accommodate[3] them.*

Use mesial-distal **size discrepancy** • **tooth-size** analysis[4]

hypo- [aɪ] *or* **oligodontia** [-dɒːnʃə] *n term*   *sim* **anodontia**[1] *n term,*
         opposite **hyperdontia**[2], **supernumerary** [uː] *or* **extra teeth**[2] *n term*

congenital[3] or acquired condition of having fewer than the normal number of teeth (i.e. missing teeth, also termed partial anodontia)

» *A 14-year-old female in oligodontia underwent implant-assisted reconstruction.*

tongue [tʌŋ] **thrust** [θrʌst] *n term*   *syn* **tongue-thrusting** *n term*

infantile [aɪ] pattern of the suckle-swallow [ɒː] movement[1] in which the tongue is placed between the incisor teeth or the alveolar ridges during the initial stage of swallowing; may result in an anterior open bite

» *Malocclusion may also result from habits such as thumb-sucking[2] [θʌm sʌkɪŋ] or tongue-thrusting.*

drift *n & v term*   *syn* **migration** [aɪ], **gression** [ʃ] *n term,*
         sim **shift**[1], **displacement**[1] *n term*

(n) unwanted change in the position of teeth; movement in which the angulation of the long axis of the tooth is altered is called tipping[2]

drifting *n term* • tip[3] *v* • sideshift[4] *n & v* • displaced *adj*

» *The adjacent first molar which had been tipped was orthodontically uprighted. This was attributed to alteration in lip support from incisal tipping. Mesial drifting of the 2nd molar had occurred [ɜː] after extraction. Shift of the adjacent teeth was prevented by a space maintainer[5].*

Use distal / mesial[6] / long-term **drift** • incisor[7] tipping • tipping force[8] / movement

bodily movement *or* **translation** *n term*   *sim* **transposition**[1] *n term*

tooth movement in which the entire tooth moves forward or backward without tipping or rotating

translate[2] *v term* • translating *n* • translational[3] *adj*

» *The cephalometric [sef-] landmarks[4] were unchanged, but marked translation movement was noted. Two molars were translated 10-12 mm mesially into an atrophic edentulous ridge[5] [dʒ].*

Use **to translate** freely • lateral **translation**

proclination *n term*   *opposite* **retroclination**[1], **retrusion**[1] *n term*

anterior coronal tilting or tipping of anterior teeth without positional variation (→ protrusion)

procline [aɪ] *v term* • proclined *adj* • retrocline *v* • inclination[2] *n*

» *Digit [dʒ] sucking[3] can cause proclination of the upper and retroclination of the lower incisors.*

Use **to deviate** [diːvɪeɪt] in[4]/correct/reduce **proclination** • angle [æŋgl] of / bimaxillary [aɪ] **proclination** • buccal [ʌ]/ lingual / mesiodistal / axial[5] / cuspal[6] **inclination** • **inclination** angle[7]

Diastema, lückige Zahnstellung

anliegend, benachbart[1] den/die P. dazu überreden[2] kieferorthopäd. Lückenschluss[3] rezidivieren[4] Diastema mediale[5]   17

Bolton-, Zahnbreitendiskrepanz

Antagonisten, Gegenzähne[1] Missverhältnis[2] nicht genügend Platz bieten[3] Bolton-Analyse[4]   18

Oligodontie, Zahnunterzahl

Nichtanlage sämtlicher Zähne, Anodontie[1] Zahnüberzahl, Hyperdontie[2] angeboren[3]
    19

Zungenpressen

Saugschluckbewegung[1] Daumenlutschen[2]

    20

Zahnwanderung; wandern

Verlagerung[1] Biegung 2. Ordnung[2] kippen[3] seitliche Verlagerung; seitl. verlagern[4] Lückenhalter[5] Mesialwanderung[6] Schneidezahnkippung[7] Kippkraft[8]

    21

körperliche Zahnbewegung, Translation

Transposition[1] verschieben[2] Translations-[3] kephalometrische Referenzpunkte[4] atrophierter Alveolarkamm[5]

    22

Vorkippung, Protrusion, Proklination

Rückneigung, -kippung, Retroinklination[1] Inklination, Kippung[2] Fingerlutschen[3] Protrusionsabweichung[4] Zahnachsenneigung[5] Höckerneigung[6] Inklinationswinkel[7]   23

retrusion [rɪtruːʒᵊn] *n term*   *opposite* **protrusion**¹ *n term or* **flaring**¹ [eə] *n clin*

backward movement, displacement or retraction of the jaw

retrusive *adj term* • retruded² *adj* • protruding/-sive³ *adj* • protrude *v*

» Excessive protrusion of the upper front teeth, so-called *flared* or *buck* [ʌ] *teeth*⁴, is by far the most common orthodontic problem and is often associated with *incompetent lips*⁵.

Use dentoalveolar / bimaxillary⁶ **protrusion** • **protruding** chin⁷ [tʃ]/ front teeth • **retruded** mandibular position / maxilla / dental appearance

Retrusion, Retroinklination
Protrusion¹ retrudiert² protrudierend³ Hasenzähne⁴ schlaffe Lippen(muskulatur)⁵ bimaxilläre Protrusion⁶ Progenie⁷

24

---

extrusion *n term*   *opposite* **intrusion**¹ *n term*

eruptive [ʌ] or orthodontic tooth movement beyond its normal position, e.g. hypereruption² (re-)intrude³ *v term* • extruded *adj* • extrusive *adj*

» With the help of fixed orthodontic appliances teeth can be *tilted*⁴, rotated, and intruded. A frequent cause of acquired malocclusion is loss of teeth with shifting of *adjacent teeth*⁵ and extrusion of *opposing teeth*⁶.

Use orthodontic / natural tooth **extrusion** • **intruded** vertically • **intrusive** force / component

Extrusion
Intrusion¹ Elongation² (re)intrudieren³ gekippt⁴ Nachbarzähne⁵ Gegenzähne, Antagonisten⁶

25

---

leveling BE **levelling** *n term*   *sim* **alignment**¹ [aɪn] *n term*

orthodontic procedure of bringing the teeth into their proper² vertical position relative to adjacent teeth

» After the arches had been orthodontically aligned and leveled, retraction was *instituted*³.

Use **leveling** wire⁴ • arch **leveling**

Nivellieren
Einreihen, Alignment¹ richtig, korrekt² begonnen³ Nivellierungsdraht⁴

26

---

torque [tɔːrk] *n & v term*   *syn* **torsiversion**, *rel* **rotation**¹[eɪ], **bend**² *n term*

(n) tooth movement centered in the tip of the crown moving the root in a buccal or labial direction

torsocclusion or torsive occlusion *n term* • rotate *v* • de-rotation³ *n* • rotational *adj* • rota(to)ry *adj*

» There were major torque and tilting forces. Firm attachment allows transverse tooth displacement and eliminates much of the transverse rotation of the tooth.

Use root / single tooth / anterior / posterior / lingual crown **torque** • **torque** control • generalized / first-order⁴ / (counter)clockwise⁵ / axis of / center of **rotation** • 30-degree transverse / long-axis⁶ / over**rotation** • **rotational** growth⁷ / forces / pattern • **rotatory** (drill) speed⁸ / movement

Torque, Biegung 3. Ordnung; torquen
Drehung (um die Längsachse)¹ Biegung² Derotation³ Biegung 1. Ordnung⁴ Drehung im/gegen den Uhrzeigersinn⁵ D. um d. Längsachse⁶ rotierendes Wachstum⁷ Drehzahl, Rotationsgeschwindigkeit⁸

27

---

traction [trækʃᵊn] *n term*   *rel* **force**¹, **pressure**² [preʃə] *n term*

drawing [ɔː] or pulling force³ applied to achieve orthodontic or orthopedic [iː] displacement of teeth or bones of the face (e.g. by elastic modules⁴ or springs⁵)

protraction⁶ *n term* • retraction⁷ *n* • retract *v* • tractional⁸ *adj*

» If less traction is applied, normal function is restored earlier. Orthodontic force was applied through the center of resistance to achieve translation in the direction of the line of force.

Use to apply / mild [aɪ] excessive / maxillomandibular⁹ / intermaxillary *or* vertical elastic / skin / force of **traction** • **tractional** forces¹⁰ • elastic / intermittent / continuous¹¹ / intraoral / extraoral / bite¹² / responsive / orthopedic¹³ / spring **force**

Extension, Zug
Kraft¹ Druck² Zugkraft³ elastische Elemente⁴ Federn⁵ Protraktion⁶ Retraktion⁷ Zug-⁸ maxillomandib. Zug(kräfte)⁹ Zugkräfte¹⁰ konstante Kraft¹¹ Kaukraft¹² kieferorthopäd. (wirksame) Kraft¹³

28

---

restrain [rɪstreɪn] *v term*   *sim* **guide**¹ [gaɪd], **retain**² [rɪteɪn] *v term*

(i) in orthodontics, to restrict or keep tooth movement under control
(ii) to restrict patient movement

restraint³ *n term* • guidance⁴ *n* • retention⁵ *n* • retainer⁶ *n*

» These appliances were used to achieve restraint and redirection of forward maxillary growth. Guide planes are orthodontic appliances designed to deflect the functional path of the mandible and alter positions of specific teeth.

Use head⁷ / wrist [rɪst] **restraint** • anterior / canine [keɪnaɪn] *or* cuspid⁸ [ʌ] **guidance** • **guide** plane⁹

(i) fixieren (ii) einschränken
steuern¹ retinieren, stabilisieren² Ein-, Beschränkung³ Führung⁴ Retention⁵ Retainer⁶ Kopfhalterung⁷ Eckzahnführung⁸ Führungsfläche⁹

29

Unit 37 Orthodontic Appliances
Related Units: 36 Orthodontic Dentistry

orthodontic appliance [aɪə] *n term*   *sim* **braces**[1] [breɪsiːz] *n clin pl*

mechanism [ek] used to apply pressure to misaligned teeth [aɪ] to produce changes in the relationship of the teeth and/or the related osseous structures

» Clues[2] indicating that the patient is not wearing [eɚ] the appliance full-time are absence of marks and frequent breakages [eɪ]. Wear your braces all the time! Use this clear wax to prevent the braces from irritating your lips or the inside of your cheeks.

Use to insert/activate/remove **the appliance** • upper removable, *abbr* URA / fixed[3] / lingual / pendulum / rapid palatal expansion[4], *abbr* RPE / extraoral **appliance** • straight [streɪt] wire / passive / active / Crozat / habit / thumbsucking [θʌmsʌkɪŋ] control[5] / pin-and-tube[6] **appliance** • to adjust[7] [ədʒʌst]/tighten [taɪtᵊn]/fit[8] **braces** • invisible **braces**[9]

kieferorthopädische(s) Gerät / Apparatur
festsitzende Zahnspange, Brackets[1] Hinweise[2] festsitzende A.[3] Gaumennahterweiterungsapparatur[4] Lutsch-Kontrollgerät[5] Stiftröhrchen-Apparatur[6] Brackets anpassen[7] B. nachstellen[8] unsichtbare Brackets[9]

1

straight wire [waɪɚ] **technique** *n term*   *rel* **edgewise (orthodontic) technique**[1] [k] *n term*

fixed, multibanded orthodontic appliance[2] [aɪə] using an attachment bracket the slot of which receives a rectangular archwire horizontally, which gives precise [saɪ] control of tooth movement in all three planes

» All patients were treated with edgewise appliances of the straight wire modification.

Use **straight wire** appliance / brackets • **edgewise** orthodontic appliance / brackets[3]

gerade Bogentechnik
Edgewise-/ Kant(en)bogen-Technik[1] Multibandapparatur[2] Edgewise-Brackets[3]

2

light wire *or* **Begg appliance** *n term*   *sim* **Begg light wire differential force technique**[1] *n term*

fixed orthodontic appliance utilizing round, small gauge[2] [geɪdʒ] labial wires with expansion and contraction loops[3] formed into it and attached to vertical slots in the bands which are fitted to individual teeth

» The round wires of the Begg appliance allow teeth to tip[4] freely, but auxiliaries[5] [ɒːgzɪl-] (elastics or springs) are required to achieve apical [eɪ] and rotational movement.

Lightwire-System
Begg-(Lightwire) Technik[1] dünn[2] Schlaufen i. Kontraktionsbögen[3] kippen[4] Hilfsgeräte[5]

3

(orthodontic) brackets *n term, usu pl*   *syn* **clip(-on) arches** *n inf*

metal attachment[1] to fasten the arch wire; bonded[2] to an orthodontic band or directly to teeth

» A composite crown was placed on the abutment[3] [ʌ] with an edgewise bracket secured[4]. These brackets have built-in hooks (wire loops[5] [uː]) to attach elastics.

Use to place[6] **brackets** • single-type / slot[7] / deltoid / twin(-wire)[8] **brackets** • plastic / tooth-colored / esthetic / ceramic [s] / metal / ribbon arch[9] / fractured **brackets** • interbracket distance • **bracket** base / wings[10] / hooks / removal

Brackets
Befestigung[1] geklebt[2] Anker[3] befestigt[4] Drahtschlaufen[5] B. setzen[6] Schlitzbrackets[7] Zwillingsbrackets[8] Ribbon-Arch Brackets[9] Bracketflügel[10]

4

arch wire [ɑːrtʃ waɪɚ] *n term*   *syn* **archwire** *n term*

metal wire attached to the brackets by small elastic donuts or ligature tie [taɪ] wires[1] which move the teeth

» Arch wires are cut off with special pliers[2] [plaɪɚz] called a distal end cutter[3]. Mesiodistal movement was achieved by sliding the teeth along the archwire.

Use rectangular[4] / flexible / stiff / superelastic / stainless steel **archwire** • nickel titanium / straight / initial[5] / finishing[6] **archwire** • **archwire** flexibility • transpalatal / fixed lingual / prefabricated[7] **arch** • segmented **archwire** technique[8] • (super)elastic / round / lingual / palatal **wire** • **wire** bending

Drahtbogen
Drahtligaturen[1] Zange[2] Distal-End Cutter[3] Vierkantbogen[4] Initial-, Nivellierungsbogen[5] Justierungsbogen[6] konfektionierter Bogen[7] Segmentbogentechnik[8]

5

leveling wire *n term, BE* **levelling**

round (cross-section) orthodontic wire of low flexural [kʃ] stiffness used in the leveling phase[1] of treatment

» Proper tooth alignment and leveling[2] of the occlusal plane must be accomplished previously[3].

Nivellierungsbogen
Nivellierungsphase[1] Ausrichtung u. Nivellierung d. Zähne[2] bereits vorher erreicht[3]

6

ligating [aɪ] **module** *n term*   *syn* **ligature** [ɪ] **(tie) wire** *n term*

small donut-shaped rubber[1] used to fix the arch wire to the brackets

ligate[2] [aɪ] *v term* • ligation[3] [laɪgeɪʃᵊn] *n*

» The device[4] [aɪ] used to place ligating modules on brackets is called a twirl [ɜː] on[5].

Use figure-of-eight[6] **ligature wire**

(elastische / Draht-) Ligatur
elastischer Ring[1] ligieren[2] Ligatur[3] Instrument[4] Ligaturenadapter[5] Achterligatur[6]

7

DENTISTRY — Orthodontic Appliances

banding *n term*   *opposite* **debanding**[1] *n, sim* **debonding**[2] *n term*

cementing orthodontic bands (metal sleeves[3] [iː] used to anchor [æŋkɚ] the ends of the arch-wires) to a tooth

band[4] *n term* • **deband** *v*

» Brackets can be secured to teeth either by bonding[5] or banding.
Use **band** becomes loose • **band** placement or fitting[6]

Bebänderung
Bänderabnahme[1] Bracketentfernung[2] Metallmanschetten[3] Band[4] Ätz-, Adhäsivtechnik[5] Anlegen / Adaptieren eines kfo. Bandes[6]   8

---

band remover *n term*   *opposite* **band sitter**[1] *n term*

special orthodontic instrument for removing bands from the teeth; they are put in place with bracket holding pliers[1] or a band sitter and bite sticks[2]

» First put the band in place, then ask the patient to bite down on the bite stick[2].

Bandabnahmezange
Bandsetzer, Band-Setzzange[1] Beissstäbchen[2]   9

---

elastic module *n term*   *sim* **elastics**[1] *n term pl*

orthodontic rubber rings[2] used in many ways to apply tension and achieve tooth movement (in)elastic *adj* • elasticity *n*

» A rubber band was stretched around the tie-wings of the bracket[3] to prevent disengagement[4] of the arch wire or auxiliary from the bracket slot[5].
Use auxiliary / heavy [e]/ light / vertical / anterior / triangular[6] [aɪ]/ asymmetrical / finishing[7] / box **elastics** • **(in)elastic** deformation[8] • **elastic** chain (module)[9] / clamping[10] / traction

Elastics
Gummizüge[1] Gummiringe[2] Bracketflügel[3] Lösen[4] Bracketschlitz[5] Delta-Züge[6] Gummiringe z. Feinabstimmung[7] elastische Verformung[8] elast. Kette[9] elast. Befestigung[10]   10

---

spring *n term*   *sim* **jumper**[1] [ʌ] *n term*

configured segment of wire included in retainers or other orthodontic appliances to–when activated–tip a tooth in a desired direction

» A spring appliance which is attached to fixed appliances to move teeth similar to a Herbst appliance[2] is termed a jumper[1]. Where palatal movement is required, a buccally [ʌ] approaching spring is necessary. Palatal finger springs are easy to adjust and activate[3].
Use to load[3]/activate/insert/(re)adjust[4] [dʒʌ] **springs** • hip / coiled[5] / Z- / T- / apron [eɪ]/ strap[6] **spring** • buccal / lingual / helical[5] / push / finger[7] / inactive **spring**

Feder
Protrusions-, Vorschubfeder[1] Herbst-Scharnier[2] (Federn) aktivieren[3] F. (neu) einstellen[4] Spiralfeder[5] Schlingenfeder[6] Fingerfeder(chen)[7]   11

---

separator *n term*   *syn* **separating module** *n term,*
   opposite **space maintainer** or **regainer**[1] *n term*

plastic wedges[2] [dʒ] inserted between teeth before banding to temporarily increase interdental spacing

» Due to premature[3] [e] loss of a primary tooth, a space maintainer was placed to hold space for the erupting permanent teeth. The separators will be removed at the banding appointment[4].

Separiergummi, Separator
Lückenhalter[1] Keile[2] vorzeitig[3] Bebänderungstermin[4]   12

---

activator *n term*   *rel* **functional** [ʌ] **appliance**[1] *n term*

removable appliance used in functional jaw [dʒɔː] orthopedics[2] to achieve growth guidance[3] [aɪ]; types include the monobloc, bionator[4], Bimler[5], Herbst and Andresen appliances[6]
activation *n term* • activating *adj*

» A bionator was placed to provide better control of the buccal musculature [ʌsk]. The Fränkel appliance[7] is an activator-type appliance intended to stimulate or inhibit jaw growth, retrain muscles [ʌsl] or widen the dental arches[8].
Use eccentric [ɪks]/ expansion **activator** • **activation** site • clip **activation** • **activating** forces • **bionator I** (to open) / **II** (to close) / to maintain • banded / crowned [aʊ]/ TMD[9] / cantilever[10] **Herbst appliance**

Aktivator
funktionelles Behandlungsgerät[1] Funktionskieferorthopädie[2] Wachstumssteuerung[3] Bionator[4] Bimler-Gebissformer[5] Andresen-Häupl-System[6] Fränkel-Funktionsregler[7] Zahnbögen erweitern[8] TMD-Gerät[9] Herbst-Scharnier[10]   13

---

twin block *n term*   *sim* **monobloc(k)**[1] *n term*

functional orthodontic appliance (URA and LRA) that serves to posture [pɔːstʃɚ] the mandible forward

» A screw was incorporated in the upper twin block to achieve expansion[2].
Use **twin block** bite block / clasp

Zwillingsblock
Monoblock[1] zur Expansion[2]   14

Orthodontic Appliances DENTISTRY 137

crib n term   sim **clasp**[1] [æ], **bar**[2], **labial** [eɪ] **bow**[3] [oʊ] n term

(i) fixed transpalatal tongue [tʌŋ] or finger interceptive appliance (ii) a wrought-wire [rɔːt] clasp[4] around a tooth

» An appliance used to control undesirable and potentially deforming tongue thrusting[5] is termed a tongue crib. No amount of adjustment will compensate for a badly made crib.

Use (anterior) tongue[6] **crib** • C / arrow[7] / Adams[8] / ball[9] **clasp** • palatal[10] **bar**

orthopedic splint [splɪnt] n term

device to stabilize teeth loosened[1] by trauma [ɔː] or a periodontal condition, or reduce[2] and stabilize fractures by applying it to both jaws and connecting it by intermaxillary wires or rubber bands

splint v term • splinting[3] n • (un)splinted adj

» A removable splint was used to temporarily relieve occlusal interferences in functional disorders of the TMJ and related musculature.

Use wire[4] / clear[5] **splint** • stabilizing / interocclusal / upper flat plane / occlusal extension[6] **splint** • **splint** fabrication

split palate n term   sim **Quad** [kwɒd] **helix** [iː]
    (expansion) appliance[1] n term

palatal expansion appliance[2] divided in the sagittal [ædʒ] plane and connected only by a jackscrew[3] which is progressively opened to widen the palate and maxillary dental arch

» Jackscrews[3] are also used for the separation of approximated teeth[4].

headgear [hedɡɪɚ] n term   syn **night brace** [breɪs] n clin & inf

removable extraoral appliance used to apply traction on teeth against the pull of rubber bands

» Extraoral headgear is the best way of obtaining anchorage for orthodontic tooth movement.

Use high-pull[1] / J-hook / Kloehn / (low) occipital[2] [ɒksɪpɪtəl] / cervical pull[3] [sɜːr]/ reverse pull or protraction[4] **headgear**

facebow [feɪsboʊ] n term   opposite **facemask**[1] n term

wire apparatus [eɪ] used to move upper molars back to create room for crowded[2] [aʊ] anterior teeth; it connects to bands or a removable appliance and to either a neckstrap[3] or a headgear and a safety [seɪfti] strap[4]

» An elastic neck band is placed around the back of the neck while the triangular cast offs on both sides of the neck band are attached to the outer bow[5] of the headgear. A plastic safety strap is placed over the neck band and onto the outer bow of the headgear.

Use **facebow** transfer

chin cap [tʃɪn kæp] n term   syn **chin cup** n term

extraoral appliance applying upward and backward pressure to the chin to prevent forward growth[1] [ɡroʊθ] in skeletal class III treatment

» Initially [ɪʃ] the skeletal profile [proʊfaɪl] was greatly improved by chin-cup therapy.

breakaway [breɪkəweɪ] n term

small plastic with an internal spring attached to a neck pad[1] used to provide force on the facebow

» The outer two curves of the facebow connect to the breakaways or high-pull headgear.

lip bumper [bʌmpɚ] n term

labial [eɪ] archwire[1] with anterior plastic pads used to push the mandibular molars back

» A lip bumper was used to move the incisors [sɪ] forward, distalize[2] the molars, and increase arch length[3].

(i) Klammer (ii) Gitter
Klammer, Anker[1] Bogen[2] Labialbogen[3] Stahldrahtklammer[4] Zungenpressen[5] Zungengitter[6] Pfeilklammer[7] Adams-K.[8] Kugelanker[9] Palatinalbogen[10]
15

orthopädische Schiene
gelockert[1] reponieren[2] Schienung[3] Drahtschiene[4] transparente Schiene[5] Extensionsgerät[6]
16

Oberkieferdehngerät
Quad-Helix[1] Gaumendehngerät[2] Dehnschraube(n)[3] engstehende Zähne[4]
17

Außenbogen, Headgear
Hochzug-Headgear[1] okkzipitaler / Hinterhauptzug-H.[2] zervikaler / Nackenzug-H.[3] Gegenzug-, Protraktionsheadgear[4]
18

Gesichtsbogen
Gesichtsmaske[1] engstehend[2] Nackenband[3] Sicherheitsband[4] Außenbogen[5]
19

(Kopf-) Kinnkappe
progenes Wachstum[1]
20

Federmodul
Nackenpolster[1]
21

Lip-Bumper
Labialbogen[1] distalisieren, nach distal verlagern[2] Zahnbogenlänge[3]
22

138 DENTISTRY — TMJ Disorders

retainer [rɪteɪnɚ] *n term*   *syn* **retaining appliance**,
                                    sim **(tooth) positioner**[1] *n term*

broad term for orthodontic appliances worn full-time or at night used to maintain space between teeth or to stabilize tooth position and prevent shifting following corrective treatment (removal of braces)

retain[2] [eɪ] *v term* • retention[3] [e] *n*

» *Retainers are routinely provided to patients after treatment to prevent relapse[4]. Compliance[5] [aɪə] with prescribed retainer wear [eə] is very important in maintaining the results of treatment. A positioner was placed for fine tuning[6] in the retention phase[7] of treatment. Lingual retainers[8] which extend between the cuspids are a variation of the lingual arch.*

Use (in)direct / Hawley[9] / continuous bar[10] / lingual **retainer** • clamp / circumferential / extracoronal[11] spring / bonded[12] **retainer** • adequate / adjustable **retention** • **retention** system

Retentionsgerät, Retainer
Positioner[1] retinieren, stabilisieren[2] Retention[3] Rezidiv[4] Compliance, Kooperation d. Patienten/-in[5] Feinabstimmung[6] Retentionsphase[7] Lingualretainer[8] Hawley-Retainer[9] fortlaufende Klammer[10] extrakoronaler Retainer[11] geklebter Retainer[12]

23

biteplate [baɪtpleɪt] *n term*   *syn* **biteplane** *n term*

orthodontic or prosthodontic device [aɪs] made of wire and plastic used for diagnostic or therapeutic [juː] purposes

» *A biteplate was used to correct her TMJ problems[1]. A flat anterior biteplate should be prescribed only if OB reduction[2] is required.*

Use Hawley[3] **biteplate** • to trim[4]/build up/remove/replace **the biteplane**

Aufbissplatte
Kiefergelenkprobleme[1] Überbissreduktion, Bisshebung[2] Hawley-Aufbissbehelf[3] Aufbissplatte einschleifen[4]

24

biteguard or **night guard** [gɑːrd] *n term*   *syn* **snoreguard** [ɔːr] *n*,
                                                    rel **mouthguard**[1] *n term*

hard or soft plastic mouthpiece to prevent damage from grinding [aɪ] teeth at night

» *Biteguards used to protect the teeth from injury during sports are called mouthguards.*

Use athletic[1] **mouthguard** • **biteguard** splint[2]

Knirscher-, Nachtschiene
Zahnschutz (für Sportler)[1] Aufbiss-, Okklusionsschiene[2]

25

Unit 38 TMJ Disorders

Related Units: 40 Restorative Dentistry, 36 Orthodontic Dentistry, 44 Oral Surgery, 45 Maxillofacial Surgery, 10 Dentition & Mastication

temporomandibular joint *n term*   *abbr* **TMJ** [tiːemdʒeɪ]

joint that connects the upper and lower jaws and controls jaw [dʒɒː] movement[1]

» *The TMJ is palpated laterally and intrameatally [ieɪ] for tenderness[2], range[3] and smoothness [uːð] of motion[4], and condylar deformity.*

Use **TMJ** disease[5] / inflammation / patient[6] / implant

Kiefergelenk, Articulatio temporomandibularis
Kiefer-, Kaubewegung[1] Druckschmerz[2] Beweglichkeit[3] Gleichmäßigkeit / Reibungslosigkeit d. Bewegung[4] Kiefergelenkerkrankung[5] Patient m. Kiefergelenkproblemen[6]

1

TMJ dysfunction [dɪsfʌŋkʃən] or **disorders** *n term*   *abbr* **TMJD**

broad term for joint and muscle [mʌsl] pain in the jaw area due to misalignment[1] [əlaɪn] of the TMJ but also related to and mimicked[2] by several other conditions (e.g. bruxism [ʌ], MPD syndrome [ɪ], depression and psychiatric [saɪkɪætrɪk] illness) more precisely termed temporomandibular pain-dysfunction syndrome[3] (abbr TMPDS)

» *In intrinsic TMJ dysfunction pain is typically exacerbated[4] [ɪgzæs-] by finger pressure on the TMJ as the patient opens the mouth. Patients with ill-fitting dentures[5] [tʃ] have an increased risk of developing TMJ dysfunction.*

Use transient[6] **TMJ dysfunction**

Kiefergelenkstörung(en), Myoarthropathie(n)
Fehlstellung[1] vorgetäuscht[2] Schmerzdysfunktionssyndrom[3] verstärkt[4] schlechtsitzende Prothesen[5] transitorische K.[6]

2

myofascial [maɪoʊfæʃəl] **pain dysfunction syndrome** *n term*
                                                   abbr **MPD syndrome**

common extrinsic cause of TMJ dysfunction (mostly habitual stress-relieving jaw clenching[1] or tooth grinding[2] [aɪ]); if untreated, it may give rise to secondary degenerative arthritis [aɪtɪs]

» *Treatment of MPD syndrome includes limited use of the jaw, a soft, nonchewy [-tʃuːi] diet[3] [daɪət], administration of analgesics[4] [dʒiː] and muscle relaxants, and use of a bite guard [ɑː] splint[5].*

myofasziales Schmerzsyndrom, Costen-Syndrom
Zahnpressen[1] Zähneknirschen[2] nicht kauzwingende Kost[3] Analgetika, Schmerzmittel[4] Aufbissschiene[5]

3

TMJ Disorders

popping *n clin*   *syn* **clicking** *n clin*

the short, sharp crepitational [eɪʃ] sound[1] that resembles the bursting[2] [ɜː] of a balloon [uː] which is typically [ɪ] observed on jaw movement in TMJ disorders

» Typical findings[3] in TMJ disorders are preauricular [priːɔːrɪkjələ˞] pain, TMJ tenderness, jaw limitation[4], and occasional clicking and popping sounds in the joint (esp. on yawning[5] [jɔːnɪŋ], chewing, etc). Clicking commonly occurs at 2-3 mm of tooth separation on opening and sometimes at closing.

Use **popping** joint sound • **clicking** ceased[6] [siː] • occasional **popping**

(jaw) locking *n clin & jar*

inability to move the jaw caused by anterior displacement[1] and entrapment[2] of the disk on translation[3] of the head of the condyle [kɒndaɪl]

» If the disk does not return to its usual location, the jaw can be locked in position.

trismus [trɪzmᵊs] *n term*   *sim* **lock-jaw** *or* **lockjaw**[1] [lɒːkdʒɒː] *n clin*

firm closure [ʒ] of the jaws due to tonic spasm of the masticatory muscles[2] resulting from a motor disturbance of the trigeminal [traɪdʒem-] nerve; also the heralding symptom[3] of general tetanus

» Palpate for signs of muscular problems (trismus, MPD syndrome), which are more common causes of limited jaw movement[4] than are joint problems (ankylosis, disk derangement[5]).

Use **trismus** of the masseter [iː] muscle [mʌsl]

masseter reflex [iː] *n term*   *syn* **chin** [tʃ] **(jerk** [dʒɜːrk]**) reflex** *or* **jaw-jerk** *n jar & clin*

spontaneous contraction of the temporal muscles after a downward tap[1] on the loosely [uː] hanging mandible[2]

» A similar increase in the masseter reflex threshold[3] [eʃ] was found when tapping on dentures.

Use to elicit *or* trigger[4] the **masseter reflex**

TMJ dislocation *n term*   *syn* **dislocated mandible** *n term*

displacement of the mandible in the TMJ

» A dislocated mandible will be fixed in a markedly open position and if the midline is deviated[1] [diːvɪeɪtɪd], the dislocation is unilateral rather than bilateral.

Use true / false[2] [ɒː]/ bilateral [aɪ]/ unilateral **dislocation** • to reduce[3] a **dislocation**

internal (disk *or* **disc) derangement** [eɪndʒ] *n term*

anterior displacement of the intra-articular disk in the TMJ caused by chronic muscle spasm, trauma [ɒː], or arthritic [ɪ] changes in the articulating surfaces[1]

» Internal disk derangements may take two forms: anterior disk displacement with reduction[2] during function (accompanied by clicking or popping sounds on opening the mouth) and without reduction, which is characterized by painful limitation of jaw movement.

Use **disk derangement** disorder • permanent / posterior **disk dislocation** • to dislocate/recapture/reposition **the disk** • TMJ / articular / anteriorly dislocated **disk** • **disk** dysfunction / position / space / adhesion [iːʒ]/ dislocation / repair / reduction / replacement

mandibular deviation [diːvɪeɪʃᵊn] *n term*
         syn **mandibular skewing** [skjʊːɪŋ] *n term*

deformity of one ramus[1] [eɪ] (e.g. due to congenital[2] [dʒe] or acquired[3] anomalies of the mandible, condyloid process[4], etc) which leads to deviation of the mandible to the affected[5] side and facial deformity[6]

» The patient had an Angle Class I facial profile with no evidence of mandibular deviation. Mandibular skewing results in severe malocclusion [uːʒ]. Condylar hypoplasia [-eɪʒ(ɪ)ə] produces facial deformity characterized on the affected side by a short mandibular body, fullness of the face, and deviation of the chin.

(Kiefer)gelenkknacken
krepitationsartiges Geräusch[1] Platzen[2] Befunde[3] eingeschränkte Kieferbeweglichkeit[4] beim Gähnen[5] Gelenkknacken ist verschwunden / hat sich gelegt[6]

     4

Kiefersperre, -klemme
Verlagerung, Verschiebung[1] Einklemmen, Festsitzen[2] Vorschubbewegung, Translation[3]

     5

Trismus, Spasmus masticatorius
Trismus; Tetanus[1] Kaumuskulatur[2] Frühsymptom[3] eingeschränkte Kieferbeweglichkeit[4] Diskusverlagerung[5]

     6

Massetterreflex
Beklopfen[1] entspannter, leicht geöffneter Unterkiefer[2] Reflexschwelle[3] Massetterreflex auslösen[4]

     7

Kiefer(gelenk)luxation, Unterkieferverrenkung
v.d. Unterkiefermitte abweichend[1] Subluxation[2] L. reponieren[3]

     8

Diskusverlagerung, -luxation
Gelenkflächen[1] Reposition[2]

     9

Unterkieferdeviation
Ramus, aufsteigender Unterkieferast[1] angeboren[2] erworben[3] Kiefergelenkfortsatz, Processus condylaris[4] betroffen[5] Gesichtsdeformität[6]

     10

TMJ Disorders

TMJ osteoarthritis [-ɑːrθrɑɪtɪs] n term
sim **degenerative** [diːdʒen-] **arthritis¹, osteoarthrosis²** n term
joint disease marked by loss or wearing down³ [eə-] of articular cartilage⁴ due to mechanical (e.g. trauma), metabolic or endocrine [aɪ] or genetic factors and by hypertrophy of bone at the articular margins and usually minimal inflammation
» Most forms of arthritis can involve⁵ the TMJ but degenerative arthritis is the most common. Secondary degenerative arthritis causes tenderness of the TMJ on lateral or intrameatal palpation.
Use primary / secondary **degenerative arthritis** • infectious [ɪnfɛkʃəs] / traumatic / erosive / rheumatic [ruːm-] **arthritis**

Kiefergelenkentzündung, -arthritis
Arthropathia deformans¹ Osteoarthrose² Abnutzung³ Gelenkknorpel⁴ betreffen, befallen⁵
11

ankylosis [æŋkɪloʊsɪs] n term
pathologic joint stiffening¹ or fixation involving fibrous [aɪ] or bony union² across the joint
» Ankylosis of the TMJ is most commonly a sequel [siːkwəl] to³ trauma or infection, though it may accompany rheumatoid arthritis or be congenital.
Use true or intraarticular / false or extraarticular⁴ **ankylosis**

Ankylose
Gelenkversteifung¹ bindegewebige od. knöcherne Verwachsung² Folge von³ unechte A., Ankylosis extraarticularis⁴
12

jaw exercises n term & clin
set of instructions for remedial¹ [iː] jaw movements and manipulation the patient is to follow² at home
» TMJ disorders are often self-limiting³ and conservative treatment with simple analgesia [dʒiː], short-wave diathermy⁴ [daɪəθɜːrmi], gentle heat and remedial exercises is effective in up to 80% of cases.
Use exercise-initiated response / habits⁵ • jaw-opening / remedial⁶ **exercises**

Kiefergelenkübungen
therapeutische, Heil-¹ durchführen soll² auch ohne Therapie abheilend³ Kurzwellentherapie⁴ eintrainierte Gewohnheiten⁵ Heilgymnastik⁶
13

splint therapy [θerəpi] n term
coverage [ʌ] with an upper or lower splint (a biteguard splint¹) to promote normal positioning of the mandible and allow for the TMJ inflammation to subside² [aɪ]
» In TMJ patients splint therapy aims at reducing bruxism [ʌ] and joint load³ and, if possible, freeing⁴ the disk by increasing the gap⁵ between condyle [-aɪl] and fossa.

Schienentherapie
Aufbiss-, Okklusionsschiene¹ abklingen² Gelenkbelastung³ entlasten⁴ Abstand⁵
14

TMJ arthroscopy n term
inspection and irrigation¹ of the upper joint space to achieve lysis² [laɪsɪs] and lavage³ [ləvɑːʒ] of adhesions⁴ [iːʒ] and synovial [ɪ||aɪ] inflammation⁵
» If anterior displacement of the disk is not self-limiting, surgical correction by arthroscopy is indicated (repositioning of the disk is generally sufficient⁶ [səfɪʃənt]).
Use video **arthroscopy**

Kiefergelenkarthroskopie
Spülung¹ Lösen, Lysis² Spülung, Lavage³ Adhäsionen, Verwachsungen⁴ Synovialitis, Entzündung d. Synovialis⁵ ausreichend⁶
15

open arthrotomy n term
» Open arthrotomy was performed for a damaged disk¹ that was beyond the scope² of arthroscopy. For anterior displacement of the disk that is not self-reducing, surgical correction by arthrotomy or arthroscopy is indicated.

chirurgische Gelenkeröffnung, Arthrotomie
Diskusläsion¹ nicht durch A. behandelbar²
16

meniscectomy [menɪsɛktəmi] n term   *syn* **discectomy** or **diskectomy** [dɪskɛkt-] n term
resection of a damaged disk in the TMJ with or without replacement by an alloplastic implant¹ or autogenous graft² [ɒtɒːdʒənəs]
» Meniscectomy was indicated as the displaced disk was not in satisfactory condition. Meniscectomy was performed and the disk replaced with an autogenous graft.
Use left TMJ / functional **discectomy** • **meniscectomy** of the temporomandibular joint / with replacement

Diskusexzision, Diskektomie
alloplastisches Interpositionsmaterial² autogenes Transplantat³

> **Note:** *Diskectomy* is commonly used to refer to intervertebral disks, whereas the term *meniscectomy* is typically used in connection with the knee joint and the TMJ (even though the articular disk in the TMJ is only rarely referred to as *meniscus*).

17

condylectomy [kɒndaɪlɛktəmi‖kɒːndᵊl-] *n term*

» *High condylectomy[1] and arthroplasty were performed for degenerative arthritis secondary to[2] persistent[3] MPD syndrome[4].*

Kondylektomie, op. Entfernung d. Kiefergelenkköpfchens
hohe Kondylektomie[1] infolge von[2] persistierend[3] myofasziales Schmerzsyndrom[4]

18

TMJ replacement surgery *n term*

arthroplasty and remodeling of the TMJ, esp. the condylar head, performed for severely ankylosed joints, comminuted fractures[1], etc.

» *Delrin and other synthetic materials might offer an alternative to metallic or other alloplastic condylar head[2] implants in TMJ replacement surgery.*

Kiefergelenkplastik
Trümmer-, Splitterfrakturen[1] Kiefergelenkkopf, -köpfchen[2]

19

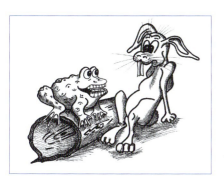

Why don't you give it a try.
Cosmetic dentistry can change your life –
just look at me!

Unit 39 Cosmetic Dentistry
Related Units: 40 Restorative Dentistry, 35 Periodontics, 42 Prosthodontics, 36 Orthodontic Dentistry, 43 Dental Implantology

cosmetic *adj*   *sim* **esthetic**[1] [esθetɪk] *adj*, **aesthetic** *BE*

preserving[2], restoring or contributing to[3] good looks

esthetics *n pl* • cosmetics *n pl*

» *During the healing phase the denture should be used for cosmetic purposes only. Great efforts were made to improve the functional and cosmetic outcome[4].*

Use **cosmetic** facade [-sɑːd]/ appearance / adjustment[5] [dʒʌ]/ and functional outcome[4] • **cosmetic** acceptability / prosthesis [iː]/ porcelain veneer [-ɪɚ] technique[6] [-iːk]/ dentistry[7] / surgery[8] • **esthetic** needs / concerns[9] / compromise[10] [-aɪz]/ zone / tooth analog[11] • poor **esthetic** quality • dental **esthetics**

kosmetisch
ästhetisch[1] erhaltend[2] beitragend zu[3] kosmetisches Ergebnis[4] kosm. Korrektur[5] kosm. Keramikveneertechnik[6] ästhetische Zahnheilkunde[7] Schönheits-, kosm. Chirurgie[8] ästhet. Bedenken[9] ästhet. Kompromiss[10] ästhet. Zahnersatz[11]

1

contour [kɒntʊɚ] *v & n term*   *sim* **facade**[1] *n*, **sculpt**[2] [ʌ] *v*, **outline**[3], **recontouring**[4] *n & v term*

(v) to shape the form, proportions and outline of teeth, lips, prostheses, etc.
(n) outline or configuration

» *This leads to unfavorable[5] [eɪ] crown contours and distorted occlusion. Tooth length, width [wɪdθ], contour, and embrasure [eɪʒ] form were evaluated. The membrane was contoured to overlap[6] the defect margin. The prosthesis served primarily as a cosmetic facade. There is no need to overfill and grind [aɪ] back[7] because the material is easy to sculpt[8].*

Use to develop/establish/finesse[9] *the contour* • **contour** line / curve / filling / amalgam • anatomic / natural-looking / chin [tʃ]/ cheek or buccal [ʌ] **contour** • facial [eɪʃ]/ palatal / gingival / crown **contours** • properly / poorly **contoured** • final / cosmetic[10] **contouring** • **contouring** pliers[11] [aɪ] • **recontoured** surfaces • tooth **recontouring** • **overcontoured** crown margins[12] [dʒ]

formen, konturieren; Kontur
Facette, Verblendung, Frontansicht[1] formen, konturieren[2] Umriss, Kontur; konturieren, umreißen[3] Rekonturierung; rekonturieren[4] ungünstig[5] überdecken[6] ab-, einschleifen[7] leicht formbar[8] Kontur optimieren[9] ästhet. Formkorrektur[10] Konturzange[11] überkonturierte Kronenränder[12]

2

Cosmetic Dentistry

profile [prəʊfaɪl] n
outline or contour of an object, body or body part, esp. of the face viewed from the side
» *The lower jaw protrudes¹ [uː] and the facial profile is convex.*
Use chin [tʃ]/ prognathic [æθ] / Angle Class I facial / labial² **profile** • **profile** view³ [vjuː]/ radiograph⁴ / analysis⁵

Profil, Seitenansicht
vorspringen¹ Lippenprofil² Profilansicht³ Profilaufnahme⁴ Profilanalyse⁵

3

Frankfort line or **plane** [eɪ] n term   syn **auriculo-infraorbital plane** n term
standard craniometric reference plane¹ marked by the right and the left porion² [pɔːrɪən] and the left orbital³
» *Position the patient's head in the cephalostat⁴ [sefəloʊstæt] so that the Frankfort plane is perpendicular⁵ to the film cassette.*
Use mental foramen [eɪ] (abbr MFP) / lingual vertical (abbr LVP) / occlusal⁶ **plane** • mandibular⁷ / nasal **line**

Frankfurter Horizontale(bene)
Bezugsebene¹ Porion² Orbitale³ Kephalostat⁴ senkrecht⁵ Okklusionsebene⁶ Mandibularlinie⁷

4

facial angle [feɪʃəl æŋgl] n term
angle between the Frankfort plane and the line between the depression at the root of the nose¹ (nasion² [neɪzɪɒn]) and the foremost³ portion of the chin (pogonion⁴)
» *The anteroposterior relation of the mandible to the upper face was established⁵ with the help of the facial angle.*
Use mandibular / nasolabial / mentolabial / gonial / opening **angle** • **angle** of the jaw / mandible

Gesichts-, Fazialwinkel
Nasenwurzel¹ Nasion² ventralste, vorderste³ Mentalpunkt, Pogonion⁴ bestimmt⁵

5

lip line n term   sim **smile line¹** n term
extent of gum [ʌ] tissue revealed by the level of the lips when the patient is in full smile²
» *In a high lip line the widest smile² reveals the gingiva [dʒ] above the upper teeth. In patients with a low lip line³ the widest smile barely reveals the bottom edges of the upper teeth and no gum tissue shows.*
Use high / medium [iː]/ low³ / even⁴ [iː] **lip line** • **lip** closure⁵ [oʊʒ]/ sucking [ʌ]/ pressure / biting⁶ • incompetent⁷ **lips** • **smile** improvement / analysis • width of / gummy⁸ [ʌ] **smile** • reverse⁹ **smile line** • **excessive gingival** show or display⁸

Lippenlinie
Lachlinie, -kurve¹ beim breitesten Lächeln² tiefe Lippenlinie³ gerade L.⁴ Lippenschluss⁵ Lippenbeißen⁶ Lippeninkompetenz, fehlender Lippenschluss⁷ Zahnfleischlächeln, Gummy smile⁸ negative Lachkurve⁹

6

gingival [dʒɪndʒɪvəl] **line** or **margin** [dʒ] n term   syn **gum** [gʌm] **line** n clin
border between the gums and the crowns
» *A normal appearing free gingival margin surrounded the implant. The gingival line over the buccal [ʌ] and lingual portions had remained unchanged.*
Use **gingival margin** discrepancy¹ • receding² [iː] **gingival margins** • **gingival** shrinkage [ʃrɪŋkɪdʒ] or recession² [se]/ stippling³ / color

Zahnfleisch-, Gingivarand, Margo gingivalis
asymmetrischer Zahnfleischverlauf¹ Gingivarezession² Zahnfleischtüpfelung³

7

height [haɪt] **of contour** n term
line encircling a tooth at its greatest bulge¹ [bʌldʒ] or diameter²
» *This bell-crowned³ tooth has a height of contour grossly [oʊ] exceeding the diameter of the neck.*
Use gingival **height of contour**

anatomischer (Zahn)äquator
Wölbung¹ Durchmesser² m. überkonturierter Krone³

8

cementoenamel junction [dʒʌŋkʃən] n term, abbr **CEJ**
                                    sim **cervical** [sɜːrvɪkəl] **line¹** n term
the line where the enamel of the crown and the cementum of the root join at the neck
» *Mean gingival recession from the CEJ was 1.9 mm. The classification of delayed² [eɪ] apical migration [aɪ] of the gingival margin depends on the relationship of the CEJ to the alveolar crest³.*
Use mucogingival⁴ [mjuːkoʊ-] **junction**

Schmelz-Zement-Grenze
Zahnhalsline¹ verzögerte² Alveolarkamm³ Mukogingivalgrenze⁴

9

biologic(al) [baɪəlɒːdʒ-] **width** [wɪdθ] n term
distance between the alveolar and the gingival crest¹
» *A zone similar to the concept of biologic width was formed around the teeth.*
Use to reestablish proper biologic² **width** • buccolingual³ / ridge **width**

biologische Breite
Gingivarand¹ adäquate biolog. Breite wiederherstellen² Bukkolingualabstand³

10

curve [kɜːrv] **of occlusion** [-uːʒən] n term
                    syn **occlusal** [uːz] **curvature** [kɜːrvətʃɚ] n term → U36-5
(i) curved surface making simultaneous contact with the major portion of the incisal and occlusal prominences (ii) the curve of the occlusal surfaces

Okklusionskurve, Spee Kurve

11

Cosmetic Dentistry

crown length [kraʊn leŋθ] *n term*   *sim* **apicocoronal** [eɪpɪ-] **height**[1] *n term*

» Tooth angulation was 70 degrees to the horizontal and the maxillary central incisor crown length was 10.5 mm.

Use clinical **crown length** • apicocoronal height deficiency [ɪʃ] • apicocoronal direction / gain / depth • esthetic **crown lengthening** surgery[2]

Kronenlänge
Wurzelkronenabstand, Apikokoronalhöhe[1] kosmet. Kronenverlängerung[2]   12

---

embrasure [ɪmbreɪʒɚ] *n term*   *rel* **(interdental) spillway**[1] *n term*

space continuous with[2] the interproximal contact area[3] produced by the curvature of adjacent teeth[4]

» Embrasure spaces[5] are checked to ensure adequate access[6] for oral hygiene.

Use buccal / gingival / lingual / occlusal / cleansable [e] **embrasure** • **embrasure** spaces *or* zones[5] / form / curve

Einziehung
Interdental-, Approximalraum[1] übergehend in[2] inter- / approximale Kontaktfläche[3] Nachbarzähne[4] Papillenräume[5] Zugang[6]   13

---

scallop [skæləp] *n & v term*

(n) series of wavy [eɪ] indentations[1] or arches on a normally smooth [uː] margin[2] of a structure, e.g. the gums

» The labial gingiva was scalloped externally. Cement lines appear thin and scalloped in form.

Use **scalloped** facial gingiva / line / appearance[3] / border

bogen-, wellenförmiger Verlauf; bogenförmig ausschneiden
Einbuchtungen, Vertiefungen[1] glatter Rand[2] girlandenförm. / gefälteltes Aussehen[3]   14

---

shade [ʃeɪd] *n term*   *sim* **blend**[1] *n & v*, **shading**[2] *n term*

quality or intensity of tooth color

» Esthetic failures were due to poor restoration shade. Color, shade, archform[3], centric relation and lip support were checked. A variety of shading is visible in this close-up view of a molar. The filling of the defect blended well with[4] that of adjacent bone.

Use to record the tooth[5] **shade** • **shade** determination[6] / selection[7] / range[8] /-matching light[9] / guide[10] [aɪ]/ scanner[11] / discrepancy • a darker[12] / lighter **shade** of white • to chose/improve **shading** • tooth / esthetic / perfect / custom[13] [ʌ]/ pontic / veneer [-ɪɚ] **shading** • **shading** paste • **blending** chart[14] [tʃ]

Note: Do not mix up *shade* and *shadow*[15].

Farbton, -nuance
(Farb)mischung; (ver)mischen, übergehen in[1] Farbabstimmung, Tönung; Schattierung[2] Zahnbogenform[3] (farblich) gut abgestimmt auf[4] Zahnfarbe nehmen[5] Farbbestimmung[6] Farbwahl[7] Tönungsbereich[8] Farbanpassungsleuchte[9] Farbring[10] (elektron.) Farbbestimmungsgerät[11] ein dunkleres Weiß[12] individuelle Farbabstimmung[13] Mischtabelle[14] Schatten, Verschattung; verschatten[15]   15

---

opacity [oʊpæsəti] *n term*   *opposite* **translucency**[1] [uː] *n term*

an area less transparent[2] [eɚ] and/or translucent[3] than surrounding tooth substance [ʌ]

opaque[4] [oʊpeɪk] *adj & v term* • **opaquer**[5] *n* • **opalescent**[6] [es] *adj*

» The framework was opaqued with a thermally cured[7] pink opaque veneer[8]. The opacities of the anterior teeth were covered up with veneering[8].

Use **opacity** period[9] • **opaque** white[10] / powder [aʊ]/ bonding dental ceramics[11] [sɪræ-] • **opalescent** dentine[12] • **opaquer** liquid / paste

Opazität, Lichtundurchlässigkeit
Lichtdurchlässigkeit, Transluzenz[1] durchsichtig, transparent[2] lichtdurchlässig, durchscheinend[3] opak; opazifizieren[4] Opaker[5] opaleszierend[6] heißpolymerisiert[7] Verblendschale, Veneer[8] Trübungsstadium[9] Deckweiß[10] opake Keramikverblendmaterialien[11] Opakdentin[12]   16

---

texture [tekstʃɚ] *n & v*

(n) the composition[1] and structure of a substance, e.g. the surface of teeth, the tongue, etc.

» The chin was deformed and presented[2] a hard, firm texture on palpation.

Use fissured[3] [ɪʃ]/ dense / rough[3] [ʌf]/ surface[4] **texture** • loosely[5] [uː] **textured** • **texturing** methods

Struktur, (Auf)bau; strukturieren
Zusammensetzung[1] wies auf[2] rissige Struktur[3] grobe/rauhe (Oberflächen)struktur[4] Oberflächenstruktur[5] locker strukturiert[5]   17

---

luster [ʌ] *n*, BE **lustre**   *syn* **sheen** [ʃiːn], **gloss**, **shine** [aɪ] *n*

natural property[1] of smooth materials (e.g. teeth or porcelain) to shine[2] with reflecting light

lustrous[3] [lʌstrəs] *adj* • **shiny**[3] *adj*

» Finally the teeth were adjusted [dʒʌ] to the opposing dentition and polished to a high luster. Controlling luster[4] is more difficult with oven [ʌ] glazing[5] [eɪz] than with hand polishing porcelain [pɔːrsəlɪn].

Use enamel-like[6] **shine** • to control[4] / to increase / level of **luster** • **gloss** intensity[7]

Glanz, Schimmer
Eigenschaft[1] leuchten, glänzen[2] glänzend[3] Glanz regulieren[4] Glanzbrand[5] perlmuttartiger Glanz[6] Glanzgrad[7]   18

Cosmetic Dentistry

bleach [bliːtʃ] n & v term   sim **tooth whitening**[1], **surface lightening**[1] n clin
  treating teeth with a strong oxidizing agent to reduce or eliminate stains[2] [eɪ]
  (over)bleaching n term • photobleaching[3] n • bleacher
» This substance inhibits bleaching of the fluorescent [es] staining. His teeth whitened up. An important step in the laser whitening process is protection of the soft tissues.
Use walking[4] [ɔːk] **bleach** • internal[4] / external[5] / vital[6] [aɪ]/ in-office / home / mouthguard[7] **bleaching** • **bleaching** agent / procedure / action / splint or tray[8] / solution / therapy • laser-assisted tooth[9] **whitening** • **whitening** time / effect / protocol / appointment

Bleichen; bleichen
Zahn-, Oberflächenaufhellung[1] Verfärbungen[2] Lichtbleichen[3] internes Bleichen[4] externes Bleichen[5] Bleichen vitaler Zähne[6] Schienenbleichung[7] Bleichschiene[8] Laserbleaching[9]   19

bonding n term
  (i) procedure in which the enamel is mildly etched [tʃ] with an acid[1] to cover up stains, improve contours or attach[2] orthodontic appliances [aɪ] or other materials (ii) chemical affinity, linkage [ɪdʒ] or adhesion [iːʒ] between two compounds[3] or materials
  bond[4] n & v term • de[5]/rebond[6] n & v • bondable[7] adj
» Loss of bond between the acrylic [ɪ] resin shell[8] and Cosmesil occurred in 12 patients. Bone can bond closely to a smooth titanium surface. The bonding agent[9] was cured[10] for 2 min before bonding the resin teeth to the denture base.
Use composite resin[11] / chemical [k]/ diffusion / dentin / adhesive[12] **bonding** • high / mechanical [k] **bond** • **bond** strength[13] • **bonding** primer[9] [aɪ]

(i) Haftung, Haftvermittlung; (ii) Bindung, Verbund
Säure[1] befestigen[2] Verbindungen[3] Bindung, Haftung; (ver)binden, (an)haften[4] Haftungsverlust; H. verlieren, (Brackets, etc.) abnehmen[5] Wiederbefestigung; -en[6] klebbar[7] Kunststoffverblendung[8] Haftvermittler[9] gehärtet[10] Befestigen m. Kompositklebern[11] Adhäsivtechnik[12] Verbundfestigkeit[13] 20

etch [etʃ] n & v → U30-19
  (v) applying an etchant solution[1] to prepare a surface for adhesive bonding
  etchant[2] n & adj term • microetching n • acid etch(ing)[3] n • frost etch v
» Acid-etched sealing composite was used. Avoid any potentially splatter[4] of the etchant.
Use enamel[5] / no-rinse self-**etching** • resin[6] **etchant** • **etch** pattern[7] / bond / technique • **etching** paste / gel[6] / acid / unit[8] / • **etched** enamel / bridge[9] / ceramics [s]

Ätzverfahren; ätzen
Ätzlösung[1] Ätzmittel; ätzend[2] (Säure-)Ätzverfahren,-technik[3] Verspritzen[4] Schmelzätzen[5] Ätzgel[6] Ätzmuster[7] Ätzstift[8] Ätz-, Adhäsivbrücke[9]   21

veneer [vəˈnɪə] n & v term   syn **laminate** n & v, sim **facing**[1] [feɪsɪŋ] n term
  (n) thin porcelain layer bonded to the tooth surface to correct imperfections[2] in color and/or shape
  veneering[3] n term • laminating[4] n • laminated[5] adj
» How about a removable labial veneer? The other side was laminated for increased stiffness. Veneer design must not contribute to food trapping[6]. This should be done prior to veneering.
Use labial [eɪ] gingival / removable[7] / laminate[8] / resin[9] **veneer** • **veneering** material[10] • porcelain[11] **laminate**

Verblendschale, Veneer; verblenden, beschichten
Facette, Verblendung[1] Mängel[2] Verblendtechnik[3] Schichtverfahren[4] schichtweise aufgebracht[5] Retention v. Speiseresten[6] abnehmbares Veneer[7] Schichtverblendung[8] Kunststoffveneer[9] Verblendmaterial[10] Keramikveneer, -verblendung[11] 22

microabrasion [maɪkroʊəbreɪʒ°n] n term
  removal of dental stains[1] [eɪ] by abrading[2] [eɪ] the tooth with mild acids

Mikroabrasion
Zahnverfärbungen[1] abtragen, -radieren[2]   23

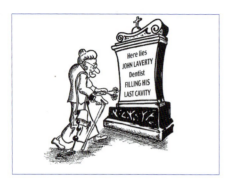

Unit 40   Restorative Dentistry
Related Units: 42 Prosthodontics, 41 Endodontics, 35 Periodontics, 43 Dental Implantology

filling n clin   sim **restoration**[1] n term

(i) a substance (amalgam, gold, etc.) used for restoring[2] cavities or missing portions removed e.g. because of tooth decay[3] [dıkeı] (ii) the process of placing a filling[4]

fill v & n term • restore[2] v • restorative[5] adj

» The internal surface is cleaned, dried and filled with a tooth-colored resin[6]. If tooth decay is extensive, placing several fillings in one tooth might undermine[7] [aı] its stability.

Use **to fill** a cavity/defect / and vibrate[8] [aı] • defect[9] **fill** • tooth / root / amalgam[10] / composite[11] **fillings** • tooth-colored[12] / discolored or stained[13] [eı] **fillings** • **filling materials**[14] / wax / gold • **restorative** dentistry[15]

Füllung(stherapie)
Restauration[1] restaurieren[2] Karies[3] eine Füllung legen[4] zahnerhaltend, wiederherstellend[5] Kunststoff[6] untergraben, beeinträchtigen[7] einrütteln[8] Defektauffüllung[9] Amalgamfüllungen[10] Kompositfüllungen[11] zahnfarbene F.[12] verfärbte F.[13] Füllungsmaterialien[14] Zahnerhaltung, konservierende Zahnheilkunde[15]   1

---

cavity debridement [dıbriːdmənt‖mɒː] n term → U28-12
                    syn **cavity toilet** [tɔılət] n jar & clin

final step of cleansing [e] and removing all debris[1] [dəbriː] from the prepared cavity before placing the restoration

» Mild pulpitis [aı] may occur secondary to[2] mechanical [k] debridement [3] of a cavity.

Use access[4] [ækses] **cavity**

Kavitätenreinigung
Gewebereste, -trümmer, Rückstände[1] infolge von[2] mechanische Reinigung[3] Zugangskavität[4]
                                                                2

---

cavity liner [laınɚ] n term   sim **lining**[1] [laınıŋ] n term

thin sealant [iː] lining[2] with antibacterial action to promote the health of the pulp

Use **cavity liner** cures [kjuːɚz] rock hard[3] • **lining** materials[4]

Kavitätenlack, -liner
Auskleidung[1] Versiegelung[2] K. wird steinhart[3] dünnschichtige Unterfüllungen[4]
                                                                3

---

cavity base [beıs] n term

used for dentin replacement to minimize bulk[1] [ʌ] of restorative material or to block undercuts[2]

Use to place[3] a **base** • **base** and liner technique [tekniːk]

Unterfüllung
Masse, Volumen[1] Unterschnitte[2] unterfüllen[3]
                                                                4

---

resin-modified glass ionomers [aıə] n term   abbr **RMGIs**

glass polyalkenoate admixed[1] with resin mainly used as fast-setting[2] liners and restorative cements; a similar material is Compomer (combines the fluoride-releasing [iː] properties[3] of GIs and the abrasion [eı] resistance[4] of composite)

» RMGIs make excellent bases and liners because they can adhere[5] [ɪɚ] to both tooth and resin. Glass ionomers are relatively brittle[6] which limits their use to non-load-bearing[7] [eɚ] situations.

lichthärtende / kunststoff-modifizierte Glasionomerzemente
beigemischt[1] schnellhärtend[2] fluoridfreisetzende Eigenschaften[3] Abrieb-, Abrasionsfestigkeit[4] haften an[5] brüchig[6] nicht tragend[7]   5

---

indirect pulp [ʌ] **capping** n term or **cap** n jar

small layer of softened [sɒːfnd] dentin[1] left in place at the base of a deep cavity to maintain[2] pulp vitality

» If elimination of all caries would risk exposure[3] [oʊʒ] of vital pulp an indirect pulp cap[4] is indicated.

Use dental / direct[5] **(pulp) capping** • **pulp capping** agent [eıdʒənt]

indirekte Pulpaüberkappung
aufgeweichtes Dentin[1] erhalten[2] Freilegung, Eröffnung[3] Pulpakappe[4] direkte (Pulpa)überkappung[5]
                                                                6

---

step n term

projection[1] [dʒek] prepared into the surface of a cavity to prevent displacement[2] of the filling by mastication[3]

» When contouring[4] [ʊɚ] the cavity, steps are essential for adequate resistance to wear[5] [weɚ].

Kavitätenstufe, Retentionsform
Vorsprung[1] Verlagerung, Dislokation[2] Kauen[3] Ausformen[4] Abrieb-, Verschleißfestigkeit[5]   7

---

shoulder [ʃoʊldɚ] n term

ledge[1] [ledʒ] formed by the junction[2] [dʒʌŋkʃ[ə]n] of the gingival and the axial wall in extracoronal restorative preparations

» Displacement of the right crown shoulder[3] increased with loading[4] [oʊ].

Use **shoulder** height [haıt]/ form • to model the / supporting **shoulder**

Schulter(präparation)
Stufe[1] Verbindung[2] Kronenschulter[3] Belastung[4]
                                                                8

butt [bʌt] *v term*

to connect two parts with flat surfaces without any overlap, e.g. placement of a restoration directly against and flush [ʌ] with¹ the tissues covering the alveolar [ɪə] ridge [rɪdʒ]

Use **butt** joint² [dʒɔɪnt]

stumpfstoßen, anlegen (an)
bündig / niveaugleich mit¹ stumpfer Stoß, Stumpffuge, butt joint²

9

cavity margin [mɑːrdʒɪn] *n term*

junction between natural tooth substance and the filling material or crown

» Loss of contact to the anterior [ɪə] margin of the prosthesis [θiː] was rarely a problem except in cases where the prosthesis extended forward onto¹ contours that altered² [ɒː] mouth opening.

Kavitätenrand
vorne reichen bis¹ veränderte²

10

facing [feɪsɪŋ] *n term*   opposite **backing¹** *n term*

tooth-colored material used on the visible surfaces of a metal crown to give the outward appearance [ɪə] of a natural tooth (usually plastic or porcelain² [pɔːrsᵊlɪn]) and hide the metal support³ on the lingual and palatal aspects

» On occasion⁴, distal pontics⁵ with only buccal [ʌ] facings can be employed.

Facette, Facing
Palatinal-, Lingualfläche¹ Keramik² Metallgerüst³ in Einzelfällen⁴ Brückenzwischenglieder⁵

11

overhang *n term*

excessive¹ amount of dental filling material projecting [dʒe] beyond² the cavity margin or normal tooth contour

» Excess¹ cement was difficult to remove because of overhang.

Füllungsüberschuss, -überhang
überschüssig¹ hinausragen über²

12

undercut [ʌndəˈkʌt] *n term*

(i) portion of a tooth between the height of contour¹ and the gingival margin (ii) contour of a residual ridge² or dental arch obstructing³ insertion or providing retention of a denture

» These copings can provide a 1.0 mm or greater undercut. Block out⁴ any undercuts with glass ionomer cement.

Use to form/produce/remove/avoid/block/retain by **undercut** • deep / circumferential / mechanical / labial / retentive / hard tissue **undercut**

Unterschnitt, unter sich gehende Stelle
Zahnäquator¹ verbleibende Stufe² behindern³ ausblocken⁴

13

(dentinal) pin *n term*   syn **dentin(e)** or **parapulpal** [ʌ] **pin** *n,*
                                sim **endodontic pin** or **post¹** *n term*

thin metal rod² [ɒː] which is cemented or screwed [skruːd] into a channel [tʃ] in the dentin to help retain³ filling material

» It is suggested [dʒ] that the U-shaped pin be in place⁴ during cementation. Pin retention may be necessary to support the cores of full coverage [ʌ] crowns⁵.

Use to position or place⁶/dislodge⁷ [ɒː]/shorten **pins** • self-threading⁸ [e]/ threaded⁹ / auxiliary [ɔːgz]/ guide / removable / spring-loaded¹⁰ [oʊ] **pin** • **pin** insertion / channel [tʃ]/ retention¹¹ • custom-made / prefabricated¹² / unretentive / smooth-sided / sandblasted¹³ / passive / serrated¹⁴ / screw-retained **post**

parapulpärer Stift
Wurzel(kanal)stift¹ Stift² verankern³ bereits eingebracht⁴ Hülsenkronen⁵ Stifte einbringen⁶ Stifte lockern⁷ selbstschneidender Stift⁸ Gewindestift⁹ Stift mit Schnappfeder¹⁰ Stiftverankerung¹¹ konfektionierter Stift¹² sandgestrahlter Wurzelstift¹³ geriffelter (Wurzelkanal)stift¹⁴

14

core [kɔːr] *n term*   rel **(endodontic) post¹** *n term*

(i) metal framework frequently with a post¹ in the root canal to retain an artificial crown (ii) more generally, the center or base of a structure

» This endodontically treated tooth had been restored with a post¹ and core.

Use dowel² [daʊᵊl] **core**

(i) Stift-, Stumpfaufbau
(ii) Kern, Zentrum
Wurzelstift¹ Stiftaufbau²

15

inlay [ɪnleɪ] *n term*   sim **onlay¹** *n term*

a custom-made² [ʌ] gold, porcelain, or composite filling made to fit a prepared cavity and cemented into place³; fillings supporting the chewing [tʃuːɪŋ] surface⁴ are called onlays

» Remove the temporary⁵, clean the tooth and try in the inlay carefully checking the marginal fit⁶. For onlays a minimum 1.5 mm reduction of the cusps⁷ [ʌ] is necessary.

Use porcelain fused [fjuː] to gold / composite / temporary⁸ **inlay**

Einlagefüllung, Inlay
Onlay¹ individuell angepasste² einzementiert³ Kaufläche⁴ Provisorium⁵ Randschluss⁶ Beschleifen d. Höcker⁷ provisorisches Inlay⁸

16

Endodontics DENTISTRY **147**

coping [koʊpɪŋ] *n term* → U42-9, 31-11

(i) thin metal covering, e.g. for retaining porcelain restorations (ii) cone-shaped¹ metal cap fitted over a prepared crown to serve as an abutment² [ʌ] for dentures (iii) resin or metal cap used to position a die³ [daɪ] in an impression

» A coping was cast⁴ for the left second molar. Radiographs have proved helpful to assure⁵ [əʃʊɚ] proper seating⁶ of the coping. Brittle fractures⁷ were seen on the porcelain crowns and the ceramic [s] copings.

Use prefabricated⁸ / gold alloy / ceramic⁹ *coping* • *coping* construction¹⁰ / prosthesis¹¹ [θiː]

(i) Metall-, Abdeckkappe, Coping (ii) Primärkrone, Innenteleskop (iii) Transferkappe
konusförmig¹ Verankerung² Modellstumpf³ gegossen⁴ sicherstellen⁵ Sitz⁶ Craquelierung⁷ vorgefertigtes / konfektioniertes Coping⁸ Keramikverblendung⁹ Metallgerüst¹⁰ Deckprothese¹¹   17

crown [kraʊn] *n term*   *sim* **cap¹** [kæp] *n clin & jar*

(porcelain and) metal restoration that replaces a decayed² [eɪ] or damaged natural crown (or a major portion) and is permanently cemented into place

crowning³ *n term* • crown⁴ *v* • crowned *adj*

» If the crown contour is to be optimal, the emergence [ɜːrdʒ] profile⁵ [proʊfaɪl] must be harmonious with that of the adjacent⁶ [ədʒeɪsənt] soft tissues.

Use to insert/place/trim⁷/smooth⁸ [uː]/polish *a crown* • preformed / custom-made / temporary⁹ / chairside / full(-coverage)¹⁰ / three-quarter(s) *crown* • stainless steel¹¹ / gold veneer¹² [-ɪɚ]/ cast gold / acrylic¹³ [ɪ]/ porcelain / metal-ceramic / all-ceramic¹⁴ [s] *crown* • porcelain jacket¹⁵ / post(-retained)¹⁶ / telescopic¹⁷ *crown* • *crown* margin¹⁸ / cementation

Krone
Überkappung, Krone¹ kariös² Überkronung³ überkronen⁴ Austritts-, Emergenzprofil⁵ anliegend⁶ K. beschleifen⁷ K. glätten⁸ Interims-, provisorische K.⁹ Hülsenkrone¹⁰ Stahlkr.¹¹ Verblendkr.¹² Kunststoffkr.¹³ Vollkeramikkr.¹⁴ Jacketkr.¹⁵ Stiftkr.¹⁶ Teleskopkr.¹⁷ Kronenrand¹⁸   18

chamfer [tʃæmfɚ] *n & v term*   *syn* **bevel** [bevəl] *n & v*

(n) marginal [dʒ] finishing line of extracoronal cavity preparation in which the gingival [dʒ] surface meets the external axial surface at an obtuse [tjuː] angle¹ [æŋgl] forming a curved, beveled edge²

chamfered *adj term* • beveled *adj*

» A definite chamfered finishing line should be established³ first. Incisally, the veneer⁴ can be finished to a chamfer at the incisal edge. A minimal chamfer is recommended.

Use to cut/reduce *to a chamfer* • *chamfer* preparation⁵ / ground section⁶ [aʊ]/ angle • *chamfered* surface

Randabschrägung; abschrägen
stumpfer Winkel¹ abgeschrägter Rand² fertiggestellt³ Verblendschale⁴ Hohlkehlpräparation⁵ Fasenschliff⁶   19

crazing [kreɪzɪŋ] *n term*

appearance of minute [maɪnuːt] cracks¹ on the surface of plastic or ceramic restorations (fillings, dentures, or denture bases²)

Craquelierung, Netzrissbildung
feine Risse¹ Prothesenbasen²   20

percolate [pɜːrkəleɪt] *v term*   *sim* **penetrate¹** *v term*

saliva² [aɪ] or fluids leaking [iː] into³ the interface⁴ between a restoration and the tooth structure

» Percolation⁵ was due to fissures [ɪʃ] resulting from thermal [ɜː] changes⁶. The abutment [ʌ] should be carefully examined for salivary percolation⁷.

eindringen, durchsickern
durchdringen¹ Speichel² eindringen³ Grenzfläche⁴ Perkolation⁵ thermisch bedingte Veränderungen⁶ Speichelperkolation⁷   21

Unit 41 Endodontics
Related Units: **35** Periodontics, **44** Oral Surgery

endodontic *adj term*

related to diseases of the dental pulp [ʌ], root [uː], and the tissues at the root apex¹ [eɪ]

endodontics or -ology² *n term* • endodontist or -ologist³ *n*

» Alveolar [ɪə] resorption⁴ can be prevented by retaining⁵ [eɪ] endodontically treated teeth. Endodontists may perform simple to difficult root canal treatments⁶ as well as surgical root procedures [iː].

Use **endodontic** instrumentation⁷ / treatment / complications / failure

endodontisch, Endodont-
Wurzelspitze¹ Endodont(olog)ie² Endodontologe, -in³ Alveolarkammabbau⁴ erhalten⁵ Wurzel-(kanal)behandlungen⁶ Wurzelkanalinstrumente⁷   1

pulpal [pʌlpəl] status [eɪ] n term

assessment[1] of the health and vitality [aɪ] of the pulp by checking its sensitivity[2] to stimuli, by x-ray films[3], etc.

» No pulpal reaction[4] was evident[5]. Radiography showed deep carious penetration[6] with potential pulpal involvement.
Use **pulpal** involvement / pathology[7] / inflammation[8] [eɪʃ]/ exposure[9] [oʊʒ]/ necrosis

Zustand der Pulpa
(Über)prüfung[1] Sensibilität[2] Röntgenaufnahmen[3] Pulpareaktion[4] feststellbar[5] Caries profunda[6] Pulpopathie[7] Pulpitis[8] Pulpaeröffnung[9]   2

pulpless or nonvital [aɪ] tooth n term   opposite vital tooth[1] n term

tooth with a necrotic pulp or one from which the pulp has been extirpated[2]

» False-positive results on pulp testing[3] may be obtained[4] in multi-rooted teeth[5] with vital and non-vital pulp.

marktoter / de- / avitaler Zahn
vitaler Zahn[1] entfernt[2] Sensibilitätsprüfung[3] erhoben[4] mehrwurzelige Zähne[5]   3

root canal [ruːt kənæl] n term

space in the root of a tooth that contains pulp tissue

» The majority [dʒ] of bacteria in an infected root canal are located in the coronal region.
Use fine[1] / curved[2] [ɜː]/ straight [streɪt]/ main / lateral[3] / patent[4] [eɪ]/ accessory [ksɛ] or extra[5] / calcified or sclerosed **root canal** • **canal** curvature • to debride[6] [iː] a **canal**

Wurzelkanal
enger W.[1] gekrümmter W.[2] Seitenkanal[3] gängiger / nicht obliterierter W.[4] akzessorischer Wurzelkanal[5] W. aufbereiten / säubern[6]   4

pulp chamber [tʃeɪmbɚ] n term   rel pulp cavity[1] [kævɪti] n term

portion of the pulp cavity in the crown of a tooth

» Irrigate[2] the pulp chamber and identify the root canal with an explorer[3] or a fine file[4] [aɪ].
Use **pulp** chamber floor[5] / fin or horn[6] / cap • **pulp** calcification / denticle[7] / exposure / ischemia [skiː] / tester[8]

Pulpakammer, -kavum
Pulpahöhle, Cavitas dentis[1] ausspülen[2] Sonde[3] feine Feile[4] Pulpakammerboden[5] Pulpahorn[6] Pulpastein, Dentikel[7] Pulpaprüfer, -tester[8]   5

root tip or end n clin   syn apex [eɪpeks] n term

the terminal end of the root
apical [eɪpɪkəl] adj term • periapical[1] adj

» Root-filling[2] to the apical constriction[3] provides a natural stop to instrumentation. A bony window[4] was created to visualize [ɪʒ] the apex.
Use to cut off the[5] **root end** • **root** shape • to reduce the / excessive **root length** • apical constriction[3] / foramen[6] [eɪ] • radiographic[7] **apex**

Wurzelspitze, Apex (radicis dentis)
periapikal, um die W. herum[1] Wurzel(kanal)füllung[2] apikale Konstriktion[3] Knochenfenster[4] W. abtrennen[5] Foramen apicale[6] radio-, röntgenolog. Apex[7]   6

pulpitis [pʌlpaɪtɪs] n term

inflammation[1] [eɪʃ] of the dental pulp due to exposure [oʊʒ] (mostly by caries or tooth fracture [ktʃ]) to and invasion[2] [eɪʒ] of bacteria

» Symptoms of reversible pulpitis typically include fleeting [iː] pain[3] to hot, cold or sweet foods which is immediate in onset but quickly subsides[4] [aɪ] on removal of the stimulus.
Use acute / (ir)reversible[5] / chronic **pulpitis**

Pulpitis
Entzündung[1] Eindringen[2] flüchtiger, stechender Schmerz[3] nachlassen, verschwinden[4] reversible Pulpitis[5]   7

apical granuloma n term   sim periapical abscess[1] [æbses] n term, gumboil[2] [gʌmbɔɪl] n clin

proliferation[3] of granulation tissue at the apex of a nonvital tooth usually due to severe tooth decay[4], pulpal necrosis, trauma, or gum disease[5]

» Periapical abscesses are best managed by RCT or surgical intervention.

apikales Granulom
periapikaler Abszess[1] Parulis, submuköser Abszess[2] Wucherung[3] Caries profunda[4] Zahnfleischerkrankung[5]   8

root canal therapy or treatment n term   abbr RCT

endodontic treatment including complete extirpation of the pulp[1], sterilization and filling of the canal

» Common errors in canal preparation include incomplete debridement[2], lateral and apical perforation. The working length of the root canal can be determined[3] radiographically.
Use to clean/shape[4]/sterilize/flare[5] [fleɚ]/fill/seal[6] [iː] **the root canal** • **root canal** preparation[7] / irrigation[8] / filling[9]

Wurzel(kanal)behandlung
Vitalexstirpation, Pulpektomie[1] Säuberung, Debridement[2] festgestellt[3] W. aufbereiten[4] W. erweitern[5] W. dicht verschließen / abdichten[6] Wurzelkanalaufbereitung[7] Wurzelkanalspülung[8] Wurzel(kanal)füllung[9]   9

Endodontics

access [ækses] **cavity** *n term*

preparation of the crown required to approach[1] [outʃ] the roof of the pulp chamber[2] and the root

» In anterior teeth the access cavity should be midway between[3] the incisal edge and the cingulum [s]. When completed the access cavity should have a smooth [uː] funnel [ʌ] shape[4].

Wurzelkanalzugang, Zugangskavität
Zugang erlangen[1] Pulpakammerdach[2] in der Mitte zwischen[3] glatt u. trichterförmig[4]   10

canal preparation *n term*   *sim* **chemomechanical** [kiːmoʊ-] **instrumentation**[1] *n term*

techniques of RTC preparation include the stepback[2], stepdown[3], balanced force[4] and modified crown-down technique[5]

» Emphysema [iː] rarely may follow use of compressed air during root canal preparation as air is forced into the alveolus [ɪə] of the bone and then dissects[6] along fascial [ʃ] planes.

Wurzelkanalaufbereitung
chemomechan. Aufbereitung[1] step-back Technik, konische W.[2] step-down T., koronal-apikale W.[3] balanced-force Methode[4] modifiz. crown-down Technik[5] sich ausbreiten[6]   11

working length [leŋθ] *n term*

distance from a reference point on the crown to the apical constriction[1] of the root canal

» The working length can be established[2] either radiographically or with an apex locator[3].

Arbeitslänge, Aufbereitungstiefe
apikale Konstriktion[1] festgestellt[2] Apexlokalisator[3]   12

elbow formation *n jar*

coronal narrowing usually caused by apical transportation (zipping[1]) that results in an hourglass[2] canal

» In a curved canal straightening[3] [eɪ] of the reamer [iː] can cause elbow formation.

iatrogene(r) Engstelle / Isthmus, Kanaleinengung
apikale Trichterbildung[1] sanduhrförmig[2] Rückstellung[3]   13

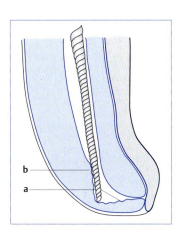

a zipping
b elbow formation

ledge [dʒ] **formation** *n term*   *syn* **ledging** *n jar*

undesirable narrow shelf[1] or spur[2] [ɜː] in the canal wall

» Ledging may cause instruments to stop short of length[3] and needs to be filed away[4]. Use to bypass[5] a **ledge**

Stufenbildung
Stufe[1] Vorsprung[2] vor dem Kanalende[3] abgefeilt[4] Stufe umgehen[5]   14

endodontic obturation *n term*   *rel* **condensation**[1] *n term*

dense filling[2] (usu. with gutta-percha [gʌtə pɜːrtʃə]) of the prepared canal to provide a hermetic seal[3] [iː] against bacteria (esp. at the apex and in the coronal region)
(micro)condenser[4] *n term* • condense[5] *v* • undercondensation[6] *n*

» The GP master point[7] must fit the apical section, then obturation of the remainder[8] [eɪ] is achieved by condensation of smaller accessory [ks] points[9].
Use poorly / densely /un**obturated** • **obturation** core / material • voids in the[10] **obturation** • cold / warm / thermomechanical[11] [k]/ lateral[12] / vertical[13] **condensation**

Wurzelkanalfüllung
Kondensation, Verdichtung[1] Aus-, Abfüllen[2] randdichter Verschluss[3] Plugger, (Wurzelkanal)stopfer[4] verdichten, kondensieren[5] unzureichende Verdichtung[6] Guttapercha-Hauptstift[7] restlicher Bereich[8] Zusatzstifte[9] Hohlräume nach Verdichten d. Füllung[10] thermomech. Kondensation[11] laterale K.[12] vertikale K.[13]   15

Endodontics

apical leakage [liːkɪdʒ] n term rel **seepage**[1] [siːpɪdʒ] n term

incomplete seal at the apex permitting influx[2] of tissue fluids that may harbor[3] bacteria

weeping [iː] canal[4] n jar

» Poorly obturated canals which contain voids[5] and therefore lack a proper seal are prone [oʊ] to[6] apical leakage.

undichter apikaler Verschluss
Sickern, Kriechen[1] Eindringen[2] beherbergen[3] undichter Kanal[4] Hohlräume[5] neigen zu[6]

16

apical perforation n term   sim **furcal** [ɜː] or **furcation perforation**[1] n term

mostly due to instrumentation errors in canal preparation (inappropriate working length, etc.)

» Apical perforation may be salvaged[2] [ɪdʒ] by vertical filling[3], if this is unsuccessful apicectomy [sek] must be performed. Lateral perforation[4] is more likely to occur if there is poor access[5].

Use root / lateral[4] / strip[6] **perforation**

Wurzelperforation i. apikalen Bereich
Furkationsperforation[1] behoben[2] vertikale Kondensation[3] (schlitzförmige) laterale Perforation[4] schlechter Zugang[5] Wurzelperforation (a. d. Innenkurvatur d. Kanalaufbereitung)[6]

17

root fracture [fræktʃɚ] n term   syn **root cracking** n jar & clin

fractures occur in the apical, middle or coronal third and may communicate with[1] the gingival [dʒ] crevice[2] [krɛvɪs]

» Fractures in the coronal third are best treated by extraction of the coronal fragment and RCT[3] of the remnant root[4].

Wurzelfraktur
in Verbindung stehen mit[1] Gingivalsulkus[2] Wurzel(kanal)behandlung[3] Restwurzel[4]

18

pulpectomy n term   sim **pulpotomy**[1] n term

complete resection of the dental pulp; removal of the coronal portion is termed pulpotomy

» If conditions are favorable pulpectomy is the treatment of choice[2] for nonvital pulps.

Use (non)vital **pulpectomy** • shallow[3] [ʃæloʊ] **pulpotomy**

Pulpektomie, Vitalexstirpation
Vitalamputation, Pulpotomie[1] Behandlung der Wahl[2] hohe Vitalamputation[3]

19

apic(o)ectomy [eɪpɪsek-‖-koʊektəmi] n term

syn **root (-end) resection** n term

removal of the apex

» Apicectomy is a second-line surgical adjunct[1] [ædʒʌŋkt] used after failure of or as a supplement to[2] [ʌ] orthograde [eɪ] endodontics[3].

Use previous [iː]/ second or revision [ɪʒ] apicectomy • apicectomy defect

Wurzelspitzenresektion
chir. Hilfsmaßnahme[1] Zusatz / Ergänzung zu[2] orthograde Wurzelkanalfüllung[3]

20

retrofilling n term   syn **root-end** or **reverse filling** n term

retrograde placement (via a periodontal approach) of hard tissue into the prepared apex to achieve a hermetic seal

over[1]/ **underfill**[2] n & v term

» An apicoectomy with retrosurgical filling[3] was performed.

Use dense / old root[4] **filling**

retrograde Wurzelkanalfüllung
Überfüllung; -füllen[1] Unterfüllung; -füllen[2] retrograde Wurzelfüllung[3] alte Wurzelfüllung[4]

21

cortical trephination [trefɪneɪʃən] n term

removal of a disk of bone with a trephine[1] [triːfaɪn], e.g. for rapid release[2] [iː] of pus[3] [ʌ] from an abscess

» Fistulative surgery[4] was used to create a release[2] by means of cortical trephination.

Knochentrepanation, Schröder Lüftung
Trepanbohrer[1] Abfluss[2] Eiter[3] Entlastungsoperation[4]

22

root amputation n term   sim **hemisection**[1], **bicuspidation**[2] [baɪkʌsp-] n term

removal of one or more roots of a multi-rooted tooth, while the remaining root canal(s) is/are treated endodontically; radectomy, radisection, radisectomy and radiectomy are dated synonyms

» Root amputation is followed by smoothing[3] [uːð], recontouring and restoration of residual[4] pulp cavities.

Wurzelamputation
Hemisektion[1] Prämolarisierung[2] Glätten[3] verbleibend[4]

23

mummification [mʌmɪfɪkeɪʃən] n term

application of fixative drugs[1] (e.g. formaldehyde [aɪ] derivatives[2]) to the residual pulp[3] following amputation of the coronal portion

» Generally, mummification is acceptable only in children in order to be able to retain[4] a deciduous tooth[5] slightly longer.

Mumifikation
Fixiermittel[1] Formaldehydderivate[2] Pulpareste[3] erhalten[4] Milchzahn[5]

24

41

Unit 42 Prosthodontics

Related Units: 40 Restorative Dentistry, 39 Cosmetic Dentistry, 43 Dental Implantology, 41 Endodontics, 35 Periodontics

prosthodontics [prɒːsθədɒːntɪks] *n term*　　syn **prosthetic** [e] **dentistry** *or* **prosthodontia** [dɒːnʃ(ɪ)ə] *n term*

restorative dentistry focused on the construction of artificial substitutes[1] for lost or missing teeth to restore function, cosmetic appearance, comfort, etc.

prosthetist [prɒːsθətɪst] *or* **prosthodontist**[2] *n term*

» The stability and longevity[3] [dʒe] of a prosthesis [iː] are key factors in implant prosthodontics[4].

Use **prosthodontic** care / aftercare / adjustment[5] [ʌ]/ design / rehabilitation / complications • removable / fixed **prosthodontics**

zahnärztliche Prothetik
künstlicher Ersatz[1] Prothetiker(in)[2] Dauerhaftigkeit[3] Implantologieprothetik[4] Prothesenanpassung[5]

1

---

dental prosthesis [-θiːsɪs] *n term, pl* -es
　　　　syn **dentures** [dentʃɚz] *n clin usu pl* → U10-8

various types of removable[1] or fixed[2], partial[3] or complete[4] replacements for teeth

(pre-)prosthetic [e] *adj term* • overdenture[5] *n*

» The design of the prostheses in these patients was changed to bar-clip retention[6].

Use to place/insert **a prosthesis** • detachable[1] [tʃ]/ maxillary / provisional[7] / permanent / 12-unit[4] **prosthesis** • cantilever(ed) [iː]/ telescopic **prosthesis** • **prosthesis** stability / retention[8] • **prosthetic** superstructure[9] / examination / substitution[10] • swinglock[11] / overlay[5] / dysjunct [dʒʌ]/ two-part[12] **denture** • **denture** wearer[13] [eɚ]

Zahnprothese, -ersatz, künstliches Gebiss
abnehmbarer Zahnersatz[1] festsitzender Z.[2] Teilprothese[3] Total-, Vollprothese[4] Deckprothese, Coverdenture[5] Stegverankerung[6] provisor. P., Interimsprothese[7] Prothesenhalt, -haftung, -retention[8] Suprastruktur, -konstruktion[9] prothetischer Ersatz[10] Schwenkriegelprothese[11] kombinierte Proth.[12] Prothesenträger(in)[13]

2

(dental) plates [eɪ] *n clin & inf usu pl*　　sim **uppers**[1] *n inf pl*

colloquial term (derived from denture plates) for a set of false teeth

» If you wear dentures, or partial dental plates, they must be removed. Dentures and plates need to fit well. Ill-fitting partial dental plates can irritate the gum tissue and the jaw bone causing ulcerations. Dental implants can be used to anchor removable dental plates or can replace them altogether.

Total-, Plattenprothese
Oberkieferprothese[1]

3

---

bridge [brɪdʒ] *n term*　　sim **bridgework**[1] *n term*

fixed or removable prosthesis replacing one or more missing crowns; anchored [k] to[2] adjacent [dʒeɪs] teeth by caps[3]

» The two key concerns[4] in bridgework are retention and support. The temporary bridge[5] was relined[6] [aɪ] at chairside[7].

Use to seat[8] [iː]/construct **a bridge** • fixed[9](-fixed) / fixed-movable/ removable / chairside / resin-bonded *or* Maryland[10] **bridge** • (direct-) cantilever[11] / spring cantilever[12] / precision [sɪʒ] attachment[13] / two-part **bridge**

Brücke
Brückenersatz[1] verankert[2] Kronen, Brückenanker[3] Hauptkriterien[4] provisorische B.[5] unterfüttert[6] am Behandlungsstuhl[7] Brücke einpassen[8] festsitzende B.[9] Adhäsiv-, Klebebr.[10] Freiend-, Extensionsbr.[11] Freiendbrücke m. Resilienzgeschiebe[12] Brücke m. Geschiebe[13]

4

---

pontic [pɒːntɪk] *n term*　　syn **dummy** [dʌmi] *n inf & jar*

artificial tooth on a partial denture which is suspended from the abutments[1]

» In direct cantilever bridges the pontic is anchored[1] at one end of the edentulous span[2] only. Ridge [dʒ] lap pontics[3] which make only minimal contact with the buccal [ʌ] ridge are most popular.

Use ridge-lap[3] / cantilevered / hygienic[4] [haɪdʒiːnɪk]/ premolar / saddle[5] **pontic**

Pontik, (Brücken)zwischenglied
durch Brückenanker befestigt[1] zahnloser Bereich[2] kammüberlappende Brückenzwgl.[3] Schwebebrückenzwischenglied, unterspülbares Zw.[4] sattelförmiges Zw.[5]

5

(denture) retainer [eɪ] *n term*　　sim **clasp**[1] [klæsp] *n term*

attachment (caps or clasps) stabilizing the pontic(s) by engaging[2] [eɪdʒ] the undercut[3] of the abutment tooth[4]

» Pontics are joined to retainers by a rigid[5] or non-rigid[6] connector[7]. Bar clasps[8] consist of two or more arms or bars[9] projecting from the connector[7] to opposite sides of the abutment; the retentive bar[10] usually terminates[11] in the gingival area of the tooth.

Use restoration / partial-coverage / free-standing / magnetic / female[12] **retainer** • infrabulge *or* roach[8] [routʃ]/ circumferential[13] / continuous[14] / extended / unsightly[15] [aɪ] **clasp** • gingivally [dʒ] approaching[16] [outʃ]/ hidden / wrought [rɒːt] gold[17] / cast cobalt[18] **clasp**

Halteelement
Klammer[1] umgreifen[2] unter sich gehender Bereich[3] Pfeilerzahn[4] starr[5] beweglich[6] Verbindungselement[7] Roachklammer(n)[8] Klammerarme[9] Halteelement[10] endet[11] Matrize[12] Ring-, E-, Akersklammer[13] fortlaufende K.[14] unästhetische K.[15] Zahnfleischkl.[16] gebogene Goldkl.[17] Kobaltgusskl.[18]

6

precision [priːsɪʒᵊn] **attachment** [ətætʃmᵊnt] *n term*
  specially designed fixation of a removable bridge hiding the attachment to the abutment teeth
  » *The restoration was held in place by a screwed[1] [skruːd] precision attachment at the dental abutment.*

cantilever (fixed) prosthesis [iː] *n term*
  restoration supported by one fixed support at only one of its ends
  » *Masticatory forces induce high bending moments in cantilever beams[1] [iː]. The prosthesis was cantilevered 20 mm from the centerline of the distal abutment. The number and distribution of cantilever occlusal contacts influences bolus[2] placement.*
  Use **cantilever** unit / joint[3] / pontic / length[4] [leŋθ]/ load / arm / extension[4]

telescopic coping [koʊpɪŋ] *n term* → U40-17
  outer crown attached to a metal thimble[1] [θɪ-] inserted on the prepared abutment tooth to anchor removable bridges, partial prostheses, etc.
  » *The design of the telescopic copings must be as parallel as possible to allow for maximum frictional retention[2]. The provisional [ɪʒ] prosthesis[3] is designed to seat and unseat[4] telescopically.*
  Use **telescopic** crown[5] / abutment / bridge[6] / anchoring [k] • (in)direct / tapered[7] [eɪ]/ square[8] **coping** • **coping** design / screw[9] / interface

abutment [ʌ] **(tooth)** *n term*
  natural tooth or implant providing anchorage[1] [æŋkɚɪdʒ] and support[2] for fixed or removable restorations
  » *A retainer is cemented to the abutments to provide retention for the prosthesis.*
  Use auxiliary [ɔːgzɪl-]/ intermediate / isolated[3] / splinted[4] / bridge / pier[5] [pɪɚ]/ terminal[6] [ɜː] **abutment** • **abutment** anchor[7] / connection / cylinder / head / screw[8] [uː]/ height [haɪt]/ length

overdenture *n term*   *syn* **bar joint** *or* **overlay denture** *n term*
  complete denture on soft tissue and natural teeth adapted and fitted with short or long copings, locking devices[1], or connecting bars[2] to optimize denture fit and retention
  » *We recommend 3-mm abutments to avoid excessive overdenture bulk[3] [ʌ].*
  Use implant-supported / interim / removable / bar-type[4] / clip-to-bar **overdenture** • **overdenture** placement / wearers / support / failure [faɪljɚ]/ abutment

tooth-borne [bɔːrn] *adj term*   *syn* **tooth-supported** *adj term*
  underlying structure or tissue bearing [eɚ] the occlusal load on the restoration
  implant-supported[1] *adj term* • tissue- *or* mucosa-borne[2] *adj*
  » *Then the tooth-borne segment of the prosthesis is removed from the preparation.*

set-up *n term*   *syn* **wax-up** [wæksʌp] *n term*   → U31-10
  arrangement of artificial teeth on a trial [traɪᵊl] denture base[1] or a wax base plate[1]
  » *The preliminary[2] set-up is tried in the mouth and adjusted for function and esthetic needs.*
  Use wax diagnostic[3] **setup**

occlusal (registration [redʒ-]**) rim** *n term*   *syn* **record rim** *n*,
                                                    rel **record base**[1] *n term*
  structure with occluding surfaces attached to permanent or temporary denture bases, used for recording[2] the relation of the maxilla to the mandible and for positioning the teeth
  » *Prosthetic teeth are placed on occlusion rims for a wax try-in appointment[3] with the patient.*
  Use to fabricate/adapt **the occlusal rim** • wax / posterior[4] **occlusal rim** • mandibular / wax-relined / well-fitting **record base**

Präzisionsverankerung, -geschiebe
verschraubt[1]
7

Freiendprothese
Freiendsattel[1] Bissen, Bolus[2] auskragendes Geschiebe / Verbindungsstück[3] Länge d. Freiendprothese[4]
8

Außen-, Sekundärkrone, Außenteleskop
Metallkappe, Innenkrone[1] Friktionshaftung[2] Interims-, provisorische Prothese[3] s. abnehmen lassen[4] Teleskopkrone[5] Teleskopbrücke[6] Konuskrone[7] parallelwandige Teleskopkrone[8] Teleskopschraube (kfo.)[9]
9

Pfeiler(zahn), Stützpfeiler, Anker
Verankerung[1] Abstützung[2] Einzelpfeiler[3] geschienter Pfeiler[4] Zwischenpfeiler[5] Endpfeiler[6] Stützanker[7] Distanzhülsenschraube (impl.)[8]
10

Deck-, Hybridprothese, Coverdenture
Verschlussmechanismen[1] Stege[2] Masse, Volumen[3] Deckprothese mit Steggeschiebe[4]
11

zahngestützt
implantatgestützt[1] schleimhautgetragen[2]
12

Wachsaufstellung
Basisplatte, individueller Abformlöffel[1] provisorisch[2] diagnostisches Set-up[3]
13

Bisswall
Bissschablone[1] Aufzeichnen[2] (Termin f.) Wachseinprobe[3] hinterer Bisswall[4]
14

try-in [traɪ ɪn] *n term*   *sim* **mock-up**[1] [mɒːkʌp] *n term*

checking the fit and esthetic appearance [ɪɚ] of a dental restoration or appliance [aɪ]

» At the try-in stage the esthetic result is more predictable and easily modified. We employ a *surgical template*[2] constructed from the original prosthetic *diagnostic try-in*[3]. *Mock-up for esthetic assessment*[4] proved helpful.

Use wax / framework[5] / final **try-in** • **try-in** procedure / appointment[6]

fit *n & v term*

(n) adaptation of inlays or dentures to the cavity preparation and denture seat [iː], respectively[1]

custom-fit[2] [ʌ] *adj term* • **press-fit**[3] *n* • *machined-fit adj*

» *Overload*[4] was due to poor interface fit between the prosthesis and the abutment. The patients found that their new dentures fit comfortably. The undercuts were adapted to allow *as snug* [ʌ] *a fit as possible*[5]. The clinical fit was satisfactory.

Use to ensure [ɪnʃʊɚ] exact **fit** • accurate / good / poor / acceptable **fit** • *tension-free*[6] / (im)proper / (non)passive / marginal[7] [dʒ] / framework[8] / friction(al)[9] [kʃ] **fit**

denture base [beɪs] *n term*

part of a complete or partial prosthesis resting on the basal seat

rebase[1] [eɪ] *v term* • baseplate[2] [eɪ] *n*

» *The role of the tongue* [tʌŋ] *is a key factor to be considered in denture base management.*

Use to fabricate/seat[3] **a base** • tooth-borne / mucosa-borne **base** • record[4] / trial [traɪəl] *or* temporary[5] / final / acrylic-resin[6] **base** • **denture base** contour / material • wax / titanium foil / preformed[7] / inert[8] [ɜː] / palatal **baseplate**

saddle *n term*   *rel* **rest area** *or* **seat**[1] [siːt] *n term*

part of a denture that rests on and covers the edentulous segment; the extensions on the abutment teeth are termed rests

» *A device*[2] [-aɪs] *that allows movement between the saddle and the retaining unit of a partial denture is termed a stress breaker*[3] [eɪ].

Use uni- or bilateral [aɪ] free-end[4] / unilateral bounded[5] [aʊ]/ anterior bounded **saddle** • occlusal / cingulum [sɪŋ-]/ lingual[6] **rest**

(denture) flange [flændʒ] *n term*

part of the denture base which extends from the dental cervix[1] [sɜːrvɪks] beyond the maximum bulbosity[2] [ʌ] of the ridge [rɪdʒ]

flanged *adj term*

» *The use of a labial flange on the overdenture helps provide adequate lip support. Dentures may be fully or partially flanged*[3] *or have no flange at all (e.g. open face crowns*[4]*).*

Use labial [eɪ]/ lingual / buccal [bʌkəl]/ removable / top **flange** • wax / denture / titanium / implant **flange** • **flange** angles [ŋg]/ design • **flanged** prosthesis / implant

anchorage [æŋkərɪdʒ] *n term*   *rel* **anchor**[1] [æŋkɚ] *n & v term*

tooth or implant which retains a fixed or removable restoration

anchoring *adj & n term* • (bone-)anchored[2] *adj*

» *Two abutments (retentive anchor*[3] *and bar abutment*[4]*) are suitable for overdentures*[5]*. Retention of the prosthesis is unsatisfactory when it cannot be anchored to residual dentition*[6]*.*

Use to provide / firm[7] / rigid [dʒ] / stable [eɪ] **anchorage** • bar[4] / screw-retained[8] / mechanical **anchorage** • retentive[3] **anchor** • **anchorage** *or* **anchoring** device / attachment[9] / band clasp[10] / screw / cap / crown / tooth[11]

An-, Einprobe

Anprobe z. ästhet. Diagnostik[1] chirurgische Schablone[2] diagnost. Wachseinprobe[3] ästhetische Diagnostik[4] Anprobe d. Prothesengerüsts[5] Einprobetermin[6]   15

Sitz, Passgenauigkeit; (an-, ein)passen, sitzen

bzw.[1] individuell angefertigt[2] Presspassung[3] Über(be)lastung[4] möglichst guten Sitz[5] spannungsfreier Sitz[6] Randschluss[7] Sitz d. Prothesengerüsts[8] Friktionspassung[9]   16

Prothesenbasis

(indirekt) unterfüttern[1] Basisplatte[2] Prothesenbasis einpassen[3] Bissschablone[4] Basisplatte, individueller Abformlöffel[5] Kunststoff-, Akrylatbasis[6] konfektionierte Basisplatte[7] biologisch inaktive Basisplatte[8]   17

Prothesensattel

Prothesenlager[1] Vorrichtung[2] Druckbrecher[3] beidseitig freiendender P.[4] einseitig begrenzter P.[5] linguale Auflage[6]

   18

(vestibulärer) Prothesenrand

Zahnhals[1] Wölbung[2] teilweise m. künstlichem Zahnfleisch versehen[3] Dreiviertelkronen[4]

   19

Verankerung, Halt

Anker; verankern[1] enossal verankert[2] Retentionszylinder, Knopfanker[3] Stegverankerung[4] Deckprothesen[5] Restgebiss[6] feste V.[7] verschraubte V.[8] Ankergeschiebe[9] Ankerbandklammer[10] Pfeiler-, Ankerzahn[11]

   20

154 DENTISTRY *Dental Implantology*

denture retention [rɪtenʃən] *n term*
fixation of a removable partial denture by the use of clasps, indirect retainers¹, or precision attachments
retain² [eɪ] *v term* • retaining *adj* • retainer³ *n* • retainerless *adj*
» This is an extracoronal slide [aɪ] attachment⁴ with a spring-activated⁵ universal joint hinge⁶ [dʒ] and adjustable retention. Long-lasting adequate retention and good serviceability are the key goals⁷ [oʊ] that should be achieved by any attachment system⁸.
Use magnet(ic) / mechanical / lingual screw / bar-and-clip / adhesive⁹ [iː]/ (in)adequate / frictional¹⁰ **retention** • lack / type / degree / loss **of retention** • **retention** base / point / device / aid / buffer [ʌ]/ groove¹¹ [uː]/ hole / clasp¹² / clip / bead¹³ [iː]

Prothesenhalt, -retention, -haftung
Sekundäranker¹ (fest)halten; erhalten² Halte-, Retentionselement³ extrakoronales Geschiebe⁴ aktivierbar⁵ Scharnier⁶ Hauptziele⁷ Ankersystem⁸ adhäsive Befestigung⁹ Friktionshaftung¹⁰ Retentionsrille¹¹ Retentionsklammer¹² Retentionsperle¹³

21

multiple-tooth splint *n term*
two or more teeth joined into a rigid [dʒ] unit¹ by means of restorations or appliances
splint² *n & v term* • splinting *n*
» The premolar and anterior teeth were splinted together with a fixed partial denture.
Use resin / acid etch cemented / anchor / cap³ / functional / interdental / wire⁴ **splint** • nonrigid / temporary⁵ **splint** • **splint** fixation / guard⁶

Zahn(verbindungs)schiene
starre / verblockte Einheit¹ Schiene, schienen, verblocken² Kappenschiene³ Draht(bogen)schiene⁴ temporäre Schiene⁵ Zahnschutz⁶

22

(dental) bar *n term*
metal segment for connecting parts of dentures
» The final overdenture may be secured¹ [sɪkjʊəd] with a bar clip², magnets, or snaps³.
Use connector / extension / parallel-sided⁴ / cantilevered / horseshoe-shaped⁵ **bar** • hand-carved⁶ / milled precision⁷ / preformed / Dolder⁸ **bar** • **bar** anchorage⁹ / splint / connector / joint¹⁰ / bridge / denture • **bar**-retained¹¹ /-borne¹¹ /-clip retention⁹ /-type superstructure

Steg
fixiert¹ Stegreiter² Retentionselemente³ parallelwandiger Steg⁴ hufeisenförm. Steg⁵ individuell gefräster Steg⁶ gefräster Präzisionssteg⁷ Dolder-Steg⁸ Stegverankerung⁹ Steggelenk¹⁰ steggestützt¹¹ 23

connector *n term*   *syn* **connecting** or **connective element** *n term*
part of a partial denture linking its components; lingual¹ and palatal bars² or plates are termed major [meɪdʒə] connectors³
» Clasps, indirect retainers, and occlusal rests⁴ linking the major connector or base of a partial denture to other units of the prosthesis are also called minor [aɪ] connectors⁵.
Use bar / female⁶ [iː]/ male⁷ [eɪ]/ major / intramobile / cantilever **connector** • **connecting** wire [waɪə]/ arm

Verbindungselement, Verbinder
(Sub)lingualbügel¹ Palatinal-, Gaumenbügel² große Verbinder³ Okklusalauflagen⁴ kleine Verbinder⁵ Matrize⁶ Patrize⁷

24

reline [*v* rɪlaɪn‖*n* rɪlaɪn] *v & n term*   *sim* **rebase**¹ [eɪ] *v & n term*
(v) to resurface² [ɜː] the tissue side of a prosthesis to achieve a more accurate fit
» Although rebasing is often used synonymously with relining, it refers to refitting dentures by replacing the base material³. Adjustment [ʌ] or reline was performed 1 month postoperatively. Two patients had the prosthesis rebased twice. Two millimeters of soft liner⁴ is sufficient to cushion⁵ [ʊ] the hard denture base.
Use wax / need for **relining** • **reline** jig⁶ [dʒɪg] • **rebase** treatment / material

direkt unterfüttern; direkte Unterfütterung
indirekt unterfüttern; indir. Unterfütterung¹ neu gestalten² Ersetzen d. Abformmasse³ Calciumhydroxid, Liner⁴ polstern⁵ Unterfütterungsgerät⁶

25

43

Unit 43   Dental Implantology
Related Units: **44** Oral Surgery, **45** Maxillofacial Surgery, **42** Prosthodontics, **21** Surgical Treatment, Plastic & Reconstructive Surgery

osseointegration *n term*
direct contact of bone to implant surface encouraging [ɜː] osteoconduction¹ [ʌ] and/or new bone formation (osteoinduction²) thus resulting in stable [eɪ] anchorage³ [æŋkərɪdʒ] of implants in the jaw [dʒɒː] bone
osseointegrate *v term* • osseointegrated *adj*
» Direct bone support of the implant body⁴ without encapsulation by connective tissue⁵ at the microscopic level is termed osseointegration, the basic concept in dental implantology.
Use **osseointegration** protocol⁶ / system / surgery • **osseointegrated** implant / surface • **fibro-osseous** integration

Osseointegration
Osteokonduktion, Einwachsen d. Knochens¹ Osteoinduktion, Knochenneubildung² stabile Verankerung³ Implantatkörper⁴ bindegewebige Einscheidung⁵ Osseointegrationstechnik⁶

1

Dental Implantology — DENTISTRY 155

dental implant *n term*   *syn* **fixture** [fɪkstʃɚ] *n jar,* ***screw-in tooth** [uː] *n*
  dental prosthesis [iː] the anchoring structure of which is surgically implanted underneath [iː] the mucosal or periosteal layer or in the jaw bone
  implant *v term* • **implantation** *n* • **implant-borne**[1] *adj* • **peri-implant** *adj*
  » Dental implants are indicated above all in edentulous [-tʃələs] patients unable to retain dentures, single anterior tooth replacement, post-cancer and trauma [ɒː] surgery.
  Use to insert[2]/load[3] **implants** • subperiosteal / osseointegrated / single-tooth[4] **implant** • ceramic [səræmɪk]/ HA-coated[5] / two-stage[6] / blade[7] [eɪ] **implant** • **implant denture**[8] [dentʃɚ]/ retention[9] / fixation[9] / material / shape[10]/ surface / healing[11] [iː]/ rehabilitation • standard / conical / self-tapping[12] **fixture** • **fixture mount**[13] / site / placement / stability / survival

Zahnimplantat, dentales Implantat, Fixtur
implantatgestützt, -getragen[1] Implantate einbringen[2] I. belasten[3] Einzelzahnimplantat[4] HA-beschichtetes I.[5] zweizeitig eingebrachtes I.[6] Blattimplantat[7] implantatgestützter Zahnersatz[8] Implantatverankerung[9] Implantatform[10] Implantateinheilung[11] selbstschneidende Fixtur[12] Einbringpfosten[13]   2

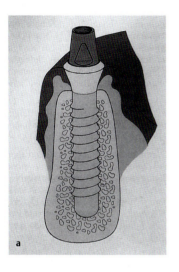
a

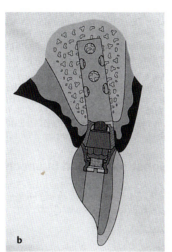
b

a screw-type implant
b two-part hollow-cylinder implant

preimplant(ation) [iː] *adj term*   *opposite* **postinsertion**[1] [-sɜːrʃən] *adj term*
  postimplantation[1] *adj term*
  » What are the effects of postimplantation drug therapy on bone ingrowth[2] into porous [pɔːrəs] implants[3]? At 8 weeks postimplantation, HA-coated implants showed calcifying deposits.
  Use **preimplant** consultation / diagnosis / procedures • **postinsertion** maintenance[4] / irradiation[5] / period / adjustment[6] [dʒʌ]/ followup[7]

Präimplantations-, vor der Implantation
nach (der) Implantation[1] Einwachsen d. Knochens[2] Implantat m. interkonnektierenden Poren[3] Implantatpflege[4] Bestrahlung nach Implantation[5] Korrekturmaßnahmen n. I.[6] Verlaufskontrolle n. I.[7]   3

endosseous [endɒːsɪəs] **(dental) implant** *n term*
  implant into alveolar bone; types of dental implants include endosseous, subperiosteal, and intramucosal fixtures[1]; among the endosseous implants the root form, blade or plate form, and the ramus frame can be distinguished
  » Increasing use of endosseous dental implants has changed the character of prosthetic surgery. An endosseous implant was inserted through the prepared root canal in order to increase effective root length.
  Use **endosseous implant** survival[2] / surface / system / placement[3] / mobility[4]

enossales Implantat
intramuköse Implantate[1] Haltbarkeit des enossalen I.[2] Implantatinsertion[3] Implantatmobilität[4]

   4

submerged [səbmɜːrdʒd] **implant** *n term*
   opposite **nonsubmerged implant**[1] *n term*
  in two-stage implant procedures[2] the submerged fixture is covered with a flap[3] for approx. 4 months, while in the 1-stage technique the implant is not submerged and a connecting bar[4] is fitted within 2 weeks
  » Exposure[5] [oʊʒ] of the submerged implant and placement of the transmucosal attachment[6] [ætʃ] was performed 4 months after implant insertion.

(ab)gedecktes Implantat
transmukosal einheilendes I.[1] zweizeitige /-phasige Implantation[2] (Schleimhaut)lappen[3] Verbindungssteg[4] Freilegung[5] Distanzhülse (z. transmukosalen Anbindung)[6]   5

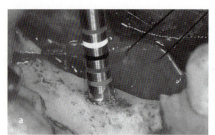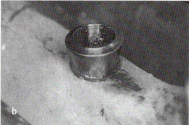

a Pretapping of the implant channel using a guide drill with a color-coded depth gauge
b Hollow-screw (HS) implant shortly after placement

screw(-type) [skruː] **implant** *n term*   *sim* **cylinder** [sɪl-] **implant**[1] *n term*
common type of implant with a round shaft which may be threaded[2] [θrɛdɪd] and hollow inside
» *The long-term success rate of two-stage endosseous screw and cylindrical implants was significantly higher and good implant-to-bone contact was achieved.*
Use implanted **screw** • cylindrical[1] / hollow-screw[3] / two-part hollow-cylinder[4] **implant** • **screw** fastening[5] [s]/ joint[6] / loosening[7] / fixation / design / breakage / failure / tap[8] / access [æksɛs] channel • healing / locking[9] / abutment[10] [ʌ]/ cover[11] **screw**

Schraubenimplantat
Zylinderimpl.[1] mit Gewinde versehen[2] Hohlschraubenimpl.[3] zweiteiliges Hohlzylinderimpl.[4] Anziehen der Schraube[5] Schraubengelenk[6] Schraubenlockerung[7] Gewindeschneider[8] Schluss-, Feststellschraube[9] Distanzhülsen-, Pfeilerschr.[10] Deckschraube[11]   6

host [hoʊst] **bed** *n term*   *syn* **implant bed** *n term*
» *Preparation of the implant bed must be performed with great care to avoid thermal [θɜːrmˀl] damage to the bony structures. Excessive bone-heating[1] was avoided by constant irrigation[2].*
Use congruent / reinnervated **host bed** • **implant bed** response[3] / preparation

Implantatbett
Erhitzen d. Knochens[1] Spülung[2] Reaktion d. Implantatbettes[3]

7

guide drill [gaɪd drɪl] *n term*   *syn* **pilot** [aɪ] **drill** *n term*
small sized drill used for preparing a pilot implant channel[1] in the alveolar bone under sterile irrigation
» *A guide drill was used to establish[2] the fixture site and evaluate cortical bone quality.*
Use **pilot** hole preparation[3] • surgical **guide** • **guide** stent[4] / template[5] [tɛmplɪt]

Führungs-, Vorbohrer
Führungs-, Pilotkanal[1] festlegen[2] Pilotbohrung[3] Führungsschiene[4] Führungs-, Bohrschablone[5]

8

axial congruency [kɒːŋgruˀnsi] *n term*   *sim* **axial parallelism**[1] *n term*
the implant bed must be prepared in proper alignment[2] [əlaɪn-] to provide proper seating[3] [iː] and relationships and avoid undesirable angulation[4] of the fixture
paralleling *adj term* • parallel to *adj*
» *For multiple implants the paralleling pin[5] is placed to obtain optimal axial congruency between implants, which are also aligned according to the adjacent [dʒeɪs] and opposing dentition[6].*
Use **axial** inclination[4] / loading[7] [oʊ]/ direction • **paralleling** guide[8] / technique[9] / pin[5]

axiale Kongruenz
Achsenparallelität[1] (Aus)richtung[2] Sitz, Halt[3] Achsenfehlstellung, -neigung[4] Parallelisierstift[5] Nachbar- u. Gegenzähne[6] axiale Belastung[7] Parallelführungshalter[8] Paralleltechnik[9]

9

depth [dɛpθ] **demarcation** *n term*
colored line markings on the drill, trephine [triːfaɪn] mill[1] and depth gauge[2] [geɪdʒ] which help determine[3] correct length
» *The osteotomies for the implants are completed at the desired angle [æŋgl], predetermined width[4] and to the demarcated depth[5]. The depth-limiting feature[6] prevented accidental intrusion of the implant into the cranium [eɪ].*
Use **depth** drill / gauge[2] / discrepancy / profile • **depth**-limiting bur[7] [bɜːr]/ feature[6] [fiːtʃɚ]

Tiefenmarkierung
Trepanfräser[1] Messlehre[2] bestimmen[3] festgelegter Durchmesser[4] markierte Bohrtiefe[5] Tiefenanschlag[6] Bohrer m. Tiefenanschlag[7]

10

Dental Implantology

tap [tæp] *n & v term* *syn* **thread** [θred] *n & v term*

(n) the process of threading or the resulting thread (v) to cut a thread into a drillhole[1] or a screw

self-tapping[2] *adj term* • pretapping *n & adj*

» Following preparation of the coronal aspect the implant channel is threaded with a thread-former[3] rotating at 50 rpm. Bottoming of the tap[4] must be prevented by all means. Implant instability may result from poor bone-tapping technique[5] or excessive countersinking[6].

Use **tapping** maneuver [uː]/ placement • full-depth / sequential[7] [-ʃəl] **tappings** • screw or threading[3] **tap** • channel[8] [tʃ] / hand **threading** • **thread** cutter[3] / profile / cleaner[9] / surface

Gewinde; G. schneiden
Bohrkanal[1] selbstschneidend[2] Gewindeschneider[3] Bodenkontakt im Bohrkanal[4] Knochenfrästechnik[5] Versenken[6] stufenweises Gewindeschneiden[7] Gewindeschneiden[8] Gewindereiniger[9]

11

insertion torque [tɔːrk] *n term* *opposite* **removal torque**[1] *n term*

force exerted on the bone bed when placing[2] and tightening[3] [taɪt-] a screw implant

» Abutments[4] [ʌ] were attached to the implants and tightened with an electric torque wrench[5] [rentʃ].

Use gentle [dʒ]/ forced / high / total / recommended tightening / undue[6] [duː]/ input[7] **torque** • **torque** wrench or driver[5] / force / gauge [geɪdʒ] / manometer / controller • **counter torque** device or driver[8]

Einbringungsdrehmoment
Entfernungsdrehmoment[1] Einbringen[2] Anziehen[3] Distanzhülsen[4] Drehmomentschlüssel[5] übermäßiges Drehmoment[6] Einbringungsdrehmoment[7] Drehmomentsperre, Gegenhalter[8]

12

healing [hiːlɪŋ] **cap** *n term* *sim* **healing abutment**[1] *n term*

implant covering placed in the postinsertion healing period[2] to promote proper tissue adaptation at the junction[3] [dʒʌŋkʃən] between the implant and the abutment in the gingiva [dʒɪndʒɪvə]

» Healing caps are placed on the abutment cylinders [sɪ] to support the tissue cuff[4] and prevent it from collapsing between postimplant appointments[5].

Use to place[6]/remove/replace **healing caps** • temporary / polymer / plastic **healing cap** • **healing** screw[7]

Heilungskäppchen, Abdeckkappe
Heilungsdistanzhülse[1] Einheilungsphase[2] Übergang[3] Gewebsmanschette[4] Kontrolltermine[5] Heilungskäppchen aufbringen[6] Abdeckschraube[7]

13

load [loʊd] *n & v term* *syn* **loading** *n term*

the force exerted on a tooth, e.g. occlusal[1], tensile[2], static, or stress loads[3]

preload[4] [iː] *n & v term* • load-bearing[5] [eə·] *adj & n* • non-loaded[6] *adj*

» Premature implant loading[7] can contribute to implant failure. Preload[4] is the force within the screw implant developed by the torque applied.

Use to apply/place/accept/withstand[8] **a load** • under[9] **load** • axial / functional / horizontal [zɒ] / vertical **load** • **load** sharing[10] / distribution[11] / capacity[12] / transfer

Belastung; belasten
Kaubelastung[1] Zugbel.[2] Druckbel.[3] Vorbelastung; vorbelasten[4] tragend; Tragkraft[5] nicht belastet[6] vorzeitige Implantatbelastung[7] einer Belastung standhalten[8] bei Belastung[9] Lastaufteilung[10] Lastverteilung[11] Belastbarkeit[12]

14

superstructure *n term* *sim* **framework**[1] [eɪ] *n term*

prosthesis [θiː] supported and retained by the implant denture substructure (metal framework, cylinder- or blade-type implant) beneath [iː] the soft tissues in contact with or embedded[2] into bone

» The superstructure is screwed on the abutments and checked for proper passive fit[3] to exclude permanent stress on the implants.

Use prosthetic [e]/ removable / cantilevered[4] [iː]/ stress-absorbing[5] **superstructure** • **superstructure** framework • implant **framework**

Suprakonstruktion, -struktur
Gerüst, Konstruktion[1] eingebettet[2] Sitz[3] freiendigende S.[4] druckabsorbierende S.[5]

15

superstructure-to-implant ratio [reɪʃ(ɪ)oʊ] *n term* *abbr* **S/I ratio** *n term*

similar to the root-to-crown ratio[1] in natural teeth; the denture-bearing area must be proportional to the prosthetic superstructure

» The S/I ratio is a valuable[2] prognostic factor if there are concerns[3] about progressive overload[4], above all in the case of ailing [eɪlɪŋ] implants[5].

Krone-zu-Implantat Quotient
Wurzel-zu-Krone Quotient[1] wertvoll, wichtig[2] Bedenken, Probleme[3] zunehmende Überbelastung[4] instabile Implantate[5]

16

biocompatibility *n term* *rel* **bioinert**[1] [baɪoʊɪnɜːrt], **bioactive**[2] *adj term*

the quality of materials (e.g. implants) of having no toxic or harmful[3] effects on the body
biocompatible[4] *adj term*

» The finding of osteocytes [saɪ] close to the implants indicates good tissue acceptance and excellent biocompatibility. The new HA material seems to be biocompatible within bone.

Use **biocompatible** materials[5] • **bioactive** coating[6] [oʊ]/ surface

Biokompatibilität
bioinert[1] bio(re)aktiv[2] schädlich[3] biokompatibel[4] Biomaterialien[5] bioaktive Beschichtung[6]

17

43

tarnish [tɑːrnɪʃ] *n & vi term*

(n) surface discoloration[1] on an implant, usually the result of oxidation

» A 3-ppm[2] solution of NaF is capable [eɪ] of tarnishing the surface of CP[3] titanium [taɪteɪniəm] implants.

Verfärbung; (sich) verfärben, anlaufen
Oberflächenverfärbung[1] parts per million[2] commercially pure[3] 18

---

pitting *or* **fretting corrosion** [-oʊʒ°n] *n term*

corrode[1] *v term* • corrosive[2] *adj* • corroding[2] *adj*

» Fluoride [flʊɚaɪd] causes fretting corrosion on titanium surfaces. Contact with gold may initiate[3] [ɪʃ] pitting corrosion in some Co-Cr alloys[4], but this phenomenon is seldom seen in vivo [iː].

Use to initiate[3] /lead to/cause/prevent **pitting corrosion** • **corrosion** resistance[5] / behavior[6] [eɪ]/ rate[7] / products • galvanic / surface / resistance to[5] **corrosion** • **corrosive** effect / medium [iː]/ layer • **corroding** solution / medium

Lochfraß
korrodieren[1] korrosiv[2] L. auslösen, zu L. führen[3] Kobalt-Chromlegierungen[4] Korrosionsfestigkeit[5] Korrosionsverhalten[6] Korrosionsgeschwindigkeit[7]

19

Unit 44 Oral Surgery
Related Units: 45 Maxillofacial Surgery, 43 Dental Implantology, 38 TMJ Disorders, 41 Endodontics, 35 Periodontics, 21 Surgical Treatment, Plastic & Reconstructive Surgery

---

oral surgeon [sɜːrdʒ°n] *n term*

dental surgeon[1] specialized in complicated extractions[2], dentoalveolar [ɪə] and preprosthetic [θe] surgery[3], etc.

» Jaw shape and bone quality were determined on a routine basis by the oral surgeon.

Use oral and maxillofacial[4] / reconstructive **surgeon** • minor / major **oral surgery** • Doctor of Dental **Surgery** (*abbr* D.D.S.)[5]

Oralchirurg(in)
Zahnarzt /-ärztin[1] erschwerte Extraktionen[2] präprothetische Chirurgie[3] Mund-Kiefer-Gesichtschirurg(in), MKG-Chirurg(in)[4] Dr. med. dent.[5]

1

---

tooth [tuːθ] **extraction** *n term*   *rel* **tooth exposure**[1] [oʊʒ], **luxation**[2] *n term*

luxation [ʌ] and removal of a tooth from its alveolus [ɪə] by application of force

extract[3] *v term* • non-extraction[4] *n* • pre-/postextraction *adj* • extracting *adj* • luxate[5] *v* • take out *v phr clin*

» Small elevators[6] were used to carefully luxate the teeth to be extracted. Extraction of malpositioned[7] teeth may require a transalveolar approach[8]. Surgical extractions involve tooth sectioning[9] [kʃ], mucoperiosteal flap reflection[10] or bone removal prior to[11] the use of elevators.

Use dental / simple / atraumatic / complicated *or* surgical / third molar **extraction** • full bony / soft tissue / serial[12] [ɪə]/ balancing *or* compensating[13] **extraction** • **extraction** socket[14] / site[aɪ]/ space[15] / forceps[16] [s]/ under antibiotic coverage[17] [ʌ] • mesial [iː]/ distal / intrusive[18] / extrusive / (in)complete **luxation** • **luxated** teeth[19] • **to take out** a tooth[20]

Zahnextraktion
Freilegung eines Zahnes[1] Zahnluxation, -lockerung[2] extrahieren, entfernen[3] Nichtextrakionsbehandlung[4] luxieren, heraushebeln[5] Hebel[6] in Fehlstellung[7] Zugang[8] Hemisektion[9] Aufklappung[10] vor[11] Reihen-, Serienextraktion[12] Ausgleichsextraktion[13] Extraktionshöhle[14] Extraktionslücke[15] Extraktionszange[16] E. m. antibiot. Abschirmung[17] Zahnintrusion[18] lose / ausgeschlagene Zähne[19] Zahn ziehen[20]

2

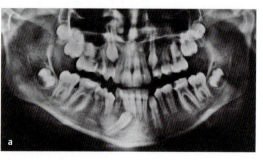

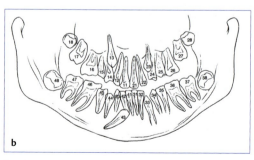

Impacted mandibular canine: **a** x-ray view **b** schematic drawing

Oral Surgery   DENTISTRY 159

impacted tooth *n term*   *opposite* **avulsed** [ʌ] **tooth**[1] *n term*

(i) tooth whose normal eruption is prevented by adjacent [dʒeɪs] teeth or bone (ii) tooth driven into the alveolar process or surrounding tissue as a result of trauma

(re)impaction[2] *n term* • impact[3] *n & v* • avulsion[4] *n*

» The left canine was submerged[5] [dʒ] and impacted in bone. Partially avulsed[6] teeth should be repositioned and stabilized [eɪ].

Use horizontal / vertical / distal / food[7] impaction • impacted third molar / canine[8] [keɪnaɪn]/ fracture / foreign body • **avulsion** socket / site • **avulsed** fragment • completely **avulsed** • chip [tʃ] fracture[9] / traumatic **avulsion** • **impact** area / load / force

impaktierter / retinierter Zahn
luxierter / ausgeschlagener Z.[1] (Re)impaktion, Reinklusion[2] Aufprall, Stoß, Auswirkung; einkeilen, beeinflussen[3] Luxation[4] versenkt[5] inkomplett luxiert[6] Impaktion v. Speiseresten[7] impaktierter Eckzahn[8] Abrissfraktur[9]   3

extraction-replantation *n term*   *syn* **re(im)plantation, intentional replantation, tooth repositioning** *n term*

elective extraction and prompt reinsertion [ɜː] of a tooth into the alveolus, e.g for retrograde filling[1]

» In adolescents[2] [es], implantation should only be considered[3] if orthodontic gap closure[4] [ʒ] or replantation is not possible.

Extraktion-Re(im)plantation
retrograde Wurzelfüllung[1] bei Jugendlichen[2] in Betracht ziehen[3] kieferorthopäd. Lückenschluss[4]   4

mucoperiosteal [mjuːkoʊperɪˈɒstɪəl] **flap** *n term*   → U50-17

flap from the hard palate[1] [pælət] or gingiva [dʒ] composed of mucosa and periosteum

» Incising the periosteum could have a negative influence on mucoperiosteal flap healing. The subperiosteal cortical layer [eɪ] was deprived [aɪ] of[2] its vascular supply[3] when the mucoperiosteal flap was elevated.

Use to raise [eɪ] or elevate[4]/mobilize/rotate/transpose/trim[5]/reflect[6] *a flap* • mucosal / gingival[7] / (buccal [ʌ]) advancement[8] / (palatal) rotation / buccal fat pad[9] *flap* • curved or semilunar / broad-based / lingual-pedicle[10] *flap* • *flap* closure / coverage[11] [ʌ]/ operation[12] / recession [se]/ sloughing[13] [slʌf-]

Mukoperiostlappen
harter Gaumen[1] abgeschnitten von[2] Blutversorgung[3] Lappen abheben / lösen[4] L. kürzen[5] L. zurückklappen[6] Zahnfleischlappen[7] Verschiebel.[8] Wangenfettl.[9] gestielter Zungenlappen[10] Lappendeckung[11] Lappenoperation, -plastik[12] Lappenabstoßung[13]   5

alveolar [ɪə] **(ridge** [rɪdʒ]**) atrophy** [æ] *or* **resorption** *n term*
rel **sulcus** [sʌlkˤs] **deepening**[1] *n term*

deterioration or loss of bone tissue in the jaws usually accompanied by gum thinning and recession [se]

atrophy[2] [ætrəfi] *v term* • atrophic [eɪtrɒfɪk] *adj*

» The patient presented with a severely atrophic mandible and was unable to wear [weə] a conventional removable denture [tʃə].

Use mandibular / maxillary / (jaw) bone / disuse[3] / senile[4] **atrophy** • **atrophic** edentulous jaw[5] (areas) / residual (alveolar) ridges[6] • extremely **atrophied** maxilla

Alveolarkammabbau, -atrophie
Sulkusvertiefung[1] atrophieren[2] Inaktivitätsatrophie[3] Altersatrophie[4] atrophierter zahnloser Kiefer[5] atrophische Alveolarkammreste[6]   6

vestibuloplasty *n term*   *rel* **frenectomy**[1] *n term*

surgical procedures to restore[2] alveolar ridge height[3] [haɪt] by lowering muscles attaching to[4] the buccal, labial, and lingual aspects of the jaws (epithelial inlay procedure[5])

» The patient underwent debulking [ʌ] of the flap[6] with vestibuloplasty and lowering of the floor of the mouth[7]. Frenectomy was performed for closure of a median diastema [daɪəstiːmə] in a tongue-tied[8] patient.

Use combined lingual[9] / mandibular / lipswitch[10] [tʃ]/ skin graft **vestibuloplasty** • preprosthetic **frenectomy**

Mundvorhof-, Vestibulumplastik
Zungenbändchenexzision, -plastik, Fren(ul)ektomie[1] wiederherstellen[2] Alveolarkammhöhe[3] ansetzen an[4] (freies) Schleimhauttransplantat, FST[5] Lappenverkleinerung[6] Mundboden[7] mit mangelnder Zungenbeweglichkeit[8] kombinierte Lippen- u. Mundvorhofplastik[9] Transposition v. Lippenrot[10]   7

alveolar ridge augmentation [ɒːgmənt-] *n term* → U49-19

alveoloplasty increasing the alveolar bone in size or volume by means of bone grafting

augment[1] *v term* • (graft)-augmented *adj*

» Implant cavity borings[2] were used for peri-implant augmentation and defect filling. The sites were augmented with PTFE barrier membranes[3].

Use sinus[4] [aɪ]/ membrane / visor [aɪ]-sandwich osteotomy[5] / guided [aɪ] bone-graft[6] (*abbr* GBGA) **augmentation** • **augmentation** material / surgery[7] / procedure[7] [-siːdʒə]/ grafting • **augmented** site / ridge / mandible

Alveolarkammaufbau, Kieferkammplastik
aufbauen, vergrößern[1] Bohrspäne[2] PTFE-Membranen[3] Sinusboden-Augmentation[4] Visierosteotomie m. Sandwichplastik[5] Augmentationsplastik m. gesteuerter Geweberegeneration[6] Augmentationsplastik[7]   8

44

160 DENTISTRY — Oral Surgery

bone grafting n term → U50-9   syn **osteoplasty** n term

bone is harvested[1] mostly from extraoral sites and grafted to the jaw for maxillary or mandibular augmentation of the resorbed alveolar ridge (inadequate height or width)

graft[2] v & n term • (post)grafting adj • grafter[3] n

» Surgical closure of the alveolar defect was performed with a bone graft and soft tissue advancement[4].

Use to harvest[5]/collect[5]/acquire[5] [əkwaɪɚ]/cut **grafting material** • block / interpositional[6] / particulate[7] **bone graft** • intraoral / extraoral / autogenous[8] [ɔːdʒ]/ corticocancellous / composite / fresh / freeze-dried[9] / delayed[10] [eɪ] **graft** • **graft** procurement[11] [kjʊɚ]/ consolidation / substitute • early **postgrafting** stage

Knochentransplantation, Osteoplastik
entnommen[1] transplantieren; Transplantat[2] Osteo-, Muko-, Dermatom[3] Weichgewebeverlagerung[4] Gewebe f. Transpl. entnehmen[5] Interpositionsknochentransplantat[6] Spanplastik, -transplantat[7] Autotransplantat[8] gefriergetrocknetes T.[9] verzögertes / mehrzeitiges T.[10] Transplantatbeschaffung[11]   9

particulate graft n term   opposite **block (bone) graft**[1] n term

cortical chips[2] and cancellous marrow shavings[3] [eɪ] are grafted to form an osteoid [ɪ] matrix[4] [eɪ]; used mainly for onlay[5], inlay[6] and interpositional grafts

particulate[7] adj & n term

» The harvested particulate graft material combines with blood to form an osseous coagulum. Differences were related to whether particulate or blocks had been used for augmentation.

Use buccal [bʌkəl] onlay / sinus-inlay **particulate graft** • **onlay** block grafting • **block**-shaped graft • combination onlay-inlay **block graft** • **particulate** bone (abbr PB)/ graft • (non)porous / metal **particulate**

Spantransplantat
Blocktransplantat[1] kortikale Knochenchips[2] Spongiosaspäne[3] knochenähnliche Gewebestruktur[4] Auflagerungs(osteo)plastik[5] Einlagerungs(osteo)plastik[6] span-; teilchenförmig; Span, Partikel[7]   10

demineralized bone matrix [eɪ] or **mix** n term, abbr **DBM**
                        sim **freeze-dried bone allograft**[1] n term, abbr **FDBA**

bone shavings[2] rich in bone morphogenic [dʒe] protein (abbr BMP) available from bone banks[3] (animal or cadaver donors[4]) which can be packed into osseous defects, around implant sites, or for augmentation procedures

» DBM acts as a scaffold[5] for bone ingrowth and promotes osseoinduction[6]. The space between the extraction socket wall and the implant was grafted with demineralized freeze-dried bone.

Use **demineralized bone** powder[7] / particles / allograft • demineralized **freeze-dried bone** allograft, abbr DFDBA

demineralisierte Knochenmatrix
gefriergetrocknetes allogenes Knochentransplantat[1] Knochenspäne[2] Knochenbanken[3] Leichenspender[4] Gerüst[5] Osteoinduktion[6] demineralisierte(s) Knochenpartikel, -mehl[7]   11

guided bone regeneration [rɪdʒen-] n term   abbr **GBR** → U35-28f

application of the principles of GTR[1] to promote[2] bone regeneration in localized bony defects

» Membrane-guided bone regeneration will potentially alter[3] the surgical technique in patients in whom implant placement[4] is performed immediately following dental extraction.

gesteuerte / membrangestützte (Knochen)regeneration
gesteuerte Geweberegeneration[1] fördern[2] verändern[3] Implantatinsertion, -einbringung[4]   12

subperiosteal tunneling [ʌ] (technique) n term
                        syn **tunnel dissection** n term

the periosteum is lifted from the underlying bone in a tunnel fashion in preparation for an onlay type graft

» The incision was extended[1] to provide access[2] [ækses] for a subperiosteal tunnel for graft insertion. For this patient it was decided to perform the osteotomy via a vertical incision using a minor [aɪ] apically [eɪ] situated buccal subperiosteal tunnel.

Use to create [krieɪt] a **tunnel**

subperiostale Tunnelmethode
erweitert[1] Zugang[2]   13

oroantral fistulation n term   rel **oroantral fenestration**[1] n term

pathological epithelium-lined[2] [θiː] tract between the mouth and the maxillary sinus (usually following extraction)

» Postextraction reflux [iː] of fluids into the nose may be a sign of oroantral fistulation. Some oroantral fistulae [iː] close spontaneously, others require sutures or placement of buccal advancement grafts.

Use **fistula** formation • oronasal / gingival **fistula** • buccolingual / bony / soft tissue / apical[3] [eɪ] **fenestration** • **fenestration** (bone) defect / repair

Antrum-, Kieferhöhlenfistelbildung
oroantrale Perforation[1] epithelial ausgekleidet[2] Wurzelspitzenfensterung, apikale Fensterung[3]   14

44

dentigerous [dentɪdʒ-] **cyst** [sɪst] n term   sim **follicular cyst**[1] n,
   rel **keratocyst**[2], **mucocele**[3] [mjʊkəsiːl], **ranula**[4] n term

cyst arising from reduced enamel epithelium surrounding the crown of an unerupted permanent tooth

» Dentigerous cysts may delay eruption [ɪrʌpʃən] and require marsupialization[5] or enucleation[6].

Use eruption / periapical or radicular[7] / gingival / retention[8] / residual[9] / solitary bone cyst • cystic mass / carcinoma

Dentitions-, Eruptionszyste
follikuläre Zyste, Zahnkeimzyste[1] Keratozyste[2] Mukoidzyste, Mukozele[3] Mundbodenzyste, Ranula[4] Marsupialisation[5] Ausschälung, Enukleation[6] radikuläre Z.[7] Retentionszyste[8] Residual-, Restzyste[9]   15

---

mandibular torus [tɔːrəs] pl **-i** n term   sim **palatine** [pælətaɪn] **torus**[1] n term

benign [bɪnaɪn] overgrowth[2] of bone (ex- or hyperostosis[3]) protruding from the lingual aspect of the mandible

» The tissue covering a torus is thin and easily traumatized [ɒː] by foods. Clinically, torus palatinus may interfere [ɪɚ] with[4] the proper fitting of dentures and require surgical removal. Tori [aɪ] can be reduced[5] under a local flap or removed with a chisel[6] [tʃ], but with a palatal torus[1] this can be risky.

Unterkieferwulst, Torus mandibularis
Gaumenwulst, T. palatinus[1] Wucherung[2] Hyperostose, Überschussbildg. v. Knochengewebe[3] beeinträchtigen[4] abgetragen[5] Meißel[6]   16

Unit 45   Maxillofacial Surgery
Related Units: 44 Oral Surgery, 43 Dental Implantology, 21 Surgical Treatment, Plastic & Reconstructive Surgery

maxillofacial [-feɪʃəl] **fractures** [fræktʃɚz] n term → U17-1 ff

include mandibular[1] (most common), midface[2], malar[3] [eɪ] and nasal fractures

» Facial fractures may give rise to dural tears[4] [teɚz] and lead to CSF leak[5] [iː]. Le Fort I may occur [ɜː] singly or be associated with other facial fractures. Infraorbital nerve paresthesia [-θiːʒ(ɪ)ə] and step deformity of the orbital rim[6] are frequently seen in these maxillofacial fractures.

Use mid(-)face / Le Fort I (horizontal)[7], II (pyramidal), III / nasal (bone) / mandibular / maxillary / orbital floor[8] **fracture** • **fractured** tooth / root [uː]/ crown / jaw [dʒɔː]/ mandible • mandibular left[9] / intracapsular[10] **condylar fracture**

Kiefer- u. Gesichtsfrakturen
Unterkieferfraktur[1] Mittelgesichtsfr.[2] Jochbeinfraktur[3] Ruptur d. Dura[4] Liquoraustritt[5] Orbitarand[6] Guérin-/Le Fort I Fraktur[7] Blow-out Fraktur[8] linke UK-Kollumfraktur[9] intrakapsuläre Kollumfraktur[10]

1

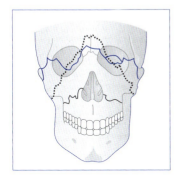

Mid-face fractures:
Le Fort I (black line), Le Fort II (dotted line), Le Fort III (blue line)

---

facial cleft n term   syn **clefting syndrome** [sɪndroʊm] n term

fissure [ʃ] or gap resulting from incomplete merging[1] [mɜːrdʒɪŋ] or fusion of embryonic processes normally uniting in the formation of the face, e.g., cleft lip (popularly known as harelip[2] [heɚlɪp]) or cleft palate

» Palato-labial [eɪ] clefts may vary from involvement[3] of only the soft or hard palate to a complete cleft of both palates, the alveolar process of the maxilla, and the lip.

Use congenital [dʒe] **cleft** palate[4] • **cleft** nose[5] / tongue[6] [tʌŋ]/ lip[7] / deformity[8] / formation / area • (unilateral) maxillary / alveolar [ɪə]/ gingival[9] [dʒ] **cleft** • (naso)maxillary / oblique [iːk] facial[10] / midline / (cranio)facial[11] / paramedian **cleft** • bilateral **clefting**

Gesichtsspalte, Prosoposchisis
Verschmelzung[1] Hasenscharte[2] Beteiligung[3] angeborene Gaumenspalte, Palatoschisis[4] Spaltnase, Nasenspalte[5] Spaltzunge, Glossoschisis[6] Lippenspalte, Cheiloschisis[7] Spaltmissbildung[8] Gingivaspalte[9] schräge Gesichtsspalte[10] mediane G.[11]

2

Maxillofacial Surgery

cleft (palate) surgery n term   sim palatoplasty n term

palatoplasty[1] plus pharyngoplasty [fərɪŋgoʊ-] to narrow the velopharyngeal [iː] opening[2]

» Surgical repair of the congenital cleft palate aims at preservation[3] of swallowing[4] [ɒː], normal dental occlusion, hearing, separation of the oral and nasal cavities and speech improvement.

(Gaumen)spaltchirurgie, -plastik
Gaumen-, Palatoplastik[1] velopharyngeale Öffnung[2] Erhaltung[3] Schluckfunktion[4]   3

craniofacial [eɪ] deformity n term   sim craniostenosis or -synostosis[1] n term

malformation that may be acquired (tumors, trauma [ɒː]) or congenital (bifid nose, microsomia, microtia[2] [maɪkroʊʃ'ə], microstomia, etc.)

» Skull deformities such as oxycephaly[3] [-sefəli], plagiocephaly[4] [pleɪdʒioʊ-], scaphocephaly[5] [skæfoʊ-] or trigonocephaly may result from premature[6] closure [ʒ] of the cranial sutures[7] [suːtʃɚz].

Use facial / condylar / unilateral / cleft lip-palate **deformity** • coronal **synostosis** • hemifacial[8] **mirosomia**

kraniofaziale Fehlbildung / Dysmorphie
Kraniosynostose, Stenozephalie[1] Mikrotie, angeborene Kleinheit d. Ohrmuschel(n)[2] Spitz-, Turmschädel, Oxyzephalie[3] Schiefschädel, Plagiozephalus[4] Kahnschädel, Skaphozephalus[5] vorzeitig[6] Schädelnähte[7] Mikrosomie / Minderwuchs einer Gesichtshälfte[8]   4

hypertelor(bit)ism [e] n term, abbr HTO   opposite hypotelorism[1] n term

abnormally increased interorbital distance[2] (abbr IOD), also termed telorbitism[3]

» It is possible to correct hypertelorbitism by moving the entire orbit after a paramedian bone resection. Hypotelorism without mental deficiency[4] [ɪʃ] is rare.

Use orbital or ocular[3] / canthal[4] [kænθ°l] **hypertelorism** • hypertelorism procedure

(okulärer) Hypertelorismus
Hypotelorismus[1] interorbitaler Abstand[2] (okulärer) Hypertelorismus[3] Intelligenzminderung[4] Telekanthus[5]   5

mandibulofacial dysostosis n term, abbr MFD   sim Treacher-Collins [iːtʃ] syndrome[1] [ɪ] n term, abbr TCS

syndrome of defective ossification characterized by palpebral [iː] coloboma[2] or notches[3] in the outer third of the lower lids, bony defects or hypoplasia [-pleɪʒ(ɪ)ə] of malar bones and zygoma [zaɪ], hypoplasia of the mandible, low-set external ears[4], atypical hair growth, macrostomia with high or cleft palate[5] and malocclusion of teeth[6]

» Treacher syndrome is an incomplete form of mandibulofacial dysostosis; in Franceschetti's syndrome[7] the same anomalies are seen in a more pronounced [aʊ] form[8].

Use **mandibulofacial dysostosis** syndrome • cranial [eɪ]/ craniofacial[9] / skeletal / metaphyseal / cleidocranial[10] [aɪ] **dysostosis**

Dysostosis mandibulofacialis
Treacher-Collins-Syndrom[1] Lidkolobom[2] Kerben, Defekte[3] tiefer Ohrmuschelansatz[4] hoher Gaumen[5] Dsygnathie[6] Franceschetti-Syndrom[7] in ausgeprägterer Form[8] Crouzon-Syndrom, kraniofaziale Dysostose[9] D. cleidocranialis, Scheuthauer-Marie-Sainton-Syndrom[10]   6

Le Fort I [ləfɔːrtwʌn] (maxillary) osteotomy n term

transverse mobilization of the lower maxilla for elevation, retrusion [uːʒ], advancement[1] or lowering of the midface in congenital, developmental[2] and posttraumatic problems osteotome[3] n term • osteotomize [-aɪz] v • osteotomized adj

» For the Le Fort I osteotomy, vestibular incision [sɪ] and reflection of the mucoperiosteal flap are followed by horizontal osteotomy, down-fracture[4] and mobilization of the maxilla.

Use subapical [eɪ]/ malar / visor-sandwich[5] [aɪ]/ posterior maxillary / Le Fort II / Le Fort III **osteotomy** • self-retained Le Fort I (abbr SRLF I) / Le Fort I ex-[6]/intrusion[7] **osteotomy** • **osteotomy** window / line • sharp / curved **osteotome**

Le Fort I Osteotomie
Vorverlagerung[1] entwicklungsbedingt[2] Osteotom, Knochenmeißel[3] "down-fracture" Technik[4] Visier-Osteotomie m. Sandwich-Plastik[5] Le Fort Verlängerungsosteotomie[6] Le Fort Verkürzungsosteotomie[7]   7

facial advancement [æ] surgery n term

release[1] [iː] of facial stenoses, mobilization and remodeling to correct malformations[2]

» In infants with Crouzon's disease suture disjunction[3] [dʒʌ] may be more important than facial advancement. In three cases only inadequate facial advancement could be achieved[4].

Use monobloc frontofacial[5] / midface or midfacial[6] / zygomatic [zaɪgoʊ-]/ forehead / frontoorbital / rotational[7] **advancement**

operative Gesichtsvorverlagerung
Beseitigung[1] Missbildungen[2] Nahtöffnung[3] erreicht[4] frontofaziales Monobloc-Advancement[5] Mittelgesichtsvorverlagerung[6] Mesialverlagerung durch Rotation[7]   8

Maxillofacial Surgery

orthognathic [ɔːrθoʊgnæθɪk] **surgery** *n term*
         syn **corrective jaw** [dʒɔː] **surgery, surgical orthodontics** *n term*
  correction of jaw malposition and the associated occlusal abnormalities by bodily repositioning of the entire mandible or maxilla or segments containing one or more teeth
  gnathic [næθɪk] *adj* • gnathologic[1] [n] *adj term* • -gnathia *comb* • gnath(o) - *comb*
» *Orthognathic surgery was delayed until after puberty to exclude interference[2] [ɪɚ] of adolescent [es] growth and reestablishment[3] of the adverse[4] pattern.*
Use to receive **orthognathic surgery** • **orthognathic** surgical technique / correction / patient • **gnathic** index[5] • **gnath**ology /graphic /dynamometer[6]

chirurgische Kieferorthopädie
gnathologisch[1] Beeinträchtigung[2] Wiederauftreten[3] ungünstig[4] Kieferindex[5] Gnathodynamometer[6]

9

prognathism [prɒgnæθɪzᵊm] *n term*   *opposite* **retrognathism**[1] [næθ] *n term*
  abnormal forward projection [dʒe] of one or both jaws beyond[2] [bɪjɒːnd] the established normal relationship with the cranial base, although the mandibular condyles [-aɪlz] are in their normal rest relationship to the TMJ[3]
  prognathic[4] *adj term* • retrognathic[5] *adj*
» *The patient appeared prognathic when speaking. Maxillary retrognathism is less prominent.*
Use **prognathic** jaw relationships / profile / occlusion • mandibular or true[6] / maxillary[7] / relative / severe / extreme **prognathism** • **retrognathic** patient / ridge [dʒ] relation

Prognathie, Progenie
Retrognathie[1] über ... hinaus[2] Kiefergelenk[3] prognath(isch)[4] retrognath(isch)[5] echte Progenie, mandibuläre Prognathie[6] maxilläre Prognathie[7]

10

segmental (alveolar) osteotomy *n term*   *syn* **visor** [vaɪzɚ] **osteotomy** *n term*
  tooth-bearing [eɚ] segments of alveolar [ɪə] bone are sectioned between and apical [eɪ] to the teeth for repositioning of individual teeth; may be combined with ostectomy[1]
» *A patient who lost the premaxilla following segmental osteotomy was successfully rehabilitated by the placement of autogenous [ɒːdʒ] bone grafts and osseointegrated implants. Orthognathic procedures include the visor or alveolar osteotomy. The malaligned [-əlaɪnd] osseointegrated implant was corrected by segmental osteotomy.*
Use mandibular (subapical) [eɪ]/ maxillary / interdental / horizontal / midline / (mandibular) body[2] / inverted L[3] / C-shaped **osteotomy** • **osteotomy** site / segment

Visier-, Segmentosteotomie
Knochenresektion, Ostektomie[1] Osteotomie des Corpus mandibulae[2] umgekehrte L-Osteotomie[3]

11

sagittal [sædʒɪtᵊl] **split osteotomy** *n term*
  transection[1] of the mandibular rami[2] [reɪmaɪ] and posterior body in the sagittal plane [eɪ] for correction of retrognathism, prognathism, and apertognathia[3]
» *For sagittal split osteotomy both an intraoral as well as an extraoral approach[4] can be used.*

sagittale Osteotomie, Unterkieferosteotomie nach Obwegeser/Dal Pont
Durchtrennung[1] aufsteigende Unterkieferäste[2] offener Biss[3] Zugang(sweg)[4]

12

sliding [aɪ] **oblique** [-liːk] **osteotomy** *n term*   *syn* **vertical osteotomy** *n term*
  extra- or intraoral vertical transection of the mandibular ramus [eɪ] from the sigmoid notch[1] [nɒːtʃ] to the angle[2] [æŋgl] to reposition the posterior mandible for correction of mandibular prognathism
» *Intra-oral vertical subsigmoid osteotomy was used to push back the mandible.*
Use horizontal / circular orbital[3] **osteotomy**

vertikale Osteotomie
Incisura mandibulae[1] Kieferwinkel, Angulus mandibulae[2] zirkuläre Orbitalosteotomie[3]

13

genioplasty [dʒiːnioʊ-] *n term*   *sim* **geniocheiloplasty**[1] [-kaɪlə-] *n term*
  plastic surgery of the chin aimed at altering its shape or size (also termed mentoplasty[2])
» *Following an intraoral incision for a genioplasty procedure the symphysis is degloved[3] [ʌ].*
Use augmentation[4] [ɒː]/ advancement[5] / intraoral / secondary **genioplasty**

Genio-, Kinnplastik, Kinnkorrektur
Kinn-Lippenplastik[1] Genioplastik[2] freigelegt[3] Kinnaugmentation, augmentierende Genioplastik[4] op. Kinnvorverlagerung[5]

14

sinus [aɪ] **lift (procedure)** *n term*
         sim **lateral wall infracture technique**[1] *n term*
  elevation of the maxillary sinus floor, usually via[2] a lateral wall osteotomy
» *The bone was ground[3] [aʊ] to a particulate size[4] [aɪ] and grafted to the left maxillary sinus via a sinus lift procedure; the bone window was infractured[5] into the sinus to create the new sinus floor.*
Use bilateral **sinus lift** • **sinus lift** graft (procedure)

Sinusbodenanhebung, -elevation, Sinuslift-Operation
Seitenwandinfraktionstechnik[1] mittels[2] zerkleinert[3] Spangröße[4] infrakturiert[5]

15

45

DENTISTRY — Maxillofacial Surgery

distraction n term

gradual[1] progressive surgical separation of two parts of a bone after it has been transected

distract[2] v term • distractor[3] n

» Total bony integration leads to the formation of a new condyle growth center provided that effective orthopedic [iː] forces are maintained to distract the condyle slightly from the glenoid fossa base.

Use skeletal / longitudinal / axial / alveolar ridge / callus[4] / joint **distraction** • **distraction of the** mandible / ramus [eɪ]/ midface • **distraction** osteotomy[5] / force / osteogenesis[6] [dʒe]/ rod / implant • extraoral / one-/ two-dimensional **distractor**

Distraktion

allmählich[1] distrahieren[2] Distraktor[3] Kallusdistraktion[4] Distraktionsosteotomie[5] Distraktionsosteogenese[6]

16

parotidectomy n term

surgical excision of the parotid gland[1] primarily performed for benign[2] [aɪn] and malignant[3] tumors

» Malignant lesions [iːʒ] of the parotid[1] require radical parotidectomy and radiotherapy; frozen section[4] may help decide whether the facial nerve can be preserved.

Use selective / superficial[5] [ɪʃ]/ total / conservative[6] **parotidectomy** • **parotid** space[7] / notch / duct[8] [ʌ]/ fascia [fæʃ(ɪ)ə]/ papilla / branch[9] / nerves / lymph [lɪmf] nodes / saliva[10] [səlaɪvə]/ abscess / tumor / adenocarcinoma

Parotidektomie

Ohrspeicheldrüse, Parotis, Glandula parotidea[1] benigne, gutartig[2] maligne, bösartig[3] Gefrierschnitt[4] subtotale Parotidektomie[5] konservative P.[6] Parotisloge[7] Parotisgang, Ductus parotideus[8] Parotisast, Ramus parotideus[9] Parotisspeichel[10]

17

ultraconservative [ʌltrə-] **dentistry** n term

minimally invasive dental surgery using endoscopic technologies[1] [k], such as TMJ arthroscopy[2], internal endoscopically assisted fracture fixation, etc.

minimal invasive Kieferchirurgie

endoskopische Verfahren[1] Kiefergelenkarthroskopie[2]

18

functional endoscopic sinus [aɪ] **surgery** n term, abbr **FESS**

biopsy [baɪəpsi], paranasal [eɪ] tissue sampling and expansion of the osteum via rigid[1] [dʒ] endoscopes with angled [ŋg] ports

» FESS with rigid endoscopes and angled viewing [vjuːɪŋ] ports[2] has proved useful in chronic sinusitis [aɪ].

funktionelle Sinuskopie, Endoskopie d. Kieferhöhle

starr[1] abgewinkelte Optiken[2]

19

craniotomy n term

opening the skull, either by attached or detached craniotomy or by trephination[1] [f]

» Access[2] to the tumor was gained by frontal-temporal craniotomy.

Use attached[3] [ætʃ] or osteoplastic[3] / sellar[4] / detached[5] **craniotomy**

Kraniotomie, Trepanation

Schädeleröffnung, Trepanation[1] Zugang[2] osteoplastische Trepanation[3] sellare T.[4] osteoklastische Trepanation[5]

20

craniofacial implants n term → U43-2

prosthetic [θe] eyes[1], ears, and noses securely fixed[2] using techniques similar to oral implants

» Violation[3] [vaɪəleɪʃ⁽ə⁾n] of the implant abutment [ʌ] epithelial [iː] interface[4] may result in tissue breakdown[5], infection, and eventual[6] failure of the craniofacial implant.

Use **craniofacial implant** placement / stability / loading[7] [oʊ]/ retention[8] / failure • **craniofacial** anomaly / rehabilitation[9] / osseointegration / microsomia[10]

kraniofaziale Implantate

Augenprothese[1] fest verankert[2] Verletzung[3] Verbindung[4] Gewebezerstörung[5] schließlich[6] Belastung d. kraniof. Implantats[7] Verankerung d. kraniof. Implantats[8] kraniof. Wiederherstellung[9] kraniof. Mikrosomie[10]

21

maxillofacial prosthesis [iː] n term, pl -ses

artificial device designed to substitute [ʌ] for[1] a diseased or missing part of the jaws or face prosthetic [e] adj term

» Auricular [ɔːrɪkjələ] prostheses[2] may be incorporated within eyeglasses or retained[3] by the creation of skin pouches[4] [paʊtʃɪz] or tunnels [ʌ]. Overlaying [eɪ] the residual alar [eɪ] cartilages[5] [ɪdʒ] had resulted in an overcontoured nasal prosthesis. A snap button [ʌ] system[6] was used for prosthetic [e] retention.

Use (cranio)facial / nasofacial [eɪ]/ nasal[7] / orbital[8] / tissue-integrated / implant-retained[9] [eɪ] **prosthesis** • **prosthetic** ear / rehabilitation

Kiefer-Gesichtsprothese, maxillofaziale Epithese

ersetzen[1] Ohrepithese[2] verankert, fixiert[3] Hauttaschen[4] Nasenflügelknorpel, Cartilagines alares[5] Druckknopfsystem[6] Nasenepithese[7] Orbitaepithese[8] implantatgestützte Prothese[9]

22

bone-anchored [æŋkəd] **hearing** [ɪə] **aid** [eɪd] n term   abbr **BAHA**

electronic device (microphone [aɪ], amplifier[1] [-aɪə], receiver [iː]) designed to convey[2] sound [aʊ] more effectively into the ear

» An implant was placed in the mastoid region for BAHA attachment.

Use **bone-anchored** implant / auricular prosthesis [iː]/ facial prosthesis[3] / support

enossal verankertes Hörgerät

Verstärker[1] übertragen[2] enossal verankerte Gesichtsprothese[3]

23

Unit 46 Basic Radiologic Terms
Related Units: 33 Dental Imaging Techniques

radiology [reɪdɪɒːlədʒi] *n term*

use of x-rays [eks reɪz], radioactive tracers[1] [eɪs] and high-energy radiation for diagnosis or treatment

radiologic(al) *adj term* • radiologist[2] *n* • radio- *comb*

» Review the radiology records[3] for recent exposure to nephrotoxic contrast agents.
Use diagnostic[4] / interventional **radiology** • **radiology** department / suite[5] [swiːt] • **radiologic** evaluation[6] / appearance [ɪɚ] / findings[7] [aɪ]/ diagnosis / sign / study / technologist[8] [knɒː] • **radio**protective clothing[9] /active rays

Radiologie
radioaktiv markierte Substanzen, Tracer[1] Radiologe/-in[2] Röntgenberichte[3] Röntgendiagnostik[4] Röntgenbereich[5] radiol. Abklärung[6] Röntgenbefund[7] radiolog. techn./ Röntgenassistent(in)[8] Strahlenschutzkleidung[9]   1

radiation [reɪdɪeɪʃᵊn] *n term*   sim **irradiation**[1] *n term*

(i) radiant energy or beam [iː] (ii) emanation[2] of rays (iii) irradiation

ray[3] [reɪ] *n term* • radiant[4] *adj* • radiate[5] [reɪdɪeɪt] *v*

» The gonads, blood cells, and cancer cells are particularly sensitive[6] to radiation. The radiation is delivered[7] in a single session.
Use background / ionizing [aɪə] / annihilation[8] / beta [eɪ‖iː]/ corpuscular [ʌ] / electromagnetic / scattered[9] / hetero-/ homogeneous [dʒiː]/ K-/ L-**radiation** • **radiation** sickness[10] / dose / dosimetry / energy /-induced / protection[11] • x- or roentgen [e]/ gamma / soft[12] / ultrahard [ʌ]/ ultraviolet **rays** • **radio**therapy[13] /biology /-labeled[14] [eɪ]/curable[15] /pharmaceuticals[16] [suː]/responsive /mimetic[17] /immunoassay

(i) & (ii) Strahlung
(iii) Bestrahlung
Bestrahlung[1] Ausstrahlung, Emanation[2] Strahl[3] strahlend[4] (aus)strahlen[5] empfindlich[6] verabreicht[7] Annihilations-,Vernichtungsstrahlung[8] Streustrahlung[9] Strahlenkater[10] Strahlenschutz[11] weiche Strahlen[12] Strahlentherapie[13] radioaktiv markiert[14] durch Strahlentherapie heilbar[15] Radiopharmaka[16] Radiomimetikum[17]   2

radiograph *n term*   syn **radio-** or **roentgenogram** *n term*, **x-ray (film)** *n clin*

record or image produced on exposed[1] and processed film by radiographic means

radiography *n term* • radiographic(ally) *adj/adv* • x-ray[2] *v* • radiographer[3] *n*, *abbr* RAD

» A followup contrast radiograph obtained 7 months later was unremarkable[4]. This lesion [liːʒᵊn] cannot be visualized by x-ray. This radiographic pattern is diagnostic of bacterial [ɪɚ] infection.
Use to take[5] **an x-ray** • AP / PA[6] / lateral[7] / **chest x-ray** • **x-ray** unit[8] / attenuation[9] / burn • GI[10] / radiographic / (lateral) skull[11] / plain[12] (abdominal) **film** • double contrast[13] **radiography** • panoramic / oblique [iːk] lateral jaw / cephalometric / bite-wing[14] / lateral decubitus[15] **radiograph** • **radiographic** studies / image / evidence[16] / features [iː] • **radiographically** benign [aɪn]/ not determined[17] / mistaken for

Röntgen(aufnahme, -bild)
belichtet[1] röntgen[2] Röntgenassistent(in)[3] unauffällig[4] Röntgenaufnahme machen[5] p.a. Aufnahme d. Thorax[6] seitliches Thoraxröntgen[7] Röntgenanlage[8] Strahlungsschwächung[9] Magen-Darm-Röntgen[10] Schädelröntgen[11] Leeraufnahme[12] Doppelkontrastdarstellung[13] Bissflügelaufnahme[14] Röntgenaufnahme in Seitenlage[15] radiolog. Nachweis[16] radiolog. nicht nachgewiesen[17]   3

irradiate [ɪreɪdɪeɪt] *v term*   sim **bombard**[1] *v term*

to expose the whole body or specific target tissues[2] to radiant energy[3]

irradiation[4] *n term* • irradiated *adj* • post-irradiation *adj*

» Irradiation alone will only produce a temporary response[5]. Lacking other options [ɒːpʃ-], the blood products from family members should always be irradiated.
Use heavily [e]/ selectively **irradiated** • **irradiated** tissue / food[6] / site / volume • elective / adjuvant / high-dose / total body[7] / grid[8] / ionizing / heavy ion [aɪən]/ beta-/ total nodal[9] (*abbr* TNI) / x-**irradiation** • **irradiation** therapy / field[10]

bestrahlen
beschießen[1] Zielgewebe[2] Strahlungsenergie[3] Bestrahlung[4] vorübergehende Wirkung[5] bestrahlte Lebensmittel[6] Ganzkörperbestrahlung[7] Siebbestrahlung[8] Bestrahlung aller Lymphknotengruppen[9] Bestrahlungsfeld[10]   4

beam [biːm] *n & v term*

(n) unidirectional emission of electromagnetic radiation or particles from the x-ray tube

beamer[1] *n term* • beam-splitter[2] *n*

» AP x-rays were taken with a horizontal x-ray beam and the patient lying on the affected side.
Use to angle [æŋgl] the[3] **beam** • x-ray / divergent [ɜːrdʒ] **beam** • **beam** quality / diameter [daɪæ-]/ restrictors[4] / hardening[5] /-splitting mirror[2] • **external beam** radiotherapy[6]

Strahl(enbündel);
(aus)strahlen
Beamer[1] Strahlentrennraster[2] Strahl richten (auf)[3] Streustrahlenraster[4] Strahlenhärtung[5] externe Hochvoltstrahlentherapie[6]   5

166 RELATED MEDICAL SPECIALTIES — Basic Radiologic Terms

collimation n term

(i) restricting the x-ray beam to a given area by elimination of scattered radiation and back-scatter[1] (ii) in nuclear medicine, restricting the detection of emitted radiation from a given area of interest

collimate[2] v term • collimator[3] n • collimated adj

» The so-called gamma knife [naɪf] delivers collimated radiation through multiple portals[4] that converge [-vɜːrdʒ] on the target.

Use x-ray / fixed cone / pinhole[5] / variable aperture[6] [æpətʃɚ] **collimator** • **collimation** system / restrictions

Strahlenfokussierung, Kollimation
Rückstreuung[1] kollimieren[2] Kollimator[3] Bohrungen[4] Einlochkollimator[5] Mehrlochkollimator[6]

6

radiation exposure [ɪkspoʊzɚ] n term   rel **radiation burn**[1] [bɜːrn] n term

short-term diagnostic, therapeutic [pjuː] or accidental contact with ionization produced by x- or gamma rays

(un)exposed adj term • expose v • overexposure[2] n

» Exposure of the whole body to approx. 10,000 rad (100 gray) causes neurologic [ʊɚ] and cardiovascular breakdown and is fatal [eɪ] within 24 hs. Though this procedure might be an atttractive alternative, radiation exposure to the fetus would be unavoidable.

Use to receive / to rule out[3] / acute / lethal [liːθəl]/ natural **radiation exposure** • massive / excessive **exposure** • **exposure** time[4] / rate / to radiation / to sunlight / to toxins • **radiation** detector[5] / absorbed dose / effects / hygiene[6] [haɪdʒiːn]/ dermatitis [aɪ]/ caries

Strahlenexposition, -belastung
akute Strahlenschädigung[1] Strahlenüberdosis[2] S. ausschließen[3] Expositions-; Durchleuchtungs-; Belichtungszeit[4] Strahlungsdetektor[5] Strahlenhygiene[6]

7

fluorescence [-esəns] n term   sim **phosphorescence**[1] n term

emission of radiation by a substance exposed to a shorter wavelength radiation as long as the stimulus is present; in phosphorescence emission persists for a time after removal of the stimulus

fluorescent adj term • fluoresce[2] [-res] v • fluoroscopic adj • fluoro- comb

» Fluoroscopic examination demonstrated a smoothly rounded outpouching[3] [aʊtʃ] in the midline. The passage of contrast material is monitored by fluoroscopy.

Use **under fluoroscopic** control or guidance[4] [aɪ] • **fluoro**scope /scopy[5] /meter /(photo)metry[6] /(radio)graphy • **fluorescent** screen[7] • videotape **fluoroscopy** • x-ray[8] **fluorescence**

Fluoreszenz
Phosphoreszenz[1] fluoreszieren[2] gleichmäßig abgerundete Ausstülpung[3] unter fluoroskop. Kontrolle[4] (Röntgen)durchleuchtung[5] Fluorometrie[6] Leuchtschirm[7] Röntgenfluoreszenz[8]

8

radiation dose [doʊs] n term

amount of ionizing radiation of the therapeutic dosage and the penetrating power[1] of x-rays

dosimetry[2] n term • dosimeter n • dosimetric adj

» The dose delivered to the target volume and the relative dose distribution[3] within the irradiated volume were measured.

Use body / threshold[4] [θreʃhoʊld]/ peak [iː]/ surface[5] / organ[6] / tissue[7] **dose** • breast [e]/ total lung / gonadal or genetically [dʒen-] significant[8] (abbr GSD) / negligible[9] [-dʒəbl] **dose** • absorbed **dose** index • **dose** rate / reduction / equivalent[10] (abbr DE) /-dependent • radiation / film **dosimetry**

Strahlendosis
Eindringtiefe[1] Dosimetrie[2] Dosisverteilung[3] Schwellendosis[4] Oberflächendosis[5] Organdosis[6] Gewebedosis[7] Gonaden-/ genetisch signifikante Dosis[8] unbedeutende D.[9] Äquivalentdosis, Dosisäquivalent[10]

9

roentgen-equivalent-man n term, abbr **rem**
    sim **(radiation) absorbed dose**[1] n term, abbr **rad**

dose of ionizing radiation producing the same effect in man as one roentgen of x- or gamma rays; in the SI nomenclature the rad has been replaced by the gray[2] (Gy; 1 rad = 0.01 Gy) and the rem by the sievert[3] (Sv; 1 rem = 0.01 Sv)

» For x-ray or gamma radiation, rems, rads and roentgen are virtually[4] [vɜːrtʃʊəli] the same, but for particulate radiation[5] emitted from radioactive materials these units may differ widely.

REM (Einheit für Äquivalentdosis)
Rad, rd (Einheit für Energiedosis)[1] Gray[2] Sv[3] nahezu[4] Teilchenstrahlung[5]

10

Basic Radiologic Terms RELATED MEDICAL SPECIALTIES **167**

radiopaque [-oʊpeɪk] or **-dense** adj term
opposite **radiolucent**[1] [-luːsənt] adj term
exhibiting relative opacity[2] [oʊpæsəti] to, or impenetrability[3] by x-rays or any other form of radiation
radiopacity[4] n term • radiodensity[4] n • radiolucency n
• hypo-/hyper-/isodense[5] [aɪ] adj
» Soft tissue films revealed a radiodense stone. The unenhanced CT scan demonstrated no radiopacity, but the urogram showed a radiolucent area surrounded by the radiopaque urine.
Use **radiopaque** dye[6] [daɪ]/ catheter / foreign body • skeletal **radiodensity** • **radiolucent** zone[7] / (filling) defect[8] / mass / band / line

strahlenundurchlässig, -dicht, radiopak
strahlendurchlässig, radioluzent[1] (Strahlen)undurchlässigkeit, Verschattung, Opazität[2] Undurchdringbarkeit[3] Strahlendichte, -undurchlässigkeit[4] hyperdens[5] radiopaker Farbstoff[6] radioluzenter Bereich[7] strahlendurchlässiger Füllungsdefekt[8]

11

visualize [vɪʒ(u)əlaɪz] v term   sim **delineate**[1], **demarcate**[2], **delimit**[2], **outline**[3] v term
visualization[4] n term • delineation[4] n • demarcation[5] n • outline[6] n
» MRI and CT can visualize neighboring [eɪ] tumor when present. Renal stones were visualized on ultrasonography. Multiple foci [foʊsaɪ] are best visualized by MRI.
Use to allow (for)/permit/provide/ensure [-ʃʊəʳ]/prevent/enhance[7] **visualization** • poor / excellent / direct / radiographic[8] / endoscopic / fetal [iː] **visualization** • adequately / clearly / readily[9] [e] **visualized** • distinctly[10] **outlined**

darstellen, sichtbar machen
umreißen, darstellen[1] ab-, begrenzen, sich abheben (von)[2] skizzieren, umreißen[3] Darstellung[4] Ab-, Begrenzung, Grenze[5] Umriss[6] Darstellung verbessern[7] Röntgendarstellung[8] gut sichtbar, deutlich dargestellt[9] scharf umrissen[10]

12

artifact also spelled **artefact** n term   rel **aliazing**[1] [əlaɪəsɪŋ] n term
an artificial finding (esp. in radiographic imaging or histologic specimens[2]) caused by the technique used rather than by the sample[3] or tissue studied
artifact-free adj term • artifactual[4] or BE artefactitious adj
» Take abdominal x-rays before performing peritoneal lavage [-ɑːʒ] as the procedure tends to produce artifacts. Sources of technical [k] artifacts[5] are collimator shifting and tube uncoupling[6] [ʌ].
Use motion or movement / muscle tension / eye twitching[7] [tʃ]/ EEG / pacemaker[8] [eɪs] **artifact** • **artifactually** distorted[9]

Artefakt
Aliasing, Umklappeffekt[1] histolog. Präparate[2] (Gewebe)probe[3] artifiziell, künstlich erzeugt[4] technisch bedingte A.[5] Röhreninstabilität[6] lidschlagbedingtes A.[7] schrittmacherbedingtes A.[8] artifiziell verzerrt[9]

13

(image) resolution n term   syn **resolving power** n term
measure [eʒ] of the degree to which the eye, lens or imaging device [-aɪs] can distinguish or display[1] detail, e.g. the perception[2] of adjacent[3] [adʒeɪsᵊnt] objects as separate
high-resolution[4] adj term
» MRI has superior [ɪəʳ] resolution and is relatively artifact-free. Problems of CT of the pituitary include artifacts due to bone and dental amalgam and limited soft tissue resolution[5].
Use to increase / high / good / contrast[6] / spatial[7] [eɪʃ] **resolution** • **resolution** matrix [eɪ]/ of borders[8] • **high-resolution** images / CT / contrast / scan / ultrasound [ʌ]

Bildauflösung, Auflösungsvermögen
(an)zeigen, darstellen[1] Wahrnehmung[2] anliegend[3] hochauflösend[4] Weichteilauflösung[5] Kontrastauflösung[6] räuml. Auflösung[7] Randschärfe[8]

14

contrast agent [eɪdʒᵊnt] n term   syn **contrast material** or **medium** [iː], pl -**ia** n term
radiopaque material (e.g. barium [eəʳ]) used to visualize soft tissues radiographically
contrast-enhanced[1] adj term • unenhanced[2] [æ] adj • double-contrast[3] adj
» CT scanning and MRI may be useful, with and without contrast. Addition of IV contrast aids recognition of pancreatic necrosis. All but[4] the smallest lesions exhibit contrast enhancement.
Use to inject/instill/excrete [iː] **contrast material** • liquid / water-soluble / IV / swallowed / iodinated[5] [aɪə-]/ radio**contrast agent** • **contrast** administration / study / radiograph[6] / enhancement[7] / substance [ʌ] / dye[8] [daɪ] / enema[9] [enɪmə] • injection of / single / double / saline [seɪlaɪn‖-iːn] bubble[10] [ʌ]/ air **contrast** • non**contrast** scan

Kontrastmittel
kontrastverstärkt[1] ohne Kontrastverstärkung[2] Doppelkontrast-[3] alle außer[4] iodiertes / iodhaltiges Kontrastmittel[5] Kontrastaufnahme[6] Kontrastverstärkung[7] Kontrastfärbemittel[8] Kontrasteinlauf[9] Kochsalzbläschen-Kontrast[10]

15

transillumination n term   syn **diaphanoscopy** or **-graphy** [daɪəfənɒː-] n term
passing light through tissues, organs or body cavities to examine them
transilluminate[1] v term • diaphanoscope[2] n • diaphano- comb
» These lesions do not transilluminate. In infants transillumination of the skull with an intensely bright light may disclose[3] subdural effusions and large cystic defects.
Use area[4] / intensity **of transillumination** • **transillumination of the** breasts [e]/ scrotum / sinuses[5] [aɪ]

Diaphanoskopie, Transillumination, Durchleuchtung
durch-, aufleuchten[1] Durchleuchtungsgerät, Diaphanoskop[2] zeigen, aufdecken[3] Durchleuchtungsfeld[4] Nebenhöhlendurchleuchtung[5]

16

46

168 RELATED MEDICAL SPECIALTIES   Basic Radiologic Terms

scintigraphy [sɪntɪ-] *n term*   *rel* **scintigram** *or* **scintiscan**[1] *n term*

imaging procedure employing IV injection of a radionuclide[2] [aɪ] with an affinity for the organ or tissue of interest to determine the distribution of the radioactivity with an external scintillation detector[3]

scintillation[4] *n term* • **scintillating** *adj* • **scinti-** *comb*

» *Serial* [ɪə] *scintiscans*[5] *of the right upper quadrant were obtained.*

Use stress[6] / rest[7] / perfusion / gated blood pool[8] / sequential[5] / thallium / lympho-/ hepatobiliary[9] **scintigraphy** • **scintigraphic** assessment / study • **scintillating** scotoma[10] • **scintillation** camera[11] / counter[3]

Szintigraphie

Szintigramm[1] Radionuklid[2] Szintillationsdetektor, -zähler[3] Szintillation, kurzlebige Lumineszenz[4] Serienszintigramme[5] Funktionsszintigraphie[6] statische Sz.[7] Blutpoolsz.[8] Chole-, Gallenwegssz.[9] Flimmerskotom[10] Gammakamera[11]   17

---

scan *n & v term*   *sim* **scanning**[1] *n term*

(n, i) short for scintiscan (ii) any image, record, or data obtained by scanning (v) to examine systematically with a sensing device[2] (e.g. an electron beam)

scanner[2] *n term* • **scanography**[1] *n*

» *Encapsulated*[3] *abscesses are characterized by a faint*[4] [eɪ] *ring on the unenhanced scan.*

Use bone / brain **scan** •(un)enhanced / perfusion (lung)[5] / total body **scan** • **scan** width[6] / field • ultrasound / (positive) radionuclide / Meckel / ventilation-perfusion / multiplanar [eɪ]/ color[7] **scan** • whole body[8] / (supercam) scintillation[9] / ultrasonic **scanner**

Scan(-Aufnahme); scannen, abtasten

Scan(ning), Abtastung, Szintigraphie[1] Abtastgerät, (Szinti)scanner[2] abgekapselt[3] blass, undeutlich[4] Lungenperfusionsszintigramm[5] Scanbreite[6] Farbszintigramm[7] Ganzkörperscanner[8] Szinti(llations)scanner[9]   18

---

tomography *n term*   *syn* **plano-, strati-, laminagraphy, sectional radiography** *n term*

taking sectional roentgenograms of serial tissue planes (slices[1]) by advancing the patient in the gantry[2] in small steps (increments[3])

tomograph *n term* • **tomographic** *adj* • **tomogram**[4] *n*

» *Tomograms should be obtained for*[5] *calcifications may be misinterpreted on plain films*[6]*.*

Use conventional / computed[7] (*abbr* CT) *or* computerized axial[7] (*abbr* CAT) / reconstruction / positron emission[8] (*abbr* PET) **tomography** • linear / pluridirectional[9] / narrow angle [g]/ focal plane **tomography** • **tomographic** film / imaging procedure

Tomographie, Schichtaufnahmeverfahren

Schichten[1] Gantry[2] Vorschüben[3] Tomogramm, Schichtaufnahme[4] denn[5] Leeraufnahmen[6] Computertomographie, CT[7] Positronenemissionscomputertomographie, PET[8] mehrdimensionale Tomographie[9]   19

---

ionization [aɪənaɪzeɪʃ(ə)n] *n term*

dissociation[1] of molecules into ions (cations[2] [kætaɪɒnz], anions[3]), e.g. by subjecting them to ionizing radiation[4]

ion [aɪən] *n term* • ionize *v* • (cat/ an/non)ionic[5] *adj* • (non)ionizing *adj*

» *Ionizing radiation has sufficient energy to ionize the irradiated material.*

Use **ionization** chamber[6] [tʃeɪ]/ density[7] / detector / dose[8] • (ultrashort) **ionizing** radiation[9] • **ionic** contrast material[10] / bond[11] • hydrogen [aɪ]/ hydroxyl / positively charged[12] [tʃɑːrdʒd] **ion** • **ion** exchange[13]

Ionisierung, Ionisation

Aufspaltung[1] Kationen[2] Anionen[3] ionisierende Strahlung[4] (nicht)ionisch[5] Ionisationskammer[6] Ionisationsdichte[7] Ionendosis[8] ultrakurze ionisierende Strahlung[9] ionisiertes Kontrastmittel[10] Ionenbindung[11] positiv geladenes Ion[12] Ionenaustausch[13]   20

---

radioactive *adj term*

spontaneously [eɪ] emitting alpha, beta [eɪ‖iː], or gamma rays

radioactivity[1] *n term*

» *These thrombi* [aɪ] *can be detected by external scanning if the fibrinogen is labeled*[2] [eɪ] *with a radioactive material such as iodine-125*[3] [aɪədɪn]*.*

Use **radioactive** implants[4] / seeds[4] [iː]/ beads[4] [iː]/ pellets[4] / (labeled) isotopes [aɪ]/ tracer [treɪsə] *or* **radio**tracer[5] / iodine (*abbr* RAI) uptake study[6] • induced **radioactivity**

radioaktiv

Radioaktivität[1] markiert[2] Iod-125[3] radioaktive Implantate[4] Radiopharmakon, Tracer[5] Radioiodtest[6]   21

---

radionuclide [-nʲuːklaɪd] *n term*   *sim* **radioisotope**[1] [-aɪsətoʊp] *n term*

artificial or natural radioactive nuclide or isotope of iodine, cobalt, phosphorus, strontium [ʃ], etc. used as tracer substances[2], e.g. to follow the course of the normal substances in metabolism

nuclide *n term* • **nuclear**[3] *adj*

» *Radionuclide imaging*[4] *is 90% sensitive, becoming positive within 2 days after the onset.*

Use **radionuclide** angiography [dʒɪɒː]/ cystogram[5] / impurity / generator • labeled **radioisotope** • **radioisotope** angiogram / renography[6] / uptake study • **nuclear** medicine[7] / electron / particle[8] / charge[9] [tʃ]/ decay[10] [keɪ]/ imaging / scanner

Radionuklid

Radioisotop[1] Tracer[2] nuklear, Kern-[3] Szintigraphie[4] Blasenszintigramm[5] Radioisotopennephrographie, Nierensequenzszintigraphie[6] Nuklearmedizin[7] Kernteilchen[8] Kernladung[9] radioaktiver Zerfall[10]   22

Basic Terms in Anesthesiology RELATED MEDICAL SPECIALTIES 169

radiosensitive [əˈnesθɪtaɪz] adj term   opposite **radioresistant**[1] adj term

readily affected[2] by the effects of radiation; self-renewing cells (e.g. sperm cells) are most susceptible[3] [səˈseptɪbl] while fixed postmitotic [aɪ] cells (e.g. neurons [ʊɚ]) are least [iː] sensitive to radiation

radiosensitivity[4] n term • **radioresistance** n • **radiosensitizing** adj

» There was no correlation between tumor grade[5] and radiosensitivity.

Use relative **radiosensitivity** • **radiosensitizing** agent or **radiosensitizer**[6]

strahlenempfindlich

strahlenresistent, -unempfindlich[1] leicht zu schädigen[2] empfänglich, empfindlich[3] Strahlensensibilität[4] Malignitätsgrad[5] Radio-, Strahlensensitizer[6]

23

Unit 47   Basic Terms in Anesthesiology
Related Units: **48** Types of Anesthesia & Anesthetics, **4** States of Consciousness, **16** Pain, **25** Perioperative Care

anesthetize [əˈnesθɪtaɪz] v term, BE **anaesthetise, -ize** [iː]
     syn **put under** v phr clin

to induce a loss of feeling or sensation by means of anesthetic drugs

put to sleep[1] phr inf • **anesthetization** [eǁiː] n term • **unanesthetized** adj

» The catheter can be placed after anesthetization. In the anesthetized arm surgery was tolerated up to 30 min. Anesthetize the skin with lidocaine [aɪ] using a 10mL syringe [dʒ] and 22-gauge [geɪdʒ] needle. The wound may be anesthetized locally with lidocaine. After full nebulized[2] lidocaine anesthetization of the pharynx and vocal cords the bronchoscope is passed through the nostrils[3].

Use deeply[4] **anesthetized** • **anesthetized** area / wound [uː]/ operative field / patient / skin / eye • **anesthetizing** needle / drugs[5]

anästhesieren, narkotisieren, betäuben

einschläfern[1] vernebelt[2] Nasenöffnungen, -löcher[3] unter starken Narkotika stehend, stark narkotisiert[4] Anästhetika, Narkotika[5]

1

anesthesia [ænəsˈθiːʒə] n term & clin   syn/rel **anesthesiology** n term

(i) informal term for anesthesiology (ii) partial or complete loss of sensation, esp. when induced by pharmacologic depression of nerve function [ʌ] to permit performance of surgery or other painful procedures

anesthetic[1] [e] adj & n term • **anesthesiologist**[2] [iː] or BE **anaesthetist**[2] n

» This procedure can be performed under local anesthesia on an outpatient basis[3]. The main objectives[4] of general anesthesia are analgesia [-dʒiːzɪə], unconsciousness, skeletal muscle relaxation and control of sympathetic nervous system responses to noxious[5] [nɒkʃəs] stimuli [aɪ].

Use prompt onset of[6] / time under / level of[7] / recovery from / surgical / standby / conduction[8] **anesthesia** • to administer/induce[9] /maintain[10]/awaken from **anesthesia** • **anesthesia** management[11] / consent / consultation / accident / hazard[12] / adjuvant • **anesthesia of the** skin / airway • **anesthesia for** abdominal surgery / children • monitored **anesthetic** care[13] • **anesthesiologist** on-call[14]

> Note: In the States the anesthetic may be administered by the anesthesiologist or another physician, a nurse anesthetist, or an anesthesia assistant. Unlike in British usage, the anesthesiologist is never referred to as the anesthetist.

(i) Anästhesie, Narkose, Anästhesiologie (ii) Betäubung, Schmerzunempfindlichkeit

anästhetisch; Anästhetikum, Narkotikum[1] Anästhesist(in), Anästhesiologe/-in, Narkosearzt /-ärztin[2] ambulant[3] Ziele[4] schädlich[5] rascher Wirkungseintritt[6] Narkosetiefe[7] Leitungsanästhesie[8] N. einleiten[9] N. aufrechterhalten[10] Narkoseführung[11] Narkoserisiko[12] anästhesiologische Überwachung[13] diensthabende(r) Anästhesist(in)[14]

2

numb [nʌm] adj & v clin   syn **blunt** [ʌ] adj & v, **dull** [ʌ], **deaden** [dedᵊn] v inf

(adj) lack or loss of sensation, e.g. because of cold, poor blood perfusion or anesthesia

numbness[1] n clin • **benumb**[2] v inf

» My face is numb. As anesthesia blunts the normal compensatory mechanisms, sudden changes in the patient's position can cause hypotension. Numbness may be used to describe a complete loss of feeling, paresthesias [- θiːʒ(ɪ)əs], or paralysis. The patient complained that his feet had a numb or wooden feeling. Frostbitten[3] parts are numb, painless, and of a white or waxy[4] appearance.

Use **numb** fingers / feeling / chin [tʃ] syndrome [ɪ] • **numbness** and tingling[5] [ŋg] • temporary / partial / subjective / facial [eɪʃ] **numbness** • nerve-**numbing** drugs[6] • **blunted** sensation / response / reflexes / affect[7] • **dulled** perception[8]

taub; betäuben, unempfindlich (machen)

Taubheit, Gefühllosigkeit[1] betäuben[2] v. Erfrierungen betroffen[3] wächsern[4] Taubheitsgefühl u. Kribbeln[5] nervenbetäubende Medikamente[6] Affektabstumpfung[7] eingeschränktes Wahrnehmungsvermögen[8]

3

47

170 RELATED MEDICAL SPECIALTIES — Basic Terms in Anesthesiology

hyp(o)esthesia [haɪpesθiːzə] *n term*   *syn* **blunted sensation** *n clin & inf*

diminished sensation[1] (hyposensitivity[1]) in reaction to stimulation (esp. touch)
hyp(o)-/ hyperesthetic *adj term* • paresthesia[2] *n* • hyperesthesia[3] *n*

» Sensory symptoms include hypesthesia (numbness or impaired feeling) or paresthesia (tingling, pins and needles[4], or a painful burning). Abnormal spontaneous sensations are generally termed paresthesias. The involved zone was hyperesthetic.

Use **hypesthetic** area • malar[5] [eɪ]/ corneal / transitory[6] **hypesthesia** • distal extremity / limb[7] [lɪm]/ facial / peri- or circumoral **paresthesias**

Hypästhesie, verminderte (Berührungs)empfindlichkeit
herabgesetzte Sensibilität[1] Parästhesie, subjektive Missempfindung[2] Hyperästhesie, Überempfindlichkeit[3] Kribbeln, Ameisenlaufen[4] Hypästhesie der Wange[5] vorübergehende H.[6] Parästhesien i. d. Extremitäten[7]   4

---

narcotics *n term usu pl, abbr* **narc**   *syn* **narcotic agent/drug** *n clin*

(i) drugs (e.g. morphine and other opium derivatives) used in moderate doses to relieve pain, dull sensation, and induce profound [aʊ] sleep that have the potential for dependence and tolerance[1] on repeated administration (ii) illegal and street drugs such as marijuana, LSD, etc.
narcotic[2] *adj & n term & clin* • nonnarcotic *adj & n term* • narcotize[3] *v* • narco- *comb*

» Increasing amounts of narcotics were required. The terms narcotics and opioids are often used interchangeably[4] for drugs whose effects mimic[5] those of morphine.

Use sedative / intravenous [iː]/ parenteral / long-acting / epidural / opioid[6] **narcotics** • **narcotic** addict[7] / effect / analgesics[8] • **narco**lepsy /hypnosis [hɪp-]/anesthesia

(i) Narkotika, Anästhetika
(ii) Rauschmittel, -gift
Gewöhnung, Toleranzentwicklung[1] Narkose-; Narkotikum, Rauschgift[2] narkotisieren, betäuben[3] synonym[4] ähnlich sein[5] Opioid[6] Rauschgiftabhängige(r)[7] narkotisch wirkende Analgetika[8]   5

---

narcosis [nɑːrkoʊsɪs] *n term*

a state of stupor[1] [stʲuːpɚ] or deep sleep rather than anesthesia produced by intoxicants[2], narcotics, or toxins

» In many people narcosis is induced at twice the legal intoxication level. Pain relief may be achieved through the judicious[3] [dʒuːdɪʃəs] use of analgesics ranging from nonnarcotics to narcotic derivatives.

Use nitrogen [aɪ] inert [ɜː] gas[4] / CO$_2$ **narcosis** • **narcotic** abuse / intoxication / poisoning / overdose / analgesia / antagonist / substitute[5] / withdrawal[6] • **narcotic**-induced /-related /-containing

> **Note:** In contrast to other languages (e.g. German), narcosis is rarely used in medical English and is hardly ever synonymous with anesthesia.

tiefe Bewusstlosigkeit, Narkose
Stupor, Reaktionsunfähigkeit[1] Rauschmittel[2] umsichtig[3] Edelgasnarkose[4] Ersatzdroge[5] Entzug von Narkotika[6]

6

---

analgesia [ænəldʒiːzɪə] *n term*   → U16-20, 48-18

a state in which painful stimuli [aɪ] are perceived[1] [iː] but are not interpreted as pain; usually accompanied by sedation without loss of consciousness
analgesic[2] [ænəldʒiːsɪk‖zɪk] *adj & n term*

» Provide analgesia as needed[3]. 10mg of epidural morphine produces satisfactory analgesia in 90% of patients for 15-16 hours.

Use to administer/give/increase **analgesia** • (in)adequate / narcotic / (non)opioid / local / patient-controlled[4] (*abbr* PCA) **analgesia** • duration / use / reversal[5] / rapid onset of **analgesia** • **analgesic** agent [eɪdʒ-]/ activity[6] / administration / compound[7] / dose / effect[6] • **analgesic** ingestion[8] [dʒ]/ lozenges[9] [lɒzɪndʒ-]/ regimen[10] [edʒ]/ properties[11] / substance / state[12] / therapy • oral / systemic / mild / simple / (non)narcotic / (non)opioid / nonaddicting[13] / urinary [jʊ]/ central-acting[14] **analgesics**

Analgesie, Aufhebung d. Schmerzempfindung
wahrgenommen[1] schmerzlindernd; Analgetikum, Schmerzmittel[2] nach Bedarf[3] patientengesteuerte A.[4] Umkehr der analget. Wirkung[5] analget. Wirkung[6] analget. Kombinationspräparat[7] Einnahme v. Schmerzmitteln[8] schmerzlindernde Pastillen[9] schmerzstillende Maßnahmen[10] analget. Eigenschaften[11] Analgesiestadium[12] nicht abhängig machende A.[13] zentral wirkende A.[14]   7

---

sedation [sɪdeɪʃən] *n term*

(i) to relax and calm down a patient especially by the administration of sedatives (ii) the state so induced
sedate[1] [eɪ] *v term* • sedative[2] [e] *adj* • presedation [iː] *adj*

» In the awake patient, neuromuscular blockade should be accompanied by sedation to blunt the noxious sensation of paralysis.

Use to be under[3] **sedation** • conscious[4] [ʃ]/ sleep[5] / intravenous / preoperative **sedation** • **sedative** effect / action of drug / narcotic • **sedated** patient

Sedierung, Beruhigung
sedieren[1] beruhigend, sedierend[2] sediert sein[3] schwache Sedierung[4] Schlafsedierung[5]

8

Basic Terms in Anesthesiology

RELATED MEDICAL SPECIALTIES

sedative [e] *n term*   *sim* **hypnotic**[1] [hɪpnɒːtɪk] *adj & n term*

drug reducing nervous excitement[2] and irritability by depressing the CNS; it has a relaxing effect and tends to produce lassitude[3]; the terms sedatives, hypnotics, anxiolytics [ɪ], antianxiety [aɪə] drugs and minor tranquilizers are often used interchangeably

» This sedative is habit-forming[4]. Heavy sedation should be avoided, but small doses of tranquilizers may be helpful in calming[5] [kɑːm-] the emotionally disturbed patient on the first few days. Sedative and hypnotic drugs often cause restlessness[6], mental confusion[7], and uncooperative behavior in the elderly. All available hypnotics involve some risk of overdosage, habituation[8], tolerance and addiction.

Use narcotic / general / cough[9] [kɒːf] **sedative** • **hypnotic** drug / effect / sedative *or* sedative hypnotic[1]

Sedativum, Beruhigungsmittel

hypnotisch; Schlafmittel, Hypnotikum[1] Erregung[2] Müdigkeit, Mattigkeit[3] zu Abhängigkeit führend[4] beruhigen[5] Unruhe[6] geistige Verwirrtheit[7] Gewöhnung, Habituation[8] Antitussivum, Hustenreiz hemmendes M.[9]

---

tranquilize [trænkwɪlaɪz] *v term, BE* **tranquillize**

to calm or quiet down anxious[1] [æŋkʃ(ə)s] or mentally disturbed patients with pacifying[2] [aɪ] or soothing[3] [uː] drugs that have no sedating or depressant effects

tranquilizer[4] *n* • tranquilizing *adj* • tranquilization[5] *n term*

» Minor [aɪ] tranquilizers are antianxiety agents[6] (e.g. Valium, Librium), whereas major [meɪdʒɚ] tranquilizers are neuroleptics[7] such as chlorpromazine (Thorazine).

Use mild [aɪ] **tranquilizer** • **tranquilizing** drugs

beruhigen, sedieren

unruhig, ängstlich[1] beruhigend[2] besänftigend[3] Tranquilizer, Sedativum[4] Beruhigung, Sedierung[5] Anxiolytika, Ataraktika[6] Neuroleptika, Antipsychotika[7]

---

paralyze [pærəlaɪz] *v term*   *rel* **paresis**[1] [iː], **palsy**[2] [pɒːlzi] *n term*

to cause a loss of motor function (usually through injury to or disease of the nerve supply [aɪ])

paralysis[2] *n term* • paralyzed *adj* • paralytic *adj* • -plegia [-iːdʒ(ɪ)ə] *comb*

» Make sure the endotracheal [eɪk] tube does not leak and the patient is well sedated or paralyzed. Paralysis denotes inability of a conscious patient to move the extremity either spontaneously or in response to commands or painful stimuli. Although paralysis by muscle relaxants decreases the need for volatile anesthetics[3], many signs of anesthesia[4] are absent in the paralyzed patient.

Use to cause/reverse[5] **paralysis** • **flaccid**[6] [ks]/ motor[7] / spastic[8] / symmetric descending[9] / total / neuromuscular / 6th nerve / periodic / progressive / impending[10] / anesthesia / facial / respiratory[11] / diaphragmatic / vocal cord[12] **paralysis** • **paralytic** disease / polio[13] / seafood poisoning • **paralytic** patient / muscle / cord / limb [lɪm]

lähmen, paralysieren

Parese, (unvollständige) Lähmung[1] Lähmung, Paralyse, Plegie[2] Inhalationsanästhetika[3] Narkosezeichen[4] Lähmung rückgängig machen[5] schlaffe L.[6] motorische L.[7] spastische L.[8] symmetr. absteigende L.[9] drohende L.[10] Atemlähmung[11] Stimmbandlähmung[12] paralytische Poliomyelitis[13]

---

anesthetic [e] **risk** *n term*

» In the preoperative [iː] anesthesia [iː] interview[1] the anesthetic risk can be estimated by a precise history[2] of the patient's previous [iː] experiences with anesthesia, eliciting[3] data on allergic reactions, delayed awakening[4], prolonged paralysis from neuromuscular blocking agents, etc.

Use overall **anesthetic risk**

Narkoserisiko

Anästhesiesprechstunde[1] Anamnese[2] erheben, erfragen[3] verzögertes Erwachen[4]

---

anesthetic induction [ʌ] *n term*

period from the start of anesthesia to the establishment of a depth of anesthesia[1] sufficient [ɪʃ] for surgery

induce[2] [ɪndʉːs] *v term* • inductive [ɪndʌktɪv] *adj*

» Unless the patient has ingested [dʒe] solid food[3], it is reasonable to allow clear fluids[4] orally up to 2 hours before induction of anesthesia. General anesthesia can be induced by IV drugs, by inhalation, or a combination of both methods. Rapid-sequence [iː] induction[5] minimizes the time during which the trachea [treɪkɪə] is unprotected.

Use **anesthetic induction** agent / regimen[6] [edʒ] • **induction** of general anesthesia • inhalation / combined intravenous-inhalation **induction**

Narkoseeinleitung

Narkosetiefe[1] einleiten[2] feste Nahrung zu sich genommen[3] Flüssigkeiten[4] kurze Anflutungszeit[5] Einleitungsschema[6]

---

anesthesia machine *n term*   *rel* **anesthetic circuit**[1] [sɜːrkɪt] *n term*

apparatus complete with flowmeters[2] [iː], vaporizers[3] [eɪ], and sources of compressed gases used for inhalation anesthesia[4]; connected with the mechanisms for elimination of carbon dioxide[5] [aɪ] and the anesthetic circuit (reservoir bag, directional valves[6] [vælvz], breathing tubes[7] [iː], CO_2 absorber)

» Malfunction of the anesthesia machine may lead to increased pressures which results in pneumothorax [nʲuː-] in the patient.

Narkosegerät, -apparat

Narkosesystem[1] Gasflussmesser, Rotameter[2] Verdampfer, -nebler[3] Inhalationsnarkose[4] Kohlendioxid[5] Richtungsventile[6] Atemschläuche[7]

RELATED MEDICAL SPECIALTIES — Basic Terms in Anesthesiology

anesthesia bag *and* **mask** n term   sim **breathing** [iː] *or* **reservoir bag**[1] n term
collapsible[2] reservoir for inhaling [eɪ] and exhaling[3] gases during general anesthesia or artificial ventilation[4]
» Check for a leak[5] [iː] between the endotracheal tube and the larynx by connecting a pressure-monitored anesthesia bag to the circuit and allow it to inflate[6] [eɪ].
Use self-refilling **bag-mask** combination / unit • **bag-valve** mask • Ambu[7] **bag**

Narkosemaske
Atembeutel[1] faltbar, zusammenklappbar[2] ausatmen[3] künstliche Beatmung[4] Leck, undichte Stelle[5] aufblasen, sich füllen[6] Ambubeutel[7]
15

infusion pump [ʌ] n term
apparatus to deliver measured [eɜ] amounts[1] [aʊ] of anesthetics or drugs over a period of time
» The dosage for adults is given as a continuous intravenous infusion[2] via[3] an infusion pump.
Use intravenous [iː]/ subcutaneous [eɪ]/ implantable[4] / constant / portable[5] / home **infusion pump**

Infusions-, Spritzenpumpe
definierte Mengen abgeben / einleiten[1] Dauerinfusion[2] mittels, über[3] implantierbare Infusionspumpe[4] tragbare Infusionsp.[5]
16

intubate [ɪntʲuːbeɪt] v term
inserting[1] an oro- or nasotracheal tube for anesthesia to prevent aspiration and/or control pulmonary [ʊ∥ʌ] ventilation
intubation n term • intubator[2] n • extubate v
» Use of sedation alone to intubate a patient in the ER[3] can be difficult and risky. If the patient has no gag reflex[4], intubate the trachea with a cuffed [ʌ] endotracheal tube[5] to protect the airway[6].
Use to facilitate **intubation** • **intubation** tube[7] • (endo-, oro-, naso-)tracheal / low-pressure cuff / blind / controlled[8] / digital[9] **intubation** • **intubated** orally *or* via the mouth / patient • experienced **intubator** • **intubator's** skill[10] / hand / finger

intubieren
einführen[1] intubierende(r) Arzt/ Ärztin[2] Notaufnahme[3] Würgreflex[4] Endotrachealtubus m. Manschette[5] Atemwege[6] Tubus, Intubationsrohr[7] Intubation unter Sicht[8] I. unter digitaler Kontrolle[9] Können d. intubierenden Arztes/Ärztin[10]
17

Esmarch [k] **tourniquet** [tɜːrnɪkət] n term   syn **Esmarch's bandage** *or* **wrap** [ræp] n term
broad elastic bandage or rubber with a chain fastener[1] [fæsənɚ] wrapped around a limb as a tourniquet[2]
» An Esmarch tourniquet was used to create a blood-free field for the procedure.
Use **Esmarch** maneuver[3] [uː] • to apply/use/release[4] [iː]/loosen[5] [uː]/remove **a tourniquet** • **tourniquet** time / ischemia [skiː]/ constriction / inflation[6] / effect

Esmarch Binde
Kettenverschluss[1] Stauschlauch, -manschette, Tourniquet[2] Esmarch-Blutsperre, -leere[3] Stauschlauch lösen[4] S. lockern[5] Aufblasen d. Staumanschette[6]
18

loading dose n term   rel **maintenance dose**[1] n term
relatively large dose given initially to induce anesthesia (or initiate [ɪnɪʃɪeɪt] drug therapy)
» A loading dose of 1mg/kg by bolus intravenous infusion[2] is followed by a maintenance dose of 1-4 mg/min by continuous intravenous infusion[3].

Initialdosis
Erhaltungsdosis[1] i.v. Schnellinfusion[2] i.v. Dauerinfusion[3]
19

depth [depθ] *or* **level of anesthesia** n term
classified in four stages (analgesia[1], delirium[2], surgical anesthesia[3] with 4 planes[4] [eɪ], overdose[5])
» Stage II anesthesia is marked by loss of consciousness and the lid reflex[6], excitement[7] of which may be associated with vomiting and laryngospasm. Complications with endotracheal intubabtion can be minimized by ensuring [ʃʊɚ] that the depth of anesthesia is adequate.
Use to monitor[8]/assess[9] **the depth of anesthesia** • adequate **depth of anesthesia** • to produce the desired **depth of anesthesia**

Narkosetiefe
Analgesiestadium[1] Exzitationsstadium[2] Toleranzstadium[3] Unterstufen[4] Asphyxiestadium[5] Lidrandreflex[6] Auslösung[7] N. überwachen[8] N. überprüfen[9]
20

emergence [ɪmɜːrdʒəns] n term   sim **recovery**[1] [ʌ] n term
return to spontaneous [eɪ] respiration, voluntary swallowing, consciousness, etc. following general anesthesia
» In children this drug can cause adverse[2] [ɜː] behavioral reactions upon emergence from sedation.
Use **emergence** delirium • postanesthesia (abbr PAR) **recovery** • **recovery** room (abbr RR) *or* area[3] / period

Aufwachphase
Erwachen (aus Narkose)[1] ungünstig[2] Aufwachraum[3]
21

anesthesia record n term
written account[1] [aʊ] of drugs administered, procedures undertaken, and cardiovascular responses during surgical or obstetric anesthesia[2]

Narkoseprotokoll
Aufzeichnungen[1] geburtshilfliche Anästhesie[2]
22

Types of Anesthesia & Anesthetics   **RELATED MEDICAL SPECIALTIES** 173

postanesthetic [e] **phase** [feɪz] *n term*
                                             syn **anesthesia** [iː] **recovery period** *n term*
period of emergence from GA during which patients are closely monitored in the RR[1]
» *The first hours immediately after the operation during which the acute reaction to surgery and the residual* [ɪ] *effects[2] of anesthesia are subsiding[3]* [aɪ] *is termed the postanesthetic observation phase of management.*
Use **postanesthetic** observation / vomiting[4] / nausea [nɒːzɪə] / hang-over[5]

Aufwachperiode
Aufwachraum[1] Restwirkungen[2] nachlassen[3] Erbrechen i.d. Aufwachperiode[4] Narkosekater[5]

23

postanesthesia care unit *n term*   *abbr* **PACU**
hospital unit equipped for meeting postoperative emergencies in which surgical patients are kept during the immediate postoperative period for care and recovery from anesthesia
» *Pulse, BP[1] and respiration of PACU patients are recorded every 15 min until stable* [eɪ].
Use **postanesthesia** nursing [ɜː]/ problems / headache / recovery area • full-intensity **PACU** care • **PACU** admission report[2] / postoperative triage [trɪɑːʒ] • discharge evaluation from **PACU** to ICU[3]

Aufwachstation
Blutdruck[1] Aufnahmebericht in der Aufwachstation[2] Entlassungsprotokoll b. Verlegung v. d. Aufwachi.d. Intensiv(pflege)station[3]

24

resuscitate [rɪsʌsɪteɪt] *v term*   *syn* **bring sb. (a)round** *phr clin*
to revive [aɪ] an unconscious person whose respirations have ceased [siːsd]
resuscitation[1] *n term* • resuscitative *adj* • resuscitator[2] *n*
» *All emergency equipment necessary to resuscitate the patient should be available. Bradycardia is a prearrest sign and necessitates aggressive resuscitation.*
Use mouth-to-mouth[3] / fluid or volume / cardiopulmonary[4] / fetus [iː]/ neonate [iː] **resuscitation** • **resuscitation** room / team / area • **resuscitative** technique [iːk]/ maneuver [uː]/ efforts

wiederbeleben, reanimieren
Reanimation[1] Beatmungsgerät; Reanimator[2] Mund-zu-Mund Beatmung[3] kardiopulmonale Reanimation[4]

25

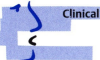
Clinical Phrases

Have you or anyone in your family ever had problems from anesthesia? Hatten Sie oder jemand in der Familie schon einmal Probleme bei einer Narkose? • Sometimes complications occur with anesthesia, but this is very rare and we will take good care of you. Sehr selten kann es im Zusammenhang mit der Narkose zu Komplikationen kommen. Aber wir werden Sie bestens versorgen! • Do you have any false teeth, removable dental caps or bridges? Haben Sie eine Zahnprothese, abnehmbare Brücken oder Kronen? • Have you had anything to eat or drink in the past 8 hours? Haben Sie in den letzten 8 Stunden etwas gegessen oder getrunken? • Now I am going to spray your throat. Ich werde jetzt Ihren Rachen einsprühen. • Then we will give you a little needle stick here and you will get numb so that you will not feel the operation. Dann werden Sie einen kleinen Stich spüren, und dieser Bereich wird sich dann taub anfühlen, so dass Sie bei der Operation keine Schmerzen haben werden. • Squeeze my hand. Hard. Harder. Drücken Sie meine Hand. Fest! Fester! • Do your legs feel numb / normal? Fühlen sich Ihre Beine taub / normal an? • Do you feel dizzy? Ist Ihnen schwindlig? • Can you wiggle your toes? Können Sie Ihre Zehen bewegen? • Do you have the taste of metal in your mouth? Haben Sie einen metallischen Geschmack im Mund?

Unit 48 Types of Anesthesia & Anesthetics
Related Units: **5** Drugs & Remedies, **20** Pharmacologic Agents, **16** Pain, **4** States of Consciousness

general anesthesia [-θiːʒə] *n term, abbr* **GA**
                                 rel **general anesthetic[1]** [e] *n term*
loss of the ability to appreciate[2] [iːʃ] pain and unconsciousness produced by anesthetic agents
» *With the patient under GA, the exteriorized bowel* [aʊ] *was rinsed[3] with Ringer's lactate solution[4]. In large amounts Midazolam (a short-acting benzodiazepine) is a general anesthetic.*
Use to undergo/require/necessitate[5]/tolerate/induce/maintain[6]/recover from/awake from **general anesthesia** • inhalation **general anesthetics** • closed manipulation / dissection[7] / rigid [dʒ] bronchoscopy / open biopsy [aɪ]/ patients **under general anesthesia**

Allgemeinanästhesie, (Voll)narkose
Anästhetikum, Narkotikum[1] empfinden[2] Darm wurde gespült[3] Ringer-Laktat-Lösung[4] (Voll)narkose erfordern[5] Narkose aufrechterhalten[6] Präparation in/unter Vollnarkose[7]

1

48

174 RELATED MEDICAL SPECIALTIES — Types of Anesthesia & Anesthetics

balanced anesthesia n term

technique of GA based on the concept that administration of a mixture of small amounts of different anesthetics summates[1] [ʌ] the advantages but not the disadvantages of the individual agents

» Following premedication[2] and induction by thiopentone [θaɪə-], balanced anesthesia was maintained by a combination of muscle relaxants, inhalational and IV anesthetic agents.

balancierte Anästhesie
vereint[1] Prämedikation[2]

[2]

local anesthesia n term, abbr LA   sim regional [riːdʒ-] anesthesia[1] n term

anesthesia of the operative site produced by direct infiltration of a local anesthetic into the area of small, terminal nerve endings or, rarely, by freezing[2] (cryoanesthesia[3] [kraɪoʊ-])

» A regional anesthetic is used when it is desirable that the patient remain conscious during the operation. If the FB[4] can be palpated, local anesthesia is given by means of submucosal and s.c. injections[5] of 0.5% bupivacaine.

Use to be a good candidate for **anesthesia** • topical[6] / periodontal / axillary / sacral [eɪ]/ girdle[7] [ɜː]/ stocking[8] [ɒː]/ glove[9] [ʌ] **anesthesia** • pharyngeal [dʒɪəl]/ segmental / unilateral / visceral [s] or splanchnic[10] [k]/ corneal / infiltration[11] **anesthesia**

Lokalanästhesie
Regionalanästhesie[1] Vereisen[2] Kälteanästhesie[3] Fremdkörper[4] subkutane Injektion[5] Oberflächen-, Lokalanästhesie[6] gürtelf. A.[7] strumpff. A.[8] handschuhförmige Anästhesie[9] Splanchnikusanästhesie[10] Infiltrationsanästhesie[11]

[3]

anesthetic [ænəsθetɪk] n & adj term   syn anesthetic agent [eɪdʒənt] n term

(n) compounds that reversibly depress nerve function and produce loss of ability to perceive[1] [iː] pain and/or other sensations; also collective term for anesthetizing agents administered to an individual at a particular time (adj, i) characterized by or capable of producing loss of sensation (ii) associated with or due to the state of anesthesia

» Most anesthetics delay[2] healing. If available, instill local anesthetic drops. All local anesthetics have CNS toxicities including confusion[3], coma, and seizures[4] [siːʒɚz].

Use to give/administer **anesthetics** • **anesthetic** medication / agent / drugs / solution / gargles[5] / ether [iː] / area / block / approach[6] / effect / properties / risk / shock / mishap or accident • short-acting[7] / long-acting **anesthetics** • general / topical / inhalation / flammable[8] / volatile[9] / gaseous[10] / intravenous [iː]/ primary / secondary / spinal / highly potent / halogenated [dʒ] **anesthetics** • delivery of[11] **anesthetics** • **anesthetic**-related complications /-induced convulsions[12] / cardiac arrest

Narkose-, Betäubungsmittel, Anästhetikum, Narkotikum; anästhesierend, betäubend, gefühllos, unempfindlich
empfinden, wahrnehmen[1] verzögern[2] Verwirrtheit[3] (Krampf)-anfälle[4] anästhesierendes Gurgelmittel[5] Anästhesieverfahren[6] Kurznarkotika[7] brennbare Anästhetika[8] volatile A.[9] Inhalationsanästhetika[9] gasförm. Narkotika, Narkosegase[10] Zufuhr von Narkotika[11] anästhesiemittelbedingte Krämpfe[12]

[4]

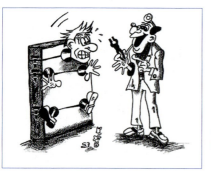

Don't worry, Mr. Pym, next week our supply of anesthetics will arrive on time again.

lidocaine [laɪdəkeɪn] (hydrochloride) [aɪ] n term
syn espBE **lignocaine** [ɪ] n term

crystalline compound[1] used as a local anesthetic with pronounced[2] [aʊ] antiarrhythmic [ɪ] and anticonvulsant [ʌ] properties[3]

» Anesthetize the skin with 1% lidocaine with the 10mL syringe and the 25-gauge [eɪ] needle. Injection of a local anesthetic such as lidocaine into the trigger point[4] site often results in pain relief. Lidocaine, tetracaine and cocaine [koʊkeɪn] are the most common choices for topical anesthesia of the airway, while procaine is too poorly absorbed to be effective topically.

Use topical / intranasal[5] [eɪ]/ 0.5% / viscous[6] [sk] **lidocaine** • **lidocaine** solution / infusion / periarticular infiltration / jelly[7] [dʒ]/ overdose / poisoning • to instill[8]/inject/administer **lidocaine**

Lidocain
Verbindung[1] ausgeprägt[2] krampflösende Eigenschaften[3] Triggerpunkt[4] intranasal verabreichtes L.[5] visköses L.[6] Lidocain-Gel[7] Lidocain einträufeln / instillieren[8]

[5]

Types of Anesthesia & Anesthetics

conduction [ʌ] or **block anesthesia** *n term*   *syn* **blockade** [-eɪd] or **blockage** [-ɪdʒ] *n term*

regional anesthesia in which a local anesthetic is injected about nerves[1] to inhibit nerve transmission; includes spinal, epidural, nerve block, and field block anesthesia[2], but not local or topical anesthesia

» Local wound [uː] infiltration or regional nerve block with 0.5% bupivacaine will help alleviate the pain. A postpartum hemorrhage is best treated by dilation and curettage using paracervical block anesthesia[3]. In patients with mitral [aɪ] valve disease conduction anesthesia is preferred to preclude[4] complications during labor[5] and delivery[6]. In a combative[7] patient, use of neuromuscular blockade provides good control of the airway.

Use sympathetic[8] / parasacral [eɪ] / pudendal[9] / caudal [ɔː] / nasopalatine / (sub)lingual nerve / saddle[10] / inferior [ɪɚ] alveolar **block (anesthesia)** • neuromuscular / ganglionic **blocking agent** or **blocker**[11] • field[2] / cholinergic[12] [kɒːlɪnɜːrdʒɪk]/ profound[13] **blockage**

Leitungsanästhesie
Nerven werden umspritzt[1] Feldblock[2] Parazervikalblockade[3] ausschließen[4] Wehen[5] Entbindung[6] aggressiv[7] Sympathikusblockade[8] Pudendusblock[9] Sattelblock[10] Ganglienblocker[11] Cholinrezeptorenblockade[12] stark ausgeprägter Block[13]

6

spinal [spaɪnᵊl] **anesthesia** *n term*   *syn* **subarachnoid** [æk] **(block) anesthesia** *n term*

anesthesia produced by injection of local anesthetics into the spinal subarachnoid space[1]

» Predisposing[2] factors of CNS infections include head and neck trauma, lumbar puncture[3] [pʌŋktʃɚ], recent neurosurgery and spinal anesthesia. Complications from epidural anesthesia are the same as those from spinal anesthesia, with the exception of headache.

Use differential / total / high[4] / low[5] / single shot / continuous[6] / intra-**spinal anesthesia**

Spinalanästhesie
spinaler Subarachnoidalraum[1] begünstigend[2] Lumbalpunktion[3] hohe Spinalanästhesie[4] tiefe S.[5] kontinuierliche S.[6]

7

epidural [epɪdʊɚᵊl] **anesthesia** or **block** *n term*
   syn **peridural anesthesia** *n term*

regional anesthesia produced by injection of a local anesthetic into the extradural space that blocks the spinal nerve roots

» Epidural anesthesia may be preferable when a low spinal level[1] is adequate for the procedure.

Use spinal[2]/ fractional [ækʃ]/ postoperative / lumbar **epidural anesthesia** • extradural **anesthesia** • epidural / spinal **block**

Epi-, Periduralanästhesie
Anästhesie im lumbalen Bereich[1] Epiduralspinalanästhesie (ESA)[2]

8

barbotage [bɑːrbətɑːʒ] *n term*

repeated alternate injection and withdrawal of fluid with a syringe[1]; for spinal anesthesia a portion of an anesthetic agent is injected into the CSF[2], and some CSF is withdrawn[3] [ɔːn] into the syringe until the entire contents of the syringe are injected; the technique is also used for gastric lavage[4]

Barbotage
Spritze[1] Liquor[2] aspiriert, abgesaugt[3] Magenspülung[4]

9

inhalation [eɪ] **anesthesia** *n term*   *sim* **insufflation anesthesia**[1] *n term*

anesthesia effected by inspiration or insufflation of volatile anesthetics (gases or vapors[2] [eɪ]) into the respiratory tract using special delivery systems[3]

» Inhalation anesthesia where the gases exhaled by the patient are rebreathed[4] [iː] as some carbon dioxide [daɪə-] is simultaneously [eɪ] removed and anesthetic gas and oxygen [ɒːksɪdʒən] are added so that no anesthetic escapes into the room is termed closed circuit anesthesia[5]. The advantage of inhalation anesthesia is that the anesthetics can be titrated[6] [aɪ] according to the patient's needs.

Use **inhalation** anesthetics[7] / induction / agents[7] • combined intravenous-**inhalation anesthesia**

Inhalationsnarkose
Insufflationsnarkose[1] Dämpfe[2] Narkosesysteme[3] wieder eingeatmet[4] geschlossenes Narkosesystem[5] titriert[6] Inhalationsanästhetika, -narkotika[7]

10

nitrous [aɪ] **oxide** [aɪ] *n term*   *syn* **(laughing** [læfɪŋ]**) gas** *n term*

colorless gas (N_2O) producing loss of sensibility to pain on inhalation which is preceded [iː] by exhilaration[1] and sometimes laughter; widely used as a rapidly acting, rapidly reversible, nondepressant and nontoxic inhalation analgesic [dʒiː] to supplement[2] [ʌ] other anesthetics and analgesics, e.g. in dentistry

» For routine delivery[3] analgesia with 40% nitrous oxide may be used as long as verbal contact with the patient is maintained. Nitrous oxide/oxygen and local anesthesia was used in 8 patients, IV sedation in 15, and no anesthetic at all in one patient. Since nitrous oxide does not provide total anesthesia, it is given in combination with a volatile anesthetic or narcotic.

Use **nitrous oxide** inhalation • oxygen-**nitrous oxide** mix[4]

Distickstoffoxid, Lachgas
Hochstimmung[1] ergänzen, verstärken[2] Entbindung[3] Sauerstoff-Lachgas-Gemisch[4]

11

48

Types of Anesthesia & Anesthetics

halothane [hæləθeɪn] n term

a widely used potent nonflammable [æ] and nonexplosive inhalation anesthetic with rapid onset and reversal; largely supplanted by[1] later-generation halogenated [dʒ] hydrocarbon[2] [aɪ] anesthetics

» The side effects of halothane include cardiovascular and respiratory depression[3], and sensitization to epinephrine-induced[4] arrhythmias [ɪ]. Anesthesia was maintained with halothane and nitrous oxide.

Use **halothane** administration / anesthesia / hepatotoxicity[5] / metabolites / reactions

Halothan
verdrängt durch[1] Halogenkohlenwasserstoff[2] Atemdepression[3] adrenalinbedingt[4] halothanbedingte Leberschädigung[5]

12

intravenous [iː] **anesthesia** n term   rel **endotracheal** [eɪk] **anesthesia**[1] n term

anesthesia produced by injection of anesthetic agents into the venous [iː] circulation

» Patients with a normal airway[2] may be intubated under intravenous anesthesia.

intravenöse Anästhesie
Endotracheal-, Intubationsnarkose[1] Atemwege[2]

13

barbiturates [ɪtʃə] n term   syn **sleeping pills** n clin

derivatives of barbituric acid (including phenobarbital [fiːnoʊ-]) that act as CNS depressants and are used for their tranquilizing[1], hypnotic[2] [ɪ], and anti-seizure[3] [iːʒ] effects; most barbiturates have the potential for abuse[4]

» Sedation can be achieved[5] by barbiturates, benzodiazepine or narcotics. Long-acting barbiturates (6-8 h) also include methobarbital, barbital, and primidone.

Use short-acting[6] / rapidly acting / IV **barbiturates** • **barbiturate** sedatives / withdrawal[7] / overdose / intoxication / poisoning / syndrome [ɪ]/ therapy

Barbiturate, Schlafmittel
sedierend, beruhigend[1] hypnotisch, schlaffördernd[2] antikonvulsiv, antiepileptisch[3] Missbrauch[4] erzielt, erreicht[5] kurzwirkende B.[6] Barbituratentzug[7]

14

basal [eɪ] **anesthesia** n term

parenteral administration of one or more sedatives to produce a state of depressed consciousness prior to[1] induction [Δ] of GA

» A patient under basal anesthesia does not respond to words but still reacts to pinprick[2] stimulation.

Basisnarkose
vor[1] Nadelstich[2]

15

muscle [mʌsl] **relaxants** n term

agents capable of relaxing striated [straɪeɪtɪd] muscle[1]; includes drugs acting at the spinal [aɪ] cord level or directly on muscle to decrease tone[2], as well as the neuromuscular relaxants

» Muscle relaxants act mainly as CNS depressants[3], inhibiting spinal synaptic reflexes, prolonging synaptic recovery time, and reducing repetitive discharges[4].

Use (non)depolarizing[5] / skeletal or striated / smooth[6] [uː] **muscle relaxant**

Muskelrelaxanzien
quergestreifte Muskulatur[1] Muskeltonus[2] zentral dämpfende Mittel[3] wiederholte Depolarisation[4] (nicht) depolarisierendes Muskelrelaxans[5] auf die glatte Muskulatur wirkendes Relaxans[6]

16

(tubo)curare [tʲuːboʊ-] n term   sim **tubocurarine**[1] [-kjʊəˈɑːrɪn] n term

toxic alkaloid (chief active constituent[2] of the arrow poison[3] curare) that produces nondepolarizing paralysis of skeletal muscle after IV injection by blocking transmission at the myoneural [aɪ] junction[4] [dʒʌŋkʃⁿn]; used clinically (e.g., as d-tubocurarine chloride [aɪ], metocurine iodide [aɪə]) to provide muscle relaxation during surgical operations

» Sedation, paralysis with curare-like agents, and mechanical ventilation[5] [kæ] are often required to control tetanus spasms.

(Tubo)curare
Tubocurarin[1] Bestandteil[2] Pfeilgift[3] motor. Endplatte, neuromuskuläre Synapse[4] künstliche Beatmung[5]

17

acupuncture analgesia n term   rel **acupressure**[1] n term

placement of acupuncture needles at specific points in the body to produce a loss of sensation of pain, e.g. for surgical procedures by blocking afferent nerve impulses

» Acupuncture anesthesia and the placebo [siː] effect may be mediated[2] [iː] in part by endorphins.

Use pressure **analgesia** • pressure[3] / acupuncture[4] **anesthesia**

Akupunkturanalgesie
Akupressur[1] vermittelt[2] Akupressuranästhesie[3] Akupunkturanästhesie[4]

18

Unit 49 Basic Terms in Plastic Surgery
Related Units: 50 Grafts & Flaps, 21 Surgical Treatment, 22 Basic Operative Techniques, 45 Maxillofacial Surgery

reconstruction n term syn **restoration** n, **repair** [rɪpeɚ·] n & v term

surgical [sɜːrdʒɪkˀl] restoration of diseased or damaged tissues

reconstruct[1] v • restore v • reconstructive adj • restorative adj

» Primary attempts to reconstruct the stellate [steleɪt] wound[2] [uː] with local flaps failed[3].

Use facial [feɪʃˀl]/ scalp / nasal [eɪ]/ ear[4] / lip / eyelid / digital[5] [dʒ] **reconstruction** • primary / secondary / one-stage / cosmetic / postablative[6] [eɪ] **reconstruction** • bladder / hernia[7] [ɜː] **repair** • **reconstructive** mammoplasty[8]

-plastik, Rekonstruktion, Wiederherstellung
wiederherstellen, rekonstruieren[1] sternförmige Wunde[2] fehlschlagen, nicht gelingen[3] Ohr-, Otoplastik[4] Fingerplastik[5] R. nach Amputation[6] Hernioplastik[7] Mammaaufbau-(plastik)[8]
1

surgical correction n term sim **replacement**[1], **rehabilitation**[2] n term

surgical procedure [prəsiːdʒɚ] that repairs or modifies traumatized [ɒː], diseased or undesirable body structures

correct[3] v term • corrective adj

» Correction may be done with simultaneous reduction or augmentation[4] [ɒː]. The defect was corrected by splenectomy. The use of implants as a foundation for prosthetic [e] replacement of missing teeth has become widespread. Geriatric [dʒ] amputees[5] [iː] were rarely rehabilitated.

Use elective **correction** • surgically **correctable** • **corrective** osteotomy[6] / procedure / repair / measures [eʒ] • **replacement** bone[7] / graft / prosthesis [iː]/ tooth • stomach[8] [k] **replacement** • facial / cardiac / oral or dental[9] / bladder / prosthetic[10] **rehabilitation** • auditory [ɒː]/ speech / (psycho)social [saɪk] / partial / postoperative **rehabilitation** • **rehabilitation** center

operative Korrektur
Ersatz, Prothese[1] Wiederherstellung[2] beheben, korrigieren[3] Aufbau, Vergrößerung[4] Amputierte[5] Korrekturosteotomie[6] Ersatzknochen[7] Ersatzmagenbildung[8] orale Rehabilitation[9] prothetische Versorgung, Protheseneinbau[10]
2

plastic surgery n term syn **reconstructive surgery** n term

surgical specialty or procedure concerned with the restoration, construction, reconstruction, or improvement in the shape and appearance [ɪɚ] of missing, defective, damaged, or mishappen[1] body structures

-plasty[2] comb • neo- [niːoʊ] comb

» Neither plastic surgery nor prosthetic rehabilitation has provided a good cosmetic outcome[3].

Use **plastic** surgeon[4] / closure [ʒ]/ repair / revision [ɪʒ] • esthetic[5] **plastic surgery** • angio[6] [ændʒɪɚ-]/ arthro/ oto[7]/ gastro/ stricture/ Z-[8]/ valvulo**plasty**[9] • **neo**bladder[10]

Wiederherstellungs-, plastische Chirurgie
missgebildet[1] -plastik, -plastie[2] kosmetisches Ergebnis[3] plast. Chirurg(in)[4] ästhetische plastische Chirurgie[5] Angioplastie[6] Ohrplastik[7] Z-Plastik[8] Valvuloplastie[9] Neoblase[10]
3

fashion [fæʃˀn] v & n term syn **shape, create** [ieɪ], **tailor** [eɪ], sim **remodel**[1] v term

preshaped[2] [iː] adj term • reshaped adj

» The flap is fashioned to avoid tension[3] [ʃ] when the wound is closed. The surgically created defects were too large and did not heal without membrane coverage [kʌvɚɪdʒ].

Use **fashioned** flap • in **a(n)** similar / stepwise[4] / retrograde / sequential[4] [-ʃˀl]/ routine / piecemeal[5] / uncontrolled / tongue-like [tʌŋ] **fashion** • poorly[6] **fashioned** • arrow[7] / wedge[8] [dʒ] / cone [oʊ]/ funnel[9] [ʌ]/ horseshoe[10] / oval / loop[11] [uː]/ L-/ acorn[12] [eɪkɔːrn]/ irregularly **shaped** • **to create** space[13] / tunnels [ʌ]/ windows / grooves[14] [uː]/ smooth [uː] surfaces / tension / flaps

formen, zurechtschneiden; Form, Art, Weise
umformen[1] vorgeformt[2] Zug vermeiden[3] schrittweise[4] Stück für Stück; stückweise[5] ungünstig geformt[6] pfeilförmig[7] keilf.[8] trichterf.[9] hufeisenf.[10] schlingen-, schleifenf.[11] eichelförmig[12] Platz schaffen[13] Furchen bilden[14]
4

coaptation [koʊæpteɪʃˀn] n term → U26-5

joining[1] or approximating[2] two structures, e.g. the lips of a wound or nerve stumps[3] [ʌ], etc.

coapt[4] v term • coapted adj

» Intraoperative factors such as proper coaptation, hemostasis [eɪ], and suture line tension[5] determine the outcome[6]. The soft tissues were coapted using the sutures of choice[7].

Use nerve / skin **coaptation** • **coaptation** suture[8]

Adaptation, Wiedervereinigung
Verbinden[1] Adaptieren[2] Stümpfe[3] adaptieren, annähern[4] Nahtspannung[5] sind entscheidend für das Ergebnis[6] Nahtmaterial der Wahl[7] Adaptationsnaht[8]
5

178 RELATED MEDICAL SPECIALTIES — Basic Terms in Plastic Surgery

anastomosis n term, pl **-ses**   sim **shunt**[1] [ʌ] n term

(i) surgical union of two hollow or tubular structures (ii) connection created by surgery, trauma, or disease between normally separate spaces or organs (iii) natural communication[2] between two blood vessels

anastomose[3] v term • anastomotic adj • anastomosed adj

» Recurrent [ɜː] anastomotic stricture[4] [-tʃɚ] is usually due to gastroesophageal [-dʒiːəl] reflux.

Use arteriovenous [iː]/ portocaval [eɪ]/ cavopulmonary / microvascular / primary / side-to-side[5] / end-to-side / end-to-end / Roux-en-Y[6] / stapled[7] [eɪ] **anastomosis** • **anastomotic** disruption / leakage[8] [liːkɪdʒ]/ failure[9] / patency[10] [eɪ]/ ulcer [ʌlsɚ]

Anastomose
Shunt, A-V Anastomose[1] Verbindung[2] anastomosieren[3] Anastomosenverengung[4] Seit-zu-Seit-A.[5] Roux-Y Operation[6] geklammerte A.[7] Anastomosenleck[8] Anastomoseninsuffizienz[9] Anastomosendurchgängikeit[10]

6

-pexy comb   sim **suspension**[1] n term

combining form referring to lifting or fixation by surgical suturing

» Contralateral orchiopexy[2] [k] is necessary because of the high incidence of recurrent torsion.

Use orchi(d)o[2] [k]/ masto/ gastropexy • uterine [ɪ‖aɪ] **suspension** • **suspension** wire[3] [waɪɚ]/ sling[4]

-fixation, -anheftung, -pexie
Aufhängung, Suspension[1] Orchi(do)pexie[2] Suspensionsdraht[3] Suspensionsschlinge[4]

7

---

plication [plaɪkeɪʃən] n term   sim **intussusception**[1] [se], **invagination**[1] [-vædʒ-] n term

procedure involving folding, ensheathing[2] [iːð], or inserting a structure within itself or another

plicated adj term • plica[3] n pl -ae [plaɪsiː‖kiː] • invaginate v • intussusceptum[4] n

» There are signs of epithelial [iː] invagination. Vaginal [dʒ] hysterectomy with anterior colporrhaphy[5] (urethral [iː] suspension, plication of the bladder neck[6], and cystocele [-siːl] repair) was indicated.

Use fundal[7] [ʌ] **plication** • **plication** suture[8] • **invaginated** ileum / epithelium

Plikation
Intussuszeption, Invagination, Einstülpung[1] Einscheiden[2] Falte, Plica[3] Intussuszeptum, Invaginat[4] vordere Kolporrhaphie[5] Blasenhals[6] Funduseinstülpung[7] Duplikatur-, Verstärkungsnaht[8]

8

---

skin coverage [kʌvɚɪdʒ] n term

spreading [e] skin grafts or flaps over exposed or denuded[1] [uː] areas

(un)cover[2] [ʌ] v term • covering[3] n • covered[4] adj

» Obtaining good skin coverage for these burns[5] will be difficult. The flap was repeatedly checked to ensure [ɪnʃʊɚ] coverage of the area without tension.

Use soft tissue / bone / flap[6] / wound[7] [uː] **coverage**

Note: The term coverage is also used as a synonym for protection, e.g. in health insurance coverage[8] or antibiotic coverage[9].

Hautdeckung
freigelegt[1] bedecken, überziehen; bloßlegen[2] Hülle, Deckschicht[3] gedeckt[4] Verbrennungen[5] Lappendeckung[6] Wundabdeckung[7] Krankenversicherung[8] antibiotische Abschirmung[9]

9

---

tissue [tɪʃuː‖tɪsjuː] **expansion** [æ] n term   rel **line of minimum tension**[1] n term

» Tissue expansion techniques should be reserved for complicated cases of decubitus ulcers[2]. An incision placed parallel to the skin lines of minimal tension will yield[3] [jiːld] the best results.

Use **tissue** expander[4] • controlled **tissue expansion**

Gewebedehnung
Linie d. geringsten Spannung[1] Dekubitalgeschwüre[2] bringen, erzielen[3] Gewebeexpander[4]

10

---

elevate v term   syn **raise** [reɪz] v term

(i) to dissect skin, etc. away from the underlying[1] [aɪ] tissue
(ii) increase (iii) lift up to a higher position

elevation[2] n term

» The middle line of the incision in a Z-plasty is made along the line of greatest tension, and triangular [aɪ] flaps are raised and transposed[3]. Seromas often follow operations that involve elevation of skin flaps.

Use **raised** margins[4] / pressure[5] / plaques[6] [plæks] • leg[7] / bite[8]-**raising** • surgical / shoulder / BP[9] / leg[7] **elevation**

(an)heben
darunterliegend[1] Heben; Erhöhung; Erhebung[2] transponiert[3] angehobene Ränder[4] erhöhter Druck[5] erhabene Plaque[6] Hochlagern d. Beins[7] Bisshebung[8] Erhöhung d. Blutdrucks[9]

11

---

harvest v & n term   sim **explant**[1] v term

(v) to collect tissue from a donor site[2] [aɪ] for transplantation

harvesting n term • explant[3] n • explantation[4] n

» Bone marrow[5] was harvested by repeated aspiration from the posterior iliac [ɪlɪæk] crest[6].

Use graft[7] / bone **harvest** • **harvest** organ[8] / tissue / technique • to be **harvested** from

(Gewebe) entnehmen; Entnahme
explantieren[1] Spenderareal[2] Explantat[3] Explantation[4] Knochenmark[5] Darmbeinkamm, Crista iliaca[6] Transplantatentnahme[7] entnommenes Organ[8]

12

Basic Terms in Plastic Surgery RELATED MEDICAL SPECIALTIES **179**

transpose v term   syn **transfer** v term

to remove tissues or organs from their anatomic position and graft them to a different site

transposable adj term • transfer[1] n • transposition(ing)[1] n

» The LD muscle[2] [s] can be detached[3] [tʃ] from its origin and transposed to the anterior chest. Avoidance of folding or kinking[4], transposition with minimal tension, and proper length-to-width ratio [reɪʃ(ɪ)oʊ] are key considerations in the technique of elevation and transposition of flaps.

Use toe-to-thumb[5] [θʌm]/ nerve / embryo / free-tissue[6] **transfer** • **transposition** flap[7] / of the great vessels • nerve[8] **transpositioning**

verpflanzen, übertragen
Verpflanzung, Übertragung[1]
M. latissimus dorsi[2] abgelöst[3]
Knicken[4] Nicoladoni-Operation[5]
freie Gewebeübertragung[6]
Transpositionslappen[7]
Nervtransposition[8]

13

transplant [trænsplænt] v, [træns-] n term

(v) to transfer or graft tissues from a donor [oʊ] to a recipient
(n) tissue or organ which is transposed

(re[1]/auto[2])transplantation n term • (non)transplanted[3] adj
• (pre/post)transplant adj

» Dialysis [daɪælɪsɪs] and renal transplantation afford[4] excellent survival in patients with ESRD[5]. Carefully selected patients in their 60s have undergone transplantation successfully.

Use **transplant** surgery / recipient[6] / patient / candidate / failure[7] / center / setting / kidney[8] • to undergo **transplantation** • **transplant-related** morbidity / complications • organ / heart / renal or kidney / bone marrow[9] (abbr BMT) / single lung **transplant(ation)** • **pretransplant** transfusion / management • **posttransplant** course / immunosuppression • **(non)transplant** patient / organ / tissue / kidney

transplantieren, Transplantat
Retransplantation[1] Autotransplantation[2] transplantiert[3] ermöglichen[4] End-stage renal disease, terminale Niereninsuffizienz[5] Transplantatempfänger(in)[6] Transplantatversagen[7] Transplantationsniere[8] Knochenmarktransplantation[9]

14

donor [doʊnɚ]n term   opposite **recipient**[1] [rɪsɪpiənt] n term

organism from whom blood, tissue, or an organ is taken for transfusion or transplantation

donate[2] v term • donation[3] n • donated adj

» Adequate amounts of donor bone were harvested from the iliac crest. Excess tissue[4] (dog ears) at the recipient site must be meticulously trimmed[5].

Use **donor** site[6] [aɪ]/ area / tissue / screening / selection[7] / marrow / hospital / (pledge [dʒ]) card[8] • heart / matched[9] / (HLA-identical) sibling[10] / universal[11] **donor** • tissue / (directed) blood / (vital or cadaver) organ[12] / replacement **donation** • **recipient** site[13]

Spender(in)
Empfänger(in)[1] spenden[2] Spende[3]
überschüssiges Gewebe[4] sorgfältig zurechtgeschnitten[5] Spenderstelle[6]
Spenderauswahl[7] Organspenderausweis[8] passende(r) Spender(in)[9]
genetisch idente(r) Geschwisterspender(in)[10] Universalspender(in)[11] Leichenorganspende[12]
Empfängerareal[13]

15

autologous [-gəs] or **autogenous** [ɒːdʒ] adj term   rel **homologous** or **homogenous**[1] adj term

referring to a transplant in which the donor and recipient areas are in the same individual

» The previously[2] harvested chips of autologous bone[3] were grafted into two implant sites.

Use **autologous** graft[4] / tissue • **homologous** insemination / serum [ɪɚ] jaundice[5] [dʒɔːndɪs]

autogen, autolog
allogen[1] vorher[2]
autologe Knochenspäne[3] Autograft[4]
homologer Serumikterus[5]

16

cadaver [æ] **donor** n term   opposite **living donor**[1] n term

a brain dead donor[2] from whom viable[3] [vaɪəbl] tissue or organs are harvested

cadaveric adj term

» These recipients of cadaver organs[4] do not benefit from[5] pretransplant transfusions.

Use **cadaver** kidney[6] (donor) / (homo)graft • **cadaveric** transplantation • (non)related[7] **living donor** • non-heart beating[8] **cadaver donor**

Leichenspender(in)
Lebendspender(in)[1] hirntote(r)
Spender(in)[2] lebensfähig[3] Leichenorgane[4] profitieren, Nutzen ziehen[5]
Leichenniere[6] verwandte(r)
Lebendspender(in)[7] Sp. m. Herz-Kreislaufstillstand[8]

17

49

implant [ɪmplænt] v [ɪmplænt] n term → U43-2

(n) biocompatible material grafted into tissues, e.g. in orthopedics [iː] metallic or plastic devices [aɪ] employed in joint reconstruction (v) to place such a device
implantation[1] n term • implantable adj • implanted adj

» An intraocular lens is routinely implanted at the time of cataract surgery. Complications include hematoma [iː], infection, and exposure, deflation[2] or rupture of the silicone implant. If implantation is delayed, patients with complete heart block require temporary pacing[3] [peɪsɪŋ].

Use **implant** material / surgeon / denture[4] [-tʃɚ] • orbital / intraocular / penile [iː]/ cochlear [k]/ inflatable[5] [eɪ]/ breast / silicone gel [dʒ] bag / radioactive seed [iː] **implant** • surgical / endosseous or endosteal[6] / magnetic / submucosal / subperiosteal / supraperiosteal / triplant **implant** • **implantation** site • pacemaker[7] [eɪs]/ post or pin[8] **implantation** • **implantable** hearing device[9] • **implanted** defibrillator [ɪ]

implantieren; Implantat
Implantation[1] Kollabieren[2] Schrittmacherunterstützung[3] implantatgestützte Zahnprothese[4] aufblasbares I.[5] enossales I.[6] Schrittmacherimplantation[7] Stiftimplantation[8] implantierbares Hörgerät[9]

18

augmentation [ɒːɡməntɛɪʃən] n term   opposite **reduction**[1] [ʌ] n term

increasing structures in size, shape, or volume by means of grafts or implants
augmented adj term • augment v • reduce [uː] v • reduced adj

» Some patients require operative augmentation of bladder capacity by enterocystoplasty[2].

Use **augmentation** procedure / mammoplasty[3] / material • patch[4] / bone[5] / alloplastic[6] / alveolar [ɪə]/ maxillary sinus[7] [aɪ] **augmentation** • **augmented** breast

Vergrößerung, Augmentation
Reduktion, Verkleinerung[1] Blasendarmplastik[2] Mammaaugmentationsplastik[3] Patch-Plastik[4] Knochenaufbau[5] alloplast. Organvergrößerung / Augmentation[6] Sinusboden-Augmentation, Sinuslift-Operation[7]

19

(bio)inert [baɪoʊɪnɜːrt] adj term   sim **biocompatible**[1] adj term

(i) not bioactive and therefore biocompatible implant material (ii) chemicals without active properties[2], e.g. inert gases[3] (iii) drugs without pharmacologic or therapeutic [juː] effect
biocompatibility n term • bioacceptance[4] n • inertness n

» A biologically inert membrane that does not allow penetration of cells was placed.
Use **inert** (plastic) materials • implant[5] **biocompatibility**

biologisch inaktiv, bioinert
biokompatibel[1] Eigenschaften[2] Edelgase[3] reizlose Akzeptanz / Gewebeannahme[4] Gewebeverträglichkeit / Biokompatibilität d. Implantats[5]

20

Unit 50 Grafts & Flaps
Related Units: 49 Basic Terms in Plastic Surgery, 44 Oral Surgery, 43 Dental Implantology, 45 Maxillofacial Surgery

graft [æ∥BE ɑː] v & n term   syn **transplant** v & n term

(v) to transplant (n) free (unattached [tʃ]) tissue, organ or synthetics (Dacron) for transplantation
grafting n term • pre/postgraft adj • engraft[1] v • engraftment n

» Avascular [eɪ] wound [uː] beds will not accept skin grafts unless viable [vaɪəbl] periosteum or perichondrium [ɒː] is present. The grafted area may shrink[2] to 50% of its original size and both the skin graft and the surrounding tissue may become distorted[3].

Use to transfer/serve as/repair with[4]/perform[4]/place[5]/accept **a graft** • tendon / corneal / fascia [ʃ]/ nerve / fat / fascicular [sɪ]/ (osteo)periosteal / mucosal[6] / omental **graft** • anastomosed / bypass / vascularized [aɪ]/ poorly functioning / avascular **graft** • augmentation[7] [ɒː]/ autodermic[8] [ɜː]/ hyperplastic / cable / composite[9] **graft** • implantation / infusion / H-/ orthotopic / syngeneic[10] [sɪndʒəniːɪk]/ cadaver[11] **graft** • **graft** take[12] / placement / bed[13] / conduit / anastomosis / closure [ʒ] rate / infection / destruction[14] • **pregraft** suppression • **postgraft** contractions • **ungrafted** body surface

> Note: Although graft and transplant are often used synonymously, graft is usually preferred with autologous transplantation of tissues while transplant is more often used with allogeneic organ transplantation.

transplantieren, verpflanzen; Transplantat
einpflanzen[1] schrumpfen[2] verschoben[3] T. durchführen[4] T. ein-, aufbringen[5] Schleimhauttransplantat[6] Augmentationsplastik[7] autogenes Hauttransplantat[8] composite graft (Haut & Knorpel)[9] syngenes T.[10] Leichentransplantat[11] Transplantatannahme[12] Transplantatbett[13] Transplantatzerstörung[14]

1

Grafts & Flaps | **RELATED MEDICAL SPECIALTIES** 181

autogeneic [-dʒəniːɪk] **graft** *or* **autograft** *n term*
syn **autologous** [-gəs] *or* **autoplastic graft** *or* **autotransplant** *n term*
tissue or an organ transferred by grafting into a new position in the body of the same individual
» *It is prudent[1] to preserve[2] the saphenous* [fiː] *vein as a venous* [iː] *autograft for vascular repair.*
Use **spleen**[3] [iː]/ adrenal [iː]/ bone marrow[4] [æ] **autotransplantation** • conjunctival[5] [kəndʒʌŋktaɪvəl] **autografting** • **autologous** transplantation / tissue / material / bone marrow

Autotransplantat, autogenes / autologes T.
sinnvoll[1] erhalten[2] autologe Milztransplantation[3] autologe Knochenmarktranspl.[4] autologe Bindehauttranspl.[5]

2

allogeneic graft *or* **allograft** *n term*
syn **homologous** *or* **homoplastic graft** *or* **homograft** *n term*
a graft transplanted between genetically nonidentical individuals of the same species [spiːʃiːz]
» *This tends to recur* [rɪkɜːr] *in renal allografts but without marked impairment[1]* [eə] *of graft function.*
Use **allogeneic** bone marrow transplantation / transplant recipients[2] • (un)related[3] **allogeneic transplants** • **allograft** survival enhancement[4] / reaction

Allograft, -transplantat, allogenes Transplantat
Beeinträchtigung[1] allogene Transplantatempfänger[2] allogene Verwandtentransplantate[3] Verlängerung der Überlebenszeit eines Allotransplantats[4]

3

syngeneic [ɪ] **graft** *or* **isogeneic** [aɪ] **graft** *n term* syn **isologous** *or* **isoplastic graft** *n term*
tissue or organ transplanted between genetically identical individuals (i.e. identical or monozygotic [zaɪ] twins[1])
» *When donor and recipient are identical twins, there is no antigenic* [dʒe] *difference and grafts are accepted without immunosuppressive therapy.*
Use twin-to-twin **graft** • **grafts** from HLA-identical siblings[2]

Syno-, Isotransplantat, syngenes / isologes T.
eineiige Zwillinge[1] Transplantate von HLA-identen Zwillingen[2]

4

animal *or* **zooplastic** [zoʊə-] **graft** *n term* syn **xenograft** [zenə‖ziːnə-], **heterograft** *or* **xenogeneic** *or* **heterologous** *or* **heteroplastic graft** *n term*
graft of tissue from an animal to a human, e.g. porcine [pɔːrsaɪn] (pig) or canine [keɪnaɪn] (dog) grafts; xenografts are tissues transferred from one species to another
» *Extensive burns[1] may be temporarily covered[2] by a biologic dressing, e.g. a porcine xenograft which is bacteriostatic and helps control pain.*
Use **heterodermic** graft[3]

Tier-, Xenotransplantat, xenogenes T.
großflächige Verbrennungen[1] (ab)gedeckt[2] heterologes Hauttransplantat[3]

5

skin graft *n term* sim **dermal graft**[1] [ɜː] *n term*
a patch[2] [æ] of skin transplanted from one part of the body to another, e.g. to resurface[3] [ɜː] a denuded[4] [uː] area; types of skin grafts include full-tickness[5] (skin & subcutaneous [eɪ] tissue) and split- or partial-thickness grafts[6] (epidermis & part of the dermis)
» *Wound* [uː] *closure with the help of a skin graft may be contemplated[7]. If the area can be skin grafted, meshed split-thickness grafts[13] are most effective (no collections of bacterial exudate).*
Use to obtain[8]/cover with/apply/accept **a skin graft** • primary **skin graft** • cutis / epidermic[9] / dermal-fat *or* adipodermal[10] **(skin) graft** • **graft donor** depth[11] / site [aɪ] • pinch[12] [tʃ]/ sieve[13] [sɪv] **graft** • free **skin grafting**

Hauttransplantat, -lappen
Dermislappen[1] Lappen[2] decken[3] entblößt, freiliegend[4] Vollhautlappen[5] Spalthauttransplantat[6] in Erwägung ziehen[7] Hautlappen entnehmen[8] Epidermistransplantat[9] Hautfettgewebetranspl.[10] Entnahmetiefe, Tiefe d. Entnahmestelle[11] Epidermisläppchen[12] Mesh-Graft[13]

6

delayed [dɪleɪd] **(skin) graft** *n term* opposite **primary** [aɪ] **(skin) graft**[1] *n term*
skin graft (first sutured [suːtʃəd] back to its bed) applied after several days so that healthy [e] granulations can form
» *The avulsed[2] [ʌ] skin was completely discarded[3] in favor of a delayed split-thickness skin graft.*

zweizeitige(s) / sekundäre(s) Hauttransplantat(ion)
primäre(s) H.[1] lose, traumatisiert, abgelöst[2] entfernt[3]

7

mesh(ed) [meʃd] **graft** *n term* syn **accordion graft** *n term*
skin graft with multiple [ʌ] perforations which can be stretched [tʃ] to cover a larger area
» *An advantage of meshed grafts is that they can be placed on an irregular, possibly contaminated wound bed[1] and will usually take[2]. Although mesh grafts can be expanded to 9 times their original size, expansion to one and a half the unmeshed size has proved most successful.*
Use **meshed** split-thickness skin graft[3]

Mesh-, Netztransplantat
verunreinigtes Wundbett[1] wächst meist ein[2] Netztransplantat[3]

8

50

182 RELATED MEDICAL SPECIALTIES — Grafts & Flaps

cancellous [kænsələs] **bone graft** n term   *opposite* **block (bone) graft**[1] n term
grafting of small chips[2] [tʃ] of spongy [spʌndʒi] bone which are packed into a bone defect, also termed filler graft
» *The patient was treated with an autologous onlay corticocancellous bone graft harvested[3] from the iliac crest[4]. All voids[5] between the block bone graft and the residual[6] mandible were packed[7] with cancellous bone chips.*
Use **onlay**[8] / **cortical**[9] / **cranial** [eɪ]/ **composite** / **freeze-dried**[10] [friːz draɪd] **bone graft**

Spongiosaplastik, -transplantat
Knochenspanplastik[1] Späne[2] entnommen[3] Beckenkamm, Crista iliaca[4] Zwischenräume[5] verblieben[6] aufgefüllt[7] Onlay-Plastik[8] Kortikalistransplantat[9] gefriergetrocknetes Knochentranspl.[10]   9

free graft or **flap** n term   *opposite* **pedicle graft** or **flap**[1] n term
graft freed completely from its bed and transplanted to the recipient site without its pedicle[2]
» *The implants were placed into free nonvascularized iliac bone grafts.*
Use **free-flap** transplantation • **free** gingival[3] [dʒɪndʒ-]/ bone / mucosal[4] **graft**

freier Lappen
gestielter Lappen[1] Stiel[2] freies Gingivatransplantat[3] freies Schleimhauttransplantat[4]   10

(pedicle) flap n term   syn **pedicle(d) graft** n term
tongue [tʌŋ] of skin and subcutaneous tissue (sometimes including muscle) only partially removed from its underlying tissue for transplantation; sustained[1] [eɪ] by a blood-carrying stem[2] or pedicle from the donor
bipedicle [aɪ] or **double pedicle flap**[3] n term
» *In periodontal surgery, pedicle flaps are used to cover a root surface by moving the attached[4] [tʃ] gingiva[5] [dʒ] to an adjacent [ədʒeɪsənt] position and suturing the free end. The vascular pedicle[2] areas of some flaps contain functional nerves which are also reattached.*
Use **to raise**[5] [eɪ]/**reflect**[6]/**debride** [iː]/**advance**[7]/**develop**[8]/**create**[8] [ieɪ]/**design**[8]/**rotate**/ (re)explore **a flap** • skin / buccal [ʌ]/ mucoperiosteal / deltopectoral / trans-rectus abdominis muscle, *abbr* TRAM / arterial / neurovascular[9] [ɚ]/ gingival / lingual or tongue **flap** • lined [aɪ]/ microvascular / sensory / motor / **composite or compound**[10] / **bilobed**[3] [oʊ]/ **cross**[11] / **free bone** / **local** / **distant**[12] / **direct or immediate**[13] [iː]/ **sickle flap** • omental / palmar-based / muscle / permanent **pedicle flap** • **pedicle flap** transfer

gestielter Lappen
versorgt[1] Gefäßstiel[2] doppelt gestielter L.[3] befestigte Gingiva, G. propria[4] Lappen heben[5] L. zurückklappen[6] L. verschieben[7] L. darstellen[8] neurovaskulärer L.[9] kombinierter L.[10] Kreuzlappen[11] Fernlappen[12] Nahlappen[13]

11

axial [æksɪəl] **(pattern)** or **arterial** [ɪɚ] **flap** n term
    opposite **random (pattern) flap**[1] n term
flap that includes a direct specific artery within its longitudinal axis
» *As they include their arteriovenous [iː] system, axial flaps may be 4 times as long as their base.*

Arterienlappen
Lappen ohne zugrundeliegende Gefäßstruktur[1]

12

(vascularized) free tissue transfer n term   syn **free flap** n term
axial flap whose neurovascular bundle[1] [ʌ] is anastomosed to that in the recipient site
» *In a free or island [aɪ] flap[2] the donor vessels are severed[3] [sevɚd] proximally and the flap is revascularized by anastomosing its supplying vessels to those of the recipient area using microsurgical techniques. Due to its long and relatively large and reliable [aɪ] vascular pedicle the latissimus dorsi [aɪ] is a popular muscle for free tissue transfer. Examples of free flaps frequently used are axial pattern skin flaps.*
Use **vascularized** compound [aʊ] transfer • microvascular [aɪ] **free flap**

freie(s) Gewebetransplantat, -übertragung
Nerven- u. Gefäßbündel[1] Insellappen[2] durchtrennt[3]

13

advancement flap n term   syn **sliding** [aɪ] or **French flap** n term
rectangular[1] flap raised in an elastic area, with its free end adjacent [dʒeɪs] to[2] a defect which is covered by longitudinally stretching the flap over it
» *Flaps used in reconstruction of the eyelids are advancement flaps, Z-plasty[3] and transposition flaps[4].*

Verschiebelappen
rechteckig[1] anliegend[2] Z-Plastik[3] Transpositionslappen[4]

14

tubed [uː] **(pedicle) flap** n term   syn **rope** [oʊ] or **Filatov(-Gillies) flap** n term
the sides of the pedicle are sutured together[1] to create a tube entirely covered by skin
» *In contrast to flat (open) flaps[2], tubed flaps are often created by joining two random flaps.*

Roll-, Rundstiellappen
miteinander vernäht[1] einseitig bedeckter Lappen[2]

15

50

Grafts & Flaps — RELATED MEDICAL SPECIALTIES

caterpillar [kætəpɪlɚ] **flap** *n term*   *syn* **waltzed** [wɒːltst] **flap** *n term*,
   sim **jump** [dʒʌmp] **flap**[1] *n term*

tubed flap transferred end-over-end in stages from the donor site to a distant recipient site

» *Jump flaps are distant flaps transferred in stages via an intermediate* [iː] *carrier; e.g., an abdominal flap is attached to the* wrist[2] [rɪst]*, then at a later stage the wrist is brought to the face.*

Wanderlappen
mehrfach transponierter Rundstiellappen[1] Handgelenk[2]

16

envelope [ɛnvəloʊp‖ɒːn-] **flap** *n term*   *syn* **wrap-around** [ræp-] **flap** *n term*

mucoperiosteal flap[1] retracted from a horizontal incision along the free gingival margin [dʒ] → U44-5

» *If the papilla between the 1st and 2nd molars has been elevated, envelope flaps may require an intraproximal suture. Envelope flaps have one,* rectangular flaps[2] *have two vertical* relaxing incisions[3]*.*

umhüllender Lappen
Mukoperiostlappen[1]
Trapezlappen[2]
Entlastungsschnitte[3]

17

buried [berɪd] **flap** *n term*   *opposite* **non-buried flap**[1] *n term*

flap denuded of both surface epithelium [iː] and superficial dermis and transferred into the subcutaneous [eɪ] tissue margin

» *Buried flaps can be effectively evaluated by means of Doppler ultrasonography.*

Unterfütterungslappen
Decklappen[1]

18

hinged [hɪndʒd] *or* **rotation flap** *n term*   *sim* **turnover flap**[1] *n term*

turnover flap transferred by lifting it over on its pedicle as though[2] [ðoʊ] the pedicle was a hinge[3]

» *A hinged flap that is turned over 180 degree to receive a second covering flap is termed a turnover flap. A lumbar* [ʌ] *periosteal turnover flap was used to* reinforce[4] *the spinal cord repair.*

Use superiorly [iː]/ nasaly [eɪ] **hinged flap** • flag **flap**

Rotationslappen
Wendelappen[1] als ob[2]
Scharnier[3] verstärken[4]

19

graft-versus-host [oʊ] **disease** *or* **reaction** *n term*   *abbr* **GVHD** *or* **GVHR**

incompatibility[1] reaction in a transplant recipient (=host) caused by T cells from grafted tissue which react immunologically against the recipient's antigens [-dʒənz] and attack the recipient tissues

» *GVHD affects especially the skin, gastrointestinal tract, and liver with symptoms including* skin rash[2] [ræʃ]*, fever* [iː]*, diarrhea* [daɪəriːə]*, liver dysfunction, abdominal pain, and* anorexia[3]*, and may be* fatal[4] [eɪ]*.*

Use to develop / oral / maternofetal [iː]/ chronic **GVHD**

GVHD, GVHR, Transplantat-gegen-Wirt Reaktion
Unverträglichkeit[1]
Hautausschlag, Exanthem[2]
Appetitlosigkeit[3] tödlich[4]

20

graft survival [səˈvaɪvəl] *n term*   *opposite* **graft rejection**[1] [rɪdʒekʃən]*n term*

satisfactory take[2] and ingrowth[3] of a viable[4] [aɪ] transplant into the recipient bed

» *The term* white graft[5] *refers to rejection of a skin allograft so acute that vascularization never occurs. A clear understanding of the* mechanisms [k] *involved in graft rejection will improve the selection of adequate immunosuppressive therapy and help* prolong graft survival[6]*.*

Use **graft survival** rate / curve • to enhance *or* extend[6] **graft survival** • improved / 1-year **graft survival** • to prevent/halt[7] [ɒː]/be responsible for **rejection** • (hyper)acute[8] [aɪ]/ chronic [k] **rejection** • organ[9] **graft rejection**

Überlebenszeit d. Transplantats
Transplantatabstoßung[1] Transplantatannahme[2] Einheilen[3] lebensfähig[4] weiße Abstoßung[5] Überlebenszeit d. T. verlängern[6] Transplantatabstoßung aufhalten[7] hyperakute Transplantatabstoßung[8] Organabstoßung, -rejektion[9]

21

Index – English

Mit Hilfe dieses Index können Sie **KWiC-Web** auch zum Nachschlagen englischer Fachausdrücke verwenden. Hier finden Sie die wichtigsten zahnmedizinisch relevanten Schlüsselwörter und deren semantisch oder morphologisch verwandte Wörter (Wortfamilie, Synonyme, Oberbegriffe etc.) in alphabetischer Reihenfolge (ca. 3000). Nominalverbindungen und feststehende Wortverbindungen sind unter dem ersten Wort zu finden (z. B. *gum line*, *inlay wax*, *informed consent*, *grinding wheel*), während Adjektiv-Komposita und Kollokationen (lose Wortverbindungen) jeweils unter dem Hauptwort gelistet sind (z. B. *hygiene, oral*; *implant, submerged*; *leakage, apical*). Bei Grenzfällen und wichtigen Termini sind jeweils beide Wörter angeführt (z. B. *lip retractor*; *retractor, lip* und *open bite*; *bite, open*). Bei Wörtern mit Mehrfachbedeutung wurde zur Verdeutlichung ein typisches Bezugswort in runder Klammer hinzugefügt, z. B. *apply (ointment)*, *thread (implant)*, *cap (crown)*. Bei Alternativformen werden bis auf wenige Ausnahmen wie z. B. *dentin(e)*, *implant, screw(-type)*, und *pedicle flap/graft*, entweder beide Formen gesondert oder die gebräuchlichere angeführt. Die britische Schreibweise wurde nicht berücksichtigt.

Verwiesen wird jeweils auf die Module (Unit) und Einträge (Zahl rechts unten in jedem Eintrag), in denen die Stichwörter vorkommen (z. B. U23 – 8,12 verweist auf die Einträge Nr. 8 und 12 in Unit 23). Zu den Units finden Sie am schnellsten über das Griffregister.

Da die Wörter in den Modulen selbst im Sinnzusammenhang bzw. in Wortfeldern dargestellt sind, bieten diese Schlüsselwörter direkten Zugang zu den Termini derselben Wortfamilie bzw. Bedeutungsfelder samt ihrem Kontext (Phrasen, Kollokationen etc.).

A

abfraction U10 – 21
ablation U22 – 13
abnormality U13 – 5
abrade U3 – 8
abrasion U3 – 8; U10 – 19
abrasive U10 – 19
abrasive paper/strip U32 – 24
abscess, endodontic-periodontal U35 – 20
–, periapical U41 – 8
absorbable U26 – 8
absorption U26 – 8
–, rate of U19 – 10
abutment (tooth) U42 – 10
accelerator U30 – 23
access cavity U41 – 10
–, surgical U21 – 6
accretion U34 – 7
ache U16 – 4
aches and pains U16 – 5
aching U16 – 4f
acid etching U30 – 19
acquired (disease) U13 – 6
acrylic resin U30 – 2
–, dental U30 – 2
action (drug) U19 – 8; U20 – 3
activate U20 – 3

activator (drug) U20 – 3
– (orthodontic) U37 – 13
active (drug) U20 – 3
activity U19 – 8
–, pharmacologic U20 – 3
acupressure U48 – 18
acupuncture anesthesia U48 – 18
Adam's apple U8 – 14
adherence (therapy) U18 – 15
– (tissue) U25 – 10
adhesiolysis U25 – 10
adhesion (tissue) U25 – 10
adhesive tape/plaster U28 – 21
adjunct U18 – 8
adjuvant U18 – 8
administration (drug) U19 – 3
advancement flap U50 – 14
adverse drug reaction U19 – 14
aerosol U20 – 14
affect U13 – 4
aftercare U18 – 14
agent U5 – 3; U20 – 2
–, anesthetic U48 – 4
–, antianxiety U47 – 10
–, antibacterial U20 – 9
–, antineoplastic U20 – 31
–, blocking U20 – 7
–, contrast U46 – 15
–, cytostatic U20 – 31

–, luting U31 – 17
–, narcotic U47 – 5
–, psychotropic U20 – 23
–, resin curing U30 – 3
agitation U4 – 12
agonist U20 – 6
aim U15 – 3
air syringe U7 – 4
airtight (seal) U34 – 16
akinetic mutism U4 – 17
alcohol U2 – 27
alert U4 – 2
alginate U30 – 15
aliazing U46 – 13
align U28 – 2
alignment U29 – 1; U36 – 26
allocation, patient U15 – 4
allograft U50 – 3
–, freeze-dried bone U44 – 11
alloy U30 – 7
–, fusible U31 – 16
–, low gold U30 – 8
–, platinum-rhodium U30 – 9
aluminum silicate U30 – 5
alveolar resorption U44 – 6
– ridge U44 – 6
– – height U44 – 7
alveolus, dental U9 – 13
amalgam, dental U30 – 1

amalgamate U30-1
amalgamation U31-14
amalgamator U30-1; U31-14
ambulation U25-13
ambulatory U25-13
amino acid U12-10
ampul U5-13
anaesthetist U23-6
analgesia U16-20; U47-7
analgesic U16-20; U47-7
analysis by intention-to-treat
   U15-20
-, life-table U14-26
-, multivariate U14-28
-, survival U14-26
anastomosis U49-6
anchor U42-20
anchorage U42-20
anesthesia U47-2
- bag U47-15
- machine U47-14
- mask U47-15
- record U47-22
- recovery period U47-23
- screen U23-7
-, balanced U48-2
-, block U48-6
-, closed circuit U48-10
-, conduction U48-6
-, depth/level U47-20
-, endotracheal U48-13
-, general U48-1
-, inhalation U48-10
-, insufflation U48-10
-, intravenous U48-13
-, local U48-3
-, regional U48-3
anesthesiologist U23-6
anesthesiology U47-2
anesthetic U47-2; U48-4
- circuit U47-14
- risk U47-12
-, general U48-1
anesthetize U47-1
angulation U17-4
animal graft U50-5
anion U46-20
ankylosis U38-12
annealer U31-15
annealing furnace U31-15
anodontia U36-19
anomaly U13-5
antacid U20-29
antagonist U20-6
antiarrhythmic U20-18
antibiotic U20-9
- coverage, prophylactic U27-13
-, antitumor U20-31
anticholinergic U20-8

anticoagulant U20-16
anticonvulsive U20-20
antidepressant U20-24
antidote U5-15
antiemetic U20-12
antiepileptic U20-20
antifungal U20-26
antihistamines U20-22
antihrombotic U20-16
anti-inflammatory (drug) U20-11
anti-ischemic U13-28
antimicrobial U20-9
antineoplastic (drug) U20-31
antiseptic U27-1
antispasmodic U20-19
antitumor (drug) U20-31
antivomiting drug U20-12
antrostomy U22-3
anxiety, presurgical U25-4
apathy U4-12
aperture, collimator U46-6
apex U41-6
- locator U41-12
aphasic U11-9
aphonia U11-23
aphtha U35-17
aphthosis U35-17
apical U41-6,17
apicectomy U41-20
apicocoronal height U39-12
apicoectomy U41-20
appetite U1-11
appliance, Begg U37-3
-, functional U37-13
-, Herbst U37-11
-, light-wire U37-3
-, orthodontic U37-1
-, palatal expansion U37-17
-, retaining U37-23
application (cream) U19-3
applicator U19-3; U24-14
apply (ointment) U19-3
appointment U6-9; U37-12
apposition U29-1; U26-5
approach, surgical U21-6
approximation U26-5; U28-2
apron, lead U33-3
arch form U36-4
- length U36-4
- shape U36-4
- width U9-9
-, dental U9-9
arches, clip(-on) U37-4
archwire U37-5
-, labial U37-22
area, hard-to-reach U34-8
armamentarium U32-1
arousal U4-2
artefact U46-13

arthritis, degenerative U38-11
arthrodesis U29-13
arthrogram U33-14
arthrography U33-14
arthroplasty U22-4
arthrotomy U38-16
articulating paper U32-25
articulation U36-3
articulator U31-1
artifact U46-13
artificial teeth U10-8
ascorbic acid U12-15
aseptic U27-1
aspirate U7-7; U22-16
aspiration U7-7; U22-16
aspirator U7-7; U22-16
assessment, nutritional U12-3
-, preoperative U25-1
assignment, patient U15-4
assistant, dental U6-4
association U14-32
atresia U13-18
atrophic U13-29
atrophy U13-29
-, alveolar ridge U44-6
attached gingiva U35-2
attachment level U35-9
- loss U35-9
-, precision U42-7
attack U16-14
attending surgeon U23-5
attire, OR U27-15
attrition U10-19
auditory U8-15
augment U44-8
augmentation U49-19
-, alveolar ridge U44-8
aural U8-15
autoclave U27-3
autocure U31-17
autogenous U49-16
autograft U50-2
autologous U49-16
autoradiograph U33-15
autotransplant U50-2
autotransplantation U49-14
auxiliaries U37-3
avulsion U17-5; U44-3
awl U24-5
axial U43-9

B

babble U11-17
baby teeth U10-2
backing U40-11
backscatter U46-6
bag, anesthesia U47-15

bag, breathing U47-15
bake U31-18
balanced force technique U41-11
balm U5-8
balsam U5-8
band U37-8
- remover U37-9
- sitter U37-9
bandage U28-20
-, Esmarch U47-18
Band-Aid® U28-22
banding U37-8
bar U37-15; U42-11
- clasp U42-6
- clip U42-23
-, connecting U43-5
-, dental U42-23
-, lingual U42-24
-, palatal U42-24
barbiturate U20-24; U48-14
bareheaded U8-1
barrier membrane U35-29
basal anesthesia U48-15
baseplate U42-17
beam, x-ray U46-5
beamer U46-5
beam-splitter U46-5
bearings U4-8
beeper U7-12
Begg appliance U37-3
- light wire differential force U37-3
bend U36-27
benumb U47-3
bevel U40-19
bias U14-18
bicuspid tooth U9-6
bicuspidation U41-23
binder U28-20
bioactive U43-17
bioactivity U20-3
bioavailability U19-10
biocompatibility U43-17
biocompatible U49-20
biodegradation U20-4
bioinert U43-17; U49-20
biologic response modifier U20-34
biological width U39-10
biopsy, cone U22-12
biostatistics U14-1
biotransformation U20-4
bisect U21-14
bite U10-11 f; U36-7
- (bit-bitten) U3-10; U10-11
- stick U37-9
-, closed U36-12
-, deep U36-12
biteguard U37-25
- splint U38-14

biteplane U37-24
biteplate U37-24
bitewing film/radiograph U33-6
biting U3-10
blabber U11-19
blackout U4-4
blade implant U43-2
bleach U39-19
bleed U3-19; U13-26
bleeding U3-19; U13-26
bleeding index, marginal U35-8
bleep U7-12
blend U39-15
blind U15-9
blockade U48-6
blockage U48-6
blocker U20-7
blocking U15-11; U20-7
blue light source U31-19
blunt U4-10; U47-3
blunted sensation U47-4
boil out (wax) U30-17
bolt U29-16
Bolton discrepancy U36-18
bombard U46-4
bond, cement U30-6
bonding U39-20
bone bank U44-11
- chisel U24-11
- grafting U44-9
- plate U29-17
- scraper U24-12
- union U17-15
bone-anchored U42-20
- - hearing aid U45-23
bone-resorptive U10-20
bone-tapping U43-11
bothersome U16-3
bowl U7-8
brace U28-26; U29-7
-, night U37-18
braces U37-1
brackets, orthodontic U37-4
braided (suture) U26-7
brain death U4-18
braze U31-16
break (broke-broken) U17-1
breakaway U37-21
breakdown U4-4
breath odor U34-20
-, bad U34-20
bridge U42-4
bridge, composite-etched U30-3
bring round U47-25
brittleness U31-15
broach U32-11
bruise U3-13
brush U34-3
-, interdental U9-22

-, polishing U32-7
bruxism U10-18; U36-11
buccal U8-5; U9-23
buccogingival U35-2
bur U32-6
burn U3-11
burnish U31-21
butt U40-9

C

cadaver donor U49-17
calcification U10-22
calculus U13-21
-, dental U34-9
-, salivary U33-13
callous U17-15
callus formation U17-15
calorie U12-4
canal preparation U41-11
-, weeping U41-16
cancellation U6-10
cancellous bone U50-9
candy U2-17
canine (tooth) U9-5
canker sore U35-17
cannula U24-6
cannulization U24-6
cantilever (fixed) prosthesis U42-8
cap (crown) U40-18
-, surgical U27-18
capsule U5-7
carbohydrate U12-5
card, medical U6-14
caries, interproximal U33-6
caries-prone U34-18
case record form U15-16
case-controlled U15-10
cast U31-4
- relator U31-1
-, dental U31-2
-, stone U30-13
castable U31-4
casting wax U30-17
catgut U26-9
catheter U22-19
cation U46-20
cauter U22-9
cauterization U22-9
caution U5-18
cavitation U34-19
cavity U34-19
- base U40-4
- debridement U40-2
- liner U40-3
- margin U40-10
- toilet U40-2
-, access U41-10

cavity, buccal U8–10; U9–23
–, oral U8–8
–, pulp U41–5
cell death U13–30
cement U30–6
–, dual affinity U30–6
cementoenamel junction U39–9
cementum U9–17
censoring U15–28
cephalometry U33–9
cephalostat U39–4
ceramic U30–4
cervical U8–13
– collar U29–9
– line U39–9
cervix U8–13
chafe U3–8
chairside U7–1
chamfer U40–19
chart U14–27
–, dental U6–14
chatter U11–19
checkup U6–15
cheek U8–5
– retractor U32–2
– tooth U9–7
cheek-biting U35–16
cheilitis U8–9
chemist U5–4
chew U10–15
chilblain U3–12
chin U8–6
– (jerk) reflex U38–7
– cap/cup U37–20
China clay U30–5
chip U17–2
– syringe U7–4
–, cortical U44–10
chip-blower U7–4
chi-square test U14–34
choke U10–16
cholinergic U20–8
cicatricial U28–10
cicatrix U28–10
circulating nurse U23–9
circumcise U21–9
circumferential wiring U29–14
clamp U24–13
clasp U37–15
–, bar U42–6
–, denture U42–6
cleanse U27–5; U34–4
cleanser, denture U10–8
clear (one's throat) U11–6
cleft U17–11
– palate U9–10
– surgery U45–3
clefting syndrome U45–2
clench U10–17

clenching, nighttime U10–17
clicking U38–4
clinical trial U15–1
clip U26–13
– applier U26–13
–, bar U42–23
clip-ligate U26–3,13
closed bite U36–12
clove oil U30–16
coagulation U20–16; U22–10
coagulator U22–10
coapt U26–5; U49–5
coaptation U49–5; U26–5
coating U30–10
cofactor U14–5
cohesive gold U30–8
cohort U14–3
col, interdental U35–18
colic U16–15
collar, cervical U29–9
collimation U46–6
colony forming unit U27–10
coma U4–14
–, irreversible U4–18
combined lesion U35–20
come in (teeth) U10–3
– to/round U4–6
comfort U16–1
committee, hospital ethics U15–24
–, steering U15–25
commotio U3–14
communication U11–8
communicative U11–8,18
comorbidity U13–2
compassionate use U15–23
compliance, patient U18–15
complication U25–9
composite resin U30–3
compress U28–25
compromise U13–4
computed tomography U33–18
concha, nasal U8–4
concretion U13–21
concussion U3–14
condensation, endodontic U32–17;
   U41–15
condenser U32–17
conduction anesthesia U48–6
condylectomy U38–18
cone biopsy U22–12
confidence interval U14–17
confirmation U15–17
confounder U14–18
confusion U4–8
congenital U13–6
congruency, axial U43–9
conization U22–12
connector U42–24
conscious U4–1

constriction U13–19
consultant U6–11
consultation U6–11
consumption U1–2
contact point, occlusal U36–9
contaminated U27–2
contamination U27–9
contour U39–2
contract U31–6
contraction, shrinkage U31–6
contracture U28–8
contra-indication U18–10
contrast agent U46–15
contrecoup U17–9
control group U15–10
contusion U3–13
convalescence U25–14
cooling U7–5
coping U40–17
–, telescopic U42–9
–, transfer U31–11
core U40–15
corona dentis U9–14
correction, surgical U49–2
corrective U31–6
correlation U14–32
corrosion, fretting U43–19
–, pitting U43–19
cosmetic U39–1
cotton ball U28–23
cough U11–6
counterdie U31–5
course (drug) U18–5
–, postoperative U25–7
covariance U14–14
coverage, antibiotic U49–9
Cox regression model U14–35
crack U17–1,11
cranial fracture U17–8
craniostenosis U45–4
craniosynostosis U45–4
craniotomy U45–20
crazing U40–20
creamy U5–8
create U49–4
crepitance U17–14
crepitation U17–14
crepitus U17–14
crest, alveolar U9–13
–, gingival U39–10
crevice, gingival U35–4
crevicular U35–4
crib U37–15
cross infection U27–11
crossbite U36–15
cross-clamping U24–13
crossover, treatment U15–14
cross-reactivity U19–11
cross-section U21–10

cross-tolerance U19–12
crowding, dental U36–16
crown U40–18
– length U39–12
– lengthening U35–25
–, dental U9–14
–, full-coverage U40–14,18
–, open face U42–19
–, porcelain jacket U40–18
crown-down technique U41–11
cry U11–3,14
cryoablation U22–13
cryoanesthesia U48–3
cryocautery U22–8
cryoprobe U22–8; U24–8
cryosurgery U22–8; U21–3
CT scan U33–18
cuff U29–8
curare U48–17
curative U18–2,9
cure U18–2
–, bench U31–8
curet U24–10; U32–14
curettage U24–10; U34–14
curing U31–19
– light U32–23
curve of occlusion U39–11
– of Spee U36–5
cusp, tooth U9–4
cuspid (tooth) U9–5
cuspidor U7–8
custom-fit U42–16
cut U3–6; U21–9
cutdown, venous U3–6; U22–18
cuticle, acquired enamel U34–10
cutoff (value) U14–24
cut-point U14–24
cutting, teeth U10–4
cyst U13–24; U44–15
–, dentigerous U44–15
cytostatic U20–32
cytotoxicity U20–32

D

dairy product U2–5
data U15–15
dazed U4–9
deaden (pain) U47–3
debanding U37–8
debond U39–20
debonding U37–8
debridement U28–12
–, cavity U40–2
–, mechanical U40–2
decalcification U10–22
decay, tooth/dental U34–17
decile U14–11

decontaminate U27–9
deep bite U36–12
deep-seated (ache) U16–4
defect, mucogingival U35–12
deflasking U31–9
deformation U13–5
deformity, craniofacial U45–4
degeneration U13–29
degrees of freedom U14–16
dehiscence, wound U28–16
delimit U46–12
delineate U46–12
delirium U4–16
demarcate U46–12
demastication U10–19
demineralized bone matrix U44–11
demulcent U20–30
dens U9–1
dens molaris U9–7
dental U9–1
– acrylic U30–2
– care U34–1
– caries U34–18
– chair U7–1
– chart U6–14
– engine U7–3
– implant U43–2
– light U7–9
– mirror U32–4
– office U6–2
– practice U6–2
– prosthesis U42–2
– surgery U6–2
– unit U7–2
dentifrice U34–4
dentigerous cyst U44–15
dentin(e) U9–16
dentist U6–1
dentistry, corrective U36–1
–, prosthetic U42–1
–, ultraconservative U45–18
dentition U10–1
–, mixed U10–1
–, permanent U10–6
–, precocious U10–1
–, residual U42–20
–, retarded U10–1
–, secondary U10–6
dentulous U10–7
denture U10–8; U42–2
– base U42–17
– wearer U42–10
–, bar joint U42–11
–, fixed U10–8
–, overlay U42–10f
–, temporary U10–8
–, transitional U10–8
–, two-part U42–10
depth demarcation U43–10

–, pocket U35–7
–, probing U35–4
de-rotation U36–27
desensitize U30–24
deviation (data) U14–13
–, mandibular U38–10
dextrose U12–7
diagram U14–27
diamond U32–6
diaphanoscopy U46–16
diastema U36–17
diathermy U22–9
die U31–5
– pin U31–12
–, female U31–5
diet, nonchewy U38–3
dietary U1–13
dietetics U1–13
dietician U1–13
digital subtraction radiography
   U33–16
dilatation U24–17
dilator U24–17
disaccharide U2–16
discectomy U38–17
disclosing paper U32–25
discomfort U16–1
discontinuation U19–6
discontinue (therapy) U19–6
discrepancy, Bolton U36–18
diseased U13–2
dish U1–8
disinfection U27–5
disk, separating U32–5
diskectomy U38–17
dislocation U3–20; U17–4
disocclude U36–7
disocclusion U36–7
disorientation U4–8
dispensary U5–5
dispense U5–5
displacement U3–20; U17–4
disposable U27–4
disposal U27–4
disruption U3–18; U17–5
disruptive U3–18
dissect (free) U21–12
dissecting microscope U21–12
– scissors U24–4
dissection U21–12
–, tunnel U44–13
distal U9–21
distance, interocclusal U10–14
distortion U3–16
– (data) U14–18
– (image) U33–5
distraction U29–3; U45–16
distractor U45–16
distress U16–2

diuretics U20-21
divide U21-14
division U21-14
dizzy U4-5
documentation U15-15
dolor U16-6
donate U49-15
donor U49-15
-, cadaver U49-17; U44-11
-, living U49-17
dosage U19-7
- form U5-6
- formulation U5-6
dose U19-7
- distribution U46-9
-, maintenance U47-19
-, radiation absorbed U46-10
dose-dependent U19-7
dosimeter U19-7; U46-9
dosimetry U46-9
double gloving U27-17
double-stapled U26-12
dowel pin U31-12
downer U20-24
drain U28-15
drainage U28-15
drape U27-7
dressing U28-17
drift U36-21
drifting U36-21
drill, dental U32-5
-, guide U32-6; U43-8
-, pilot U32-6; U43-8
drillhole U43-11
drink U2-24
drooling U10-9
dropout (study) U15-29
drops (medication) U5-11
drowsiness U4-5
drowsy U4-5
drug U5-3
- delivery U19-4
- interaction U19-11
- release U19-4
- targeting U19-4
-, anti-inflammatory U20-11
druggist U5-4
drug-induced U5-3; U19-15
drug-related U5-3
dull (ache) U16-4
dummy U42-5
dysarthric U11-9
dysesthesia U16-17
dysostosis, mandibulofacial U45-6
dysphonia U11-23

E

ear U8-15
earache U16-4
eardrum U8-15
earlobe U8-15
eat (ate-eaten) U1-1
ecchymosis U13-27
edema U3-15
edematous U3-15
edentulism U10-7
edentulous U10-7
edge, beveled U40-19
-, incisal U9-13
edgewise technique U37-2
edible U1-5
effectiveness U15-26
efficacious U15-26
efficacy U15-26; U19-9
efficiency U15-26
elastic module U37-10
elasticity U37-10
elastics U37-10
elbow formation U41-13
elective U21-5
electrocautery U22-9
- snare U22-11
electrocoagulation U22-10
electroconization U22-12
electrodessication U22-14
electrosurgery U21-3; U22-9
element, connecting U42-24
elevate U49-11; U32-15
elevation U49-11
elevator U32-15
eloquent U11-18
emanation U46-2
embed U31-8
embrasure U39-13
-, incisal U9-3
emergence (anesthesia) U47-21
emergency U21-5
emery disk U32-8
emetic U20-12
emollient U20-30
enamel cleaver U32-18
- fissures U34-15
- grooves U34-15
- pits U34-15
- porosities U34-15
-, dental/tooth U9-15
-, mottled U34-13
endodontic U41-1
endodontic-periodontal abscess U35-20
endpoint U14-20
engraft U50-1
enrollment, patient U15-4
ensnare U22-11

enunciation U11-13
epithelialization U28-6
erode U10-21
erosion U10-21
erosive U10-21
error, systematic U14-18
erupt (teeth) U10-3
eruption (teeth) U10-3
-, impeded U10-3
eschar U28-9
Esmarch's tourniquet U47-18
esthetic U39-1
estimation U14-29
etch U30-19; U39-21
etchant U30-19; U39-21
etching liquid U30-19
- solution U30-19
-, acid U30-19
eugenic acid U30-16
eugenol U30-16
evaporate U22-15
event U14-19
-, primary U14-20
evidence U15-17
examination, gingival U35-6
excavation U32-14
excavator U32-14
excise U21-9,15
excision U21-15
exfoliate (teeth) U10-5
exfoliation (teeth) U10-5
exolever U32-15
expand U31-6
expanded access U15-22
expansion, palatal U37-17
-, setting U31-6
expectorant U20-15
expectorate U20-15
experimental group U15-10
explantation U49-12
exploration U21-11
explorer U32-9
expose U46-7
exposure, surgical U21-7
extend U29-3
extension U29-3
extirpation U21-15; U22-13
extraction socket U9-13
-, tooth U44-2
extraction-replantation U44-4
extraoral U9-25
- view U33-4
extrusion U36-25
extubate U47-17
exudate U28-13
exudative U28-13
eye U8-3
-, black U3-13
eyeball U8-3

eyebrow U8-3
eyelashes U8-3
eyelid U8-3

F

facade U39-2
face U8-2
- mask U27-18; U37-19
- shield U27-18
facebow U37-19
facial U8-2
- advancement surgery U45-8
- angle U39-5
- cleft U45-2
facies U8-2
facing U39-22; U40-11
factor U14-5
factorial design U15-13
faint, to feel U4-4f
faintness U4-4
fall out (teeth) U10-5
false negative U14-22
- positive U14-22
falter U11-20
familial U13-7
fashion U49-4
fasting U1-15
fast-setting (amalgam) U30-1
fat U12-11
fatty acid, essential U12-12
fauces U8-12
feed (fed-fed) U1-3; U12-1
fester U28-14
fetor oris U34-20
fiber, dietary U12-16
fibrin glue U26-14
fibromatosis, gingival U35-22
figure-of-eight suture U26-19
filament (suture) U26-7
file (instrument) U24-12; U32-12
filling U40-1
-, retrosurgical U41-21
-, reverse U41-21
-, root-end U41-21
film, bitewing U33-6
-, fast U33-3
-, interproximal U33-6
-, plain U46-19
-, skull U33-10
-, sticky U34-8
-, ultraspeed U33-7
-, x-ray U33-2
fire U31-18
fissure U17-11
fistula U13-25
-, inflammatory U35-21
fistulation U13-25

-, oroantral U44-14
fistulization U13-25
fit U42-16
fixator U29-4
fixture U43-2
-, intramucosal U43-4
flange, denture U42-19
flap, advancement U50-14
-, arterial U50-12
-, axial (pattern) U50-12
-, bipedicle U50-11
-, buried U50-18
-, caterpillar U50-16
-, envelope U50-17
-, Filatov(-Gillies) U50-15
-, free U50-13
-, French U50-14
-, hinged U50-19
-, mucoperiosteal U44-5
-, nonburied U50-18
-, random (pattern) U50-12
-, rope U50-15
-, rotation U50-19
-, sliding U50-14
-, tubed (pedicle) U50-15
-, turnover U50-19
-, waltzed U50-16
-, wrap-around U50-17
flaring U36-24
flask, casting/denture U31-9
flinch U16-12
floss, dental U34-5
fluorescence U46-8
fluoride, stannous U34-13
fluoroscopic U46-8
flush (away) U34-6
focus U13-3
foil, gold U30-8
-, occlusal U32-25
-, platinum U30-9
folacin U12-14
folate U12-14
folic acid U12-14
follicular cyst U44-15
followup U6-15; U18-14
-, postoperative U25-15
fomentation U28-25
food U1-6
- additive U2-22
- exchange list U2-21
- substitute/replacer U2-21
- trapping U39-22
-, solid U1-6
force U36-28
-, chewing U10-15
forceps U24-14
-, dental U32-15
-, extracting U32-15
-, film-holding U33-2

-, grasping U24-13
-, sponge U24-18
-, suture U24-15
formulate (drug) U5-6
fractile U14-11
fracture U17-1
- fixation U29-4
-, chip U17-5
-, closed U17-3
-, comminuted U17-7
-, compression U17-6
-, contrecoup U17-9
-, fatigue U17-13
-, fissured U17-11
-, hairline U17-11
-, impacted U17-6
-, linear U17-11
-, maxillofacial U45-1
-, simple U17-3
-, skull U17-8
-, splinter(ed) U17-7
-, stress U17-13
fragment U17-2
fragmentation U17-2
framework U43-15
Frankfort line/plane U39-4
free U21-12
- tissue transfer, vascularized U50-13
freeway space U10-14
freeze-dried bone allograft U44-11
frenectomy U44-7
frenulum U9-11
frenum U9-11
frequency distribution U14-12
freshening (wound) U28-12
frit U30-21; U31-18
fritting U30-21
frostbite U3-12
frostnip U3-12
fulguration U22-14
functional endoscopic sinus surgery U45-19
fungal U20-26
fungicidal U20-26
furcation defect U35-23
- perforation U41-17

G

gag U10-16
gangrene U13-30
gantry U46-19
gap closure, orthodontic U44-4
gargle U11-7
gauge, depth U43-10
gauze, surgical U28-18
gel U5-8

generic U19-2
genial U8-6
geniocheiloplasty U45-14
genioplasty U22-4; U45-14
giggle U11-2
gingiva U9-12
-, attached U35-2
-, free U35-2
gingival crest U35-3
- crevice U35-4
- index U35-7
- line U39-7
- margin U35-3
- sulcus U35-4
gingivectomy U22-1; U35-25
gingivitis U35-13
-, acute (necrotizing) ulcerative U35-14
gingivoplasty U35-26
glaze U31-20
gloss U39-18
glossal U8-11
gloves, disposable U27-17
glove-wearing U27-17
gloving U27-17
gluconate U12-7
glucosamine U12-7
glucose U12-7
gnathic U45-9
gnathologic U45-9
gold annealing U30-8
- foil U30-8
-, cohesive U30-8
gouge U24-11
gown (OR) U27-15
-, total body exhaust U27-16
gowning U27-15
graft U50-1
- rejection U50-21
- survival U50-21
-, accordion U50-8
-, allogeneic U50-3
-, autogeneic U50-2
-, autologous U50-2
-, autoplastic U50-2
-, block (bone) U50-9
-, cancellous bone U50-9
-, delayed (skin) U50-7
-, dermal U50-6
-, free U50-10
-, heterologous U50-5
-, heteroplastic U50-5
-, homologous U50-3
-, homoplastic U50-3
-, inlay U44-10
-, isogeneic U50-4
-, isologous U50-4
-, isoplastic U50-4
-, mesh(ed) U50-8

-, onlay U44-10
-, particulate U44-10
-, primary (skin) U50-7
-, skin U50-6
-, split-thickness U50-6
-, syngeneic U50-4
-, xenogeneic U50-5
-, zooplastic U50-5
graft-augmented U44-8
graft-versus-host disease /reaction U50-20
granulate U28-7
granulation tissue U28-7
granuloma, apical U41-8
graph U14-27
grasper U24-13
graze U3-8
gression U36-21
grind (ground-ground) U10-18
grinding wheel U10-18
groan U11-4
guidance U36-29
-, canine U9-5
guide U36-29
- drill U43-8
guided bone regeneration U44-12
- tissue regeneration U35-28
gum disease U41-8
- knife U24-3
- line U39-7
gumboil U41-8
gummy U9-12
gums U9-12
gutta-percha point U30-14
gypsum U30-12

H

habit, grinding U10-18
habit-forming U47-9
habituation U47-9
hair U8-16
hairline (fracture) U17-11
hairy U8-16
half-life, biologic U20-5
- - , pharmacologic U20-5
halitosis U34-20
halothane U48-12
handpiece, dental U32-5
harm U28-1
harness U29-8
harvest (tissue) U49-12
hazard U25-5
head U8-1
- halter U29-9
headache U8-1; U16-4
headgear U37-18
heal (up) U18-2; U28-4

healing U28-4
- abutment U43-13
- cap U43-13
health freak U1-17
healthful U1-12
healthy U1-12
heave U10-16
height of contour U39-8
hematoma U3-13; U13-26
hemisection U41-23
hemorrhage U3-19; U13-26
hemostasis U22-10
herbal U2-20
hereditary U13-7
heredity U13-7
hermetic seal U41-15
heterograft U50-5
high-potency U19-9
high-resolution U46-14
high-risk U25-5
hiss U11-21
hoe U32-18
holder, needle U24-15
homogenous U49-16
homograft U50-3
homologous U49-16
hook, electrosurgical U24-9
hospital stay, postoperative U25-11
hospital-acquired U13-6; U27-12
hospitalization U25-11
host bed U43-7
hunger U1-11
hurt (hurt-hurt) U3-1; U16-3
hygiene, oral U34-1
hygienist, dental/oral U34-1
hyperactivity U4-12
hyperdense U46-11
hyperdontia U36-19
hyperemia U13-28
hyperesthesia U16-17; U47-4
hypernasal U11-22
hyperplasia U13-15
hypertelorbitism U45-5
hypertelorism U45-5
hypertrophy U13-15
hypesthesia U47-4
hypnotic U47-9
hypodense U46-11
hypodermic needle U7-6
hypodontia U36-19
hypoesthesia U47-4
hyponasal U11-22
hyposensitivity U47-4
hypotelorism U45-5
hypothesis, alternative U15-19
-, null U15-19

I

iatrogenic U13 – 9; U19 – 15
idiopathic U13 – 8
imaging, 3 D U33 – 19
–, radionuclide U46 – 22
imbed U31 – 8
immobile U29 – 5
immobilization U29 – 5
immunomodulator U20 – 34
impact U17 – 6; U44 – 3
impaction U17 – 6; U44 – 3
impairment U13 – 4
impenetrability U46 – 11
implant U43 – 2; U49 – 18
– bed U43 – 7
– loading U43 – 14
– placement U44 – 12
–, blade U43 – 2
– body U43 – 1
–, craniofacial U45 – 21
–, cylinder U43 – 6
–, dental U43 – 2
–, endosseous (dental) U43 – 4
–, nonsubmerged U43 – 5
–, porous U43 – 3
–, screw(-type) U43 – 6
–, single-tooth U43 – 2
–, submerged U43 – 5
–, titanium U30 – 10
implantable U49 – 18
implantation U49 – 18
implant-borne U43 – 2
implant-supported U42 – 12
impression post U31 – 12
– tray U31 – 3
–, alginate U30 – 15
–, dental U31 – 2
–, full arch U30 – 15
–, preliminary U31 – 2
in vitro U15 – 18
in vivo U15 – 18
inaccessible U21 – 6
inactive control treatment U15 – 8
inborn U13 – 6
incidence U14 – 7
incise U21 – 9
incision U3 – 6; U21 – 9
incisor tooth U9 – 3
inclination U36 – 23
increment U46 – 19
incurable U18 – 2
index, caries U34 – 21
–, Dean's fluorosis U34 – 13
–, gingival U35 – 7
–, marginal bleeding U35 – 8
–, oral hygiene U34 – 21
–, periodontal disease U35 – 7
–, sulcus bleeding U35 – 8

indication U18 – 10
indicator U18 – 10
indolent U16 – 6
induction room U23 – 3
–, anesthetic U47 – 13
induration U13 – 14
inedible U1 – 5
inefficient U15 – 26
inelastic U37 – 10
inert U49 – 20
infection U27 – 9
infiltration U13 – 13
inflammation U13 – 11
information U15 – 15
informed consent U25 – 3
infusion cannula U24 – 6
– pump U47 – 16
–, bolus intravenous U47 – 19
–, continuous intravenous U47 – 19
ingest U1 – 1
ingestion U1 – 1
ingrowth, bone U43 – 3
inhalant U20 – 14
inhalation U20 – 14
inhaler U20 – 14
inherited U13 – 7
inhibitor U20 – 7
injure U3 – 1; U28 – 1
injurious U3 – 2
injury U3 – 1 ff
injury-free U3 – 2
inlay U40 – 16
inlay wax U30 – 17
inoperable U21 – 1
insertion torque U43 – 12
–, implant U43 – 2 ff
insignificant, statistically U14 – 21
insoluble U5 – 11
inspection U21 – 11
instability U29 – 4
institutional review board U15 – 24
instrument U24 – 1; U32 – 1
– cart U23 – 19
– cupboard U7 – 11
– stroke U32 – 1
– table U7 – 11
–, blunt U32 – 1
instrumentation U24 – 1; U32 – 1
–, chemomechanical U41 – 11
insufflation anesthesia U48 – 10
insurance coverage U49 – 9
intact U21 – 13
intake U1 – 1
–, food U1 – 6
–, oral U25 – 12
intensity (pain) U16 – 9
intention-to-treat analysis U15 – 20
interact U19 – 11
interappointment U6 – 9

interarch distance U10 – 14
intercom U7 – 13
intercuspidation, maximum
  U36 – 13
interdental col U35 – 18
internal derangement U38 – 9
interocclusal U36 – 7
– distance U10 – 14
– record U36 – 2
– registration U36 – 2
interproximal U9 – 22
– film U33 – 6
intolerance U19 – 12
intonation U11 – 11
intractability U18 – 13
intractable U18 – 13
intraoperative U21 – 2
intraoral U9 – 25
– view U33 – 4
intrusion U36 – 25
intubation U47 – 17
intubator U47 – 17
intussusception U49 – 8
invagination U49 – 8
invest U31 – 8
investigation U15 – 2
investing machine U31 – 8
investment U31 – 8
– material, refractory U31 – 8
involvement U13 – 4
–, furcal U35 – 23
ion U46 – 20
ionize U46 – 20
ionomer, resin-modified glass
  U40 – 5
irradiate U46 – 4
irradiation U46 – 2
irrigation U7 – 5; U22 – 17
irrigator U22 – 17
irritability U13 – 10
irritant U13 – 10
irritation U16 – 3; U13 – 10
ischemia U13 – 28
isodense U46 – 11

J

jackscrew U37 – 17
jaw U8 – 7
– exercises U38 – 13
– locking U38 – 5
jawbone U8 – 7
jaw-jerk U38 – 7
joint stiffening U38 – 12
joule U12 – 4
juice U2 – 25
jumper U37 – 11

junction, cementoenamel U35-3;
 U39-9
-, dentoenamel U9-16

K

kaolin U30-5
keloid, gums U35-22
keratocyst U44-15
knife U24-3
knot U26-6
knot-tying U26-6

L

labial U8-9; U9-23
- bow U37-15
laceration U3-7
lactin U12-8
lactose U12-8
lallation U11-17
laminagraphy U46-19
laminate U39-22
lamp, annealing U31-15
landmark U21-8
-, cephalometric U36-24
laser U22-7
lateral wall infracture technique
 U45-15
laugh U11-2
laughing gas U48-11
lavage U28-11
Le Fort I osteotomy U45-7
lead shield U33-3
leaflet, patient instruction U5-17
-, practice U6-8
leakage, apical U41-16
ledge formation U41-14
ledging U41-14
leeway (space) U36-6
lens, magnifying U22-6
lesion U3-5; U13-3
-, combined U35-20
lethargy U4-12
leveling U36-26
- wire U37-6
leverage U32-15
liberate U21-12
lid U8-3
lidocaine U48-5
life-preserving U21-13
ligament, periodontal U35-23
ligating module U37-7
ligation U26-3; U37-7
ligature U26-3
- (tie) wire U37-7
light wire appliance U37-3

light-curing U30-3
light-headedness U4-5
lignocaine U48-5
likelihood U14-31
line of minimum tension U49-10
-, central venous U22-19
lingua U8-11
lingual U8-11; U9-23
lining U40-3
lip U8-9
- bumper U37-22
- line U39-6
- retractor U32-2
lipid U12-11
lips, incompetent U36-24
lipstick U8-9
lisp U11-21
load U43-14
load-bearing U43-14
loading U43-14
- dose U47-19
loca(liza)tion (pain) U16-10
locator, apex U41-12
lockjaw U38-6
logopedics U11-9
long-range U14-15
loop U24-9
-, contraction U37-3
-, wire U37-4
lotion U5-10
loupe, magnifying U22-6
lozenge U5-14
lucid U4-3
lump U13-16
luster U39-18
lustrous U39-18
lute U31-17
luting agent U31-17
- composite U30-3
luxation (joint) U17-4
- (tooth) U44-2

M

machined fit U42-16
macronutrient U12-2
magnetic resonance imaging
 U33-12
magnification U22-6
magnify U22-6
maintenance dose U47-19
malalignment U29-1
malformation U13-5
malnourishment U12-1
malocclusion U10-13; U36-8
-, class III U36-14
malunited (bone) U17-15
management U18-1

- plan U6-13
mandible, dislocated U38-8
manipulation U29-2
marginal bleeding index U35-8
mass U13-16
masseter reflex U38-7
mastication U10-15
masticatory U10-15; U38-6
- muscles U38-6
matrix retainer U32-21
maxillofacial U9-26
maxillomandibular registration
 U36-2
meal U1-7
mean U14-10
median U14-10
medical U5-1
- card U6-14
medicate U5-1
medication U5-1
medicine U5-1
melting point U31-16
meniscectomy U38-17
mentoplasty U45-14
mentum U8-6
mercury vapor U31-14
mesial U9-21
microabrasion U39-23
microcondenser U41-15
microdissect U22-5
microneurosurgery U22-5
micronutrient U12-17
micropetechiae U13-27
micropin U29-15
microscissors U24-4
microsurgeon U22-5
microsurgery U21-3; U22-5
migration U36-21
milk U2-4
- sugar U12-8
- teeth U10-2
mill U36-10
-, trephine U43-10
milled-in curves/paths U36-10
minimum tension, line of U49-10
mini-plate U29-17
moan U11-4
mobile U29-5
mobility U29-5
mobilization U25-13; U29-5
mock-up U42-15
modality, therapeutic U18-3
model, proportional hazard U14-35
module, elastic U37-10
molar (tooth) U9-7
-, first U9-7
-, third U9-8
mold U31-3f
molding U31-4

monitor U25-8
monobloc U37-14
monofilament U26-7
monosaccharide U2-16
morbid U13-2
morbidity U13-2; U18-12
- rate U14-9
morsel U10-12
mortality U14-9
mount U31-7
mounting (cast) U31-7
mouth U8-8
- gag U32-3
- mirror U32-4
-, roof of the U9-10
-, trench U35-14
mouthful U8-8
mouthguard U37-25
mouthwash U8-8
movement, bodily U36-22
mucocele U44-15
mucogingival defect U35-12
mucolytic U20-15
mucosa, oral U35-17
mucosa-borne U42-12
multifactorial U14-5
multifilament (suture) U26-7
multifocal U13-3
multiplanar reconstruction U33-19
multiple-tooth splint U42-22
multivariable analysis U14-28
multivariate U14-5
multivitamin U12-13
mumble U11-15
mummification U41-24
munch U10-15
murmur U11-15
muscle relaxant U48-16
muscles, masticatory U38-6
mutter U11-15
myofascial pain dysfunction syndrome U38-3

N

nail U29-16
nape U8-13
narcosis U47-6
narcotic agent/drug U47-5
narcotics U47-5
narcotize U47-5
nasal U8-4
nasion U39-5
neck U8-13
neckline U8-13
necrosis U13-30
necrotizing U13-30
needle holder U24-15

-, hypodermic U7-6
-, surgical U24-5
neoadjuvant U18-8
nibble U10-11
night brace U37-18
- guard U37-25
nitrous oxide U48-11
nodosity U13-16
nodular U13-16
nodulation U13-16
nodule U13-16
noncompliant U18-15
noncrossover (treatment) U15-14
nonedible U1-5
nonexfoliated (teeth) U10-5
non-extraction U44-2
non-loaded U43-14
nonnarcotic U47-5
nonobstructive U13-18
nonprescription U19-1
non-proprietary U19-2
nonrandomized U15-5
nonresponder U18-11
non-sterile U27-2
nonsubmerged (implant) U43-5
nontoxic U19-13
nontransplanted U49-14
nose U8-4
nosebleed U3-19; U8-4
nosocomial U19-15; U27-12
nourish U1-3; U12-1
nourishment U12-1
nucha U8-13
nuclear U46-22
nuclide U46-22
numb U47-3
numbness U47-3
nurse anesthetist U23-6
-, circulating U23-9
-, recovery room U23-17
-, registered U23-6
-, surgical U23-8
nurture U12-1
nutrient U12-2
nutritional supplement U2-22
nutritious U12-2
nutritive U12-2

O

objective U15-3
obliteration U13-18
observation, postanesthetic U25-8
obstructing U13-18
obstruction U13-18
obtunded U4-10
obturation U13-18
-, endodontic U41-15

occlude U10-13, U36-7
occlusal U9-24; U10-13
- (registration) rim U42-14
- curvature U39-11
- foil U32-25
- trauma U35-19
occlusion (teeth) U36-7; U10-13
- (vessel) U13-18
-, balanced U36-7
-, centric U10-13
-, torsive U36-27
odor, breath U34-20
ointment U5-8
- cannula U24-6
oligodontia U36-19
on-call, anesthesiologist U23-6
onlay U40-16
ooze U13-26
opacity U39-16
opalescent U39-16
opaque U39-16
open bite, anterior U36-12
operate on (patient) U21-1
operating light U7-9
- microscope U22-6
- room U23-1
- table U23-10
- team U23-4
- theatre U23-1
operation U21-1
operative U21-2
- permit U25-3
operator U23-5
operator-dependent U23-5
option, therapeutic U6-13
OR technician U23-9
oral cavity U8-8
- Hygiene Index U34-21
- intake, postoperative U25-12
- surgeon U44-1
order U19-1
organic U26-10
organ-sparing U21-13
oriented, well U4-8
orthodontic appliance U37-1
orthodontics U36-1
-, surgical U45-9
orthognathic surgery U45-9
orthopedics, dental U36-1
-, dentofacial U36-1
orthosis, cervical U29-9
osseointegration U43-1
osteoarthrosis U38-11
osteorrhaphy U29-12
osteosuture U29-12
osteosynthesis U29-4,12
osteotome U24-11
osteotomy, sagittal split U45-12
-, segmental U45-11

osteotomy, sliding oblique U45-13
-, vertical U45-13
-, visor U45-11
outcome U15-27
-, cosmetic U49-3
-, primary U14-20
-, surgical U15-27
outlier U14-12
outline U39-2; U46-12
overbite U36-13
- reduction U37-24
overbleaching U39-19
overdenture U42-11
overdose U19-7
overeat U1-1
overexposure U46-7
overfill U41-21
overhang U40-12
overjet U36-14
overjut U36-14
overlap, vertical U36-13
overlay denture U42-10f
overnourishment U12-1
overtone U11-11

P

pack U28-24
package U5-16
- insert U5-17
packet U5-16
packing U28-24
pad U28-19
padding U28-19
pager U7-12
pain U16-6
- killer U16-20
- relief U16-19
- threshold U16-18
-, character/nature U16-7
-, duration U16-8
-, gnawing U16-7
-, intensity U16-9
-, nagging U16-8
-, shooting U16-7
-, site/location U16-10
-, stabbing U16-7
pain-free U16-6
painful U16-11
palatable U1-5
palatal U9-10,23
palate U9-10
-, cleft U9-10
-, hard U9-10
-, soft U9-10
-, split U37-17
palatine U9-10
palatoplasty U45-3

palliation U16-19; U18-9
palliative U18-9
- therapy U16-19
palsy U47-11
pan U33-5
panoramic radiograph U33-5
papilla, gingival U35-5
-, interdental U35-5
paralleling pin U43-9
parallelism, axial U43-9
paralysis U47-11
paralyze U47-11
parameter U14-5
parasigmatism U11-21
parasympatholytic U20-8
paresis U47-11
paresthesia U16-17; U47-4
parotidectomy U45-17
paroxysm U16-14
particulate (bone graft) U44-10
- radiation U46-10
pass out U4-6
paste U5-8
-, dental (protective) U30-24
-, desensitizing U30-24
pastille U5-14
pathogen U13-1
pathologic U13-1
pathology U13-1
patient instruction leaflet U5-17
pedicle flap U50-11
- graft U50-10f
pegged tooth U9-1
pellet U5-9
pellicle, acquired (oral) U34-10
penetrate U40-21
penicillin U20-10
percentage U14-8
percentile U14-11
percolate U40-21
perforation, apical U41-17
-, furcal U41-17
periapical U41-6
perio U35-1
periodicity, pain U16-8
periodontal U35-1
- (disease) index U35-7
- ligament U35-23
periodontics U35-1
periodontist U35-1
periodontitis U35-15
periodontology U35-1
perioperative U21-2
permit, operative U25-3
pernio, erythema U3-12
persistent vegetative state U4-17
personnel U6-3
pestle U31-14
petechia U13-27

pharmaceutics U20-1
pharmacology U20-1
pharmacy U5-4
pharyngeal U8-12
- reflex U10-16
pharynx U8-12
phial U5-13
phlegm loosener U20-15
phonation U11-10, 13
phonetic U11-13
phosphorescence U46-8
photobleaching U39-19
physiotherapy, oral U34-1
pill U5-7
pilot drill U43-8
pin U29-15
-, dentinal U40-14
-, paralleling U43-9
-, parapulpal U40-14
pinning U29-15
pinprick U29-15
pins-and-needles U16-17
place U23-11
placebo U15-8
plane, auriculo-infraorbital U39-4
-, occlusal U39-4
planography U46-19
plaque, calcified U34-9
-, dental U34-8
plaque-disclosing tablet U34-12
plaster (of Paris) U30-12
- cast U29-6
plastic surgery U49-3
plates U10-8
-, dental U42-3
plating U29-17
platinum foil U30-9
pledget U28-23
plica U49-8
plication U49-8
pliers U32-16
-, bracket holding U37-9
plot U14-27
plotter U14-27
plugger U32-17
-, cement U30-6
plugging U32-17
pocket elimination U35-24
- reduction U34-14
-, periodontal U35-11
pocketing U35-11
pogonion U39-5
polish U31-21
polishing, air-abrasive U34-11
polymerization shrinkage U31-6
pontic U42-5; 40-11
popping U38-4
population U14-3
porcelain U30-4

porcelain, powder U30-21
position U23-11
-, dorsal recumbent U23-12
-, dorsosacral U23-14
-, flank U23-16
-, lateral decubitus U23-16
-, lateral recumbent U23-15
-, semiprone U23-15
positioner, tooth U37-23
post, endodontic U40-15
-, impression U31-12
postanesthesia care unit U47-24
- recovery area U23-17
postanesthetic phase U47-23
postburn U3-11
postconcussion U3-14
postextraction U44-2
postgraft U50-1
postimplantation U43-3
postinsertion U43-3
postirradiation U46-4
postoperative U21-2
posttransplant U49-14
postulate U15-19
potency U19-9
potent U19-9
poultice U28-25
powder U5-9
power, penetrating U46-9
practice leaflet U6-8
practitioner, dental U6-1
precarious U34-18
precaution U5-18
precision attachment U42-7
prediction U14-29
predictive U14-29
predictor U14-29
preextraction U44-2
pregraft U50-1
preimplant U43-3
preload U43-14
premolar U9-6
preoperated U21-1
preoperative U21-2
prep U27-14
- room U23-3
preponderance U14-8
preprosthetic U42-2
prescribe U19-1
prescription U19-1
presedation U47-8
preservation U21-13
preserve U21-13
preshaped U49-4
press-fit U42-16
pressure U36-28
pretapping U43-11
pretransplant U49-14
prevalence U14-7

prevention U18-6
preventive U18-6
prick U3-10
probability U14-31
probe U24-8; U32-9
probing U24-8
- instrument U32-1
procedure, surgical/operative U21-4
-, two-film U33-2
proclination U36-23
profile U39-3
prognathism U45-10
prolabium U8-9
prolapse U13-22
prominence, laryngeal U8-14
pronounce U11-13
pronunciation U11-13
proof U15-17
prophy U34-2
prophylactic U18-6; U34-2
prophylaxis U18-6
-, antibiotic U27-13
-, dental U34-2
proportion U14-8
proprietary U19-2
prospective U15-6
prosthesis, auricular U45-22
-, dental U42-2
-, maxillofacial U45-22
-, provisional U42-9
prosthetic U45-22
- dentistry U42-1
prosthetist U42-1
prosthodontics U42-1
protein U12-9
proteolytic U12-9
protocol U15-7; U18-5
protraction U29-3; U36-28
protrusion U36-24
provitamin U12-13
proximal U9-22
pseudocyst U13-24
psychoactive substance U20-23
ptosis U13-22
ptyalography U33-13
puffiness U3-15
puffy U3-15
pull (muscle) U3-17
pulp cap(ping), indirect U40-6
- cavity U41-5
- chamber U41-5
- tester U32-20
-, dental U9-18
pulpal status U41-2
pulpectomy U41-19
pulpitis U41-7
pulpotomy U41-19
pumice, flour of U30-18

puncture U3-10
purulent U13-12; U28-14
pus U13-12
put to sleep U47-1
- under U47-1

Q

Quad helix appliance U37-17
quadrant U9-20
quartile U14-11

R

radiant U46-2
radiate (rays) U46-2
radiating pain U16-10
radiation burn U46-7
- dose U46-9
- exposure U46-7
radioactive U46-21
radioactivity U46-21
radioautogram U33-15
radioautography U33-15
radiodense U46-11
radiogram U46-3
radiograph U46-3
-, periapical U33-7
-, skull U33-10
radiographic film U33-2
radiography U46-3
-, sectional U46-19
radioisotope U46-22
radiologic U46-1
radiology U46-1
radiolucency U46-11
radiolucent U46-11
radionuclide U46-22
radiopacity U46-11
radiopaque U46-11
radioresistant U46-23
radiosensitive U46-23
radiosensitivity U46-23
radiotracer U12-17
radiovisiography U33-15
radix dentis U9-19
raise (flap) U49-11
random U15-5
randomization U15-5
range, therapeutic U14-15
ranula U44-15
rasp U24-12
raspatory U24-12; U32-12
rate U14-8
ratio U14-8
-, risk-benefit U25-5
ray U46-2

realignment U29-2
reamer U32-11
reappoint U6-9
reapproximate U26-5; U28-2
reattachment, periodontal U35-27
rebake U31-18
rebase U42-17,25
rebond U39-20
recalcitrant U18-13
recall U6-15
recede U35-10
receding gums U9-12
reception room U6-7
receptionist U6-6
recession, gingival U35-10
recipient U49-15
reconstruction U49-1
reconstructive surgery U49-3
recontouring, gingival U35-26
record base U42-14
- rim U42-14
-, interocclusal U36-2
recovery U25-14
- (anesthesia) U47-21
- room U23-17
- - bed U23-18
recruitment, patient U15-4
recuperation U25-14
redisplacement U17-4
redress U28-17
reduction U49-19
- (fracture) U29-2
reexplore U21-11
reference plane U39-4
referral U6-12
refire U31-18
reflex threshold U38-7
-, pharyngeal U10-16
refractory U18-13
refracture U17-1
regimen U18-5
registration, interocclusal U36-2
-, maxillomandibular U36-2
regression U14-33
rehabilitation U49-2
reimpaction U44-3
reimplantation U44-4
reintrude U36-25
relapse U37-23
relation(ship) U14-32
relaxant, muscle U48-16
reliability U14-30
reline U42-25
remedial U5-2
remediation U5-2
remedy U5-2
remodel U49-4
removal torque U43-12
repackaging U5-16

repair U49-1
replacement U2-21; U49-2
replantation U44-4
reposition U23-11
reproducibility U14-30
research U15-2
resectable U21-15
resection U21-15; U22-13
-, root-end U41-20
reservoir bag U47-15
reshaped U49-4
resin, acrylic U30-2
-, composite U30-3
resin-modified glass ionomer
 U40-5
resistance U18-13
-, wear U30-3
resolution, image U46-14
-, soft tissue U46-14
resolving power U46-14
resorption U10-20; U26-8
-, alveolar U44-6
respond (therapy) U18-11
response U18-11
responsive U4-7
rest area U42-18
resterilize U27-2
restoration U40-1; U49-1
restorative U40-1; U49-1
restrain U36-29
resuscitation U47-25
resuture U26-1
retain U36-29
retainer U37-23; U42-21
-, denture U42-6
retarder U30-23
retch U10-16
retention U36-29; U37-23
-, bar-clip U42-2
-, denture U42-21
-, frictional U42-9
retract U32-2; U36-28
retractability U32-2
retraction U24-16; U29-3; U32-2
retractor U24-16
-, cheek U32-2
retransplantation U49-14
retroclination U36-23
retrocline U36-23
retrofilling U41-21
retrognathism U45-10
retrospective U15-6
retruded U36-24
retrusion U36-23f
return to normal activity U25-14
reusable U27-4
reverse filling U41-21
rhinoplasty U22-4
ridge, alveolar U9-13

rinse U27-5; U34-6
risk, operative U25-5
roentgen-equivalent-man U46-10
roentgenogram U46-3
rongeur (forceps) U24-11
root (tooth) U9-19
- amputation U41-23
- apex U9-19
- canal U41-4
- - therapy U41-9
- - treatment U41-9
- coverage U35-12
- cracking U41-18
- curettage U24-10
- dentine U9-16
- exposure U35-12
- fracture U41-18
- planing U34-14
-, remnant U41-18
root-end filling U41-21
rotation U36-27
roughage U12-16
route, surgical U21-6
rubber dam U32-19
rugine U24-12
rupture U3-18; U13-23

S

saccharide U12-6
saccharin U12-6
saddle U42-18
safety specs/goggles U7-10
sagittal split osteotomy U45-12
saliva U10-9
- ejector U7-7
salivary U10-9
salivation U10-9
salt U2-18
salve U5-8
sample U14-4
sampling U14-4
sandblasting U30-11
sanitization U34-2
scab U28-9
scald U3-11
scale U14-6
scaler U32-13
scaling U34-14
scallop U39-14
scalpel U24-3
scan U46-18
scanner U46-18
scanography U46-18
scar U28-10
scarring U28-10
schedule U19-1
scintigram U46-17

scintigraphy U46-17
scintillation U46-17
scintiscans, serial U46-17
scissors U24-4
scoop U24-10
score U14-6
–, raw U14-6
–, scaled U14-6
–, standard U14-6
scrape U3-9
scratch U3-9
scream U11-14
screw U29-16
screw-in tooth U43-2
scrub nurse U23-8
– suit U27-6,15
scrub-up U27-6
sculpt U39-2
seal U26-11; U34-16
–, hermetic U41-15
sealant U26-11; U34-16
sealer U34-16
sear off (gutta-percha) U30-14
seat U42-18
sectio U21-10
section U21-10
secure U26-4
sedation U47-8
sedative U47-8f
seepage U41-16
selection, patient U25-2
self-curing (resin) U30-3
self-medication U5-1
self-tapping U43-11
semi-comatose U4-14
semi-starvation U1-14
semi-stuporous U4-11
sensation, blunted U47-4
sensitivity (test) U14-23
separator U37-12
septic U27-1
sequel(a) U25-9
series U14-3; U15-12
setting U29-2
– expansion U31-6
set-up U42-13
shade U39-15
shading U39-15
sham treatment U15-8
shape U49-4
sharps U24-2
shavings, bone U44-11
shears U24-4
shed (teeth) U10-5
sheen U39-18
shift U36-21
shine U39-18
shiner U3-13
shiny U39-18

shoulder (crown) U40-8
shout U11-14
shriek U11-14
shrink (shrank-shrunken) U31-6
shrinkage contraction U31-6
–, gingival U35-10
–, polymerization U31-6
shunt U49-6
sialography U33-13
side effect U19-14
sideshift U36-21
sigh U11-4
sigmatism U11-21
significance U14-21
significant, statistically U14-21
sinus lift (procedure) U45-15
skeletal traction U29-3
skewing, mandibular U38-10
skewness U14-13
skin coverage U49-9
– preparation, preoperative U27-14
skull film U33-10
– fracture U17-8
– radiograph U33-10
slash U3-6
slice U3-6
sliding flap U50-14
sling U29-8
slipknot U26-6
slope U14-33
slot, bracket U37-4
smile line U39-6
–, full/widest U39-6
snare U22-11
sneeze U11-6
snore U11-5
snoreguard U37-25
snort U11-5
sob U11-3
socket, tooth U9-13; U30-16
solder U31-16
solubility U5-11
solution U5-11
solvent U5-11
somnolence U4-13
sonography U33-11
sopor U4-13
sore U13-17; U16-11
soreness U16-11
sound (instrument) U24-8; U32-9
– (tone) U11-11
space closure, orthodontic U36-17
– maintainer U32-22
–, embrasure U39-13
–, freeway U10-14
–, interproximal U9-22
spaced out U4-9
spacing U36-16

spare U21-13
spasmolytic U20-19
speak (spoke-spoken) U11-8
specificity U14-23
spectacles, protective U7-10
Spee curve U36-5
speech U11-8
spillway, interdental U39-13
spit U10-10
spitoon U7-8; U10-10
splint U29-7; U42-22
– therapy U38-14
–, biteguard U38-14
–, multiple-tooth U42-22
–, orthopedic U37-16
splinter U17-2
splinting U29-7; U37-16; U42-22
split U21-14
– palate U37-17
split-thickness graft U50-6
sponge, surgical U24-18
spoon U24-10
spot, colored U34-11
spreader U32-17
–, gutta-percha U30-14
–, hand U32-17
spring U37-11
sprue pin/former U30-20
stabilization U29-4
stable U29-4
staff U6-3
stain U34-11
staining U34-12
stammer U11-20
stannous fluoride U34-13
stapler U26-12
starch U12-5
starving U1-14
statistician U14-1
statistics U14-1
status, gingival U35-6
stenosis U13-19f
stenotic U13-20
stent U22-20
step (preparation) U40-7
stepdown technique U41-11
stereoroentgenography U33-2
sterile U27-2
sterility U27-2
sterilization U27-2
–, dry heat U27-2
–, saturated steam U27-2
– chamber U27-2
Steri-strip® U28-21
stiffening, joint U38-12
stilette U24-7
sting (stung-stung) U3-10
stinging (pain) U16-7
stitch U26-1

stitch (pain) U16-13
stockinet U29-10
stomatitis U35-16
stone U13-21
- breakage U31-19
-, artificial U30-13
-, dental U30-13
-, die U30-13; U31-5
stop condition U15-30
stopping rule U15-30
storage U5-19
straight wire technique U37-2
straining U3-17
strand (suture) U26-7
strap U29-11
strapping U29-11
stratigraphy U46-19
strenuous U3-17
stress breaker U42-18
stricture U13-19
strip, abrasive U32-24
student's test U14-34
study U15-1
- manual of operations U15-7
stunned U4-9
stupefaction U4-11
stupor U4-11
stutter U11-20
stylet U24-7
subconsciousness U4-1
subgroup U14-3
subject U14-2
subluxation U17-4
subperiosteal tunneling U44-13
subset U14-3
substitution U2-21
successor tooth/teeth U36-6
suction U22-16
- cannula U24-6
suffer U16-2
sugar U2-16; U12-6
suite, (pre)surgical U23-2
-, operating U23-2
sulcular U35-4
sulcus bleeding index U35-8
- deepening U44-6
-, gingival U35-4
sunburn U3-11
superstructure U43-15
superstructure-to-implant ratio U43-16
supplement U2-22
suppository U5-12
suppuration U28-14
suppurative U28-14
supragingival U35-2
surface lightening U39-19
surgeon U21-3; U23-5
-, attending U23-5

-, dental U6-1
-, oral U44-1
surgery U21-3
-, corrective jaw U45-9
-, facial advancement U45-8
-, functional endoscopic sinus U45-19
-, orthognathic U45-9
-, reconstructive U49-3
surgical U21-2f
- correction U49-2
- gloves U27-17
- nurse U23-8
- team U23-4
surveillance U18-7
surveyor U32-10
survival U14-25
survivorship U14-25
suspend U29-3
suspension U29-3; U49-7
suture U26-1
- forceps U24-15
- material U26-7
-, figure-of-eight U26-19
-, interlocking U26-16
-, interrupted U26-15
-, lock-stitch U26-16
-, mattress U26-17
-, over-and-over U26-15
-, purse-string U26-18
-, quilt(ed) U26-17
-, running U26-16
sutureless U26-1
suture-ligate U26-3
suturing U26-1
swab U28-23
swathe U29-8
swell (swelled-swollen) U3-15
swelling U3-15; U13-16
syllable U11-12
syllable-stumbling U11-12
sympatholytic U20-27
sympathomimetics U20-27
syncope U4-4
syndrome, myofascial pain dysfunction U38-3
synthetic U26-10
syringe U7-6
-, chip U7-4
-, water U7-5
syrup U5-11
systemic U19-5

T

t- test U14-34
table (statistical) U14-27
-, operating U23-10

tablet U5-7
-, plaque-disclosing U34-12
tabulation U14-27
tack U26-4
tailor U49-4
take in (food) U1-1
take out (tooth) U44-2
tampon U28-24
tap (screw) U43-11
- (suction) U22-16
taping U29-11
tapping (suction) U22-16
target tissue U46-4
tarnish U43-18
tartar U34-9
task light U7-9
tear U3-7
tear (tore-torn) U3-18
tearing U3-18
technician, dental (laboratory) U6-5
-, radiologic U33-2
technique, stepback U41-11
-, surgical/operative U21-4
teeth U9-1
- grinding U10-18
-, baby U10-2
-, buck U36-24
-, crowded U37-19
-, deciduous U10-2
-, extra U36-19
-, false U10-8
-, flared U36-24
-, front/anterior U9-2
-, milk U10-2
-, permanent U10-6
-, posterior U9-2
-, secondary U10-6
-, successor U36-6
-, supernumerary U36-19
-, well-spaced U36-16
teether U10-4
teething U10-4
telescopic coping U42-9
temper U31-15
template, surgical U31-13
temporomandibular joint U38-1
tenaculum U24-16
tenderness U16-11
tenorrhaphy U26-2
teratogen U20-33
teratogenicity U20-33
termination U15-30
texture U39-17
therapeutic U18-4
- modality U18-3
- range U19-13
therapy U18-1,4
-, expectant U18-7

therapy, palliative U16–19
–, splint U38–14
thimble, metal U42–9
thirst U1–11
thread (implant) U43–11
– (suture) U26–7
threshold U14–24
–, pain U16–18
–, reflex U38–7
throat U8–12
thrombolytic U20–16
tie U26–6
tie off U26–3
tincture U5–10
tipping U36–21
tissue expansion U49–10
–, granulation U28–7
tissue-borne U42–12
titanium U30–10
TMJ arthroscopy U38–15
– dislocation U38–8
– dysfunction/disorder U38–2
– osteoarthritis U38–11
– replacement surgery U38–19
tolerance U19–12
–, pain U16–18
tomogram U46–19
tomograph U46–19
tomography U46–19
tone (voice) U11–11
tongue U8–11
– depressor U32–3
– thrust U36–20
tongue-tied U44–7
tonsil, palatine U9–10
tool, therapeutic U6–13
tooth U9–1
– cement U9–17
– decay U34–17
– exposure U44–2
– extraction U44–2
– sectioning U44–2
– whitening U39–19
–, adjacent U9–1
–, avulsed U44–3
–, bicuspid U9–6
–, cheek U9–7
–, cutting U9–3
–, eye U9–5
–, impacted U44–3
–, incisal U9–3
–, incisor U9–3
–, multi-rooted U9–19; U41–3
–, nonvital U41–7
–, opposing U9–1
–, pegged U9–1
–, pulpless U41–7
–, screw-in U43–2
–, vital U41–7

–, wisdom U9–8
toothache U16–4
tooth-borne U42–12
toothbrush U34–3
toothless U10–7
toothpick U34–3
tooth-size discrepancy U36–18
tooth-supported U42–12
topical U19–5
torn U3–7
torque U36–27
– wrench U43–12
–, insertion U43–12
torsion U3–16
torsional U3–16
torsive occlusion U36–27
torsiversion U36–27
torsocclusion U36–27
torus, mandibular U44–16
–, palatal U44–16
tourniquet, Esmarch U47–18
toxic level U19–13
– range U19–13
toxicity U19–13
toxicology U19–13
trace element U12–17
– metal U12–17
– mineral U12–17
tracer U46–21; U12–17
tract, fistulous U35–21
traction U36–28
–, skeletal U29–3
trait U14–5
trance U4–15
tranquilizer U47–10
transect U21–14
transection U21–14
transfer U49–13
– coping U31–11
transfix U29–4
transgingival U35–2
transillumination U46–16
translation, bodily U36–22
translucency U39–16
transplant U49–14; U50–1
transpose U49–13
transposition U36–22; U49–13
transudate U28–13
trauma U3–2,4
traumatize U3–4; U28–1
tray, impression U31–3
Treacher-Collins syndrome U45–6
treatment U18–1
– arm U15–12
– block U15–11
– card U6–14
– group U15–10
– lag U15–21
– modality U18–3

– plan U6–13
–, sham U15–8
Trendelenburg, reverse U23–13
trephination, cortical U41–22
trephine mill U43–10
trismus U38–6
triturate U31–14
trocar U24–7
try-in U42–15
T-Scan U33–8
tube, endotracheal U47–17
tubocurare U48–17
tumescence U3–15
tumor U13–16
tungsten carbide U30–11
tunnel dissection U44–13
tunneling, subperiosteal U44–13
tweezers U24–13f
twin block U37–14
twinge U16–13
twirl on U37–7

U

ulcer U13–17
ultraconservative dentistry U45–18
ultrasonography U33–11
ultrasound U33–11
unaffected U13–4
unbiased U14–18
unblind U15–9
uncomfortable U16–1
uncomplicated U25–9
unconfirmed U15–17
unconscious U4–1
uncorrelated U14–32
uncoupling, tube U46–13
uncover U49–9
underbite U36–14
undercondensation U41–15
undercut U40–13
underfeeding U1–3
underfill U41–21
undertone U11–11
undisplaced U3–20
undocumented U15–15
unerupted (tooth) U10–3
uneventful U25–9
unexposed U21–7; U46–7
unhurt U3–1
uninjured U3–1
union, bony U17–15
univariate U14–5
unpalatable U1–5
unreliable U14–30
unresponsive U4–7
unresponsiveness U18–11
unruptured U3–18

unscarred U28-10
unset (bone) U29-2
unsplinted U37-16
unstable U29-4
unstrapped U29-11
untaped U29-11
untoward effect U19-14
ununited (bone) U17-15
uppers (dentures) U42-3
urgent U21-5
utter U11-1

V

valid U14-30
validation U14-30
validity U14-30
vaporize U22-15
variability U14-14
variable U14-5
variance U14-14
variation U14-14
varnish U30-22
vasoconstriction U20-17
vasodilation U20-17
vasopressor U20-17
vault, palatal U9-10
vegetarian U1-16
veneer U39-22
veneering, ceramic U30-4
venepuncture U22-18
venipuncture U22-18
ventilation system U27-8
-, artificial U47-15
-, mechanical U48-17
verify U15-17

vertical dimension U36-3
vestibule, oral U8-10
vestibuloplasty U44-7
vial U5-13
videosubtraction U33-16
view, intraoral U33-4
vigil coma U4-17
vigilance U4-2
visit U6-9
visualize U46-12
vitalometer U32-20
vitamin U12-13,15
vocal U11-10
voice U11-10
void U41-16

W

waiting room U6-7
waiver, informed U25-3
watchful waiting U18-7
wax U30-17
wax-up U31-10; U42-13
wedge U32-22
- apart (teeth) U35-14
weep (wept-wept) U11-3
weep (wound) U28-13
wheel, rubber U34-2
whisper U11-16
wholefood U1-12
wholesome U1-12
wince U16-12
wing, bracket U37-4
wire U29-14
-, figure-of-eight U29-14
wiring U29-14

-, circumferential U29-14
withdraw (drug) U19-6
withdrawal (study) U15-29
working length U41-12
workup, preoperative U25-1
wound U3-1,3f
wound care U28-1
- closure U28-3
- contraction U28-8
- healing U28-5
- irrigation U28-11
- management U28-1
- repair U3-3; U28-5
wrap U28-20
-, Esmarch U47-18
wrench, torque U43-12

X

Xbite U36-15
xenograft U50-5
xero(radio)graphy, dental U33-17
x-ray U46-3
- film U33-2
- tube U33-1
-, skull U33-10

Y

yell U11-14

Z

zipping U41-13

Index – Abbreviations

Hier finden Sie alle im Text enthaltenen englischen Abkürzungen und Akronyme in alphabetischer Reihenfolge mit einem Verweis auf das Modul und den betreffenden Eintrag.

a.c. U19–1
AA U12–10
ACE U20–7
ADE U5–3
ADH U20–21
ADR U5–3; U19–14
alt.noct. U19–1
ANOVA U14–14
ANUG U35–14
AOB U36–12
AUC U14–27
AUG U35–14
b.i.d. U19–1
BAHA U45–23
BBQ U2–23
BCAA U12–10
BMP U44–11
BMT U49–14
BP U47–24
BPH U13–15
BSS U26–10
cal U12–4
CAT U33–18; U46–19
CEJ U39–9
cfu U27–10
CI U14–17
CRF U15–16
CRP U12–9
CSF U12–7
CT U33–18
CTAT U33–18
CV U14–14
DC U24–10
D.D.S. U44–1
DBM U44–11
DE U46–9
DEF, def U34–21
df U14–16
df U34–21
DFDBA U44–11
dmfs U34–21
DSMB U15–15
DT U4–16
EAA U12–10

EFA U12–12
ENT U8–14
ER U21–5
f/u, F/U U25–15
FB U22–16
FBS U12–6
FDBA U44–11
FESS U45–19
Frx U17–1
GA U48–1
GBGA U44–8
GBR U44–12
GCF U35–4
GI U35–7
GSD U46–9
GTF U12–7
GTR U35–28
gtt. U5–11
GVHD U50–20
GVHR U50–20
Gy U46–10
h.s. U19–1
HTO U45–5
i.a. U19–3
i.m. U19–3
i.v., IV U19–3
ICC U15–25
IDE U15–2
IMF U29–4
IND U5–3; U15–2
INDA U15–2
IOD U45–5
IOTN U36–1
IRB U15–24
J U12–4
LA U48–3
LD U19–7
Liq. U5–11
LSD U14–21
LVH U13–15
LVP U39–4
MANOVA U14–28
MAO U20–7
MBI U35–8

MFD U45–6
MFP U39–4
MPD U38–3
MRI U33–12
narc U47–5
NEAA U12–10
NPO U8–8
NSAID U20–11
o.h. U19–1
o.n. U19–1
OB, o/b U36–13
OD U19–7
OHI U34–21
OHI-S U34–21
oint U5–8
OJ, o/j U36–14
OR (stat.) U14–8
OR (surg.) U23–1; U21–2
OT U23–1; U21–2
OTC U5–3
P value U13–31
p.o. U19–3
P.O.P., POP U29–6; U30–12
p.r.n. U19–1
PACU U47–24
PAR U47–21; U23–17
PB (graft) U44–10
PB (phon.) U11–13
PBI U12–9
PCA U47–7
PDI U35–7
PDL U35–1
PET U46–19
Pl U30–9
PND U16–14
PVS U4–17
q.d. U19–1
q.h. U19–1
q.l. U19–1
q.p. U19–1
q.r.s. U19–1
q4 U19–1

rad U46–10
RAD U46–3
RAI U46–21
RCT U41–9
RDFT U34–21
REC U15–25
rem U46–10
RMGI U40–5
ROC U14–27,34
RPE U37–1
RR U47–21; U23–17
R_x U19–1
s.c. U19–3
S/I ratio U43–16
SBI U35–8
SC U15–25
SD U14–13
SDM U14–13
SEM U14–10
SFFR U35–4
SMR U14–9
SRLFI U45–7
SS U14–34
sub-q U19–3
Sv U46–10
t.i.d. U19–1
tab U5–7
TC U30–11
TCS U45–6
Ti U30–10
TMJ U38–1
TMJD U38–2
TMPDS U38–2
TNF U13–30
TNI U46–4
TPN U12–3
TRAM U50–11
TSD U36–18
T_x U18–1
UNG U5–8
URA U37–1
US U33–11
W/N U12–1

Index – Deutsch

Mit Hilfe des Index können Sie **KWiC-Web** auch zum Nachschlagen von Fachausdrücken verwenden. Hier finden Sie die deutschen Fachtermini in alphabetischer Reihenfolge. Umlaute werden dabei nicht gesondert berücksichtigt, d. h. **ä, ö, ü** werden wie **a, o, u** behandelt. Adjektiv-Verbindungen finden Sie unter dem Hauptwort (z. B. *harter Gaumen* unter *Gaumen*). Da auch viele fachspezifische Verben und Adjektive sowie allgemeinsprachliche Wortverbindungen im Index enthalten sind, wurde die Wortbedeutung in fraglichen Fällen durch ein typisches Bezugswort (in runder Klammer) verdeutlicht, z. B. *absetzen (Therapie), pressen (Zähne), erhärtet (Amalgam), anziehen (Schraube)*. Bei Alternativformen wurden bis auf wenige Ausnahmen wie z. B. *Arznei(mittel)* beide Formen oder die jeweils gebräuchlichere angeführt.

Verwiesen wird auf die Module (Unit) und Einträge (Zahl rechts unten in jedem Eintrag), in denen die Fachwörter vorkommen (z. B. U23–8,16 verweist auf die Einträge Nr. 8 und 16 in Unit 23). Zu den Modulen finden Sie am schnellsten über das Griffregister. Die halbfette Markierung des Moduls (z. B. **U23**–8) zeigt an, dass der Terminus im ersten Eintrag als Schlüsselwort aufscheint.

Aus Platzgründen war es nicht möglich, sämtliche in **KWiC-Web** enthaltenen deutschen Fachwörter im Index aufzulisten. Da aber die Wörter in den Modulen im Sinnzusammenhang dargestellt sind, findet man Termini derselben Wortfamilie bzw. Bedeutung jeweils im gleichen Eintrag, z. B. *Drainage* bei *Drain*, *Entkeimung* bei *entkeimen*, *hufeisenförmiger Zahnbogen* bei *Zahnbogenform*, *druckschmerzempfindlich* bei *druckschmerzhaft* usw. Weiterhin wurde der Index auf die zahnmedizinisch relevanten Stichwörter beschränkt, die dem Benutzer einen sehr spezifischen Zugang zu den insgesamt ca. 40.000 englischen Fachtermini und deren Kontext ermöglichen.

A

Abbau **U10**–20
abbaubar, biologisch U20–4
abbauen (Stoffwechsel) U1–6; U26–8
abbeißen U10–11
Abbindeexpansion **U31**–6
Abbindekontraktion U31–6
abbinden **U26**–3; U30–6
abbrechen (Therapie) **U19**–6; U15–30
abdecken, steril **U27**–7
Abdeckfolie (OP) U27–7,14
Abdeckkappe **U40**–17; **U43**–13
Abdeckschraube U43–13
Abdecktuch, steriles **U27**–7; U7–10
abdichten **U26**–11
Abdichtung U30–6; U34–16
Abdichtungsmasse U34–16
Abdichtungsmittel U26–11
Abdruck **U31**–2; U36–2
Abdrucklöffel **U31**–3
Abdrucknahme U6–9
Abdruckpfosten U31–2,12
abfeilen U41–14
abfließen **U28**–15
Abfluss U41–22

Abflussstörung **U13**–18
abformen U31–2
Abformgips U30–13
Abformkappe, konische U31–2
Abformlöffel **U31**–3,19,2; U30–2
–, individueller U42–13,17
–, perforierter U31–3
Abformlöffelhalter U31–3
Abformmasse U31–3; U42–25
Abformung **U31**–2; U36–2
Abformwachs U30–17
abfüllen U41–15
Abgabe (Arznei) U19–1
abgegrenzt (Läsion) U13–3
abgekapselt U46–18
abgeklemmt und ligiert U26–3
abgelagert U34–7
abgenutzt U10–19
abgesaugt U48–9
abgesondert U28–13
abgestorben U28–12
abgestumpft **U4**–10
Abgrenzung (Gewebe) U46–12
– (Sterilbereich) **U23**–7
abhalten (Wange) U32–2
abhängig (Droge) U5–3
Abhängigkeit U47–9
abheben (Gewebe) U32–15

abheilen U18–2; U28–4
Abkauung U10–19
abklären (Symptom) U16–18; U23–16
Abklärung, dringende U21–5
–, medizinische U6–11; U25–1
–, radiologische U46–1
abklemmen **U26**–13; U24–13
abklingen (Entzündung) U38–14
Ablagerungen U10–22; U34–9
Ablatio **U22**–13
Ablauf, biochemischer U20–32
Ablaufdatum U1–5
ableiten **U28**–15
ablösen U28–6
Ablösung U22–13
abmischen U5–5
abnehmbar (Teilprothese) U32–10
Abneigung (Speisen) U1–6
abnorm U13–5
Abnützung U3–18; U10–19; U38–11
abpräparieren U24–12; U21–12
abradieren U10–19; U39–23
Abrasion **U3**–8; U10–19
Abrasionsfestigkeit U30–3; U40–5
Abrasivpartikel U32–24
abraspeln U32–12

abreiben U3–8; U10–19; U27–6
abreißen U17–5
Abrieb U3–8; **U10**–19
Abriebfestigkeit U40–5,7
Abrissfraktur **U17**–5,2; U3–16; U44–3
Abruf, auf U6–12
absaugen **U22**–16,19
Absaugvorrichtung **U27**–16; U7–7
Abschabung U3–8
abschieben (Gewebe) U24–12
Abschirmung, antibiotische U20–9; U44–2; U49–9
abschleifen **U10**–18; U32–8
abschneiden U3–6
Abschnitt **U21**–10
abschnüren U35–5
abschrägen **U40**–19; U24–11
Abschürfung **U3**–8
abschwellendes Mittel U20–17
absetzen (Medikament) U19–6,14; U20–23
– (Therapie) **U19**–6; U18–11
– zw. Clips U26–13
– zw. Klammerreihen U21–14
– zw. Ligaturen U21–10
Absonderung, wässrige U28–13
absplittern U17–2
absprengen U32–18
Absprengungsfraktur U17–2
abspülen U27–5
Abstand, interorbitaler U45–5
absterben U13–30
Abstoßung, weiße U50–21
Abstrich U24–18
Abstützung U42–10
Abszedierung U13–12
Abszess, submuköser U41–8
abtasten **U46**–18
Abtastgerät U46–18
abtöten U20–25
abtragen U10–19,21; U30–11 f; U39–23; U44–16
Abtragung **U22**–13; U3–8
abtrennen U21–14
abtupfen U28–23
abwehrgeschwächt U13–4
Abweichung (Mittelwert) **U14**–13; U13–5
ACE-Hemmer U20–7
Achsenfehlstellung U17–4
Achsenknickung U17–4
Achsenneigung U43–9
Achsenparallelität U43–9
Achsenstellung **U29**–1
Achterdraht U29–14
Achterligatur U37–7; U29–14
Achternaht **U26**–19
Achtertourenpflasterverband U29–11

ad axim verschoben U17–4
Adamsapfel **U8**–14
Adams-Klammer U37–15
Adaptation **U49**–5; U28–2; U29–1
Adaptationsnaht **U49**–5; U26–1
Adaptationsschiene U29–7
adaptieren **U26**–5; **U28**–2; U49–5
– (kfo. Band) U37–8
Aderer Zange U32–16
adhärent U25–10
Adhäsiolyse U25–10
Adhäsion **U25**–10; U38–15
– (Entzündung) U13–11
Adhäsivbrücke U30–19; U42–4
Adhäsivtechnik U37–8
Adipositas U13–2
Adiuretin U20–21
adjustiert (Rate) U14–8
Adjuvans **U18**–8
adjuvant **U18**–8,4
Adrenalin U20–27
adrenalinbedingt U48–12
Aerosol **U20**–14
Affektabstumpfung U47–3
Agens **U20**–2
agitiert U4–12
Agonist U20–6
Ahle U24–5
Akersklammer U42–6
Akrylat **U30**–2; U31–2,11
Akrylatbasis U42–17
Akrylsäure U30–2
Aktivator **U37**–13; U20–3
aktivierbar U42–21
aktivieren U20–3
– (Feder) U37–11
Aktivität, biologische **U20**–3
Aktivkohle U5–9; U20–3
Akupressur U48–18
Akupressuranästhesie U48–18
Akupunkturanalgesie **U48**–18
Akupunkturanästhesie U48–18
Akzeptanz, reizlose U49–20
Alabastergips U30–13; U31–6
Alginat **U30**–15
Alginatabformlöffel U30–15
Alginatabformung U30–15
Alginatlack U30–15
Alginsäure U30–15
Aliasing U46–13
Alignment (Zähne) U36–26
alimentär U12–3
Alkohol **U2**–27
Alkoholdelir U4–16
Alkoholtupfer U24–18
Alkylans U20–2
Allgemeinanästhesie **U48**–1
Allgemeinbevölkerung U14–3
Allheilmittel U28–4
allogen U49–16

Allograft **U50**–3
Allotransplantat **U50**–3
Alternativhypothese **U15**–19
altersadjustiert (Inzidenz) U14–7
Altersatrophie U13–29; U44–6
Altersbeschwerden U16–5
altersentsprechend U14–11
Altersgrenze U14–24
Altersgruppe U14–3
Alterspercentile U14–11
Alveolarfortsatz U9–13
Alveolarkamm U10–7; U32–2; U39–9
–, atrophierter U36–22
Alveolarkammabbau **U44**–6; U41–1; U10–20
Alveolarkammatrophie **U44**–6
Alveolarkammaufbau **U44**–8
Alveolarkammhöhe U44–7
Alveolarkammreste U44–6
Alveole **U9**–13; U32–14
Amalgam **U30**–1; U31–14
Amalgamator U30–1
Amalgamfeilung U30–1
Amalgamfüllung U30–1; U40–1
amalgamieren U31–14
Amalgamierungsverhältnis U31–14
Amalgamintoxikation U30–1
Amalgamkern U30–1
Amalgammischgerät U30–1; U31–14
Amalgampistole U30–1
Amalgamstopfer U32–17
Amalgamträger U30–1; U31–4
Amalgamvibrator U31–14
Ambubeutel U47–15
ambulant U25–1,13; U47–2; U18–14
Ameisenlaufen U16–17; U47–4
Amelogenese U9–15
Aminoazidämie U12–10
Aminosäure, verzweigtkettige U12–10
Aminosäurelösung U12–10
Aminosäuren **U12**–10
Ammoniak U30–15
Ammonium U30–15
Amnesie U3–14
Ampulle U5–13
Ampullenflasche **U5**–13
Amputation U49–1
amputieren U22–13; U49–2
Analgesie **U47**–7; U16–20
–, patientengesteuerte U47–7
Analgesiestadium U47–7,20
Analgetika-Nephropathie U16–20
Analgetikum **U16**–20; U38–3; U47–7
Analyse, bivariate U14–28
–, Intention-to-treat **U15**–20

Analyse, kephalometrische U33–9
–, multivariate **U14**–28
Anamnese **U25**–1 f; U47–12
Anästhesie **U47**–2
–, balancierte **U48**–2
–, intravenöse **U48**–13
anästhesiemittelbedingt U48–4
Anästhesiesprechstunde U47–12
Anästhesieverfahren U48–4
Anästhesiologie **U47**–2
Anästhesist **U23**–6; U47–2
Anästhetikum **U47**–5,1; **U48**–4,1; U25–8
Anastomose **U49**–6
Anastomosendurchgängigkeit U49–6
Anastomoseninsuffizienz U49–6
Anastomosenleck U49–6
Anastomosenstriktur U13–19
Anastomosenverengung U49–6
Anatomie U13–2
Anbindung, transmukosale U43–5
anbrünieren **U31**–21
Andresen-Häupl-System U37–13
aneinanderlegen U26–5; U29–1
Aneurysma U16–7; U21–12
Anfall **U16**–14
–, epileptischer U20–20
Anfangsdosis U19–7
anfärben **U34**–11 f
Anflutungszeit U47–13
anfrischen (Wundränder) U22–17; U28–2
angeboren **U13**–6 f
angehoben (Wundränder) U49–11
Angehörige U25–3
angelagert U34–7
angespannt U11–20
angewinkelt U23–12
Angiographie, selektive U25–2
Angioplastie U22–4; U49–3
Angle Klasse U36–8
angreifen (Gesundheit) **U13**–4
Angstabbau U25–4
ängstlich U47–10
Angstzustände U4–16
Angulus mandibulae U8–7; U45–13
angurten U23–2
anhaften U34–9; U35–9; U39–20; U40–5
Anhaltung U25–10
anheben **U49**–11; U24–9; U32–15
anheften U26–4; U29–15
Anheftung **U49**–7; U35–9
Anionen U46–20
Anker **U42**–10,20; U37–4,15
Ankerbandklammer U42–20
Ankergeschiebe U42–20

Ankersystem U42–21
Ankerzahn U32–10; U42–20
Ankleiden (OP) U27–15
Ankyloglossie U8–11
Ankylose **U38**–12; U29–13
Ankylosis extraarticularis U38–12
Anlagerung U26–5; U29–1
Anlassen **U31**–15
anlaufen **U43**–18
Anleitung U19–1
anliegend **U40**–9; U29–1; U36–17; U40–18
Anmeldung U6–6
anmischen **U31**–14
annähen **U26**–1
annähern **U28**–2; U26–5; U49–5
Annahme (stat.) U15–17
Annihilationsstrahlung U46–2
Anodontie U36–19
Anomalie **U13**–5
anordnen (Therapie) U19–1
anpassen (Prothese) **U42**–16; U37–1
Anprobe **U42**–15
Anprobetermin U6–10
anregen U20–3
Anreicherung (Nahrungsmittel) U1–6
ansammeln U22–16
Ansammlung U28–15; U34–7
Ansatz, therapeutischer U18–4
Ansatzstück U7–3
anschlingen U22–11; U24–9
anschnallen U29–11
anschwellen U13–27
Anschwellung **U3**–15
ansetzen (OP) U19–1
ansetzen an (Muskel) U44–7
anspannen (Muskel) U16–12
ansprechbar **U4**–7
ansprechen (Medikament) **U4**–7
– (Therapie) **U18**–11
Anstaltsapotheke U5–4 f
Anstaltspackung U5–16
Anstrengung U3–17
Antagonist (Wirkstoff) **U20**–6
– (Zahn) U9–1; U10–13; U36–18,25
Antazidum **U20**–29; U19–2
Antiarrhythmikum **U20**–18
Antibiogramm U20–9
Antibiotika, zytostatische U20–31
Antibiotikaprophylaxe **U27**–13,10; U18–6
Antibiotikaresistenz U20–9
Antibiotikum **U20**–9
anticholinerg U20–8
Antidepressivum **U20**–24
Antidiarrhoikum U20–13

Antidiuretika U20–21
Antidot **U5**–15
Antiemetikum U20–12
antiepileptisch **U20**–20; U48–14
Antihistaminika **U20**–22
Antihormon U20–31
Antikoagulanzien **U20**–16
antikonvulsiv U48–14
Antikonvulsivum **U20**–20
antikörpervermittelt U20–32
Antimetabolit U20–31
Antimykotikum **U20**–26
Antioxidans U12–15
Antiphlogistika **U20**–11; U13–11
–, nichtsteroidale U20–11
Antipsychotikum **U20**–2; U47–10
Antischaummittel U20–2
Antisepsis U27–1
Antiseptikum U27–1
Antithrombosestrümpfe U29–10
Antithrombotika **U20**–16
Anti-Trendelenburglage U23–13
antiviral U20–9
Antriebslosigkeit U4–12
Antrumfistelbildung **U44**–14
Antrumraspel U24–12
ANUG **U35**–14
anwachsen U30–17
Anwendung (Medikament) U5–2; U19–3,5
Anwendungsweise U5–17
Anxiolytika U20–23; U47–10
Anzeichen **U18**–10; U4–14; U35–21
anzementieren U30–6
anziehen (Schraube) U43–6
Aortenstenose U13–20
apallisches Syndrom **U4**–17
Apathie U4–12
Apex radicis dentis **U41**–6
–, radiologischer U41–6
Apexlokalisator U41–12
aphasisch U11–11
Aphonie **U11**–23
Aphthe **U35**–17; U13–17
Aphthose U35–17
apikal U41–6,12; U44–14
Apikokoronalhöhe U39–12
Apotheke **U5**–4
Apparatur, kfo. **U37**–1
Appetit **U1**–11,6
Appetitlosigkeit U1–11; U50–20
Appetitzügler U1–11
Applikation **U19**–4,3
–, konjunktivale U20–17
Applikationsart U19–3
Applikator U19–3; U24–14
applizieren U19–4; U20–12
Apposition U29–1; U26–5

Approximalbereich U9 – 22
Approximalkaries U33 – 6
Approximalraum U39 – 13
Äquator, anatomischer **U39** – 8
Äquivalentdosis U46 – 9
Arbeit, wissenschaftliche U47 – 3
Arbeitsende U32 – 17
Arbeitshypothese U15 – 19
Arbeitslänge **U41** – 12
Arbeitsmodell U31 – 2
Arbeitsraum (OP-Feld) U21 – 7
Arbeitsseite (Kauen) U36 – 12
Arbeitstrokar U24 – 7
arbeitsunfähig U13 – 4
Armamentarium **U32** – 1
Armstütze U23 – 12
Arousal U4 – 2
Arrhythmie U20 – 18
Artefakt **U46** – 13
Arterienlappen **U50** – 12
Arthrodese U29 – 13
Arthrogramm U33 – 14
Arthrographie **U33** – 14
Arthropathia deformans U38 – 11
Arthroplastik U22 – 4
Arthropneumographie U33 – 14
Arthrose U13 – 29
Arthrotomie **U38** – 16
Articulatio temporomandibularis **U38** – 1
artifiziell verzerrt U46 – 13
Artikulation **U36** – 3; U8 – 11; U9 – 1; U11 – 1,13
Artikulationsfolie U36 – 3
Artikulationspapier **U32** – 25
Artikulationsstörung U11 – 17,22
Artikulator **U31** – 1; U6 – 11
artikulieren U11 – 1
Arznei(mittel) **U5** – 1 ff
Arzneibuch U5 – 5; U20 – 1
Arzneidroge U5 – 1
Arzneiform **U5** – 6; U19 – 11
arzneimittelbedingt **U19** – 15
Arzneimittel-Codex U5 – 5
Arzneimittelhandel U5 – 3
arzneimittelinduziert **U19** – 15
Arzneimittelinteraktion **U19** – 11
Arzneimittellehre **U20** – 1
Arzneimittelresistenz U18 – 13
Arzneimittelunverträglichkeit U19 – 12
Arzneimittelwechselwirkung **U19** – 11
Arzneimittelwirkung **U20** – 3
–, unerwünschte **U19** – 14; U5 – 3
Arzneistofffreisetzung U19 – 4
Arzneistoffinkompatibilität U5 – 3
Arzneizubereitung U5 – 6
Arzt im Praktikum U23 – 5

–, praktischer U25 – 15
Arztbesuch U6 – 10
Ärztebedarf U5 – 4
Arztelement **U7** – 2
ärztlich U5 – 1
Ascorbinsäure **U12** – 15
Asepsis U27 – 1
aseptisch **U27** – 1
Asphyxiestadium U47 – 20
Aspirat U7 – 7; U22 – 16
Aspiration **U22** – 16
Aspirationsbiopsie U22 – 16
Aspirator U22 – 16
aspirieren U22 – 16,19; U48 – 9
Assistent, radiolog. techn. U46 – 1
ästhetisch U39 – 1
Asthmatiker U20 – 27
Atem anhalten U34 – 20
– holen U34 – 20
Atembeutel U47 – 15
Atemdepression U48 – 12
Atemgeräusch, pfeifendes U11 – 23
Atemlähmung U47 – 11
Atemnot U16 – 2
Atemschläuche U47 – 14
Atemwege U47 – 17; U48 – 13
– freihalten U32 – 3
Atemwegsobstruktion U13 – 18
Äthanol-Wassergemisch U5 – 10
Atherom U13 – 24
Ätiologie U13 – 8
atraumatisch (Instrument) U32 – 1
Atresie U13 – 18
Atrophie U13 – 29
atrophieren U44 – 6
Attachment level **U35** – 9
Attachmentverlust U35 – 9
Attacke U16 – 14
Attrition **U10** – 19; U35 – 7
Ätzbrücke U30 – 19
ätzen **U39** – 21
ätzend U22 – 9; U30 – 24
Ätzflüssigkeit U30 – 19
Ätzgel U30 – 19; U39 – 21
Ätzlösung U39 – 21
Ätzmittel **U30** – 19,21; U39 – 21
Ätzmuster U30 – 19; U39 – 21
Ätzschorf U28 – 9
Ätzstift U39 – 21
Ätztechnik U37 – 8
Ätzverfahren **U39** – 21,19
auditiv U8 – 15
Aufbau **U39** – 17; U49 – 2
aufbauen (Alveolarkamm) U44 – 8
aufbereiten (Wurzelkanal) U41 – 11
Aufbereitungstiefe **U41** – 12
Aufbissaufnahme U33 – 4
Aufbissplatte **U37** – 24

Aufbissschiene U10 – 12; U37 – 25; U38 – 3,14
aufblasen (Wangen) U8 – 6
Aufbrennen U31 – 18
aufdehnen U24 – 17
aufeinanderfolgend U20 – 4
auffällig U18 – 13
aufgedunsen U3 – 15
aufgehen (Klammer) U26 – 12
aufgerissen U3 – 7, U17 – 5
aufgespalten U12 – 8
Aufhängung U29 – 3; U49 – 7
aufklappen (Lappen) **U44** – 2
Aufklärung (Patient) U25 – 3
Auflage, linguale U42 – 18
Auflagerung **U34** – 7; U29 – 1
Auflagerungs(osteo)plastik U44 – 10
Auflagetablett U7 – 11
auflegen (Instrumente) U23 – 8
aufleuchten U46 – 16
auflösen (Thrombus) U20 – 16
Auflösung, räumliche U46 – 14
Auflösungsvermögen **U46** – 14
Aufnahme (Nahrung) U1 – 1
– (Studie) U15 – 4
–, intraorale U33 – 4
–, periapikale **U33** – 7
Aufnahmebericht (Aufwachstation) U47 – 24
Aufnahmekriterien U15 – 4
aufplatzen (Wunde) U28 – 16
Aufprall U3 – 14; U44 – 3
aufquellen (Nahtmaterial) U24 – 18
aufscheuern U3 – 8
aufschlitzen U3 – 6
aufschneiden **U21** – 9; U3 – 6
Aufspaltung U46 – 20
aufstechen U3 – 10
Aufstellkalotte **U31** – 13
Aufstellungshilfe U31 – 13
auftragen (Salbe, Lack) U5 – 8; U19 – 3; U30 – 22
Auftreibung, ballonförmige U13 – 23
Auftreten, familiäres U13 – 7
Aufwachbett **U23** – 18
Aufwachperiode **U47** – 23; U23 – 17
Aufwachphase **U47** – 21
Aufwachprotokoll U23 – 17 f
Aufwachraum **U23** – 17; U47 – 21,23
Aufwachschwester U23 – 17
Aufwachsen U31 – 10
–, diagnostisches U30 – 17
Aufwachspinsel U31 – 10
Aufwachstation **U47** – 24
Aufwachstechnik U30 – 17; U31 – 10
aufwecken U4 – 2
Aufzeichnungen U47 – 22
Aufzementieren U30 – 6
Augapfel U8 – 3

Auge **U8**-3
-, blaues U3-13; U13-26
Augenhöhle U8-3
Augenklappe U28-25
Augenkompresse U28-19
Augenprothese U45-21
Augensalbe U5-8
Augenwässer U5-11
Augenzahn **U9**-5
Augmentation **U49**-19
Augmentationsplastik U44-8; U50-1
augmentierend (Plastik) U45-14
ausatmen U47-15
Ausbettmeißel U30-13
Ausbettung U31-9
ausblocken (Unterschnitt) U40-13
ausbrechen (Schmelz) U10-21
ausbreiten, sich U13-3
Ausbruch (Krankheit) U13-7
ausdehnen U31-6
Ausdehnung U29-3
ausdrücken, sich **U11**-9,1
auseinandergekeilt U35-14
Auseinanderklaffen U28-16
auseinanderspreizen U24-16
Auseinanderweichen U28-16
Ausfall (Gerhirnfunktion) U4-18
-, irreversibler U4-18
ausfallen (Zähne) **U10**-5
Ausfallsrate U15-29
Ausformen U40-7
Ausgangsdroge U5-3
Ausgangswert U15-15
ausgebrüht U30-17; U31-9
ausgegossen U30-15
ausgehärtet U31-19; U32-17,23
ausgeprägt U11-13; U48-5
ausgeschlagen (Zahn) U17-5; U44-2,3
ausgestanzt U35-6
ausgewählt U25-2
ausgießen **U31**-4
Ausgleichsextraktion U44-2
Ausgussstein U13-21
Aushärtelicht **U32**-23
aushärten U31-6
Ausheilung **U13**-14
aushelfen U6-6
aushusten U11-6; U20-15
auskleiden (Epithel) U44-14
Auskleidung U35-8; U40-3
-, epitheliale U13-24; U44-14
auskragend (Geschiebe) U42-8
auskratzen (Kürette) **U24**-10
auslösen (Ereignis, Kolik) U14-19; U16-15; U20-2
auspiepsen U7-13
Ausprägung (Variable) U14-5

ausräumen (Wurzelkanal) U32-11
Ausreißer U14-12
Ausrichtung **U29**-1; U43-9
- (Zähne) U37-6
Ausriss, knöcherner **U17**-5
Ausrissfraktur **U17**-5
Ausrissverletzung U17-5
Ausrüstung **U32**-1; U24-1
ausschaben (Kürette) U24-3,10
ausschälen (Kürette) U44-15
ausscheiden (Studie) U15-29
Ausscheidung U20-1
Ausschlag U8-2,15; U13-14
ausschließen (Komplikationen) U48-6
ausschneiden U21-9
- (Wunde) U28-12
Ausschuss, ständiger U15-25
Außenbogen **U37**-18,19
Außenteleskop **U42**-9
Äußerung, verbale U11-1
Aussprache **U11**-13; U9-1; U8-11
aussprechen U11-1,13,23
ausspucken **U10**-10
ausspülen **U34**-6; U7-8; U10-10; U27-5; U34-6; U41-5
- (Wunde) U28-11
Ausspülung **U22**-17
ausstellen (Rezept) U19-1
ausstrahlen **U46**-5; U46-2
- (Schmerz) U16-16
Ausstrahlung U46-2
ausstrecken (Arm) U29-3
Ausstülpung (Wundränder) U26-17
Austastung **U21**-11; U24-8
Austritt (Blut) U13-23 ff
Austrittsprofil U31-18; U40-18
Auswahlkriterien U25-2
auswaschen (Wunde) **U28**-11
auswerfen (Schleim) U20-15
Auswirkung U17-6; U19-8
Ausziehdraht U29-14
autogen (Transplantat) **U49**-16; U38-17
Autograft U49-16
Autoklav **U27**-3
autoklavierbar U27-3
autolog **U49**-16
Autopolymerisation U31-19
autopolymerisierend U30-3; U31-17
Autoradiographie **U33**-15
autosomal (Erbgang) U13-7
Autotransplantat **U50**-2; U44-9
Autotransplantation U49-14
A-V Anastomose U49-6
axial (Belastung) U43-9
Azidität U20-29

B

babbeln U11-17
Backe **U8**-5
Backenzahn **U9**-6,2
-, großer **U9**-7
Bäder U28-13
Bajonettfehlstellung U17-10
Bajonettstellung U29-1
Bakterienstamm U27-11
bakterizid U20-9
balanced-force Methode U41-11
Balkendiagramm U14-27
Ballaststoffe **U12**-16; U20-2
Ballondilatation U24-17
Ballonkatheter U22-19
Balsam U5-8
Band U32-24
-, diamantiertes U32-13
-, kfo. U37-8
Bandabnahmezange **U37**-9
Bandage **U28**-20; U29-8
bandagieren U29-11
Bändchen **U9**-11
Bänder U3-16
Bänderabnahme U37-8
Bänderriss U3-18
Bandscheibe U17-5
Bandsetzer U37-9
Band-Setzzange U37-9
Barbiturat **U48**-14; U20-24
Barbituratentzug U48-14
Basisnarkose **U48**-15
Basisplatte U42-13,17
Bauchkrämpfe U16-15
Bauchlage U23-16
Bauchpresse U3-17
Bauchschmerzen U16-4
Baumwolle U26-10; U28-18
Baumwollschlauch **U29**-10
Bausch **U28**-23
Beamer U46-5
Beanspruchung, starke U11-14
Beatmung, künstliche U47-15; U48-17
Beatmungsgerät U47-25
Bebänderung **U37**-8
Bebänderungstermin U37-12
Beckenkamm **U50**-9
Bedarf, bei/nach U20-27; U47-7
bedecken (Defekt) U49-9
Bedenken U39-1; U43-16
bedrückt sein **U16**-2
beeinträchtigen U13-4; U23-11
Beeinträchtigung U29-7; U45-9; U50-3
Beendigung U15-30
Befall U13-4
befallen **U13**-4; U38-11; U25-4

befangen U4–1; U14–18
befestigen U26–3; U32–7; U39–20
Befestigung U30–6; U37–4
–, adhäsive U42–21
–, elastische U37–10
–, intraorale U9–25
Befestigungskomposite U30–3
Befestigungsmaterial U9–17
Befestigungszement **U30**–6
–, Zinkoxid-Eugenol- U30–16
befeuchten U5–12; U24–18
befolgen U18–15
Befund U38–4
–, intraoperativer U21–2
Befunderhebung, kfo. U36–1
Befundkarte U35–1
Befundung, kephalometrische U33–9
Begg-Lightwire Technik U37–3
Beginn (Krankheit) U13–7
beginnend U13–10
Begleiterkrankung U13–2; U25–9
begrenzen U8–10,14; U46–12
Begrenzung U27–8
begünstigen U48–7
Behälter U5–13
behandeln mit U20–20
Behandlung **U18**–1 ff; U5–2
– der Wahl U18–1; U41–19
–, ambulante U18–14
–, chirurgische U21–3
–, experimentelle U15–2,22
–, medikamentöse U5–3,4
–, stationäre U25–11; U27–12
–, teilstationäre U18–14
Behandlungsdauer U7–1
Behandlungseinheit **U7**–2
Behandlungsfeldleuchte **U7**–9
Behandlungsgerät, funktionelles U37–13
Behandlungsgruppe U15–10
Behandlungsmethode **U18**–3 f
Behandlungsmöglichkeiten U6–13; U15–22; U18–3
Behandlungsplan **U6**–13,10; U15–7; U18–5
Behandlungsprotokoll U15–7; U18–5
Behandlungsschema **U18**–5
Behandlungsstuhl **U7**–1; U6–4; U42–4
Behandlungstermin **U6**–10
Behandlungsziel U15–27; U18–9
Behandlungszyklus U18–1,5
beharren auf U11–8
beherbergen (Keime) U26–7; U41–16
behindern U13–4; U35–22
beimischen U40–5

Beipackzettel **U5**–17
beißen **U10**–11; U3–10
Beißring U10–4
Beissstäbchen U37–9
bekämpfen U20–28
beklopfen U32–4; U38–7
bekömmlich **U1**–12
Belag **U34**–7,9,2
–, farbiger **U34**–11
Belastbarkeit U43–14
Belastung **U43**–14; U3–17
– (Implantat) U45–21
–, axiale U43–9
–, emotionelle U25–4
–, vorsichtige U25–13
Beleg **U15**–17
belegen U15–15
Belegschaft **U6**–3
belegt U32–8
Beleibtheit U12–16
Beleuchtung (OP) U23–9
belichtet U46–3
Belichtungszeit U46–7
Belüftungsanlage **U27**–8
benachbart U9–21; U36–17
benigne U45–17
Benommenheit U4–5,9,11; U5–18
Beobachtung U25–8
–, abgebrochene **U15**–29; U14–18
–, zensierte **U15**–28
Beobachtungsstrategie **U18**–7; U15–7
Beobachtungsstudie U15–1
Beratung, ärztliche **U6**–9
Beratungskomitee U15–25
beredt **U11**–18
Bereich **U14**–15
Berstungsfraktur U17–8
berufsbedingt U13–6
beruhigen U18–2; U28–13; U47–8 ff; U48–14
beruhigend **U20**–30
Beruhigung **U47**–8 ff
Beruhigungsmittel **U47**–9; U20–23 f
Berührungsempfindlichkeit **U47**–4
besänftigen U47–10
beschichten **U39**–22; U31–20; U32–25
beschichtet (Draht) U29–14
– (Film) U33–2
Beschichtung U30–10
Beschichtungsmaterial U34–16
beschießen (Bestrahlung) U46–4
beschlagen (Spiegel) U32–4
beschleifen U32–8; U40–16
Beschleuniger U30–23
beschmutzen U7–10
beschränkt auf U13–3

Beschränkung U36–29
Beschwerdeausschuss U15–25
Beschwerden, körperliche **U16**–1
beseitigen (Gewebe) U22–7
Beseitigung (Zahnfleischtaschen) **U35**–24; U27–4
besorgt (Angehörige) U16–2
bessern **U5**–2
Besserung U5–2; U16–8; U25–14
Bestandteil U12–5; U48–17; U19–1
bestätigen U4–15; U11–8
Bestätigung U15–17
Besteck, chirurgisches U24–1
Bestrahlung **U46**–2,4; U43–3
Bestrahlungsfeld U46–4
Beta-Blocker U20–7
Beta-Laktamase U20–10
betäuben **U47**–1 f
betäubt (Schlag) **U4**–9
Betäubung U4–11
Betäubungsmittel **U48**–4; U5–3
Beteiligung U13–4; U45–2
Betonung U11–13
betreffen **U13**–4; U9–14
bettlägrig U25–13
Bettruhe U25–13
Bettwäsche U27–5,9
betupfen U28–23
beugen U3–17
beunruhigen **U16**–2; U25–9
beurteilen U14–20
bevölkerungsbasiert U14–3
Bevölkerungsstatistik U14–1
bevorstehend U4–5
beweglich U8–13; U29–11; U42–6
Beweglichkeit U29–5; U35–7; U38–1
Bewegungsgips U29–7
Bewegungsschiene U29–7
Bewegungsschmerz U16–11
Beweis **U15**–17
Beweismaterial U15–17
Bewilligung U15–23
bewirken U15–26
bewusst **U4**–1
bewusstlos U4–1,6
Bewusstlosigkeit U4–14
–, tiefe **U47**–6
Bewusstsein U4–1
–, bei **U4**–3
Bewusstseinslage U4–1
Bewusstseinstrübung U4–1; U16–20
Bewusstseinsveränderung U4–1
Beziehung U14–32
Bezugsebene U39–4
Bezugspunkt **U21**–8
–, kephalometrischer U33–9

Bias **U14**–18
biegsam U29–14
Biegung **U36**–27,21
Bikuspidat **U9**–6
Bildauflösung **U46**–14
Bimler-Gebissformer U37–13
Bimsstein **U30**–18
Bimssteinbehälter U30–18
Binde **U28**–20; U29–8
–, elastische U28–20; U29–10
Bindegewebe U35–27
Bindung **U39**–20
Binokularmikroskop U22–6
bioaktiv (Beschichtung) U43–17
Bioäquivalenz U19–10
bioinert **U49**–20,17
biokompatibel U49–20
Biokompatibilität **U43**–17
biologisch verfügbar U19–10
biologische Breite **U39**–10
Biomaterialien U43–17
Bionator U37–13
Biopsienadel U24–5
Biopsiezange U24–14
bioreaktiv U43–17
Biostatistik U14–1
Biotransformation **U20**–4
Biotransformationsrate U20–4
Bioverfügbarkeit **U19**–10
Bisquitbrand U31–18
Biss **U3**–10; **U10**–12
–, offener **U36**–12
Bissanomalie U36–1
Bissebene U9–24
Bissen **U10**–12; U1–4,6; U8–8
Bissflügel U10–12
–, umgekehrter U33–6
Bissflügelaufnahme **U33**–6;
  U9–22; U46–3
Bisshebung U37–24; U49–11
Bisshöhe U10–12
Bisskeil U36–7
Bissnahme U10–12
Bissschablone U30–2; U42–14,17
Bissverhältnisse, normale **U29**–1
Bisswachs U30–17
Bisswall **U42**–14; U36–10
Bisswunde U3–10
Bittersalz U20–13
bivariat (Analyse) U14–28
Blackout U4–4
Bläschenbildung U17–9
blass werden U28–10
Blässe U3–12
Blattgold U30–8
Blattimplantat U43–2
Bleichen **U39**–19
Bleichschiene U39–19
Bleigummiabdeckung **U33**–3

Bleischürze U33–3
blind **U15**–9
Blindversuch U15–9
blinzeln U8–3
Blisterpackung U5–16
blitzartig U22–14
Blockanlage U15–11
Blockbildung U15–11
Blockdiagramm U14–27
Blocker **U20**–7
Blocktransplantat U44–10
bloßlegen U49–9
Blow-out Fraktur U17–8; U45–1
blubbern U11–7
Blutaustritt U3–19
Blutdruck U47–24
blutdrucksenkend U19–8; U20–17
Bluter U3–19
Bluterguss **U3**–13; **U13**–26
Blutfülle U13–27
Blutgerinnung U12–9; U20–10,16
blutig-serös U28–13
Blutkörperchen, weißes U20–34
Blutleere **U13**–27
Blutpoolszintigraphie U46–17
Blutspender U15–6
Blutstillung **U22**–10; U26–11
Blutstillungsmeißel U24–11
Blutung **U3**–19; U13–26
blutunterlaufen U8–3
Blutvergiftung U27–1
Blutversorgung U44–5
B-Mode Darstellung U33–11
Bogen, konfektionierter U37–5
bogenförmig **U39**–14
Bogentechnik, gerade **U37**–2
Bohrdraht **U29**–15, 14
Bohrer **U32**–6
Bohrkanal U43–11
Bohrlochosteitis U29–15
Bohrschablone U43–8
Bohrspäne U44–8
Bohrstaub U7–4
Bohrstift **U29**–15
Bohrstück U32–6
Bohrtiefe U43–10
Bolton-Analyse U36–18
Bolton-Diskrepanz **U36**–18
Bolus U1–6; **U42**–8
Bolzung U29–16
Borsten U34–4
bösartig U45–17
Brace U29–7
Bracketentfernung U37–8
Bracketflügel U37–4,10
Brackets **U37**–4,1; **U39**–20
–, Ribbon-Arch U37–4
Bracketschlitz U37–10
Branchen U24–13; U32–15

Brand U13–30
Brandführung U31–18
Brandwunde **U3**–11
brauseförmig U20–29
Brausetablette U5–7
brechen (Knochen) **U17**–1
Brechreiz **U10**–16
Breikost U1–13
Breitbandantibiotikum U18–6;
  U20–9; U27–13
Breite, biologische **U39**–10
–, therapeutische U14–15; U19–13
Breiumschlag U28–25
brennbar U48–4
brennen **U31**–18; U35–16
Brennen, schmerzhaftes U3–10f;
  U16–17
Brennkammer U31–18
Brennschwund U31–18
Brennwert U12–4
Bridenstriktur U13–19
Broca-Aphasie U11–11
Bronchialstimme U11–16
Bronchodilatatoren U20–14
Bronchophonie U11–16
Bruch **U3**–18; **U13**–23; **U26**–18
–, geschlossener **U17**–3
Bruchende U28–2
Bruchfragment U29–2
brüchig U40–5
Bruchkerbe U5–7
Bruchspalt U17–1
Bruchstelle U17–14; U3–20
Bruchstück **U17**–2
Brücke **U42**–4
Brückenanker U42–4f
Brückenersatz U42–4
Brückenzwischenglied **U42**–5;
  U40–11
brummen U11–5,15
brünieren **U31**–21
Brünierer U31–21
Brustschmerz, stechender U16–13
Brustverletzung U3–2
Bruxismus **U36**–11; U10–18
Bucca **U8**–5
bücken, sich U3–17
bukkal U8–5; U9–23
Bukkolingualabstand U39–10
Bulldogklemme U24–13
bündig U40–9
bürsten (Zähne) **U34**–4
Bürstenkopf U34–4
Büschelbürste U34–4
Butt joint U40–9

C

Calciumhydroxid U42–25
Callositas U17–15
Callus luxurians U17–15
Camouflage U36–1
Caput **U8**–1
Carbo medicinalis U5–9; U20–3
Caries acuta U34–17
– florida U34–17
– profunda U34–18; U41–2,8
Caro luxurians U28–7
Cartilagines alares U45–22
Cartilago cricoidea U8–14
Catgut **U26**–9
Cavitas **U34**–19
– dentis U41–5
– oris U8–8
Cavum **U34**–19
Cementum **U9**–17
Cerumen U8–15
– obturans U17–6
Chancenverhältnis U14–8
Checkbiss **U36**–2; U10–12
Cheilitis U17–9
Cheiloschisis U45–2
Chemie, pharmazeutische U20–1
Chemoprophylaxe U18–6
Chemotherapie U18–4
Chi²-Test **U14**–34
Chinidin U19–12; U20–18
Chirurg **U23**–5; U21–3
–, behandelnder U23–5
Chirurgie **U21**–3
–, minimal invasive U25–14
–, plastische **U49**–3
chirurgisch **U21**–2
Chlorid U12–17
cholinerg U20–8
Cholinergikum **U20**–8,2
Cholinrezeptorenblockade U48–6
Chromkatgut U26–9
Cicatrix **U28**–10
Clavicula U8–12
Clip **U26**–13
Clip-Applikator U26–13
Clip-Magazin U26–13
clippen U26–3
Clipzange U26–13
Cluster-Analyse U14–28
Cluster-Stichprobe U14–4
Col **U35**–18
Collum **U8**–13
Collyria U5–11
Coma vigile **U4**–17
Commotio **U3**–14
Compliance **U18**–15,21; U37–23
composite graft U50–1

Computertomographie **U33**–18; U46–19
Concha nasalis U8–4
Congelatio **U3**–12
Contrecoup-Hirnprellung U17–9
Contusio cerebri U3–13
Coping **U40**–17
Corona dentis **U9**–14
Corpus mandibulae U45–11
Costa cervicalis U8–13
Costen-Syndrom **U38**–3
Coverdenture **U42**–11,2
Cox Regression **U14**–35
Craquelierung **U40**–20,17
Creeping attachment U35–9
Creme U5–8
Crepitatio **U17**–14
Crista iliaca U49–12; U50–9
Crossover **U15**–14
Crossover-Studie U15–14
Crouzon-Syndrom U45–6
crown-down Technik U41–11
CT **U33**–18; U46–19
CT-Schichtaufnahmen U33–18
Cuff (Tubus) U4–10
Curare **U48**–17
Cuspis dentis **U9**–4
Cuticula dentalis **U34**–10
Cutoff **U14**–24

D

D cur U19–7
Dachziegelverband U29–11
Dämmerzustand U4–1
Dampf U3–11; U22–15; U48–10
dämpfen (Empfindung) U4–10; U30–24
– (Stimme) U11–9
Dampfsterilisation U27–2
Darmbeinkamm U49–12
Darmentleerung, präoperative **U25**–6
Darmspülung U22–17; U25–6; U48–1
Darmtätigkeit U12–16
Darreichungsform **U5**–6
darstellen **U46**–12,14; U33–12
Darstellung **U21**–7; U32–4; U33–11
– (OP-Feld) U23–11
–, B-Mode U33–11
–, graphische U14–27
darunterliegend U49–11
Datenerhebung U15–15
Datenmaterial **U15**–15
Datenschutz U15–15
Dauerdrainage U28–15

Dauerhaftigkeit U42–1
Dauerinfusion U47–16,19
Dauermedikation U5–1; U19–3
Dauerzug U29–3
Daumenlutschen U36–20
Dean-Fluorose-Index U34–13
Debridement **U28**–12; U41–9
Decklappen U50–18
Deckprothese **U42**–11,2,20; U40–17
Deckschicht U49–9
Deckschraube U43–6
Deckweiß U39–16
deep scaling U32–13; U34–14
Defekt, kariöser U34–17
Defektauffüllung U40–1
Defektbildung U34–19
Deformität U13–5
Degeneration U13–29
degenerativ **U13**–29
Dehner **U24**–17
Dehnschraube U37–17
Dehnsonde U24–17
Dehnung U29–3
Dekalzifikation **U10**–22
Dekubitalgeschwür U3–5; U13–17
Dekubitus U28–19
Delirium **U4**–16
Delta-Züge U37–10
Demastikation U10–19
demineralisiert (Knochenpartikel) U44–11
Demulzenzium U20–30
Dens **U9**–1
– caninus **U9**–5
– incisivus **U9**–3
– molaris **U9**–7
– praemolaris **U9**–6
– serotinus **U9**–8
Dentalamalgam **U30**–1
Dentalfluorose U34–13
Dentalhygieneassistent U6–8; U34–1
Dentalkunststoff **U30**–2
Dentalplaque **U34**–8
Dentes **U9**–1
Dentikel U41–5
Dentin **U9**–16
–, aufgeweichtes U40–6
Dentinkanälchen U9–16
Dentinoblasten U9–16
Dentitio difficilis U10–3
– praecox U10–1
– tarda U10–1
Dentition **U10**–1
Dentitionszyste **U44**–15
Depolarisation U20–20; U48–16
Depotpräparat U5–3; U19–4
Dermatom U44–9

Dermislappen U50–6
Derotation U36–27
Desensibilisierungspaste **U30**–24
Design, faktorielles **U15**–13
–, gruppensequentielles U15–13
Desinfektion **U27**–6; U23–19
–, präoperative U27–5f
Desinfektionsmittel U20–2; U27–5
desinfizieren **U27**–5f
Desmodont U9–13; U35–1,9,23
Desorientiertheit **U4**–8
destruktiv (Verhalten) U3–18
deutlich artikuliert U11–1,8
devital (Zahn) U9–1
Dextrose **U12**–7
Dezile U14–11
Diagnostik **U25**–1; U42–15
Diagramm U14–27
Diamant, mittelkörniger U32–6
Diamantschleifkörper U32–6
Diaphanoskop U46–16
Diaphanoskopie **U46**–17
Diastema **U36**–17
– mediale U36–17
Diät **U1**–13; **U18**–5
Diätempfehlung U1–13
Diathermie U22–9
Diathermieschlinge U22–7,11; U24–9
Diathermiestift U22–9
Diätvorschrift U19–1
dichotom (Variable) U14–5,19
Dichtungsmittel U26–11
diensthabend U5–4; U23–6; U47–2
Diffusionsvermögen U20–4
Dilatator **U24**–17
Diplom-Krankenschwester U23–6
Disaccharid U12–6
Diskektomie **U38**–17
diskludieren U36–7
Disklusion U36–8
Diskriminanzanalyse U14–28
Diskusexzision **U38**–17
Diskushernie U13–22
Diskusläsion U38–16
Diskusluxation **U38**–9
Diskusverlagerung **U38**–9,6
Dislokation U3–20; U17–4; U40–7
Disposition, familiäre U13–7
Dissektion U21–12
disseminiert U13–27
distal U9–21
Distalbisslage U36–7
Distal-End Cutter U37–5
distalisieren U37–22
Distalokklusion U36–7
Distanzhülse U43–5,12

Distanzhülsenschraube U42–10; U43–6
Distickstoffoxid **U48**–11
Distorsion **U3**–16
distrahieren U29–3; U45–16
Distraktion **U45**–16
Distraktionsosteogenese U45–16
Distraktionsosteotomie U45–16
Distraktor U45–16
Diuretika **U20**–21
DMF Flächenindex U34–21
DMFS-Index U34–18
Dokumentation U15–15
Dolder-Steg U42–23
dopaminerg U20–3
Doppelbindung U12–11
Doppelblindversuch U15–9
Doppelhandschuhe U27–17
Doppelkinn U8–6
Doppelkontrastarthrogramm U33–14
Doppelkontrastdarstellung U46–3
doppellumig (Drain) U28–15
Doppler-Sonographie U33–11
Dorn (Stift) U29–15
dösen U23–2
Dosieraerosol U5–6
Dosierinhalator U20–14
Dosierung **U19**–7; U5–17
Dosierungsschema U18–5
Dosimetrie U46–9
Dosis **U19**–7
–, genetisch signifikante U46–9
dosisabhängig U19–7
Dosisäquivalent U19–7; U46–9
Dosisverteilung U46–9
Dosis-Wirkungs-Kurve U19–7
Doublieren U31–13
Dowel pin **U31**–12
down-fracture Technik U45–7
Dr. med. dent. U44–1
Dragee U5–7
Draht(schneide)zange U32–16
Drahtbogen, kfo. **U37**–5; U26–3; U29–14
Drahtbogenschiene U42–22
Drahtligatur **U37**–7,5
Drahtnaht U29–14
Drahtosteosynthese U29–14
Drahtsäge U29–14
Drahtschiene U37–16
Drahtschlaufen U37–4
Drahtschlinge U22–11; U24–9
Drahtschneideschere U24–4
Drahtumschlingung **U29**–14
Drain **U28**–15
–, Penrose- U28–15
Drainage, Spül-Saug- U28–15
Drainagerohr U28–15

Drehbruch U17–1
Drehfehlstellung U3–16
Drehmoment U32–5
Drehmomentschlüssel U43–12
Drehmomentsperre U43–12
Drehung U3–16
– um Längsachse U36–27
Drehzahl U36–27
Dreieckstuch U28–20; U29–8
Dreifachzucker U12–6
Dreikantspitze U24–7
Dreiviertelkrone U42–19
dringend (Abklärung) U21–5
Droge **U5**–3
–, pflanzliche U5–2
drogenabhängig U5–3
Drogeneinfluss, unter U4–9
Drogenikterus U5–3
Drogentoter U5–3
Drogerie U5–4
Drogist U5–4f
drohend (Kollaps) U4–5
Drop-out Rate U15–29
Druck U36–28
– mindern U28–19
druckabsorbierend U43–15
Druckbelastung U43–14
Druckbrecher U42–18
Druckgeschwür U3–5
Druckknopfsystem U45–22
Drucknekrose U13–30
Druckschmerz U16–11; U38–1
druckschmerzhaft **U16**–11; U13–14
Druckschmerzhaftigkeit U17–13
Druckspülung U22–17
Druckstelle (Gips) U13–17; U29–6
Druckverband U28–17
Drug targeting U19–4
Dsygnathie U45–6
dualhärtend U30–6; U31–19
Dübel U29–15
Dublieren U31–13
Ductus parotideus U45–17
dünnschichtig U40–3
Duplikaturnaht U49–8
Dura, Ruptur U45–1
durchbeißen U10–11
durchbrechen (Zahn) **U10**–3; U9–6,23
durchführbar U21–4
durchgängig (Gefäß) U22–19; U28–15
Durchhärtungstiefe U31–19
Durchleuchtung **U46**–17,8
Durchleuchtungsfeld U46–16
Durchleuchtungszeit U46–7
Durchmesser U24–17; U39–8
durchmischt mit U26–14
durchscheinend U39–16

durchschneiden, quer **U21**–14,9
durchschnittlich U14–10
Durchschuss U3–3
durchsichtig U39–16
durchsickern **U40**–21
Durchspülung **U22**–17
durchstechen U3–10; U24–2
durchstoßen U24–2
durchtrennen **U21**–10,9; U26–5
–, quer **U21**–14
Durchtrennung U21–14; U45–12; U50–13
Durchuntersuchung U25–1
durstig U1–11
Düsenaerosolgerät U19–3
Dysarthrie U11–11
Dyslalie U11–17,20
Dysmorphie, kraniofaziale **U45**–4
Dysosthosis cleidocranialis U45–6
– mandibulofacialis **U45**–6
Dysphemie **U11**–20
Dysphonie U11–23

E

Ebene U33–18 f
Echolalie U11–17
Echtzeitsonographie U33–11
Eckzahn **U9**–5
Eckzahnführung U9–5; U36–29
Eckzahnspitze U9–5
Edelgas U49–20
Edelgasnarkose U47–6
Edelmetalllegierung U30–7
Edelstahlscaler U32–13
Edgewise-Brackets U37–2
EEG, isoelektrisches U4–18
Effektivität **U15**–26; U19–9
Effizienz U15–26
Eigenschaft U13–6; U30–7
einartikulieren **U31**–7,1
einatmen U20–14
einbetten **U31**–8 f
Einbettgerät U31–8
Einbetthilfe U31–8
Einbettmasse U31–8
Einbettmassemodell U31–8
Einbettung U30–13; U31–8
Einbrennen U31–18
Einbringpfosten U43–2
Einbringungsdrehmoment **U43**–12
Einbuchtungen U39–14
eindringen **U40**–21; U41–7,16
Eindringtiefe U46–9
Einengung U13–19
einfädeln U24–5
Einfädler (Zahnseide) U34–5
Einfluss U17–6

einführen (Tubus) U47–17; U5–12
eingebettet U30–20; U35–1; U43–15
eingehüllt U27–3
eingeschränkt U4–11
Eingeweide U27–17
eingewendelt (Naht) U26–16
eingipsen U29–6
Eingriff U25–6; U22–5
–, chirurgischer **U21**–3,1 f
–, nervschonender U21–13
–, offenchirurgischer U21–1
–, therapeutischer U15–27
Einhaltung U18–15
einheilen (Transplantat) U50–21
Einheilungsphase U43–13
Einheit, koloniebildende **U27**–10
–, verblockte U42–22
einhergehen mit U4–5; U13–3
Einkeilung U17–6; U44–3
einklemmen U38–5; U13–23
Einlagefüllung **U40**–16
Einlagerungs(osteo)plastik U44–10
einleiten (Narkose) U47–13
Einleitung U18–10
Einleitungsschema U47–13
Einlochkollimator U46–6
Einmalabdecktücher **U27**–4
Einmaldiamantschleifkörper U32–6
Einmalhandschuhe U27–4,17
Einmalskalpell U24–3
Einnahme (Medikament) U1–1; U19–7; U20–12
einnehmen (Mahlzeit) **U1**–1
einpassen U42–16
einpflanzen U50–1
einpinseln U27–5
Einprobe **U42**–15
Einprobetermin U6–10; U42–15
einpudern **U5**–9
Einreibemittel U5–10
einreihen (Zähne) U36–26
einrichten (Bruch) U28–2,4; U29–1 f
Einrichtung (Ausrüstung) **U32**–1
– (Fraktur) **U29**–2; U17–1
Einriss U3–7,18
einrütteln U40–1
einsatzbereit U4–2
einschätzen U35–7
einscheiden U49–8
Einscheidung, bindegewebige U43–1
einschläfern U4–13; U47–1
einschleifen **U10**–18; U36–10; U37–24
einschließen U27–16
Einschlusskriterien U14–3
einschneiden U3–6; **U21**–9

Einschnitt U3–6; U21–9
Einschnürung U13–19
einschränken **U36**–29; U13–4
Einschränkung U14–16; U36–29
einstellen (Feder) U37–11
Einstich U3–10
Einstichstelle U7–6; U24–5
einstufen U35–7
Einstülpung U49–8
eintauchen U30–21
einträufeln U5–11; U48–5
einwachsen (Knochen) U43–1,3; U50–8
einwickeln **U28**–24,17,20
Einwilligung(serklärung) **U25**–3
Einwilligung, aufgeklärte U15–4
Einwilligungsformular U25–3
Einwohner U14–8
Einzeldosis U19–7
Einzeldosisampullen U5–13
Einzeldosispackung U5–16
Einzelfall U40–11
Einzelgabe U19–7
Einzelknopfnaht **U26**–15
Einzellaut U11–12
Einzelpfeiler U42–10
einzelstehend U13–3
Einzelzahnimplantat U43–2
einzementieren **U30**–6; U40–16
Einziehung (Zahn) **U39**–13; U9–3
Eisen U12–17
Eispackung U28–24
Eiter **U13**–12; U28–14; U35–20
Eiterableitung U13–12
Eiteransammlung U13–12
Eiterbildung U13–12; U28–14
eitern **U28**–14
Eiterung U13–12
eitrig U35–3
eitrig-serös U28–13
Eiweiß **U12**–9
eiweißabbauend U12–9
Ekchymose U13–27
E-Klammer U42–6
Elastics **U37**–10
elastische Elemente (kfo.) U36–28
elektiv **U21**–5
Elektiveingriff U21–3,5; U25–6
Elektrochirurgie **U22**–9
Elektrodesikkation U22–14
Elektrokauterisation U22–9
Elektromotor **U7**–3
Elevatorium **U32**–15
Elimination U20–1
Eliminationshalbwertzeit U20–5
Elongation U36–25
emaillieren **U31**–20
Emanation U46–2
Emergenzprofil U31–18; U40–18

Emetikum **U20** – 12; U5 – 11
Emollienzium **U20** – 30
Empfänger U49 – 15
Empfängerareal U49 – 15
empfinden (Reiz) U16 – 18; U48 – 1,4
empfindlich **U16** – 11; U46 – 23
– (Zahn) U9 – 1
– reagieren U32 – 20
Empfindlichkeit, verminderte **U47** – 4
Empfindung U16 – 6
emulgierend U5 – 8
Enamelum **U9** – 15
En-Bloc Resektion U21 – 15
Endodontie U41 – 1
endodontisch **U41** – 1
Endodontologe U41 – 1
Endo-Paro-Läsion **U35** – 20
Endoprothese **U22** – 20
Endoskopie (Kieferhöhle) **U45** – 19
Endotrachealnarkose U48 – 13
Endotrachealtubus U47 – 17
Endpfeiler U42 – 10
Endplatte, motorische U48 – 17
Endpunkt **U14** – 20
Energiedosis U46 – 10
eng werden U13 – 20
Engstand **U36** – 16; U37 – 17
Engstelle, iatrogene **U41** – 13
enossal U42 – 20; U45 – 23; U49 – 18
Entartung U13 – 29
Entblößung U35 – 10
entfernen (Gewebe) U22 – 16; U32 – 16
Entfernung (Zahn) U33 – 13
–, operative **U21** – 15,3; **U22** – 1,13
Entfernungsdrehmoment U43 – 12
entgegenwirken U5 – 15
Entgiftungsmittel U12 – 15
Enthaarungscreme U27 – 14
Entkalkung **U10** – 22
entkeimen U27 – 2,5
Entlassung (Krankenhaus) U25 – 11
Entlassungsprotokoll U47 – 24
Entlastungsnaht U26 – 1; U29 – 3
Entlastungsoperation U41 – 22
Entlastungsschnitt U21 – 9; U50 – 17
Entnahmestelle U50 – 6
Entnahmetiefe U50 – 6
entnehmen (Gewebe) **U49** – 12; U24 – 11; U50 – 9
– (Organ) U44 – 9; U49 – 12
Entschäumer U20 – 2
Entseuchung U27 – 5
entsorgen U5 – 13; U24 – 2; U27 – 4
entwicklungsbedingt U45 – 7
Entzug (Narkotika) U19 – 6; U47 – 6
Entzugsdelir U4 – 16
entzündet U16 – 11; U28 – 14

Entzündung **U13** – 11; U20 – 11; U41 – 7
entzündungshemmend **U20** – 11
Entzündungsherd U13 – 3
Entzündungszeichen U13 – 11
Enukleation U44 – 15
Enzym U12 – 9
Epidermisläppchen U50 – 6
Epidermistransplantat U50 – 6
Epithelbrücke U28 – 6
epithelial ausgekleidet U44 – 14
Epithelisierung **U28** – 6
Epithese, maxillofaziale **U45** – 22
Erbgang, X-chromosomaler U13 – 7
erblich **U13** – 7
Erbrechen U9 – 14; U20 – 12; U47 – 23
Erbrochenes U1 – 6
Erdbeerzunge U8 – 11
Ereignis, statistisches **U14** – 19,3
–, wiederkehrendes U14 – 19
–, zufallabhängiges U14 – 19
ereignisabhängig U14 – 19
Erfassungssystem U33 – 8
erforschen U15 – 2
Erfrierung **U3** – 12,2; U47 – 3
erfroren U3 – 10
ergänzen U12 – 15; U48 – 11
Ergebnis, zensiertes U15 – 27
ergebnislos U21 – 11
Ergebnisparameter, binärer U15 – 27
Erguss, eitriger U13 – 12
erhaben (Läsion) U13 – 3
– (Plaque) U49 – 11
erhalten (Organ) **U21** – 13; U23 – 5; U40 – 6; U41 – 24
Erhaltung U21 – 13; U45 – 3
Erhaltungsdosis U19 – 7; U47 – 19
erhärten (Amalgam) U30 – 1
– (Verdacht) U4 – 15
erheben (Anamnese) U47 – 12
Erhebung, prospektive U15 – 6
erhitzen U43 – 7
Erhöhung (Blutdruck) U49 – 11
Erinnerungslücke U3 – 14
erleichtern U18 – 9
Erleichterung U11 – 4; U22 – 14
erleiden U16 – 2; U25 – 5
Ermüdungsbruch **U17** – 13
ernähren **U1** – 3; **U12** – 1
Ernährung U1 – 3
–, künstliche U25 – 12
Ernährungsberater U1 – 13
Ernährungsberatung U12 – 3
Ernährungsgewohnheiten U12 – 3
Ernährungslehre **U12** – 3; U1 – 13
Ernährungsstatus U25 – 1
Ernährungszustand U28 – 5
ernsthaft erkrankt U19 – 14

erodieren U10 – 21
eröffnet (Pulpa) U30 – 16
Eröffnung, OP **U22** – 2; U21 – 9; U40 – 6
Erosion **U10** – 21; U13 – 17
Erreger **U20** – 2; U13 – 1; U27 – 9
–, opportunistischer U27 – 9
Erregung U4 – 2,16; U47 – 9
Ersatz, künstlicher U42 – 1
–, prothetischer U42 – 2
Ersatzdroge U47 – 6
Ersatzknochen U49 – 2
Erschöpfung U16 – 5
Erschöpfungsdelirium U4 – 16
Erschöpfungszustand U16 – 5
Erschütterung **U3** – 14
–, seelische **U3** – 4
ersparen (Operation) U21 – 13
Erstabformung U31 – 2
Erstarrungskontraktion U31 – 6
ersticken U10 – 16
Erstlot U31 – 16
ertragen (Schmerzen) U16 – 18
Eruptionszyste **U44** – 15
erwachen (Narkose) U47 – 12,21
– (Schlaf) U4 – 2
erwartet U14 – 4
erwartungstreu U14 – 18
Erweiterer **U24** – 17
erweitern (Kanal) U24 – 17
erworben (Krankheit) U13 – 6
erwünscht U19 – 11
Erythem U35 – 13
erzielen U14 – 6
Esmarch Binde **U47** – 18; U28 – 20
Esmarch-Blutleere U13 – 27
Esmarch-Blutsperre U47 – 18
essbar U1 – 5
essen U1 – 1f
Essen **U1** – 6,7
Essensgelüste U1 – 6
essentiell **U13** – 8
Essgewohnheiten U1 – 1,7
Essigumschlag U28 – 25
Essstörung U1 – 1
Etagennaht U26 – 1
Ethikkommission **U15** – 24f
etikettieren U5 – 5; U23 – 8
Eugenol **U30** – 16
Eugenol-Abformpaste U30 – 16
eugenolfrei U30 – 16
evident U15 – 17
Exanthem U13 – 11,13; U50 – 20
–, hämorrhagisches U13 – 26
Exitus U15 – 27
Exkavator **U32** – 14
–, beilförmiger U32 – 14
–, hauenförmiger U32 – 14
Exkoriation U3 – 8

expandieren U31–6
Expansion, thermische U31–6
Expektorans **U20**–15
expektorieren U20–15
explantieren U49–12
Exploration **U21**–11; U24–8
Explosionstrauma U3–2
Expositionszeit U46–7
Exstirpation U22–13
Exstirpationsnadel U32–11
exstirpieren U21–15
Exsudat **U28**–13
Extension (Fraktur) **U29**–3
– (kfo.) **U36**–28
Extensionsbrücke U42–4
Extensionsgerät U37–16
Extensionsschiene U28–26; U29–3
extrahieren U44–2
Extraktion U33–13; U44–1 f
Extraktion-Re(im)plantation **U44**–4
Extraktionshöhle U9–13; U44–2
Extraktionslücke U44–2
Extraktionswunde U30–16
Extraktionszange U32–15; U44–2
extraoral U9–25; U33–4
Extremitätenischämie U13–27
Extremwert U14–15
Extrusion **U36**–25
exzentrisch (Kontakte) U36–9
exzidieren U21–9,15
Exzision **U21**–15, **U22**–1
Exzitationsstadium U47–20

F

Facette **U40**–11; U39–2,22
Facies U8–2
Facing **U40**–11
Faden U26–7; U34–5
fadenförmig U8–16
Fadenpinzette U24–14
Fadenschere U24–4
Fadenstärke U26–7
fahrbar U23–19
Fakten (Studie) U15–15
Faktor, statistischer U14–5
–, verfälschender U15–9
–, verzerrender U14–18
Fall U14–2
Fall-Kontroll-Studie U15–1
Fallstudie U14–2
falsch-positiv **U14**–22
Falte U49–8
Fältelung U13–29
Faltenzunge U8–11
familiär U13–7
Farbabstimmung U39–15
Farbanpassungsleuchte U39–15

Farbbestimmung U39–15
Farbbestimmungsgerät U39–15
Färbemittel U34–11
färben **U34**–11
Färbetechnik U34–11
Farbmischung U39–15
Farbnuance **U39**–15
Farbring U39–15
Farbstoff U32–25; U34–11
Farbstofflaser U22–7
Farbszintigramm U46–18
Farbton **U39**–15
Farbwahl U39–15
Fasenschliff U40–19
Fasergips U30–13
fassen U24–9,13
Fassinstrument U32–16
fassungslos **U4**–9
Fasszange U24–13
fasten **U1**–14 f
Fauces U8–12
faulen U34–18
Fazialislähmung U8–2
Fazialwinkel **U39**–5
Feder **U37**–11; U36–28
Federmodul **U37**–21
Fehlbildung **U13**–5; U11–21
–, kraniofaziale **U45**–4
Fehler, systematischer **U14**–18
fehlerhaft U14–12
Fehlernährung U12–3
fehlschlagen U49–1
Fehlstellung U3–20; U17–4,15; U29–1; U38–2
– (Zahn) U9–1; U36–8
Feile **U32**–12 f; U24–12
–, feine U41–5
Feinabstimmung U37–10,23
feinmaschig U28–18
Feinnadelbiopsie U22–16
Feldblock U48–6
Feldspat U30–4; U31–18
Feldversuch U15–7
Fenster, therapeutisches U18–4
Fensterung, apikale U44–14
Fernlappen U50–11
Fertigung U30–9
fest U32–23
festhaken **U24**–9
Festigkeit U30–5
Festigung **U13**–14
festschnallen U29–11
festsitzen (Diskus) U38–5
feststellen (Status) U32–20
Feststellschraube U43–6
Festwerden U13–14
Fett **U12**–11
Fette, einfach ungesättigte U12–12
Fetteinlagerung U12–11

Fettgewebe U12–11
fetthaltig **U12**–11
fettig U5–8
fettleibig **U12**–11
Fettpolster U12–11
Fettsäure, essentielle **U12**–12
–, mehrfach ungesättigte U12–11
Fettsucht U13–2
fettsüchtig **U12**–11
feucht U27–18
Feuchtigkeit U32–19
Feuchtigkeitscreme U5–8
feuerfest (Einbettmasse) U31–8
Fibrinkleber **U26**–14,11; U22–10
Fibrinolytika U20–16
Fibrinschaum U26–14
Fibromatosis, gingivale **U35**–22
Fieberbläschen U3–5
Fieberdelir U4–16
Fieberkurve U23–18
fiebersenkend U20–11
Filmhalter U33–2
Filmkassette U33–2
Filmschwärzung U33–2
Filmtablette U5–7
Filmverband U28–17
Fingerfederchen U37–11
Fingerlutschen U36–23
Fingerplastik U49–1
Fingerplugger U32–17
Fingerstopfer U32–17
Finierer U32–6
Fissur **U17**–11,1
Fissurenversiegler U34–16
Fistel U13–25
–, entzündliche **U35**–21
–, oroantrale U35–21
Fistelbildung **U13**–25; U35–21
Fistelexzision U35–21
Fistelgang U13–25; U35–21
Fistelmaul U13–25
Fistelmund U13–25
Fixateur externe U29–4
Fixation (Fraktur) **U29**–4
–, chirurgische **U49**–7
–, mandibulomaxilläre U29–4
fixieren **U36**–29; U29–15; U30–6
Fixiermittel U41–24
Fixierschraube U29–4
Fixtur **U43**–2
Flachmeißel U24–11
Flachzange U32–16
Flammenlötung U31–16
Flankenschmerz U16–10,15
Flaschenkaries U34–17
Fleck, blauer **U3**–13; U13–26
Fleisch, wildes U28–7
Flimmerskotom U46–17
Fluor U12–17

Fluoreszenz U46-8
Fluoridaufnahme U34-13
fluoridfreisetzend U40-5
Fluoridgehalt U34-13
fluoridhaltig U34-2
Fluoridierung U34-13
Fluoridintoxikation U34-13
Fluoridlack U30-22; U34-13
Fluoridsalz U34-13
Fluorometrie U46-8
Flussdiagramm U14-27
Flüssigkeit U47-13
Flüssigkeitsabsonderung U13-11
Flüssigkeitsansammlung U3-15
Flüssigkeitszufuhr U25-12
Flussmittel U31-4,16
Flusssäure U30-19
flüstern **U11**-16
Flüsterprobe U11-16
Flüsterstimme U11-16
Foetor ex ore **U34**-20
fokal U13-3
Fokus **U13**-3
Folat U12-14
Folge **U15**-27
Folgeerscheinung U25-9
Folsäure **U12**-14
Folsäureantagonist U20-6
Folsäuresalz U12-14
Folsäuresupplementierung U12-14
Foramen apicale U41-6
– mentale U8-6
förderlich U24-1
fördern U12-15; U44-12
Formaldehydderivat U41-24
formbar U39-2
Formbeständigkeit U31-4
formen **U31**-4; **U39**-2; **U49**-4
Formkorrektur U39-2
Forschung U15-2
Forschungsstadium U15-2
forte (Tablette) U5-7
Fortlaufnaht U26-16
Fortschritte (Genesung) U25-7
Fragment **U17**-2
Fragmentation U17-2
Fraktile U14-11
Fraktur U17-1 ff; U3-20
–, Contrecoup **U17**-9
–, dislozierte U3-20; U17-4
–, Gegenstoß- **U17**-9
–, Guérin- U45-1
Frakturausläufer U17-11
Fraktureinrichtung U29-1
Frakturheilung **U17**-15,1
frakturieren **U17**-1; U3-20
Frakturlinie U17-7
Franceschetti-Syndrom U45-6
Fränkel-Funktionsregler U37-13

Frankfurter Horizontale **U39**-4
Fräse U36-10
Freiendbrücke U42-4
Freiendprothese **U42**-8; U10-7
Freiendsattel U42-8
freigelegt U30-16; U49-9
Freiheitsgrade **U14**-16
freilegen U21-7 ff; U32-2
Freilegung **U21**-7; U35-10; U40-6
– (Zahn) U44-2
freiliegend U35-12; U50-6
Freipräparierung **U21**-7,12
freisetzen U19-4
Freiwilliger U15-10
Fremdkörper U24-9; U28-12
Fremdkörperaspiration U22-16
Fremdprotein U12-9
Frenektomie U44-7
Frenulum **U9**-11
– labii U8-9
Fresssucht U1-1
Friktionshaftung U42-9,21
Friktionspassung U42-16
frischoperiert U21-1
Fritte **U30**-21
Frontansicht U39-2
Frontzähne **U9**-2
Frontzahnstufe, sagittale **U36**-14
–, vertikale **U36**-13
Frontzahnüberbiss U36-13
Frostbeule U3-12
Frühbehandlung, kfo. U36-1
Frühkontakte U36-9
Frühmobilisation U25-13; U29-5
Frühsymptom U38-6
FST U44-7
führen (zu) U28-8
Führungsbohrer **U43**-8
Führungsdraht U29-14
Führungsfläche, selbsteingeschliffene **U36**-10,29
Führungshohlsonde U24-8
Führungskanal U43-8
Führungsschablone, chirurgische U31-13
Führungsschiene U26-5; U43-8
Fulguration **U22**-14
füllen (Wurzelkanal) U41-15
Füllung **U40**-1; U30-6
Füllungsdefekt, strahlendurchlässiger U46-11
Füllungsmaterialien U40-1
Füllungsüberhang **U40**-12
Füllungszement, Zinkoxid-Eugenol- U30-16
Funda U28-20
Fungizid U20-26
Funken U22-14
Funkenerosion U10-21

Funktion, mentale U3-14
Funktionserhaltung U21-13
Funktionsgips U29-7
Funktionskieferorthopädie U37-13
Funktionsszintigraphie U46-17
furchenförmig U35-4
Furkation, tunnelierte U35-23
Furkationsbefall **U35**-23
Furkationsdefekt **U35**-23
Furkationsperforation U41-17
Furkationsplastik U35-23
Fußschalter U7-3
Fußstütze U23-11
Fußtieflage U23-13
füttern **U1**-3; U12-1

G

Gabe **U19**-3,7
gähnen U9-9; U38-4
Gammakamera U46-17
Ganglienblocker U20-7; U48-6
Ganglioplegikum U20-7
Gangrän U13-30
Gantry U46-19
Ganzkörperbestrahlung U46-4
Ganzkörperscanner U46-18
Gasbrand U13-30
Gasbrenner U31-15
Gaumen **U9**-10; U8-8
–, harter U44-5
–, weicher U10-16; U11-5
Gaumenbogen U9-10
Gaumenbügel U42-24
Gaumendehngerät U37-17
Gaumenmandel U9-10
Gaumennahterweiterungsapparat U37-1
Gaumenplastik U45-3
Gaumensegel U9-10
Gaumenspaltchirurgie **U45**-3
Gaumenspalte U9-10; U17-11; U44-2
Gaumenwulst U44-16
Gauß-Verteilung U14-12
Gaze **U28**-18; U5-8; U24-18
–, paraffingetränkte U28-18
Gazekissen U24-18
Gazestreifen U28-18
Gazetampon U28-18
Gazetupfer U28-18
Gebiss **U10**-1
–, bleibendes **U10**-6
–, künstliches **U10**-8; **U42**-2
Gebissanomalie U36-8
gebogen U24-9
gebrannt (Gips) U30-13
– (Porzellan) U31-18

gebrochen U17–1
Gebühr U6–8
gebündelt (Strahlen) U33–3
gedämpft (Bewußsein) **U4**–10f; U13–13
– (Stimme) U11–10
gedeckt (Hautdefekt) U49–9
Gefahr U25–5
gefährden U13–4
gefältelt U39–14
Gefäßbündel U50–13
Gefäßchirurg U21–3
Gefäßclip U26–13
Gefäßerweiterung U20–17
Gefäßklemme U22–10; U23–19; U24–13f
Gefäßnadel U24–5
Gefäßpinzette U24–14
Gefäßplastik U22–4
Gefäßruptur U3–7
Gefäßstiel U26–3; U50–11
gefäßverengend U20–17
geflochten U26–7
geformt U5–7
gefriergetrocknet U44–9,11; U50–9
Gefrierschnitt U21–10; U45–17
gefühllos **U48**–4
Gefühllosigkeit U47–3
Gegenanzeige U5–17; U18–10
Gegengift **U5**–15
Gegenguss U31–5
Gegenhalter U43–12
Gegenmittel **U5**–15
Gegenquadrant U9–20
Gegensprechanlage **U7**–12
gegenüberstehen **U8**–2
Gegenzähne U9–1; U36–18,25
Gegenzug U29–3
Gegenzugheadgear U37–18
gegossen U30–14
gehämmert (Goldlegierung) U30–7
gehärtet U32–23; U39–20
gehemmt U4–1
gehfähig U25–13
Gehirnerschütterung U3–14
Gehörgang U8–15
Gehörknöchelchen U8–15
gekerbt (Modellstift) U31–12
gekippt U36–25
geklebt U37–4
Gekrätz U30–9
Gel U5–8
Gelbsucht, chronische U13–8
Gelenk **U36**–3
Gelenkbelastung U38–14
Gelenkeröffnung, chirurgische **U38**–16
Gelenkersatz U22–4
Gelenkfläche U38–9

Gelenkfraktur U17–1
Gelenkknacken **U38**–4
Gelenkknorpel U38–11
Gelenkreiben U17–14
Gelenkschiene U29–7
Gelenkversteifung U29–13; U38–12
gelötet U30–7
gemahlen, fein U30–3
Genauigkeit U18–15
genehmigen U15–24
geneigt U23–13
generisch U19–2
Genesung U25–14
Genesungszeit U18–14; U25–14
genetisch U13–6
genießbar U1–5
Genioplastik **U45**–14; U8–6; U22–4
genuin **U13**–8
gepolstert U23–13; U28–19
gepresst (Tablette) U5–7
gerastert (Film) U33–2
Gerät U24–1; U31–1; U36–1
–, kfo. **U37**–1
Geräte, optische U24–1
Geräusch U11–10
gereizt (Stimmung) U13–10
Gereiztheit U4–12
geriffelt U40–14
geringfügig U19–14
gerinnen U22–10
Gerinnungshemmer **U20**–16
Gerinnungsstörung U13–1; U22–10
Gerüst U31–10,17; U43–15; U44–11
Gerüsteiweiß U12–9
Gerüstkonstruktion U30–7
Gesamtinzidenz U14–7
Gesamtrisiko U25–5
Gesäß U16–16; U23–14
geschädigt U13–4
Geschiebe U42–4,21
–, auskragendes U42–8
geschient (Pfeiler) U42–10
Geschlechtsperzentile U14–11
geschliffen (Fläche) U10–18
Geschmacksorgan U8–11
geschmeidig (Narbe) U28–10
geschützt, patentrechtlich **U19**–2
geschwächt U27–12
Geschwisterspender U49–15
Geschwulst U13–16
Geschwür **U13**–17; U3–5; U16–6
Geschwürabheilung U28–4
Gesicht **U8**–2
–, verzerrtes U3–16
Gesichts- u. Kieferchirurg U6–1

Gesichtsausdruck U8–2
Gesichtsbogen **U37**–19
Gesichtsdeformität U38–10
Gesichtsfraktur **U45**–1
Gesichtsmaske U37–19
Gesichtsprothese U45–23
Gesichtsspalte **U45**–2; U11–22; U17–11
Gesichtsvorverlagerung, operative **U45**–8
Gesichtswinkel **U39**–5
Gesichtszüge U8–2
gespalten U17–11
gespickt U29–14
gesprächig U11–8,18
gespreizt U23–12
gesteigert U20–28
gestielt (Lappen) U44–5; U50–10f
– (Polyp) U22–11
gestopft (Guttapercha) U30–14
gestört (Befinden) U13–2
– (Okklusion) U10–13
Gestotter U11–20
gesund **U1**–12; U23–16
Gesunder U15–10
Gesunderhaltung U21–13
gesundheitsbewusst U4–1
gesüßt U12–6
getapet U29–11
Getränk **U2**–24
–, alkoholisches **U2**–27
Gewebeannahme U49–20
Gewebedehnung **U49**–10
Gewebedosis U46–9
Gewebeeinschmelzung U13–12
Gewebeexpander U24–13f
Gewebefasszange U24–13f
Gewebeprobe U23–8; U46–13
Geweberegeneration, gesteuerte **U35**–28; U44–8,12
Gewebereste U40–2
Gewebeschrumpfung U13–30
Gewebeschwund U13–29
Gewebetransplantat, freies **U50**–13
Gewebetrümmer U13–30; U40–2
Gewebeübertragung, freie **U50**–13; U49–13
Gewebeverhärtung U13–13
Gewebeverträglichkeit U49–20
Gewebezerstörung U45–21
Gewebsmanschette U43–13
Gewebstod **U13**–30
Gewichtszug U29–3
Gewinde **U43**–11
Gewindereiniger U43–11
Gewindeschneider U43–6,11
Gewindestift U40–14
gewissenhaft U4–1; U16–6
Gewohnheit, eintrainierte U38–13

gewohnheitsmäßig U10-17
Gewöhnung U47-5
gezahnt (Arbeitsende) U32-16f
gießen **U31**-4,2
Gießfähigkeit U31-4
Gießküvette U31-4,8
Gießtemperatur U31-4
Gift U5-15; U19-12
Giftigkeit U19-13
Giftstoff U5-15
Gingiva **U9**-12; U34-14
- propria U35-2
-, freie **U35**-2
-, interdentale U35-5
-, marginale **U35**-2
Gingivaatrophie U13-29
Gingivafasern U35-3
Gingivaindex **U35**-7
Gingivalsaum U35-2
Gingivalsulkus **U35**-4; U41-18
Gingivarand **U35**-3,2; **U39**-7,10
Gingivarandschräger **U32**-18; U35-3
Gingivaretraktion U35-10
Gingivarezession **U35**-10; U39-7
Gingivasaum **U35**-3
Gingivaspalte U45-2
Gingivastatus **U35**-6
Gingivatransplantat, freies U50-10
Gingivektomie U35-25
Gingivitis **U35**-13
- ulcerosa **U35**-14
Gingivoplastik **U35**-26
Gingivostomatitis herpetica U35-17
Ginvivaindices U35-6
Gips **U30**-13; U31-2
Gipsabbindebeschleuniger U30-13
Gipsabdruck U30-13
Gipsbinde U29-10
gipsen U29-6
Gipsexpansion U30-13
Gipshandschuh U29-6
Gipshülse U29-6
Gipsmeißel U30-13
Gipsmodell U30-13; U31-5
Gipsschale U29-7
Gipsschere U24-4
Gipsschiene U29-7
Gipsspat U30-13
Gipsverband **U29**-6; U28-20
Gipsvorwall U30-13
girlandenförmig U39-14
Gitter (Krankenbett) U23-18
- (Zunge) **U37**-15
Glandula parotidea U45-17
Glanz **U39**-18
-, perlmuttartiger U39-18
Glanzbrand U31-20; U39-18

glänzen **U31**-20; U39-18
glanzgebrannt U31-18
Glanzgrad U39-18
Glanzlack U31-20
Glanzlackpinsel U31-20
glanzpolieren U31-21
Glasgow-Komaskala U4-14
glasieren **U31**-20
Glasionomerzement **U40**-5
Glasur **U31**-20; U30-21
Glasurmasse U31-20
glatt (Muskel) U20-19; U48-16
glätten **U31**-21; U32-8,12; U24-12; U41-23
Glattflächenkaries U34-17
gleichaltrig U14-3
Gleichgewicht U8-15
Gleichgültigkeit U4-12
gleichverteilt U14-12
Gleitlochschraube U29-16
Gleitmittel U20-30; U27-17
Gliederschmerzen **U16**-5
Glossa **U8**-11
Glossitis U8-11
Glossoschisis U45-2
Glukonat U12-7
Glukosamin U12-7
Glukose **U12**-7
Glukoserest U12-5
Glukoseschwelle U12-7
Glukosespiegel U12-7
Glukosetransporter U12-7
Glukosurie U12-7
Glykogen U12-7
Gnathodynamometer U45-9
gnathologisch U45-9
goldarm (Legierung) U30-8
Goldfolie U30-8
Goldgerüst U30-8
Goldgussfüllung U30-8
Goldinlay U30-8
Goldklammer U30-8; U42-6
Goldknopfzähne U30-4
Goldlegierung U30-7
-, gehämmerte U30-7
Goldlot U31-16
Goldrand, sichtbarer U30-8
Goldspäne U30-8
Goldvergütung U30-8
Gonadenbelastung U33-3
Gonadendosis U46-9
Gonadenschutz U33-3
Granula, gefriergetrocknete U5-9
granulär U28-7
Granulat U5-9
Granulationsgewebe **U28**-7
-, überschießendes U28-7
Granulom, apikales **U41**-8
Graph U14-27

Grauschleier U33-2
Grauwertsonographie U33-11
Gray U46-10
Grenzdifferenz U14-21
Grenzfläche U40-21
Grenzwert **U14**-24
grenzwertig (Signifikanz) U14-21
Griff U24-2; U32-18; U34-4
Grit U32-24
grob (Oberfläche) U39-17
Grobfeile U32-12
grobkörnig U13-30
Größe U13-15
großlumig U22-18; U24-5; U7-6
Grübchenbreite U34-15
Grundkrankheit U18-9
Grundleiden U13-1
gründlich U3-11; U28-11
Gründlichkeit U34-12
Guérin-Fraktur U45-1
Gültigkeit U14-30
Gültigkeitsprüfung U14-30
Gummipolierer U34-2
Gummiring U37-10
Gummizüge U37-10
Gummy smile U9-12; U39-6
Gurgelmittel U8-12; U48-4
gurgeln **U11**-7; U34-6
Gurt U23-10; U29-8,11
Gusseigenschaft U31-4
Gussform U30-20; U31-3,13
Gussgerät U31-4
Gusshohlform U31-4
Gusskanal U30-20
Gusskegel U30-20
Gussmaschine U32-1
Gussmuffel U31-4,8
Gussreservoir U30-20
Gussspannung U31-4
Gussstift **U30**-20
Gussstück U31-2f
Gusswachs **U30**-17; U31-4
gutartig U45-17
Guttae **U5**-11
Guttapercha-Hauptstift U41-15, U30-12
Guttaperchastift **U30**-12
guttural U8-12
Gutturallaute U11-2
GVHR **U50**-20

H

H1-Antihistaminika U20-22
H1-Rezeptorenblocker U20-22
Haar **U8**-16
Haaransatz U8-15f
Haarbruch **U17**-11

Haarzunge U8-11
HA-beschichtet U43-2
Haftung **U39**-20
Haftungsverlust U39-20
Haftvermittler **U31**-17; U39-20
Haftvermittlung **U39**-20
Haken **U24**-9
Hakendraht U29-14
Hakenscaler U32-13
Halbhydrat, α **U30**-13
–, β U30-12f; U31-6
halbjustierbar U31-1
Halbwertbreite U20-5
Halbwertzeit **U20**-5
Haloextension U29-9
Halo-Fixateur U29-9
Halogenkohlenwasserstoff U48-12
Halothan **U48**-12
halothanbedingt (Leberschädigung) U48-12
Hals **U8**-12f
Halskrause **U29**-9; U8-13
Halskrawatte U29-9
Halsrippe U8-13
Halsschmerzen U8-12; U11-7; U16-11
Halsspülung U8-12
Halswirbelsäule U8-13
Halt **U42**-20
Haltbarkeit U5-19; U43-4
Halteelement **U42**-6,21
Haltenaht U26-1; U32-2
Haltung, schlechte U3-17
Hämatom U13-26; U3-13
Hämophiler U3-19
Hämorrhagie **U3**-19; U13-26
Hämostase **U22**-10
Hämostatikum U22-10
Hämostyptikum U22-10
Händedesinfektion **U27**-6
Handelsname U19-2
Händereinigung, chirurgische U23-2
Handfläche U17-10; U23-12
Handgelenk U50-16
Handgriff U29-2
Handschuh, OP U27-15
Handspreader U32-17
Handstück **U32**-5; U7-5
Handtuch U28-24
Handzerstäuber U20-14
Harnausscheidung U20-21
Harnsäure U20-28
harntreibend U20-21
hart U31-19; U32-23
Härte U30-5
Härtegrad U31-15
härten **U31**-19
Härter U31-19

Hartgips **U30**-14
Hartgipsbruch U31-19
Hartgipsmodell U30-14
Hartlöten U31-16
Hartlötnaht U31-16
Hartmetallbohrer U30-11; U32-6
Hartmetallknochenfräse U30-11
hartnäckig **U18**-13
Hasenscharte U8-9; U45-2
Hasenzähne U36-24
hässlich (Narbe) U28-10
Haue U32-18
Häufigkeitsverteilung **U14**-12
Häufung, familiäre U13-7
Hauptindikation U18-10
Hauptkriterien U42-4
Hauptnahrung U1-13
Hauptveranwortung U23-17
Hauptziel U25-4
Hausarzt U25-15
Hausbesuch U6-8,10
Hauskrankenpflegerin U28-1
Hausmittel U5-2
Hautabschürfung U28-13
Hautausschlag U50-20
Hautblutung U13-27
Hautdeckung **U49**-9
Hautdesinfektion **U27**-14
Hautdesinfektionsmittel U27-1
Hautfettgewebetransplantat U50-6
Hautirritation U16-3
Hautjucken U20-22
Hautlappen **U50**-6
Hautläsion U3-5; U13-17
Hautschnitt U21-9
Hauttasche U45-22
Hauttransplantat **U50**-6 f,1,5
–, sekundäres **U50**-7
–, zweizeitiges **U50**-7
Hautverletzung U28-22
Hawley-Aufbissbehelf U37-24
Hawley-Retainer U37-23
Headgear **U37**-18
Hebel **U32**-15; U17-4; U44-2
Hebelwirkung U32-15
heben **U49**-11
heften U29-15
Heftnaht U26-4
Heftpflaster **U28**-21 f,3; U29-11
Heftpflaster-Verband U28-21
heikel (Essen) U1-1
heilbar U5-2
Heilbarkeit U18-2
heilen **U5**-2; **U18**-2; **U28**-4
Heilerde U28-4
Heilgymnastik U38-13
Heilkräuter U5-1
Heilmittel **U5**-2; **U18**-2; U11-5
Heilung **U18**-2; U21-4; U28-4

Heilungsabsicht U18-2
Heilungsaussichten U18-2
Heilungsdistanzhülse U43-13
Heilungskäppchen **U43**-13
Heilungsprozess U28-4
Heilungsrate U14-8; U18-2
heiser U8-12
Heiserkeit U11-23
Heißluftsterilisation U27-2
heißpolymerisiert U31-19; U30-2; U39-16
Heizkissen U28-19
helfen (bei) U11-7
hell (Bewusstsein) **U4**-3
hellwach U4-2
Hemisektion U41-23; U44-2
hemmen U20-6f; U27-5
Hemmer **U20**-7
Hemmstoff **U20**-7
heraushebeln U17-4; U32-15; U44-2
Herbst-Scharnier U37-11,13
Herd **U13**-3
Herdinfektion U13-3
Herdläsion U3-5
hereditär **U13**-7
Herpes simplex U3-5; U13-17
Herstellung U30-9
hervorbringen (Laute) **U11**-1
hervorrufen U20-2
hervortreten U13-23; U28-16
Herzhypertrophie U13-15
Herzkatheter U22-19
Herzminutenvolumen U20-21
Herzmonitor U25-8
Herzversagen U20-18
Heuschnupfen U5-3
Heuschnupfenpatient U16-2
Hilfe benötigen U16-2
Hilfe, unsterile **U23**-9
Hilfsgeräte, kfo. U37-3
Hilfsmittel U18-3; U31-13
Hilfspersonal U6-3
Himbeerzunge U8-11
hindeuten auf U25-7
hineinbeißen U10-11
Hinterhauptzug-Headgear U37-18
hinunterschlingen **U1**-4
Hinweis U37-1
hinweisen (auf) U11-8
hinzuziehen (Kollegen) U6-9
Hirnprellung U3-13
Hirnstammschädigung U4-17
Hirntod **U4**-18; U49-17
Hirntoddiagnose U4-18
Histaminantagonist **U20**-22
Histopathologie U13-1
hitzegehärtet U31-19
Hitzeriss U31-18

HLA-ident (Zwillinge) U50-4
HNO U8-12
hochauflösend U46-14
hochdosiert U18-4; U19-7
Hochdrucksterilisator U27-3
hochempfindlich (Film) U33-7
hochlagern (Beine) U49-11
Hochlagerung U8-1; U29-10
Hochstimmung U48-11
hochtourig U32-6
Hochvoltstrahlentherapie,
  externe U46-5
hochwirksam U19-5,9
Hochzug-Headgear U37-18
Höckerneigung U9-4; U36-23
Höckerspitze U9-4,23; U36-5
Höckerwinkel U9-4
höckrig U9-4
Höhle **U34**-19
Hohlkehlpräparation U40-19
Hohlmeißel U24-11
Hohlnadel **U24**-6,5
-, großlumige U7-6
Hohlorgan U22-3
Hohlraum U41-15f
Hohlschraubenimplantat U43-6
Hohlsonde U32-9
Hohlzylinderimplantat U43-6
Honorar U6-8
Hörgerät **U45**-23; U49-18
Hormon, antidiuretisches U20-21
Hormonantagonist U20-31
Hormonentzugstherapie U22-13
Hornhautabschabung U3-8
Hörschwelle U8-15
HRCT U33-18
hufeisenförmig U9-9; U36-4;
  U42-23
Hülle U49-9
Hülsenkrone U40-14,18
Hunger U1-11
hungern **U1**-14f
Husten U11-2,6; U21-4
Hustenanfall U16-14
Hustenpastille U5-14
Hustensaft U5-11
Hybridprothese **U42**-11
Hygieneindex, oraler **U34**-21
Hypästhesie **U47**-4
Hyperaktivität U4-12
Hyperämie U13-27
Hyperästhesie U47-4
hyperdens U46-11
Hyperdontie U36-19
hypernasal **U11**-22
Hyperostose U44-16
Hyperplasie U13-15
Hypertelorismus, okulärer **U45**-5
hypertroph (Narbe) U28-10

Hypertrophie **U13**-15
Hypervitaminose U12-13
Hypnotikum U20-23; U47-9
hypnotisch U48-14
Hypokaliämie U20-21
hyponasal U11-22
Hyponasalität U11-22
Hypophyse U22-5
Hypotelorismus U45-5

I

iatrogen **U13**-9; U19-15
idiopathisch **U13**-8
Ikterus U13-8
imitieren U20-27
Immobilisation **U29**-5
Immobilisationsdauer U29-5
Immunantwort U18-11
Immunmodulatoren **U20**-34
Immunreaktion U18-11
immunsupprimiert U27-9
impaktiert (Weisheitszahn) U9-8
Impaktion U17-6
- (Speisereste) U44-3
Impfstoffe U7-6
Impfung U18-10
Implantat **U49**-18
-, dentales **U43**-2ff
-, enossales U49-18
-, gelockertes U33-7
-, intramuköses U43-4
-, kraniofaziales **U45**-21
-, radioaktives U24-7; U46-21
Implantatbelastung U43-14
Implantatbett **U43**-7
Implantateinbringung U44-12
Implantateinheilung U43-2
Implantatform U43-2
implantatgestützt U42-12
implantatgetragen U43-2
Implantatinsertion U43-4; U44-12
Implantation U49-18
-, vor der **U43**-3
Implantatkörper U43-1
Implantatmobilität U43-4
Implantatpflege U43-3
Implantatverankerung U43-2
implantieren **U49**-18
Implantologieprothetik U42-1
Impressionsfraktur U17-8
Impulsechoverfahren U33-11
in vitro **U15**-18
in vivo U15-18
inaktiv U15-8
-, biologisch **U49**-20; U26-10
Inaktivitätsatrophie U13-29;
  U44-6

Incisura mandibulae U45-13
Index U14-5
-, Papillen-Blutungs- U35-8
-, Sulkus-Blutungs- **U35**-8
Indikation **U18**-10
Indikator U14-5; U18-10
individuell angefertigt U42-16
- angepasst U40-16
indiziert U18-10
indolent U16-6
Induration **U13**-13
ineffizient U15-26
Infektion U27-9
Infektionserreger U20-2
Infektionsquelle U23-4
Infektpseudarthrose U17-15
Inferenzstatistik U14-1
Infiltrat U13-14
Infiltration U13-14
Infiltrationsanästhesie U48-3
Informationen U15-15
Informationsplakette, mediz. U4-2
infrakturiert U45-15
Infusionskanüle U24-6
Infusionspumpe **U47**-16
Infusionsständer U23-18
Inhalat **U20**-14
Inhalation U20-14
Inhalationsanästhetika U47-11;
  U48-4,10
-, volatile U32-3
Inhalationsmittel **U20**-14
Inhalationsnarkose **U48**-10;
  U47-14
Inhalator U20-14
Inhibitor **U20**-7
Initialbogen U37-5
Initialdosis **U47**-19; U19-7
Initialkaries U34-17
Injektion, subkutane U48-3
Injektionskanüle U7-6
Injektionsnadel **U7**-6; U24-5
Injektionsspritze U7-6
Inklination U36-23
Inklinationswinkel U36-23
Inlay **U40**-16
Inlaywachs U30-17
Innenkrone U42-9
Innenkurvatur U41-17
Innenohr U8-15
Innenteleskop **U40**-17
inoperabel U21-1
Insektenstich **U3**-10
Insellappen U50-13
Inspektion (Untersuchung) U21-11
Instabilität U29-4
instillieren U5-11; U48-5
Instrument **U24**-1f; U32-1
-, atraumatisches U32-1

Instrument, stumpfes U32–1
Instrumentarium U24–1; U32–1
Instrumentation U32–1
Instrumentbewegung U32–1
instrumentell U24–1
Instrumentenbestand U24–1
Instrumentensatz U24–1
Instrumentenschale U24–1
Instrumentenschrank U7–11
Instrumententisch **U7**–11
Instrumentenwagen **U23**–19
Instrumentieren U6–4; U24–1
Instrumentierschwester **U23**–8
Insufflationsnarkose U48–10
Insult, hämorrhagischer U13–26
Intelligenzminderung U45–5
Intensivstation U47–24
Intensivtherapie U25–8
Intention-to-treat Analyse **U15**–20
Interaktion, pharmakokinetische U19–11
Interdentalbürstchen U9–22; U34–4
Interdentalkeil U32–22
Interdentalpapille **U35**–5
Interdentalraum U9–22; U36–16; U39–13
Interdentalstimulator U34–1
Interferenzen, okklusale U36–7
Interimskrone U40–18
Interimsprothese U10–8; U42–2,9
interkurrent (Erkrankung) U15–29
Interkuspidation, maximale U36–13
Interkuspidationskontaktpunkte U36–9
Intermediärkallus U17–15
intern gekühlt U32–6
Interokklusalabstand **U10**–14; U36–7
interorbital U45–5
Interpositionsknochentransplantat U44–9
Interpositionsmaterial U38–17
interproximal (Kontakt) U39–13
Interventionssialographie U33–13
Interventionsstudie U15–1
Interzeptivbehandlung U36–1
Intimaruptur U17–5
Intoleranz U19–12
Intonation U11–10
Intoxikationszeichen U19–13
intramukös (Implantat) U43–4
intranasal verabreicht U48–5
intraoral **U9**–25; U33–4
Intrusion U36–25
Intubationsnarkose U48–13
Intubationsrohr U47–17
intubieren **U47**–17

invasiv (OP) U21–4
Inzidenz **U14**–7
inzidieren **U21**–9f
Inzisalpunkt U9–3
Inzision U3–6; U21–9
Iod U12–17; U46–21
Iodsalbe U5–8
Iodtinktur U5–10
Ion, positiv geladenes U46–20
Ionenaustausch U46–20
Ionenbindung U46–20
Ionendosis U46–20
Ionisation **U46**–20
Ionisationsdichte U46–20
Ionisationskammer U46–20
ionisierend U46–20
Ionisierung **U46**–20
Irrigation **U22**–17
Irrigator U22–17; U27–2
Irritabilität U13–10
Irritans U13–10
Irritanzien U20–14
Irritation **U13**–10; U16–3
irritieren U16–3
Ischämie **U13**–27
Isoliermittel (Alginat) U30–15
Isotransplantat **U50**–4
Isthmus, iatrogener **U41**–13

J

Jacketkrone U40–18
5-Jahresrate U14–8
jammern U11–3
Ja-Nein Quotient U14–35
Jochbein U8–5
Jochbeinfraktur U45–1
Joule **U12**–4
jucken U3–9; U13–10; U20–30
Juckreiz U3–9
Jugulariseröffnung U22–18
justierbar U31–1
Justierungsbogen U37–5

K

Kahnschädel U45–4
Kalium U12–17
Kallus U17–15
Kallusbildung U17–15
Kallusdistraktion U45–16
Kalorie U12–4
kalorienarm U12–4
Kalorienbedarf U12–4
kalorienbewusst U12–4
Kalorienverbrauch U12–4
Kalorienzufuhr, empfohlene U12–4

kalorisch (Wert) U12–4
Kalotte **U31**–13
Kalottenartikulation U31–13
Kalottenaufstellung U31–13
Kalottenfraktur U17–8
Kälteablation U22–13
Kälteanästhesie U48–3
Kältebehandlung U22–8
Kältesonde U22–8; U24–8
Kalzifikation U10–22
Kalzium U12–17
Kalziumantagonist U20–7
Kalziumblocker U20–7
Kammer, feuchte U28–5
kammüberlappend U42–5
Kanal, undichter U41–16
Kanalaufbereitung U41–17
Kanaleinengung **U41**–13
Kanalende U41–14
Kanalerweiterer **U32**–11
Kant(en)bogen-Technik U37–2
Kantenbiss U36–12
Kanüle **U24**–6
Kaolin **U30**–5
Kaplan-Meier Diagramm U14–27
Kappenschiene U42–22
Kapsel U5–7
kardiopulmonal (Reanimation) U47–25
Karies **U34**–**17**f; U9–18
kariesanfällig U10–22; U34–18
kariesbefallen U34–17
kariesfördernd U34–17
Kariesprophylaxe **U34**–2,17
Kariesrezidiv U34–17
kariös **U34**–18,17; U13–3
Kariostatikum U34–17
Karteikarte **U6**–14,13
Karton U5–16
Kasuistik U14–2
Kataplasma U28–25
Katgut **U26**–9,8
Katheter **U22**–19,18
Katheterisierung U22–19
Katheterspitze U22–19
Kationen U46–20
Kaubelastung U10–15; U43–14
Kaubewegung U10–15; U36–10; U38–1
kauen **U10**–15; U40–7
Kaufläche U9–24; U40–16
Kaukraft U9–7; U10–15; U36–28
Kauleistung U10–15
Kaumuskulatur U38–6
kaustisch U22–9; U30–24
Kautablette U5–7
Kautelen, aseptische U23–9; U27–1
Kauterisation U22–9

Kauvorgang U10–15
kauzwingend U38–3
Kauzyklusdauer U10–15
Kavität **U34**–19,17
Kavitätenbohrer U34–19
Kavitätenlack **U40**–3; U30–22; U34–19
Kavitätenliner **U40**–3
Kavitätenpräparation U34–19
Kavitätenrand **U40**–10; U34–19
Kavitätenreinigung **U40**–2; U34–19
Kavitätenstufe **U40**–7
Kavitätenumriss U34–19
Kavitätenwand U34–19
Kavitation U34–19
Kegel U22–12
Kegelbohrer U32–6
kegelförmig U5–12; U35–5
Kehle **U8**–12
Kehlkopf U8–14; U11–10
Kehllaute U11–2
Keil **U32**–22; U37–12
keilen (Gips) U29–6
keilförmig U24–11; U32–22
Keilresektion U21–15
Keim U27–8
keimfrei **U27**–2,14
Keimfreiheit U27–1 f
keimtötend U27–1,3
Keimverschleppung **U27**–9
Keloid U28–10
Kenngröße **U14**–5
Kennziffer U14–5
Kephalometrie **U33**–9
Kephalostat U33–9; U39–4
Keramik **U30**–4,2; U40–11
Keramikfacettenkrone U30–4
Keramikglasur U30–4
Keramikinlay U30–4
Keramikmantel U30–4
Keramikmasse U30–21
Keramikofen U31–20
Keramiküberzug U30–4
Keramikveneer U39–22
Keramikverblendmaterialien U39–16
Keramikverblendung U30–4
keramisch U30–4
Keratozyste U44–15
Kern **U40**–15
Kernladung U46–22
Kernspintomographie **U33**–12
Kette, elastische U37–10
Keuchen, krampfartiges U11–3
Kiefer **U8**–7
Kieferaufnahme, laterale U33–4
Kieferbeweglichkeit U38–4,6
Kieferbewegung U38–1

Kieferbruch U3–20
Kieferbruchschiene U29–7
Kieferchirurgie, minimal invasive **U45**–18
Kieferfraktur **U45**–1
Kiefergelenk **U38**–1; U31–1; U45–10
Kiefergelenkarthritis **U38**–11
Kiefergelenkarthroskopie **U38**–15; U45–18
Kiefergelenkentzündung **U38**–11
Kiefergelenkerkrankung U38–1
Kiefergelenkfortsatz U38–10
Kiefergelenkknacken **U38**–4; U8–7
Kiefergelenkköpfchen **U38**–18 f
Kiefergelenkluxation **U38**–8
Kiefergelenkplastik **U38**–19
Kiefergelenkposition, zentrische U36–2
Kiefergelenkproblem **U37**–24; U38–1
Kiefergelenkstörung **U38**–2
Kiefergelenkübungen **U38**–13
Kiefer-Gesichtsprothese **U45**–22
Kiefer-Gesichtsprothetik U9–26
Kieferhöhlenensterung U22–3
Kieferhöhlenfistelbildung **U44**–14
Kieferhöhlensonde U24–8; U32–9
Kieferindex **U45**–9
Kieferkammplastik **U44**–8
Kieferklemme **U38**–5
Kieferknochen U8–7
Kiefer-Lid-Phänomen U8–7
Kieferluxation **U38**–8
Kieferorthopäde **U36**–1; U6–1
–, chirurgische **U45**–9
Kieferregulierung **U36**–1
Kieferrelation U8–7
Kieferrelationsbestimmung **U36**–2; U31–2
Kiefersperre **U38**–5
Kieferwinkel U8–7; U45–13
Kieferzyste U13–24
kieselsteinartig U35–22
kindersicher U5–16
Kinderzahnarzt U6–1
Kinn **U8**–6
Kinnaugmentation U45–14
Kinnkappe **U37**–20; U8–6
Kinnkorrektur **U45**–14; U22–4
Kinn-Lippenplastik U45–14
Kinnplastik **U45**–14
Kinnstütze U8–6
Kinnvorverlagerung U45–14
kippen U36–21; U37–3
Kippkraft U36–21
Kippung U36–23
Kirschner-Bohrstift U29–14
Kirschnerdraht-Fixation U29–15

Kissen **U28**–19
klaffen (Wunde) U3–3; U28–16
klagen U11–3 f
Klammer **U37**–15; U42–6
–, fortlaufende U37–23
Klammerarm U42–6
Klammerjustierzange U32–16
klammern U26–4
Klammernaht **U26**–12 f
Klammernahtgerät U26–12
Klang **U11**–10
klar (Verstand) **U4**–3
Klarheit U4–3
klebbar U39–20
Klebeband **U28**–21,3; U29–11
Klebebrücke U42–4
Kleber **U31**–17; U30–6
Klebestreifen U29–11
Klebezement U30–6
Klebstoff **U31**–17
Kleeblattschädel U17–10
Klemme **U26**–13; **U24**–14,13
Klemmzange U24–13
Klinge U24–2 f
Klingenhalter U24–3
Klinikapotheke U5–4 f
Klinikpackung U5–16
klinisch (Studie) U15–1
Klumpen-Stichprobe U14–4
knabbern U10–11
knicken U49–13
knirschen (Zähne) **U10**–18; U36–11
Knirscherschiene **U37**–25
Knirschhabit U36–11
Knirschunart U36–11
Knisterrasseln **U17**–14
Knochenabbau U10–20; U35–12
Knochenabsprengung U17–5
Knochenapposition, höhengleiche U29–1
Knochenaufbau U49–19
Knochenbank U44–11
Knochenbruch U17–1,5; U3–20
Knochenchip, kortikaler U44–10
Knochenfeile U24–12; U32–12
Knochenfenster U41–6
Knochenfissur U17–1
Knochenfragment **U17**–2
Knochenfraktur U17–1; U3–20
Knochenfräse U32–12; U36–10
Knochenfrästechnik U43–11
Knochenheilung **U17**–15
Knochenmark U49–10
Knochenmarkinfiltration U13–14
Knochenmarktransplantation U49–14; U50–2
Knochenmatrix, demineralisierte **U44**–11
Knochenmehl U44–11

Knochenmeißel U24-11
Knochennagel **U29**-15
Knochennaht U29-12
Knochenneubildung U43-1
Knochenpartikel, demineralisierte U44-11
Knochenplatte **U29**-17
Knochenregeneration, gesteuerte **U44**-12
Knochenresektion U45-11
Knochenschere U24-4
Knochenschraube U29-16
Knochenspan U49-16; U44-11
Knochenspanplastik U50-9
Knochensplitter U17-2
Knochentasche, infraalveoläre U35-11
Knochentransplantat U44-11; U50-9
Knochentransplantation **U44**-9
Knochentrepanation U41-22
Knochenzange **U24**-11
Knopfanker U42-20
Knopfnaht U26-15
Knopfsonde U32-9
Knorpel U8-14
Knorpelfragment U17-2
Knötchen **U13**-16
Knoten **U13**-16
–, chirurgischer **U26**-6,1
–, indurierter U13-13
–, schmerzhafter U16-11
Knotenbildung U13-16
Knotentechnik U26-6
Koagulation U20-16; U22-10
Koagulator U22-10
koagulieren U20-16
Koagulopathie U13-1; U22-10
Koaptation U26-5
Kobalt-Chromlegierung U43-19
Kobaltgussklammer U42-6
Kochenanbau U29-1
Kochsalz, fluoridiertes U34-13
Kochsalzbläschen-Kontrast U46-15
kochsalzimprägniert U28-18
Kochsalzlösung U5-11; U11-7
Kofaktor U14-5
Kofferdam **U32**-19
Kofferdamklammer U32-19
Kofferdam-Klammerzange U32-19
Kofferdam-Lochzange U32-19
Kohäsionskraft U31-15
Kohlendioxid U47-14
Kohlenhydrate **U12**-5
Kohorte U14-3; U15-11
Kohortensterbetafel U14-26
Kohortenstudie U15-11
Kolik **U16**-15
kolikartig U16-7,15

kollabieren U49-18
Kollaps U4-4
Kollimation **U46**-6
Kollimator U46-6
kollimiert (Strahlen) U33-3
Kollumfraktur U45-1
Koma **U4**-14
komatös U4-14
Kombinationstherapie U18-3
kommen, zu sich U4-6
kommunizieren U11-8
Komorbidität U13-2; U14-9
Kompensation, dentoalveoläre U36-1
Komplikation **U25**-9
komplikationsfrei U25-7
Komplikationsrate U25-9
Komposit **U30**-3
Kompositadhäsivbrücke U30-3
Komposit-Dentin-Verbundfestigkeit U30-3
Kompositfüllung U40-1
Kompositkleber U30-3,6; U39-20
Kompositveneer U30-3
Kompositverblendschale U30-3
Kompresse **U28**-19; **U28**-25
Kompressionsfraktur U17-6
Kompressionsosteosynthese U29-17
Kompressionsplatte, dynamische U29-17
Kompressionsstrümpfe U29-10
Kompressionsverband U28-20
Kompromiss, ästhetischer U39-1
Kondensation U41-15,17
kondensieren U32-17
Kondylektomie **U38**-18
Kondylenschraube U29-16
konfektioniert U30-7
Konfidenzgrenze U14-17
Konfidenzintervall **U14**-17
Konfidenzniveau U14-17
konfluierend U13-27
kongenital U13-6
Kongruenz, axiale **U43**-9
Konisation **U22**-12,5
Konkrement **U13**-21
Konkremententfernung U32-13; U34-14
konsekutiv (Serie) U14-3; U15-11
Konsequenz U18-15
Konservierung U21-13
Konservierungsmittel U1-6
Konsiliarius U6-9
Konsonant U11-12
Konstriktion U13-19
–, apikale U41-6,12
Konstruktion U43-15
Konsultation **U6**-9

konsumieren **U1**-2
Kontakte, exzentrische U36-9
–, funktionelle U36-9
–, okklusale U33-8
Kontaktfläche U31-21; U35-5; U36-9
–, interproximale U39-13
Kontaktführung U36-9
Kontaktpunkt, okklusaler **U36**-9
Kontaminant U27-9
Kontamination **U27**-9; U23-7
kontaminiert U27-2; U28-12
Konter U31-5
Kontingenztafel U14-27
Kontinuität U3-18
kontrahieren U31-6
Kontraindikation U5-17; U18-10
Kontraktionsbögen U37-3
Kontraktur U13-19; U28-8
Kontrastauflösung U46-14
Kontrastaufnahme U46-15
Kontrastfärbemittel U46-15
Kontrastmittel **U46**-15,20; U33-13
Kontrastverstärkung U33-16; U46-15
Kontrolle U6-15
–, unter fluoroskopischer U46-8
Kontrollgruppe **U15**-10; U14-22
Kontrollperson U14-2; U15-10; U25-5
Kontrolltermin U6-10; U43-13
Kontrolluntersuchung **U6**-15; U18-14
Kontur **U39**-2
konturieren U39-2
Konturzange U32-16; U39-2
Kontusion **U3**-13
Konusbiopsie U22-12
konusförmig U40-17
Konuskrone U42-9
Konzentration U5-13
kooperativ U18-15
Kopf **U8**-1
Kopfbedeckung U8-1
Kopfbiss U36-12
Kopf-Brust-Gipsverband U29-9
Kopfhalterung U29-3,9; U36-29
Kopfhaut U8-16
Kopfhautverletzung U3-5
Kopf-Kinnkappe **U37**-20
Kopfschmerzen U16-4
Kopfstütze U7-1; U8-1
Kornährenverband U28-20
körnig U28-7
Körnung U32-24
koronardilatatorisch U20-17
Körperabsonderungen U27-16
Körpergröße U14-11
Körperkreislauf U19-10

Körperverletzung U3–2f
Korrektur, operative U22–4; U49–2
Korrekturmaßnahme U43–3
Korrekturosteotomie U49–2
Korrelation U14–32
Korrosionsfestigkeit U43–19
Korrosionsgeschwindigkeit U43–19
Korrosionsverhalten U43–19
Kortikalistransplantat U50–9
kosmetisch U39–1; U49–3
Kost U1–7,13,16
Kovarianzanalyse U14–28
Kraft, kfo. wirksame U36–28
Kräfte, okklusale U33–8
Krallenhebel U32–15
Krampfanfall U20–20; U48–4
krampfartig U16–4
krampflösend U20–19f; U48–5
kranial U23–13
Kraniosynostose U45–4
Kraniotomie U45–20
krank U13–2
Krankenblatt U23–2
Krankengymnastin U18–4
Krankenhaus U27–12
Krankenhausaufenthalt U25–11
Krankenhauspersonal U27–11
Krankenkost U1–13
Krankenschwester U23–6
Krankenversicherung U49–9
krankhaft U13–1f
Krankheitserreger U13–1; U20–2
Krankheitshäufigkeit U13–2
Krankheitsherd U13–3
Krankheitsursache U13–8
kratzen U3–9
Kratzspuren U3–9
Kratztest U3–9
Krebszelle U20–31
Kreisdiagramm U14–27
Kreislauf U19–10
Krepitation U17–14
krepitationsartig U38–4
Kreuzbiss U36–15,7
–, transversaler U36–15
Kreuzinfektion U27–11
Kreuzkorrelation U14–32
Kreuzlappen U50–11
Kreuzreaktion U19–11
Kreuzschmerzen U16–10,16
Kreuztoleranz U19–12
Kribbeln U16–17; U47–3f
Kriechen U41–16
Krone U9–14; U40–18; U42–4
–, wachsmodellierte U30–17
Kronenlänge U39–12
Kronenrand U39–2; U40–18
Kronenschulter U40–8

Kronenverlängerung U35–25; U39–12
Krone-zu-Implantat Quotient U43–16
Krücken U25–13
Kruste (Wunde) U28–9,6
Kryoablation U22–13
Kryochirurgie U22–8; U21–3
Kryokauter U22–8f
Kryosonde U24–8
Kryotherapie U22–8
Kugelanker U37–15
Kugelstopfer U32–17
Kühlmittel U7–5
Kühlsalbe U5–8
Kühlung U7–5
–, interne U32–6
–, Wasser U7–5; U32–19
Kummer U16–2
künstlich U42–1,19
Kunststoff U30–2; U31–2,11,19
Kunststoff-Abformlöffel U31–3
Kunststoffbasis U42–17
Kunststoffhärter U30–3
Kunststoffkrone U40–18
Kunststoffschablone U31–13
Kunststoffschlauch U22–20
Kunststofftrimmer U30–2
Kunststoffveneer U39–22
Kupfer U12–17
Kur U18–2,1,5; U5–1
kurativ U18–2,9
Kürettage U34–14
Kürette U24–10; U32–14
–, scharfe U24–2
kurieren U5–2
Kurort U18–2
Kurvenschreiber U14–27
Kurznarkotika U48–4
Kurzwellendiathermie U22–9
Kurzwellentherapie U38–13
Küvette U31–9,3
Küvettenbügel U31–9
Küvettenpolymerisation U31–9
Küvettenpresse U31–9
Küvettenschluss U31–9

L

labial U9–23; U8–9
Labialbogen U37–15,22
Labialfläche U9–23
Labiallaut U8–9
Labium U8–9
Laborbericht U15–16
Lächeln U39–6
lachen U11–2
lächerlich U11–2

Lachgas U48–11
Lachkurve U36–5; U39–6
Lachlinie U39–6
Lack U30–22
Lackzunge U8–11
Ladung, elektrische U12–17
Lage U23–11
Lageanomalie U13–2
Lagedrainage U28–15
Lagerung U5–19; U23–10f
lähmen U47–11
Lähmung U47–11
Laktose U12–8,6
Laktosemangel U12–8
Lallen U11–17
Lallphase U11–17
Lalophobie U11–17
Laminar-Flow-System U27–8
Laminektomie-Stanze U24–11
Landkartenzunge U8–11
langfristig U14–15
Langlochplatte U29–17
Längsschnittstudie U15–1
Längsteilung U21–14
Langtubus, IO Aufnahme U33–4
Langzeitergebnis U14–20
Langzeitfolgen U25–9
Langzeitimmobilität U29–5
Langzeitmorbidität U18–12
Langzeitnachbetreuung U18–14
lanzinierend U16–7
Lappen U26–4; U50–6
– ohne Gefäßstruktur U50–12
–, einseitig bedeckter U50–15
–, freier U50–10
–, gestielter U50–11
–, umhüllender U50–17
Lappenabstoßung U44–5
Lappendeckung U49–9
Lappenplastik U44–5
Lappenverkleinerung U44–7
Laryngospasmus U11–9
Larynx U8–14
Laser U22–7
Laserablation U22–13
Laserbleaching U39–19
Lasersonde U22–7
Laserstrahl U22–7
Laservaporisation U22–7
Läsion U3–5; U13–3; U28–17
–, Endo-Paro- U35–20
–, kariöse U13–3; U34–18
Lastverteilung U43–14
Laut U11–10,12
Lautbildung U11–9,13
Lautsatz U11–10
Lautunterscheidung U11–10
Lavage U28–11; U38–15
Le Fort I Fraktur U45–1

Le Fort I Fraktur, Osteotomie **U45**–7
Lead-time Bias U14–18
Lebendspender U49–17
lebensbedrohlich U19–14; U25–5,9
lebenserhaltend U21–13; U19–6
Lebenserwartung U14–18
lebensfähig U35–27; U49–17; U50–21
lebensgefährlich U14–15
Lebensmittel U1–6
Lebensqualitätsstudie U14–20
lebensrettend U21–4
Lebenszeitwahrscheinlichkeit U14–31
Lebertoxizität U19–13
Leck U26–11; U47–15
lecker U1–11; U8–8
lederartig U35–22
Leeraufnahme U46–3,19
Leermedikament **U15**–8
Leeway Space **U36**–6
legen (OP-Tisch) **U23**–11
Legierung U30–7,1
–, edelmetallreduzierte U30–7
–, goldarme U30–8
–, goldfreie U30–8
–, Platin-Iridium U30–9
–, schmelzbare U31–16
Legierungsbasis U30–7
Leichenorgan U49–17
Leichenorganspende U49–15
Leichenspender **U49**–17; U44–11
Leichentransplantat U50–1
Leiden **U16**–2
leise (sprechen) U11–16
Leistenbeuge U16–15
Leistungsfähigkeit U15–26
Leiter (Institut) **U8**–1
Leitungsanästhesie **U48**–6; U9–25; U47–2
Leitungsaphasie U11–11
Leitungswasser U3–11; U28–25
letal (Ausgang) U14–20
– (Dosis) U19–7
Lethargie **U4**–12
leuchten U39–18
Leuchtschirm U46–8
Leukozyt U20–34
Lichtbleichen U39–19
Lichtdurchlässigkeit U39–16
lichthärtend U30–3; U31–19
Lichtofen U31–19
lichtpolymerisiert U31–19
lichtstarr U4–7
lichtundurchlässig U39–16; U19–9
Lid U8–3
Lidkolobom U45–6
Lidocain **U48**–5
Lidocain-Gel U48–5

Lidrandreflex U47–20
lidschlagbedingt U46–13
Lidschwellung U3–15
Ligand U12–17; U20–4
Ligatur **U26**–3
–, elastische **U37**–7; U26–3
Ligaturclip U26–13
Ligaturenadapter U37–7
Ligaturendraht U26–3
Ligaturschere U24–4
Ligaturschlinge U26–3
Lightwire-System **U37**–3
ligieren **U26**–3; U37–7
ligiert und durchtrennt U3–6
lindern U5–2; U20–18; U30–24
lindernd **U18**–9; **U20**–30
Linderung U16–19; U18–9
Liner U30–22; U42–25
Lingua **U8**–11
lingual U9–23
Lingualbügel U42–24
Lingualfläche U40–11
Lingualhöcker U9–23
Lingualkippung U9–23; U36–13
Lingualnerv U9–23
Lingualretainer U37–23
Linolsäure U12–12
Lip-Bumper **U37**–22
Lipid **U12**–11
Lippe **U8**–9
Lippen vorstülpen U8–6
Lippenbalsam U8–9
Lippenbändchen U8–9
Lippenbeißen U39–6
Lippenentzündung U8–9
Lippenhalter **U32**–2; U8–9
Lippeninkompetenz U8–9; U39–6
Lippenlinie **U39**–6
Lippenmuskulatur, schlaffe U36–24
Lippenplastik U44–7
Lippenprofil U8–9; U39–3
Lippenrot U8–9
–, Transposition von U44–7
Lippensaum U8–9
Lippenschluss U8–9; U39–6
Lippenschlusslinie U8–9
Lippenspalte U8–9; U45–2
Lippenwulst U8–9
Liquor U48–9
Liquoraustritt U45–1
Liquorrhoe U17–8
Liquorzuckerspiegel U12–7
lispeln **U11**–21
Loch (Zahn) **U34**–19
Lochfraß **U43**–19
locker U10–12
lockern, sich U10–5
Lockerung U9–1; U35–15,19
Löffel, scharfer U24–3,10

Löffelexkavator U32–14
Löffelmasse U31–3
Logopäde U11–8; U18–4
Logopädie U11–11
Logorrhoe U11–11
Logrank-Test U14–34
lokal **U19**–5
Lokalanästhesie **U48**–3
Lokalanästhetikum U19–5
Longitudinalstudie U15–1
lose (Zähne) U10–12; U44–2
lösen (Befestigung) U37–10
Losgelöstsein U4–15
Löslichkeit U5–11
L-Osteotomie, umgekehrte U45–11
Lösung U5–11
Lösungsmittel U5–11
Lösungstablette U5–7
Lot **U31**–16
Löteinbettmasse U31–16
Löten U31–16
Lötfuge U31–16
Löthilfe U31–16
Lotion U5–10
Lötkolben U31–16
Lötlampe U31–15
Lötofen U31–16
Lötstelle U31–16
Löttemperatur U31–16
Lötverfahren U30–9
Lückenhalter U32–22; U36–21; U37–12
Lückenschluss, kfo. U36–17; U44–4
lückig (Gebiss) U10–2
Luer-Zange **U24**–11; U32–12
Luftbläser **U7**–4
luftdicht (Verschluss) U19–9; U26–11
Luftmotor **U7**–3
Luftströmung U27–8
Lüftung, Schrödersche **U41**–22
Lumbalpunktion U3–10; U22–16; U48–7
Lumineszenz, kurzlebige U46–17
Lungenperfusionsszintigramm U46–18
Lupenbrille U22–6
Lust (Essen) U1–11
lutschen U5–14
Lutsch-Kontrollgerät U37–1
Lutschtablette **U5**–14
Luxation **U3**–20, **U17**–4
–, offene U17–3
Luxationsfraktur U3–20; U17–4
luxieren U3–20; U17–4
luxiert (Zahn) U44–3
Lymphadenektomie U21–12
Lymphdrainage U28–15
Lymphknotenbefall U13–4

Lymphknotendissektion U21–12
Lysis U38–15

M

Magen-Darm-Röntgen U46–3
– – Trakt U34–20
Magengeschwür U13–17
Magenreizung U13–10
Magensaft U2–25; U20–29
Magenschmerzen U16–4
Magentropfen U5–11
Magnetresonanztomographie **U33**–12
mahlen **U10**–18
Mahlzahn **U9**–7
Mahlzeit **U1**–7
Maisstärke U12–5
makroskopisch U15–17
maligne U45–17
Malignitätsgrad U46–23
Malokklusion **U36**–8; U10–13
Mandibula U8–7
Mandibularlinie U39–4
mandibulomaxillär U29–4
Mandrel U32–5
Mandrin U24–7
Mangan U12–17
Mangelernährung U1–13; U12–3
Mangelkrankheit U12–13
Mangelzustände U1–6
Manipulation U29–2
Manschette U29–7f
Manteltablette U5–7
Margo gingivalis **U35**–3; **U39**–7
Marienglas U30–13
Markierung, autoradiographische U33–15
Marsupialisation U44–15
Masse U12–16
Masseterreflex **U38**–7; U8–6f
Maßnahme, therapeutische **U18**–5f
Maßstab U14–6
Matratzennaht **U26**–17
Matrize U32–21; U42–6,24
Matrizenband U32–21
Matrizenhalter **U32**–21
Matrizenspanner **U32**–21
Mattigkeit U4–12; U47–9
Maul (Zange) U24–13; U32–15
–, gezahntes U32–16
Maxilla U8–7
maxillofazial **U9**–26
Meatus acusticus U8–15
Median U14–10
Medianschnitt U21–9
Medikament **U5**–1; **U5**–3
Medikation **U5**–1

medizinisch U5–1
Medizinprodukt, neues U15–2
Mehrfachapplikator U26–13
Mehrfachentnahmeflasche U5–13
Mehrlochkollimator U46–6
mehrwurzelig U9–19; U41–3
mehrzeitig (Transplantat) U44–9
Meißel U44–16
Meistermodell U31–2,5
Melanodontie U34–11
Melanoglossie U8–11
Membrana tympani U8–15
mental U3–14
Mentalpunkt U39–5
Mentum **U8**–6
Merkmal U14–5
Mesh-Graft U50–6
Meshtransplantat **U50**–8; U26–4
mesial **U9**–21
Mesialbiss U36–7
Mesialverlagerung U45–8
Mesialwanderung U36–21
Messer, chirurgisches **U24**–3
Messerspitze U24–3
Messlehre U31–13; U43–10
Messwert **U15**–15; U14–12
metabolisiert U20–4
Metabolismus U12–7
Metall-Abformlöffel U31–3
Metallgerüst U40–11
Metallkappe **U40**–17; U42–9
Metallkeramik U30–4
Metallmanschette U37–8
Metallplatte U29–17
Metastasenherd U13–3
Metastasierung U13–4
Methode der Wahl U18–3
–, operative **U21**–4
Mikroabrasion U39–23
Mikrochirurgie **U22**–5
mikrochirurgisch U22–5
Mikroelement **U12**–17
–, essentielles U12–17
Mikromanipulator U22–5
Mikroorganismen U27–8
Mikroschere U24–4
Mikrosomie, Gesichtshälfte U45–4
–, kraniofaziale U45–21
Mikrosonde U22–5
Mikrotie U45–4
Mikro-Zahnbürste U34–3
Milch **U2**–4f
Milcheckzähne U36–6
Milchgebiss **U10**–2
Milchprodukte U1–2
Milchsäure U12–8
Milchzähne **U10**–2; U41–24
Milchzucker **U12**–8,6
mildern (Schmerz) U16–19

Mimik **U8**–2
mindestens haltbar bis U1–2
Mineralsalz U34–9
Minerva-Gips U29–9
Miniplatte U29–17
mischen U5–5; U19–1
Mischgebiss U10–1
Mischtabelle U39–15
Missbildung U13–2,5; U20–33; U45–8; U49–3
Missbrauch U48–14
Missempfindung, subjektive **U16**–17; U47–4
Missverhältnis U36–18
Mitella U29–8
mitteilsam U11–8,18
Mittel (Arznei) **U5**–3; **U20**–2
– (Erkältung) U5–2
– der Wahl U5–3
–, einhüllendes U20–30
–, entzündungshemmendes **U20**–11
–, erweichendes U20–30
–, gefäßerweiterndes **U20**–17
–, schmerzstillendes **U16**–20
–, wassertreibendes **U20**–21
Mittelgesichtsfraktur U45–1
Mittelgesichtsvorverlagerung U45–8
Mittelohr U8–15
Mittelohrentzündung, eitrige U28–14
Mittelwert **U14**–10
Mixtur U5–6
MKG-Chirurg U6–1; U9–26; U44–1
Mobilisation **U25**–13; U29–5
Mobilität U29–5
Modell U30–14; U31–1f
–, aufgewachstes **U31**–10
Modellgips U30–14; U31–5
Modellherstellungsverfahren U31–5
modellieren **U31**–4
Modellierwachs **U30**–17
Modellmontage **U31**–7,1
Modellstift **U31**–12
Modellstumpf **U31**–5,10,12; U40–17
Molar **U9**–7f
Molkeeiweiß U12–9
Molkereiprodukte **U2**–4
Monitor U25–8
Monoaminooxidasehemmer U20–24
Monobloc-Advancement U45–8
Monoblock U37–14
monofil U26–7
Montage U31–7

Montagegips U31–7
Montagehilfe U31–7
Montageplatte U31–7
montieren U31–1
morbid **U13**–2
Morbidität **U18**–12; U13–2
Morbiditätsrate **U14**–9
Mörser U31–14
Mörserkolben U31–14
Mortalitätsquotient U14–9
Mortalitätsrate U14–9
Mortalitätsstatistik U14–1
Moskitoklemme U24–14
Mucilago U20–30
Müdigkeit U4–12; U47–9
Muffel U31–4
Mukogingivaldefekt U35–12
Mukogingivalgrenze U35–2;
  U39–9
Mukoidzyste U44–15
Mukoperiostlappen **U44**–5;
  U35–23; U50–17
Mukotom U44–9
Mukozele U44–15
Mullbinde U28–18
Mullkompresse U28–18,20
Multibandapparatur U37–2
multifil U26–7
multivariat U14–5,28
Mumifikation **U41**–24
Mund **U8**–8
– spitzen U8–6
Mund-Antrum-Verbindung U35–21
Mundatmung U8–8
Mundboden U44–7
Mundbodenzyste U44–15
Munddusche U22–17; U34–1
mundgerecht U10–12
Mundgeruch, übler **U34**–20
Mundhöhle U8–8; U34–19
Mundhygiene **U34**–1
Mundhygienekontrolle U34–1
Mundhygienikerin U34–1
Mund-Kiefer-Gesichtschirurg
  U9–26; U44–1
Mundmilieu U9–25
Mundschleimhaut U35–17
Mundschleimhautentzündung
  U8–8
Mundschutz **U27**–18
Mundsperrer **U10**–16; **U32**–3
Mundspiegel **U32**–4
Mundspülbecher U7–8
Mundspülbecken U7–8
Mundspülung U34–6
Mundvorhof **U8**–10; U9–23;
  U17–9
Mundvorhofplastik **U44**–7
Mundvorhoftiefe U8–10

Mundwasser U11–7; U34–4,20
Mundwinkel U8–8
Mund-zu-Mund Beatmung U47–25
murmeln **U11**–15
Musculus latissimus dorsi U49–13
Muskelhartspann U16–16
Muskelkater U16–11
Muskelkrampf, anfallsartiger
  U16–14
Muskelmasse U12–16
Muskelrelaxanzien **U48**–16
Muskelriss U17–5
Muskelschmerzen U16–21
Muskeltonus U48–16
Muskelverspannung U16–16
Muskelzerrung U3–17
Muskelzucken U16–12
Muskulatur, glatte U20–19
–, quergestreifte U48–16
Mutismus, akinetischer U4–17
Myalgie U16–21
myelotoxisch U20–32
Myoarthropathie **U38**–2

N

Na-Alginat U30–15
nach Bedarf U47–7
Nachbarherd U13–3
Nachbarzahn U9–1; U36–25;
  U39–13
Nachbehandlung **U18**–14
Nachbehandlungsplan U18–14
Nachbildung U31–2
Nachblutung U3–19; U13–26
nachbrennen U31–18
nachgefärbt U33–15
Nachkomme U13–7
Nachlot U31–16
nachpolymerisieren U31–3
Nachsorge **U18**–14; **U25**–15;
  U6–15; U21–2
Nachsorgetermin U6–10
nachstellen (Brackets) U37–1
nachstoßen (Zähne) U36–6
Nachtangst U11–14
Nachtschiene **U37**–25; U11–5
Nachuntersuchung **U25**–15;
  U6–15; U18–14; U21–2
Nachuntersuchungstermin U25–15
Nachuntersuchungszeitraum
  U18–14; U14–10
Nachweis **U15**–17; U14–1; U46–3
nachweisbar U12–17
Nachwirkung U15–26
Nacken **U8**–13
Nackenband U37–19
Nackenpolster U37–21

Nackensteifigkeit U8–13
Nackenzug-Headgear U37–18
Nadel **U29**–15
–, chirurgische **U24**–5; U22–6
Nadel-Faden-Kombination U24–5
Nadelhalter **U24**–15
Nadelstich U29–15; U48–15
Nadelstichverletzung U3–2
Nagel **U29**–15
Nägelkauen U10–11
Nagelung U29–15f
nähen **U26**–1; U24–5
Nahlappen U50–11
Nähnadel U24–5
nähren **U1**–3; **U12**–1
nahrhaft **U12**–2,1
Nährlösung U12–2
Nährstoff **U12**–2
Nährstoffanreicherung U2–22
Nährstoffaufnahme U12–2
Nährstoffzufuhr U25–12
Nahrung **U1**–3,6,13; U12–1f
–, feste U47–13
–, flüssige U25–12
Nahrungsaufnahme **U25**–12;
  U1–1,6; U19–6
Nahrungskarenz U1–15; U18–11;
  U21–2
Nahrungsmittel U1–6,16
Nahrungsmittelersatz **U2**–21
Nahrungszufuhr, empfohlene
  U1–13
Nährwert U1–6; U12–2
Naht, chirurgische **U26**–1f
–, eingewendelte U26–16
–, fortlaufende **U26**–16
Nahtlinie U31–21
Nahtmaterial **U26**–7; U49–5
Nahtöffnung U45–8
Nahtschere U24–4
Nahtschlinge U24–9
Nahtspannung U49–5
Narbe **U28**–10
Narbenbildung U13–19; U25–10;
  U28–5,8,10
Narbenbruch U3–18; U13–23;
  U21–9
Narbenretraktion **U28**–8
Narbenschrumpfung **U28**–8
narbiges Gesicht U28–10
Nares U8–4
Narkose **U47**–2,6; **U48**–1
Narkoseapparat **U47**–14
Narkosearzt **U23**–6; U47–2
Narkoseeinleitung **U47**–13
Narkoseführung U47–2
Narkosegas U48–4
Narkosegerät **U47**–14
Narkosekater U47–23

Narkosemaske U47-15
Narkoseprämedikationsraum U23-3
Narkoseprotokoll U47-22
Narkoseraum U23-3
Narkoserisiko U47-12,2
Narkoseschwester U23-6
Narkosesystem U47-14; U48-10
Narkosetiefe U47-20,2,13; U23-6
Narkosezeichen U47-11
Narkotikum U47-5,1f; U48-4,1; U5-3
narkotisieren U47-1
Nase U8-4
Nase putzen U11-6
näseln (Sprache) U11-17,22
Nasenbluten U3-19; U28-23
Naseneingang U8-10
Nasenepithese U45-22
Nasenflügelknorpel U45-22
Nasenhöhle U8-4
Nasenloch U47-1
Nasenraspel U24-12
Nasensekret U11-6
Nasenspalte U45-2
Nasentamponade U28-24
Nasenwurzel U39-5
Nasion U39-5
nässen (Wunde) U28-13
Natrium U12-17
natriumhaltig U5-1
Naturgips U30-13
Nebenhöhlen U8-4
Nebenhöhlendurchleuchtung U46-16
Nebenwirkung U19-14,11,13; U5-3,17; U20-24
Nebulisator U20-14
neigen zu (Krankheit) U13-27; U16-13; U41-16
Nekrose U13-30
nekrotisch U13-30; U28-12
Nelkenöl U30-16
neoadjuvant U18-8
Neodym-YAG-Laser U22-7
nephrotoxisch U20-32
Nervenadaptation U26-5
Nervenbündel U50-13
Nervennaht U26-2
Nervensystem, autonomes U20-8
Nervenwurzelreizung U13-10
nervös U11-20
nervschonend (Eingriff) U21-13
Nervtransposition U49-13
Nervus lingualis U9-23
Netzrissbildung U40-20
Netztransplantat U50-8
Neubildung (Parodontalgewebe) U35-27

Neuerkrankungsrate U14-7
Neuroleptikum U20-2,23; U47-10
Nichtanlage (Zähne) U36-19
Nichtansprechbarkeit U3-14
Nichtextrakionsbehandlung U44-2
Nierenbeteiligung U13-4
Nierendurchblutung U20-21
Nierenkolik U16-15
nierenschädigend U20-32
Niesanfall U11-6
niesen U11-6,2; U23-4
Niesreflex U11-6
Niesreiz U11-6
niveaugleich U40-9
Nivellieren U36-26
Nivellierungsbogen U37-6,5
Nivellierungsdraht U36-26
Nivellierungsphase U37-6
Nodositas U13-16
Nodulus U13-16
Nonokklusion U36-7
Noradrenalin U20-27
Normalverteilung U14-12
Normotoniker U14-22
nosokomial U27-12; U13-6; U19-15
Not(lage) U16-2
Notamputation U21-5
Notarzt U21-5
Notaufnahme U21-5; U23-19; U47-17
Notfall U21-5
Notfallbehandlung U6-15
Notfallversorgung U18-1
Notfallwagen U23-19
notleidend U16-2
Notmaßnahmen U21-5
Notoperation U21-3
NSA U20-11
nüchtern U1-15; U8-8; U16-13; U25-6
Nüchternblutzucker U1-15; U12-6f
Nüchternschmerz U1-11; U16-7
Nuklearmedizin U46-22
Nullhypothese U15-19
Nulllinien-EEG U4-18
Nullzeitpunkt U14-26
nuscheln U11-15

O

Obduktion U14-2; U21-12
Oberfläche U31-20
Oberflächenanästhesie U48-3
Oberflächenaufhellung U39-19
Oberflächendosis U46-9
Oberflächenstruktur U39-17

Oberflächenverfärbung U43-18
Oberkiefer U8-7
Oberkieferdehngerät U37-17
Oberkieferprothese U42-3
Oberlippengrübchen U8-9
Oberschenkel U23-15
Oberschenkelbeuger U16-13
Oberschenkelgurt U23-13
Oberschenkelkopf U8-1
Obliteration U13-18
Obstipation U20-13
obstipiert U1-1
Obstruktion U13-18
Odds Ratio U14-8
Ödem U3-15
Odontoblasten U9-16
offen (Drain) U28-15
- (Wunde) U17-3
offenchirurgisch U21-1
offenhalten (Drain) U22-20
Öffnung, op. angelegte U22-3
-, velopharyngeale U45-3
OHI U34-21
Ohnmacht U4-4ff
ohnmächtig U4-4,6
Ohr U8-15
Öhr (Nadel) U24-5
Ohrepithese U45-22
Ohrfluss U8-15
Ohrmuschelansatz U45-6
Ohrpinzette U24-14
Ohrplastik U49-3
Ohrspeicheldrüse U45-17
Okkludator U31-1
okkludieren U10-13; U36-7
okklusal U9-24; U33-8
Okklusalauflage U42-24
Okklusalaufnahme U33-4
Okklusion U36-7; U13-18
-, balancierte U36-7,12
-, gestörte U10-13
-, traumatische U35-19
-, zentrische U10-13; U36-13
Okklusionsausgleich U36-7
Okklusionsbefund U10-12
Okklusionsdiagnostik U10-12
Okklusionsebene U10-13; U36-7; U39-4
Okklusionsfolie U32-25
Okklusionskurve U39-11
Okklusionspapier U32-25
Okklusionsschiene U37-25; U38-14
Okklusionsstörung U36-8,7; U10-13
Okklusionsverband U28-5,17
Okular U8-3
Oligodontie U36-19
Omega-3-Fettsäure U12-12

Onlay U40–15
Onlay-Plastik U50–9
opak U39–16
Opakdentin U39–16
Opaker U39–16
OP-Anzug **U27**–15f
Opazität **U39**–16; U46–11
OP-Bedarf U23–9
OP-Einrichtung U23–1
Operateur **U23**–5,3
Operation **U21**–2f,1
–, explorative U21–3
–, zweizeitige U21–4
Operationsangst **U25**–4
Operationsassistent U23–4
Operationseinwilligung U21–2; U25–3
Operationsergebnis U15–27; U21–3
Operationsfeld U21–2
Operationshandschuhe **U27**–17
Operationskleidung U27–6
Operationsleuchte U7–9
Operationsmikroskop **U22**–6
Operationsnarbe U21–2
Operationsrisiko **U25**–5
Operationssaal **U23**–1; U21–2
Operationssitus U21–2
Operationsteam **U23**–4
Operationstechnik **U21**–4
Operationstisch **U23**–10
Operationstrakt U23–2
Operationsvorbereitung U21–2
Operationsweg **U21**–6
operativ **U21**–2
operieren **U21**–1
OP-Gehilfe U23–9
OP-Handschuh U27–15
OP-Haube U27–18
Opioid U47–5
Opiumtinktur, benzoesäurehaltige U5–10
OP-Kleidung **U27**–15; U23–1f
OP-Mantel **U27**–15
opportunistisch (Erreger) U27–9
OP-Saal **U23**–2
OP-Schleuse, Wartebereich vor U23–2
OP-Schürze U27–15
OP-Schwester **U23**–8; U27–6
Optik, abgewinkelte U45–19
Optikusatrophie U13–29
optisch U24–1
OP-Tisch U21–2
oral U8–8
Oralchirurg **U44**–1; U6–1
Orbita U8–3
Orbitaepithese U45–22
Orbitale U39–4

Orbitalosteotomie U45–13
Orbitarand U45–1
Ordination **U21**–3
Ordinationszeit U6–2,15
Organdosis U46–9
organerhaltend U21–13
organisch U26–10; U34–9
Organrejektion U50–21
organrettender Eingriff U21–4
Organspenderausweis U49–15
Organtoleranzdosis U19–12
Organvergrößerung U49–19
orientiert (Zeit, Raum, Person) U4–8
Orientierung **U4**–8
Orientierungspunkt **U21**–8
oroantral U35–21; U44–14
Orthetiker U29–9
Orthodontie **U36**–1
orthograd (WK-Füllung) U41–20
Os zygomaticum U8–5
Ösophagotrachealfistel U13–25
Ösophagusstimme U11–8
Osseointegration **U43**–1
Ossicula auditus U8–15
Ostektomie U45–11
Osteoarthrose U38–11
Osteoinduktion U43–1; U44–11
osteoklastisch U45–20
Osteokonduktion U43–1
Osteoplastik **U44**–9; U35–26
osteoplastisch U45–20
Osteosynthese **U29**–12; U29–4,12
Osteotom U24–11; U44–9
Osteotomie **U44**–11 ff
–, Le Fort I **U45**–7
Östrogenbehandlung U18–5
Otoplastik U49–1
Otorrhoe U8–15
Overbite **U36**–13
Overjet **U36**–14
Oxyzephalie U45–4

P

Packung **U5**–16; **U28**–24
–, feuchtwarme U28–24
Packungsbeilage **U5**–17
palatal U9–23
Palatinalbogen U37–15
Palatinalbügel U42–24
Palatinalfläche U40–11
Palatoplastik U45–3
Palatoschisis U45–2
Palatum **U9**–10
palliativ U18–9
Palliativoperation U18–9
Palliativtherapie U16–19

Palliativum U16–19
Panoramaaufnahme **U33**–5
Panorama-Röntgengerät U33–5
– Schichtaufnahme U33–5
– Vergrößerungsaufnahme U33–5
Papierstreifen U32–25
Papillae linguales U8–11
Papille U35–5
Papillen-Blutungs-Index U35–8
Papillenhyperplasie U35–5
Papillenräume U39–13
Pappkarton U5–16
Paradontitis **U35**–15
paraffingetränkt (Gaze) U28–18
Parallelführungshalter U43–9
Parallelisierstift U43–9
Parallelisierungshilfe **U32**–10
Parallelisierungsspiegel **U32**–10
Paralleltechnik U43–9
parallelwandig (Steg) U42–23
Paralyse **U47**–11
Parameter **U14**–5,19
–, prädiktiver U14–29
paraphasisch U11–11
Parästhesie **U16**–17; U3–12; U47–4
parasympatholytisch U20–8
parenteral U12–1ff; U19–3
Parese **U47**–11
Parodont **U35**–1
Parodontalindex **U35**–7
Parodontalprophylaxe U35–1
Parodontalsonde U35–1
Parodontalstatus **U35**–6,1
Parodontalverband U35–1
Parodontitis marginalis U35–15
Parodontologe U35–1
Parodontopathie U35–1
Parotidektomie **U45**–17
Parotis U45–17
Parotisast U45–17
Parotisgang U45–17
Parotisloge U45–17
Parotisspeichel U45–17
Paroxysmus **U16**–14
Partikel (Knochen) U44–10
Parulis U41–8
Passgenauigkeit **U42**–16
Paste U5–8; U30–16
Pastille **U5**–14
Patch-Plastik U49–19
pathogen U13–1
Pathologie U13–1
pathologisch **U13**–1f
Patient U16–2
Patientenbogen **U6**–14
Patienten-Compliance **U18**–15
Patientenerhebungsbogen **U15**–16

patientengesteuert (Analgesie) U47-7
Patienteninformation **U6**-8
Patientenreihe, konsekutive U15-11
Patientenrekrutierung **U15**-4
Patientenselektion **U25**-2
Patientenserie U15-11; U14-3
Patientenstuhl **U7**-1
Patrize U42-24
pausbäckig U8-5
PBI U35-8
Pellet U5-9
Penicillamin U20-10
Penicillin **U20**-10
Penicillinderivat U20-10
Penizillinase U20-10
penizillinresistent U20-10
Penrose-Drain U28-15
Perforation, oroantrale U44-14
–, schlitzförmige U41-17
periapikal U41-6,8
Periodenprävalenz U14-7
Periodontalbefundung U6-14
Periostelevatorium U32-15
Peristaltik U12-16
Peritoneum U28-14
Perkolation U40-21
Perkussion U32-4
perkutan U19-3; U22-20; U29-14
perkutieren U22-16
perlmuttartig U39-18
Pernio U3-12
peroral U19-3
persistieren U16-6; U18-11; U38-18
Personal **U6**-3
–, steriles U27-6
Personaleinstellung U6-3
Perzentile **U14**-11
Perzentilenrang U14-11
PET U46-19
Petechie **U13**-27
Pfählungsverletzung U3-2
Pfeiler, geschienter U42-10
Pfeilerschraube U43-6
Pfeilerzahn **U42**-10,6,20; U32-10
pfeilförmig U49-4
Pflaster **U28**-21 f,3; U19-3; U29-11
–, wasserabweisendes U28-21
Pflasterbinde, elastische U29-11
Pflasterverband **U29**-11
Pflege, häusliche U18-1,9
Phänomen U14-5
Phantomschmerz U16-10
Pharmakodynamik U20-1; U19-8
Pharmakogenetik U20-1
Pharmakognosie U20-1
Pharmakokinetik U20-1; U19-11

Pharmakologie **U20**-1
Pharmakopoe U20-1
Pharmazeutik **U5**-4; U20-1
Pharmazie **U5**-4; U20-1
Pharynx **U8**-12
Philtrum U8-9
Phlebotomie **U22**-18
Phonasthenie U11-9
Phonem U11-12
Phoniatrie U11-9
phonieren U11-13
phonisch U11-9
Phosphoreszenz U46-8
Physiotherapie U18-4
Piepser **U7**-13
Pille U5-7
Pilotbohrer U32-6
Pilotbohrung U43-8
Pilotstudie U15-1
Pilz U20-26; U1-1
pinseln U27-5
Pinzette U24-14,13
Pistill U31-14
Placebogruppe U14-3
Placeboresponder U15-8
Plagiozephalus U45-4
Planstopfer U32-17
Plaque **U34**-8
Plaquebefall U34-11
plaquebehaftet U35-13
Plaquebeseitigung U34-8
Plaquebildung U34-8
Plaque-Färbemittel U34-8
Plaquefärbetabletten **U34**-12
Plaquehemmstoff U34-8
Plaque-Hemmung U34-7
Plaqueindex U34-8
Plaque-Indikator U34-8
Plastik (Chirurgie) **U22**-4; **U49**-1
Plastik, V-Y U21-4
Platinfolie **U30**-9
Platinfolienabdruck U30-9
platinhaltig (Gekrätz) U30-9
Platinkrampon U30-9
Platinrhodiumlegierung U30-9
Platinstift U30-9
Platte (Osteosynthese) **U29**-17
Plattenepithelbildung U28-6
Plattenosteosynthese U29-17
Plattenprothese **U42**-3
Platzangebot U36-16 ff
Platzdiskrepanz, OK/UK U36-4
platzen **U3**-18; U13-23; U38-4
Platzhalter U32-22
Platzwunde **U3**-7
Plaut-Vincent Angina U35-14
Plazebo **U15**-8
Plazeboresponder U18-11
Plegie U47-11

Plica U49-8
Plikation **U49**-8
Plugger **U32**-17; U41-15
Pneumarthrographie U33-14
Pogonion U39-5
polierbar U31-21
Polierbürste **U32**-7
polieren U31-21; U34-11
Poliergerät U31-21
Poliermaschine U31-21
Polierpaste U10-19; U31-21
Polierrad, bimssteinhaltiges U30-18
Poliersatz U31-21
Polierscheibe U32-8
Polierstreifen **U32**-24
Politur U31-21
polstern **U28**-19; U42-25
Polsterung U28-19; U29-9
Polsterwatte U28-19
Polyesternaht U26-10
Polymerisation **U31**-19
Polymerisationsleuchte **U32**-23; U31-19
Polymerisationsschrumpfung U31-6
polymerisieren U31-6; U32-23
Polytrauma U3-4
Pontik **U42**-5
Population **U14**-3
Poren, interkonnektierende U43-3
Porion U39-4
porös U34-17
Porzellan **U30**-4
Porzellanerde **U30**-5
Position **U23**-11
Positioner U37-23
Positionierungshilfe U31-2
Positionswechsel U23-11
Positronenemissionscomputer- tomographie U46-19
Postulat U15-19
potenzieren U20-24
Power (Statistik) U14-1
ppm U43-18
Prädiktion **U14**-29
Prädisposition U13-7; U19-15
Prädispositionsfaktor U14-5
Präkanzerose U3-5
Prämedikation U5-1; U25-4; U48-2
Prämolar **U9**-6
Prämolarisierung U41-23
präoperativ U25-6
Präparat U5-1; U46-13
Präparation U21-12; U48-1
Präparierbesteck U24-1
präparieren **U21**-12
Präparieren, scharfes U24-2

Präpariermikroskop U21-12
Präparierschere U24-4
präprothetische Chirurgie U44-1
Prävalenz U14-7
Prävalenzrate U14-7
Prävalenzstudie U15-1
präventiv **U18**-6
Präventivmedizin U18-6
Praxis **U21**-3; U6-2
Praxisalltag **U6**-2
Praxisleuchte U32-1
Praxismanagement **U6**-2
Präzisionsgeschiebe **U42**-7
Präzisionssteg U42-23
Präzisionsverankerung **U42**-7; U32-10
Prellung **U3**-13
Pressen U11-2
– (Zähne) U36-11
Presspassung U42-16
prickeln U16-17
Pricktest U3-10
Primärbehandlung U18-1
Primärheilung U28-4; U29-1
Primärkrone **U40**-17
Primärnaht U26-1; U28-3
Proband **U14**-2
Probeexzision U21-9
Probepunktion U21-11
Processus condylaris U38-10
Profil **U39**-3
Profilanalyse U39-3
Profilansicht U39-3
Profilaufnahme U39-3
progen (Wachstum) U37-20
Progenie **U45**-10; U36-8,24
Prognathie **U45**-10; U36-8
Proklination U36-23
Prolabium U8-9
Prolaps **U13**-22
Proliferation U20-9
Prominentia laryngea **U8**-14
prophylaktisch **U18**-6; U34-2
Prophylaxe U18-6
– postexpositionelle U18-6
Prophylaxehelferin U34-1
Prosoposchisis **U45**-2
prospektiv **U15**-6
Prostration U16-5
Protease U12-9
Protein **U12**-9
Protein-Energie-Mangelsyndrom U12-3
Proteinurie U12-9
Proteoglykan U12-9
proteolytisch U12-9
Prothese U49-2
–, implantatgestützte U45-22
–, provisorische U42-9

–, schlechtsitzende U38-2
Prothesenanpassung U42-1
Prothesenbasis **U42**-17; U10-8; U32-23; U40-20
Protheseneinbau U49-2
Prothesengerüst U42-15f
Prothesenhaftung **U42**-21
Prothesenhalt **U42**-21,2
Prothesenhärtung U31-19
Prothesenlager U42-18
Prothesenrand **U42**-19, U9-23
Prothesenreiniger U10-8
Prothesenretention **U42**-21,2
Prothesensattel **U42**-18
prothesentragend U10-8
Prothesenträger U42-2
Prothetik, zahnärztliche **U42**-1
Prothetiker U42-1
prothetisch U42-2
Protokoll **U15**-7
Protraktion U29-3; U36-28
Protraktionsheadgear U37-18
Protrusion U36-23f
–, bimaxilläre U36-24
Protrusionsabweichung U36-23
Protrusionsfeder U37-11
Protrusionsstellung U36-1
Protuberantia mentalis U8-6
provisorisch U42-13
Provisorium U40-16
Provitamin U12-13
proximal **U9**-22
Prozentsatz U14-8
Prüfvariable U15-10
Pruritus U20-22
Pseudarthrose U17-15
Pseudotasche U35-11
Pseudozyste U13-24
Psychopharmakon **U20**-23; U5-3
PTFE-Membran U44-8
Ptose U13-22
Puder **U5**-9,8
Pulpa (dentis) **U9**-18
Pulpaeröffnung U41-2
Pulpaextraktor U32-11
Pulpafreilegung U9-18
Pulpahöhle U41-5
Pulpahorn U41-5
Pulpakammerboden U41-5
Pulpakammerdach U41-10
Pulpakappe U40-6
Pulpakavum **U41**-5; U9-18
Pulpaprüfer **U32**-20; U41-5
Pulpareaktion U41-2
Pulparest U41-24
Pulpastein U41-5
Pulpatester **U32**-20; U41-5
Pulpaüberkappung **U40**-6; U9-18
Pulpektomie **U41**-19

Pulpitis **U41**-2,7
Pulpopathie U41-2
Pulpotomie U41-19
Puls, schwacher U4-4
pulssynchron spritzen U3-19; U13-26
Pulver **U5**-9
pulverisiert U5-9
Pulverstrahlgerät U34-11
Pumex **U30**-18
Punkteschema U14-6
Punktezahl U14-6
Punktion U3-10; U22-16; U24-5
Punktionsflüssigkeit U22-16
Punktionsnarbe U7-6
Punktionsstelle U24-5
Punktprävalenz U14-7
Punktschmerz U16-11
Pupille U8-3; U4-7,14
Pupillen, lichtstarre U4-7
–, stecknadelkopfgroße U4-14
purpuraartig U13-27
purulent U13-12; U28-14
Pus **U13**-12
Pusteln U28-9
Putzbewegungen U34-4
putzen (Zähne) **U34**-4,3
Putzläsionen U34-4
Putzrillen U34-15
p-Wert U14-21
Pylorusstenose U13-20

Q

Quad-Helix U37-17
Quadrant **U9**-20
Quadratsummen U14-34
qualvoll (Schmerzen) U16-9
Quartile U14-11
Quecksilber U30-1
Quecksilberaustritt U30-1
Quecksilberdampf U31-14
quellen U24-18; U26-7
Querfraktur U17-1
quergestreift (Muskel) U48-16
Querhiebbohrer U32-6
Querinzision U21-9
Querschnitt U21-10,14; U33-18
Querschnittfläche U21-10
Querschnittstudie U15-1
Quetschung **U3**-13,2
Quetschwunde U3-13
Quotient U14-8
–, Krone-zu-Implantat **U43**-16

R

Rachen **U**8–12
Rachenabstrich U8–12
Rachenmandel U8–12
rad U46–10
radioaktiv **U**46–21,1 f ; U24–7
– markiert U46–1 f
Radioaktivität U46–21
Radioiodtest U46–21
Radioisotop U46–22
Radioisotopennephrographie U46–22
Radiologe U46–1
Radiologie **U**46–1
radioluzent U33–7; U46–11
Radiomimetikum U46–2
Radionuklid **U**46–22,17
radiopak **U**46–11
Radiopharmakon U46–2,21
Radiosensitizer U46–23
Radiovisiographie U33–15
Radix dentis **U**9–19
– linguae U8–11
Raffnaht **U**26–18
Ramus U38–10
– parotideus U45–17
Rand U33–12
Randabschrägung **U**40–19
randdicht (Verschluss) U41–15
randomisiert U15–12
Randomisierung **U**15–5
Randsaum U35–17
Randschärfe U46–14
Randschluss U40–16; U42–16
Randulkus U13–17
Ranula U44–15
rasend (Schmerzen) U16–9
Raspatorium U24–12; U32–12
Raspel **U**24–12
Rasur, präoperative U27–14
Rate **U**14–8
–, adjustierte U14–8
–, rohe U14–8
rauh (Oberfläche) U39–17
– (Stimme) U8–12
Raumforderung U13–3; U18–8
raumfüllend U12–16
Rauschdroge **U**5–3
Rauschgift **U**47–5
Rauschmittel **U**47–5 f; U5–3
räuspern, sich U8–12; U11–6
Reagenzglas U15–18
Reagibilität U4–7
reagieren (Stimulus) **U**4–7
– (Therapie) U18–11
reagieren auf U4–7
Reaktion **U**18–11
Reaktionsfähigkeit U4–7

Reaktionsunfähigkeit **U**4–11; U47–6
Reamer **U**32–11
Reanimation U21–1; U47–25
–, kardiopulmonale U47–25
reanimieren **U**47–25
Reattachment **U**35–27
Recallsystem U6–15
Receiver-Operating-Characteristic Kurve U14–34
Rede U11–8
Rededrang U11–11
Redeflussstörung U11–16
redegewandt U11–18
Redressionsgips U29–6
redselig U11–18
Reduktion U49–19
Reduktionskost U1–13
reduzieren (Dosis) U19–6
Referenzbereich U14–15
Referenzpunkte, kephalometrische U33–9; U36–22
Reflexschwelle U38–7
Reformkost U1–6
refraktär U18–13
Refraktärzeit U18–13
Refraktur U17–1
rege **U**4–2
Regeneration (Gewebe) **U**44–12; U35–27
Regenerationsmembran **U**35–29,28
Regionalanästhesie U48–3
Regression **U**14–33
Regressionsanalyse, logistische U14–33
Regressionsgerade U14–33
Regressionskoeffizient U14–33
Regressionsmodell, lineares U14–35
Rehabilitation, orale U49–2
Reibegeräusch **U**17–14
reich an (Nährstoffen) U1–12; U26–14
reichlich vorhanden U12–17
Reihe (Patienten) U14–3
Reihenextraktion U44–2
Reihenuntersuchung U34–21
Reimpaktion U44–3
reinigen U27–5; U28–1; U34–3 f
Reinigung, mechanische U40–2
Reinigungslotion U5–10
Reinigungsmittel U27–5
Reinklusion U44–3
reintrudieren U36–24 f
reißen U13–23
Reizbarkeit U13–10
Reizmittel U20–14
Reizung U13–10; U16–3
Rekonstruktion **U**49–1

Rekonturierung U39–2
Rekonvaleszenz U18–14; U25–7,14
Rekrutierungschance U15–5
Relaxans U48–16
Reliabilität **U**14–30,23
–, Inter-Beobachter- U14–30
REM **U**46–10
Remission U16–8
Remodellierung U33–16
Reoperation U21–1; U25–10
Reparaturlot U31–16
reponieren U28–2,26; U37–16; U38–8;
Reposition (Fraktur) **U**29–2; U3–20; U17–1; U28–2 f; U38–9
–, geschlossene U17–3
Reproduzierbarkeit U14–30
Resektion **U**21–15; U22–13
Resektoskop U21–15
resezieren U21–15
Residualzyste U44–15
Resilienzgeschiebe U42–4
resistent U18–13
Resistenz U18–13
Resonanzkörper U11–10
resorbierbar **U**26–8
Resorption **U**10–20
Resorptionsgeschwindigkeit U19–10
Resorptionszeit U26–8
Restauration U40–1
Restbeschwerden U16–1
Restgebiss U42–20
Restriktion U14–16
Resttumor U24–7
Restwirkungen U47–23
Restwurzel U41–18
Restzyste U44–15
Resultat **U**15–27
Retainer **U**37–23; U36–29
Retardpräparat U5–3,6f; U19–4
Retention U36–29; U37–23
Retentionselement U42–21,23
Retentionsform **U**40–7
Retentionsgerät **U**37–23
Retentionsklammer U42–21
Retentionsperle U42–21
Retentionsphase U37–23
Retentionsrille U42–21
Retentionsstelle U34–8
Retentionszylinder U42–20
Retentionszyste U44–15
Retest-Stabilität U14–30
retinieren U9–8; U36–29; U37–23
retrahieren U32–2
Retraktion U29–3; U36–28
Retraktionsfähigkeit U32–2
Retransplantation U49–14
Retrognathie U45–10

Retroinklination **U36**–24
retrospektiv U15–6
Retrusion **U36**–24,8
Rezept (Arznei) U19–1
rezeptfrei U5–2; U19–1
Rezeptionsassistentin **U6**–6
Rezeptorenblocker, H1- U20–22
Rezeptorstellen U19–11
rezeptpflichtig U5–3; U19–1
Rezession, parodontale U35–12
Rezidiv U3–5; U5–1; U37–23
rezidivieren U36–17
Rezidivrate U14–8
Rhinolalie U11–17,22
Rhinophonie U11–17
Rhythmusstörung U20–18
Ribbon-Arch Brackets U37–4
richten auf (Strahl) U46–5
richtig negativ U14–22
Richtungsventil U47–14
Riemen U28–26; U29–11
Ring, elastischer U37–7
Ringer-Laktat-Lösung U48–1
Ringklammer U42–6
Ringknorpel U8–14
Rippenraspatorium U24–12
Risiko **U25**–5
Risiko-Nutzen-Verhältnis U25–5
Risikopatient U25–5
Risikopersonen U14–2
Riss **U3**–18,7; U17–1,5,11; U13–23
Risswunde **U3**–7
ritzen (Haut) U24–5
Roachklammer U42–6
Röhrengehäuse U33–1
Röhreninstabilität U46–13
Röhrenschutzhaube U33–1
Rohwert U14–6
Rollbinde U28–20
Rolllappen **U50**–15
röntgen U46–3
Röntgenanlage U46–3
Röntgenassistent U6–5; U33–3; U46–1,3
Röntgenaufnahme **U33**–2,4,9; **U46**–3; U41–2
Röntgenbefund U46–1
Röntgenbereich U46–1
Röntgenbild **U33**–2; **U46**–3; U6–14
Röntgenbildbetrachter U33–4
Röntgendarstellung U46–12
Röntgendiagnostik U46–1
Röntgendurchleuchtung U46–8
Röntgenfilm **U33**–2
Röntgenfluoreszenz U46–8
Röntgenröhre **U33**–1; U3–20
Röntgenschablone U31–13
Röntgenstereographie U33–2

Röntgenstrahler U33–1
Rosenbohrer U32–6
rostfrei (Stahl) U26–12
Rotameter U47–14
Rotationsgeschwindigkeit U36–27
Rotationslappen **U50**–19
Rotationsstellung U29–1
Rötung U35–6,13
Rückbildung U3–11
Rückenlage **U23**–12,11,13,16
Rückenlehne U7–1
Rückenmarkerschütterung U3–14
Rückenmarkverletzung U3–2
Rückfall U5–1
Rückkippung U36–23
Rückneigung U36–23
Rückstände U40–2
Rückstellung U41–13
Rückstreuung U46–6
Ruf U11–1
rufen **U11**–14
Ruhelage (Kiefer) U10–14
Ruheschmerz U16–7
Ruheschwebe U10–14; U36–12
Ruhigstellung **U29**–5
Rumpf U23–12
Rundlochplatte U29–17
Rundstiellappen **U50**–15 f
Ruptur **U3**–18,7; U13–23; U17–5

S

sabbern U10–4,9
Saccharide **U12**–6
Saccharin U12–6
Saccharose **U2**–16
Sagittalschnitt U33–19
Salbe **U5**–8; U30–24
Salbenkanüle U24–6
Salivation **U10**–9
sandgestrahlt U40–14
Sandstrahlen U30–11
sanduhrförmig U41–13
Sandwich-Plastik U45–7 f
Sattel, interdentaler **U35**–18
Sattelblock U48–6
sattelförmig U42–5
Satzmelodie U11–10
Säuberung U41–9
Sauerstoff-Lachgas-Gemisch U48–11
Saugdrainage U22–16; U28–15
saugen (Aspiration) **U22**–16; U7–7
Säugetiermilch U12–8
Saugflasche U1–3
Saugkanüle **U7**–7; U24–6
Säugling U1–3
Säuglingsernährung U12–3

Säuglingsnahrung U1–6
Saugschluckbewegung U36–20
Saugvorrichtung U22–16; U28–15
Säulendiagramm U14–27
Saumepithel U35–3
Säure U39–20
Säureätzverfahren U30–19; U39–21
säurebindend **U20**–29; U19–2
Säuregrad U20–29
Scaler **U32**–13; U34–9
Scan **U46**–18
Scanbreite U46–18
Scanner U46–18
Schabeisen **U24**–12; U32–12
schaben **U3**–9
Schablone **U31**–13
–, chirurgische U42–15
Schädel U8–1
Schädelbasisbruch U17–1,8
Schädelbruch **U17**–8
Schädeldachfraktur U17–8
Schädeleröffnung U45–20
Schädelfraktur **U17**–8
Schädelimpressionsfraktur U17–3
Schädelnähte U45–4
Schädelröntgen **U33**–10; U8–1; U46–3
schaden U3–3; U13–11
Schädigung **U3**–5; U13–3 f
schädlich U3–2; U19–11 f; U27–9; U43–17
Schadstoff U27–9
Schaft U32–18
Schale **U1**–8
Schall U11–10
Schallsonde U24–8
Schalltrauma U3–4
Schallwellen U33–11
Schanz-Krawatte **U29**–9
scharfkantig U24–2
Scharnier U32–16; U42–21; U50–19
Schattierung U39–15
Schätzfunktion U14–18
Schätzwert U14–29
Schaumpolster U28–19
Schaumstoff-Halskrawatte U29–9
Schaumstoffpolster U29–10
Scheibe U3–6
Scheibenträger U32–5
Scheinfütterung U15–8
Scheinmedikament **U15**–8
Schema U14–6
Schere **U24**–4
Scheuthauer-Marie-Sainton-Syndrom U45–6
Schicht U33–18; U46–19
Schichtaufnahme **U46**–19

Schichtnaht U26-1
Schichtrekonstruktion, 3 D- **U33**-19
Schichtverblendung U39-22
schichtweise (Wundverschluss) U28-3
Schiebeknoten U26-6
Schiefe U14-13
Schiefschädel U45-4
schielen U8-3
Schiene **U29**-7; U17-3; U28-26; U42-22
-, gepolsterte U28-19
-, orthopädische **U37**-16
schienen **U22**-20; U23-10; U30-2
Schienenbleichung U39-19
Schienentherapie **U38**-14
Schienung U37-16; U29-7
Schifferknoten U26-6
Schimmer **U39**-18
Schlaf, hypnotischer U4-15
Schläfe U8-2
Schläfenbeinfraktur U17-8
schlaff U28-26
schlaffördernd U48-14
Schlaflosigkeit U18-13
Schlafmittel **U48**-14; U4-13; U20-23; U47-9
Schläfrigkeit U4-5; U5-18
Schlafsedierung U47-8
Schlaf-Wach-Rhythmus U4-16
Schlag U3-13; U17-9
Schlaganfall U16-2
Schlankheitsdiät U1-13
Schlaufen (Kontraktionsbögen) U37-3
schlechtsitzend (Prothese) U38-2
schleichend U13-18
schleifen **U10**-18
schleifenförmig U49-4
Schleifinstrument U32-5
Schleifkörper U32-5
Schleifmittel U3-8
Schleifpapier U10-19
Schleifscheibe **U32**-8
Schleifverfahren U30-20
Schleim U11-6; U20-15,30
Schleimhaut U8-11; U20-30
-, mastikatorische U10-15
schleimhautgetragen U42-12
Schleimhautlappen U43-5
schleimhautprotektiv U20-29
Schleimhautreizung U16-3
Schleimhauttransplantat U44-7, U50-1,10
schleimlösend **U20**-15,2
Schleudertrauma U3-2
Schleuderverband U28-20
Schlinge (Knoten) U26-6,17
- (Verband) **U29**-8; U28-20

-, elektrische **U22**-11; U24-9
Schlingenelektrode U22-9
Schlingenfeder U37-11
schlingenförmig U49-4
Schlitzbrackets U37-4
schluchzen **U11**-3
Schluck U8-8
Schluckbeschwerden U16-6
schlucken U1-4; U8-11; U10-15; U11-10
-, ganz U5-14
-, unzerkaut U5-7; U19-3
Schluckfunktion U45-3
Schlund **U8**-12
Schlundenge U8-12
Schlussdesinfektion U27-5
Schlüsselbein U8-12
Schlüsselwert U15-16
Schlussschraube U43-6
schmackhaft U1-5
Schmelz **U9**-15
Schmelzätzen U39-21
Schmelzbildung U9-15
Schmelz-Dentin-Grenze U9-16
schmelzen U5-12
Schmelzfissuren U34-15
Schmelzfurchen **U34**-15
Schmelzgrübchen U34-15
Schmelzmeißel **U32**-18
Schmelzmesser **U32**-18
Schmelzoberhäutchen **U34**-10; U9-15; U10-9
Schmelzporositäten U34-15
Schmelzpulver U9-15
Schmelzpunkt U31-16
Schmelz-Zement-Grenze **U39**-9; U9-17; U35-3
Schmerz **U16**-3ff, **U16**-21
-, flüchtiger U41-7
-, klopfender U9-1
-, stechender **U16**-13
Schmerzattacke U16-14
Schmerzbahn U16-20
Schmerzdauer **U16**-8
Schmerzdysfunktionssyndrom U38-2
schmerzempfindlich U13-13
Schmerzempfindung **U47**-7; U16-20
Schmerzen verursachen U16-18
schmerzerfüllt U16-6
schmerzfrei U16-20
schmerzhaft **U16**-11,4,6
Schmerzintensität **U16**-9
schmerzlindernd U30-24; U47-7
Schmerzlinderung **U16**-19
Schmerzlokalisation **U16**-10
schmerzlos U16-6

Schmerzmittel U4-10; U38-3; U47-7
Schmerzqualität **U16**-7
Schmerzschwelle **U16**-18
schmerzstillend **U16**-20; U47-7
Schmerzsyndrom, myofasziales **U38**-3
Schmerztoleranzgrenze U16-18
Schmerzunempfindlichkeit **U47**-2; U16-6
schmerzverzerrt U16-6,12
schmierig U5-8
Schmirgel U32-8
Schnabeltasse U1-3
Schnappfeder U40-14
Schnarchen **U11**-5
Schneidblätter U24-4
Schneide U24-3; U32-18
Schneidekante U9-3
schneiden **U3**-6
Schneidezahn **U9**-3
Schneidezahnkippung U36-21
schnellabbindend U30-13
Schnellaufnahme (Film) U33-3
schnellhärtend U40-5
Schnellinfusion U47-19
Schnitt **U21**-10, **U22**-2; U3-6; U21-9
Schnittfläche **U21**-10
Schnittkonisation U22-12
Schnittrand U3-6; U26-12
-, chirurgischer U21-3
Schnittverletzung U3-9
Schnittwunde **U3**-6
Schock, septischer U27-1
schonen **U21**-13
Schönheitschirurgie U39-1
Schonkost **U1**-13
Schorf **U28**-9,6
Schorfbildung U8-9
Schrägfraktur U17-1
Schramme **U3**-8f
Schraubenbolzen U29-16
Schraubengelenk U43-6
Schraubenimplantat **U43**-6
Schraubenkopf U8-1
Schraubenlockerung U43-6
schreien **U11**-14
schrittweise U49-4
Schröder Lüftung **U41**-22
schrumpfarm U31-6
Schrumpfausgleich U31-6
schrumpfen U28-8; U50-1
Schrumpfung U30-13
Schulterpräparation **U40**-8
Schulterstütze U23-13
Schuppenepithelbildung U28-6
Schürfwunde **U3**-8
Schüssel **U1**-8

Schüttelfrost U16-14
Schüttelmixtur U5-10
Schutz U24-2; U33-3
Schutzbrille **U7**-10
Schutzhandschuhe U27-17
Schutzschicht U30-22
Schutzvorrichtung U27-15
Schwabbel U31-21
schwach **U4**-4
Schwächegefühl U4-4
Schwächung U13-4
Schwammgold U30-8
schwammig U35-6
schwanken U14-15
Schwebebrückenzwischenglied U42-5
schweigsam U11-18
Schwellendosis U46-9
Schwellenwert **U14**-24
Schwellung **U3**-15f
Schwenkarm U7-9
schwenken U5-9
Schwenkriegelprothese U42-2
Schweregrad U20-20
schwerstbehindert U11-18
schwerverdaulich U1-7
schwerwiegend U19-14
schwerzugänglich U34-8
Schwindelanfall U16-14
schwindlig U4-5
Schwindung U30-13; U31-6
Schwund (Zahnfleisch) U9-12
Score U14-6,16
Screeningaufnahme U33-2
Sechsjahrmolaren U9-7
Second-look-Operation U21-1
Sedativum **U47**-9f; U20-23
sedieren **U47**-10,8
sedierend U20-22; U48-14
Sedierung **U47**-8ff
Segmentbogentechnik U37-5
Segmentosteotomie **U45**-11
Sehkraft U8-3
Sehne U3-16
Sehnennaht U26-2
Sehnenriss U3-7,18
Sehnenruptur U3-7
Sehnenschmerz U16-21
Sehnervenatrophie U13-29
Sehprobentafel U8-3
Sehvermögen U13-4
Seide U26-10
Seite, gesunde U23-16
Seitenansicht **U39**-3
Seitenbandzerrung U3-16
Seitenkanal U41-4
Seitenlage **U23**-16,11
Seitenwandinfraktionstechnik U45-15

seitlich (verlagern) U36-21
Seit-zu-Seit-Anastomose U49-6
Sekret, wässriges U28-13
Sekretolytikum **U20**-15
Sektion U14-2; U21-12
sekundär (Heilung) **U50**-7; U28-5
Sekundäranker U42-21
Sekundärkallus U17-15
Sekundärkrone **U42**-9
selbsthärtend U30-3; U31-21
Selbstlaut U11-12
selbstschneidend U40-14; U43-2,11
Selbstverstümmelung U3-2
Selektionskriterien U25-2
Selen U12-17
Senkung U13-22
Sensibilität U16-19;U41-2; U47-4
Sensibilitätsprüfung U9-18; U32-20; U41-3
Sensibilitätsstörung U3-12
Sensitivität **U14**-23
Separator **U32**-22; **U37**-12
Separiergummi **U37**-12
Sepsis U27-1
sepsisbedingt U18-12
Sequenztherapie U18-5
Serienextraktion U44-2
Serienschnitt U21-10
Serienszintigramme U46-17
Serotoninaktivität U20-3
Serumikterus U49-16
Set-up, diagnostisches U42-13
seufzen **U11**-4
sezernieren U28-13
sezieren **U21**-12
Seziermesser U24-3
Shunt U49-6
Sialographie **U33**-13
Sialolith U13-21; U33-13
Sicherheitsband U37-19
Sicherheitsnadel U29-15
Sicherheitsvorkehrung U5-18; U24-5; U27-1
sichern **U26**-4
sicherstellen U15-24
Sicherung U24-2
Sicht, unter U33-14; U47-17
Sichtbarmachung **U46**-12; U32-4
Sichtkontrolle U24-8
Sichtschutz (Anästhesiebereich) **U23**-7
Sickerblutung U3-19; U13-26
sickern U41-16
Siebbestrahlung U46-4
siedend (heiß) U3-11
Siegelwachs U34-16
Sigmatismus **U11**-21
signalfrei U33-12

signifikant, statistisch **U14**-21
Signifikanzniveau U14-21
Signifikanztest U14-34
Silbe **U11**-12
Silbenstolpern U11-12,20
Siliciumcarbid U32-24
Silizium U12-17
Sinus paranasales U8-4
Sinusbodenanhebung **U45**-15
Sinusboden-Augmentation U44-8; U49-19
Sinuskopie, funktionelle **U45**-19
Sinuslift-Operation **U45**-15; U49-19
Sirup U5-11
Situationsnaht U26-1
Sitz **U42**-16; U40-17; U43-15
Sitzung U6-10
Skala U14-6
Skalpell **U24**-3
Skaphozephalus U45-4
smile, gummy U9-12; U39-6
solitär U13-3
Solitärknoten U13-16
Solitärläsion U3-5
Somnolenz **U4**-13
Sonde **U24**-8; **U32**-1,9; U41-5
Sondenernährung U1-3
Sondenspitze U32-9
sondieren **U24**-8,3; U32-9; U35-3; U11-11
Sondierungstiefe U35-4
Sonogramm U33-11
Sonographie **U33**-11
Sopor **U4**-13
sorgfältig U16-6
Spalt U17-11
Spaltchirurgie **U45**-3
spalten U3-18; U14-27; U21-9,14
Spalthauttransplantat U21-14; U50-6
Spaltmissbildung U45-2
Spaltnase U45-2
Spaltplastik **U45**-3
Spaltzunge U8-11; U21-14; U45-2
Span (Knochen) U44-10; U50-9
Spanbläser **U7**-4
Spangröße U45-15
Spanngummi **U32**-19
spannungsfrei U42-16
Spannweite **U14**-15
Spanplastik U44-9
Spantransplantat **U44**-10
Spasmolytikum **U20**-19
Spasmus masticatorius **U38**-6
Spätkomplikation U25-9
Spätmorbidität U18-12
Spätschmerz U16-8

Spearman'scher Rangkorrelations-
  koeffizient U14–32
Spee Kurve **U36**–5; **U39**–11
Speibecken U10–10
Speichel U34–8; U40–21
Speichelbildung **U10**–9
Speicheldrüse U33–13
Speichelfluss **U10**–9
Speichelperkolation U40–21
Speichelsauger **U7**–7
Speichelstein U13–21; U33–13
Speischale **U7**–8
Speise **U1**–8
speisen U1–4,2
Speisereste U1–6; U17–6; U34–6
Spender (Organ) **U49**–15,17
Spenderareal U49–12
Spenderauswahl U49–15
Spender-Empfänger-Auswahl
  U25–2
Spenderstelle U49–15
Spezialhartgips **U30**–14; **U31**–12
Spezialhartgipsmodell U31–2
Spezialzahnseide U34–5
Spezifität U14–23
Spica U28–20; U29–6
Spickdraht **U29**–15
Spickung U29–4,14f
–, perkutane U29–14
Spiralbruch U17–1
Spiralfeder U37–11
Spitzgaumen U9–10
Spitzschädel U45–4
Splint **U22**–20
Splitter U17–7
Splitterfraktur U17–7; U38–19
Splitterpinzette U24–14
Splitterzange U24–14
Spongiosa U17–6
Spongiosaplastik **U50**–9
Spongiosaspäne U17–2; U44–10
Spongiosatransplantat **U50**–9
Spontanfraktur U17–1
Spontanheilung U25–14; U28–4
Spontanluxation U17–4
Spontanruptur U3–18
Sporen U27–2
Sprachäußerungen U11–17
Sprache **U8**–11; U11–8
–, skandierende U11–8
Sprachentwicklung U11–8
Sprachmelodie U11–10
Sprachproduktion U11–11
Sprachstörung U11–8,11
Sprachverständnis U11–8
Spraywasser (Kühlung) U7–5;
  U32–19
Spreader U30–12; U32–17
Sprechangst U11–17

sprechen **U11**–8,1,11
–, deutlich U11–8
–, fließend U11–8
Sprechhilfen U11–8
Sprechlautbildung U11–1
Sprechstimme U11–9
Sprechstörung U11–8,11
Sprechstunde U6–9
Sprechstundenhilfe **U6**–6
Sprechweise U11–1,8
Spreizer (Guttapercha) U30–12;
  U32–17
Spritze U5–11; U27–2; U48–9
Spritzenpumpe **U47**–16
Spritzgussverfahren U31–4
Sprödigkeit U31–15
Sprühverband U28–17
Sprung U17–1
spucken **U10**–10
Spülbecken **U7**–8
spülen U11–7; U22–17; U30–19;
  U27–5
Spülflüssigkeit U22–17; U28–11;
  U34–6
Spülkanüle U24–6
Spülung **U22**–17; U28–1,11;
  U34–6; U7–5
Spurenelement **U12**–17
Stab U29–16
stabil U29–4
stabilisieren U36–29; U37–23
Stabilisierung (Fraktur) **U29**–4
Stabilisierungsstab U29–4
Stabilität U5–19
Staging-Operation U21–4
Stahl, rostfreier U26–12
Stahldrahtklammer U37–15
Stahleinlage U28–26
Stahlkrone U40–18
Stammeln U11–20
Standardabweichung U14–13
Standardfehler U14–18
–, Mittelwert U14–10
Standardwert **U14**–6
stanzen U24–5
stärkehaltig U12–5
Stärkezucker U12–5
starr U42–6,22; U45–19
Station, chirurgische U21–3;
  U23–17
stationär (Behandlung) U25–11;
  U27–12
Stationsschwester U23–2
Statistik **U14**–1
Statuserhebung U25–1
Staubinde U28–20
Stauchungsbruch **U17**–6
Staumanschette U47–18
Stauschlauch U47–18

Stauungshyperämie U13–27
Stauungsödem U13–19
Stechampulle **U5**–13
stechen **U16**–13; U3–10
Stecknadel **U29**–15
Steg **U42**–23,11
–, parallelwandiger U42–23
Steggelenk U42–23
Steggeschiebe U42–11
steggestützt U42–23
Stegreiter U42–23
Stegverankerung U42–2,20,23
Steigung U14–33
Steilgaumen U9–10
Stein **U13**–21
steinbedingt U13–21
steinfrei U13–21
steinhart U40–3
Steinleiden U16–15
Steinmann-Nagel U29–15
Stelle, opake U34–13
–, unter sich gehende **U40**–13
–, wunde U13–17
Stellung **U23**–11
–, korrekte U29–1
Stenose U13–20,19; U28–10
Stenozephalie U45–4
Stent **U22**–20
Stentverlegung U22–20
step-back Technik U41–11
Sterbetafel U14–26
Sterbetafelmethode U14–29
Sterblichkeit U14–9
steril **U27**–1f,7
Sterilisation U27–2
Sterilisator U27–2
Sterilisierbehälter U27–2
Sterilisiertrommel U27–2
Sterilität U27–2
Sterilzone U27–8
Sternfraktur U17–8
steuern U36–29
Stich **U3**–10; **U16**–13
Stichinzision U21–9
Stichprobe **U14**–4
Stichprobenerhebung U14–4
Stichprobenumfang U14–4
Stichprobenverfahren U14–4
Stichwunde U3–3,7
Stickstoff, flüssiger U22–8
stickstoffhaltig U12–10
Stiel U50–10f
Stift **U29**–15f,14; U32–10; U40–14
–, parapulpärer **U40**–14
Stiftaufbau **U40**–15
Stiftfixation U29–4,15f
Stiftimplantation U49–18
Stiftkrone U40–18
Stiftröhrchen-Apparatur U37–1

Stiftverankerung U40-14
stillen (Blutung) U13-26
– (Säugling) U1-3; U12-1; U20-31
Stimmbänder U11-9
Stimmbandlähmung U47-11
Stimmbildung U11-9,13
Stimme **U11**-9f,23
stimmhaft U11-9
Stimmklang U11-8
Stimmlippen U11-9
Stimmlippenknötchen U11-14
Stimmlosigkeit **U11**-23
Stimmritzenkrampf U11-9
Stimmschwäche U11-9
Stimmstörung U11-23
Stimmung, gereizte U13-10
Stimulanzien U20-23
Stippling U35-6
Stirn U8-2
Stirnfräse U32-6
Stirnlampe U7-9
Stirnspiegel U8-1
stocken (Sprechen) U11-12,20
Stockzahn **U9**-6
Stoffauflage U28-25
Stoffwechsel U12-7
Stoffwechseldefekt U13-6
Stoffwechselprozess U20-5,11
stöhnen U11-4
Stoma **U22**-3
Stomatitis **U35**-16f; U8-8
stopfen (Amalgam) U30-1
Stopfer **U32**-17; U41-15
Stopfgold **U30**-8
Stopfgoldfolie U31-15
Stopp, okklusaler U36-7
stören U16-3
Störgröße U14-18
Störung U13-4
Stoß U3-13f; U17-9; U44-3
–, stumpfer U40-9
Stoß-auf-Stoß-Naht U26-5
Stoßherd U17-9
stottern **U11**-20,12
Strahl richten auf U46-5
Strahl(enbündel) **U46**-5,2
Strahlenbelastung **U46**-7
strahlendicht **U46**-11
Strahlendosis **U46**-9
strahlendurchlässig U33-7; U46-11
strahlenempfindlich **U46**-23
Strahlenexposition **U46**-7
Strahlenfokussierung **U46**-6
Strahlenhärtung U46-5
Strahlenhygiene U46-7
Strahlenkater U46-2
Strahlennekrose U13-30

strahlenresistent U46-23
Strahlenschädigung U46-7
Strahlenschutz U46-2
Strahlenschutzkleidung U46-1
Strahlenschutzplakette U33-2
Strahlensensibilität U46-23
Strahlensensitizer U46-23
Strahlentrennraster U46-5
Strahlenüberdosis U46-7
strahlenundurchlässig **U46**-11
Strahlung **U46**-2
–, ionisierende U46-20
–, ultrakurze U46-20
Strahlungsdetektor U46-7
Strahlungsenergie U46-4
Strahlungsschwächung U46-3
Strategie, abwartende U18-7
Streckung U29-3
Streckverband U29-3
Streifen U32-24
Streudiagramm U14-27
Streupuder U5-9
Streustrahlenraster U46-5
Streustrahlung U46-2
Stridor U11-23
Striktur **U13**-19
Strom, elektrischer U22-9
Struktur **U39**-17
Strukturprotein U12-9
Struma U13-16
Studie, klinische **U15**-1f
Studienabbruch **U15**-29
Studienabbruchbedingung U15-30
Studienabbruchbestimmung U15-30
Studienanleitung U15-7
Studienbegleitkommission **U15**-25
Studiendesign U15-7
Studienprotokoll **U15**-7
Studienteilnehmer U15-4
Stufe U40-8; U41-14
Stufenbildung **U41**-14
Stuhl(gang) U12-6; U16-15; U25-6
Stuhlassistenz U7-1
Stuhlentleerung U20-13
stumm U4-11
Stumpf U26-5; U49-5
– (Fraktur) U28-2
stumpf (Spitze) U24-4
– (Verletzung) U17-3
– (Winkel) U40-19
Stumpfaufbau **U40**-15
Stumpffuge U40-9
Stumpflack U31-5
Stumpfmodell **U31**-5
stumpfstoßen **U40**-9
Stupor **U4**-11; U47-6
stuporös U4-11

Stützanker U42-10
Stützapparat U29-9
stützen U23-10; U28-26; U29-7
Stützklebeband U28-21
Stützkorsett U28-26; U29-7
Stützpfeiler **U42**-10
Stützstrumpf U29-10
Subarachnoidalraum U48-7
Subklaviapunktion U22-18
Sublingualbügel U42-24
Subluxation **U17**-4; U38-8
Substanz, antineoplastische **U20**-31
–, psychotrope **U20**-23
–, schädliche U20-12
Substrat U20-32
Subtraktionsradiographie, digitale **U33**-16
Suchtgift **U5**-3
süchtig U5-3
Sulcus gingivalis **U35**-4
Sulkus-Blutungs-Index **U35**-8
Sulkusepithel **U35**-4
Sulkusfklüssigkeit **U35**-4
Sulkusflüssigkeits-Fließrate U35-4
Sulkusformer **U35**-4
Sulkusvertiefung U44-6
Superhartgips U30-14
Suppositorium **U5**-12; U20-12
Suppuration U28-14
Suprakonstruktion **U43**-15; U42-2
Surveillance **U18**-7; U14-3; U15-7
Suspension U5-8; U29-3; U49-7
Suspensionsdraht U29-3; U49-7
Suspensionsschlinge U49-7
süßen **U2**-16
Süßigkeiten **U2**-17
Süßstoff U12-6
Sutura **U26**-1
Sympathikusblockade U48-6
Sympatholytika U20-27
Sympathomimetika **U20**-27
Synalgie U16-10
Synapse, neuromuskuläre U48-17
Syndrom, postkommotionelles U3-14
Synergismus U20-6
Synergist U20-6
Synkope U4-4
Synotransplantat **U50**-4
Synovialis U38-15
Synovialitis U38-15
synthetisch **U26**-10
systemisch U19-5
Szintigramm U46-17
Szintigraphie **U46**-18,22
Szintillation U46-17
Szintillationsdetektor U46-17
Szintiscanner U46-18

T

Tabakbeutelnaht **U26**–18
tabellarisch U14–27
Tabelle **U14**–27
Tablette **U5**–7
Tafel **U14**–27
Tafelmethode U14–29
Tagesklinik U21–3
Taille U23–16
Talgzyste U13–24
Tampon U28–24
tamponieren **U28**–24
Tapen U28–21
Tape-Verband **U29**–11; U28–21
Tasche U26–16
Taschenbildung U35–11
Taschenreduktion U34–14
Taschentiefe U35–7
tastbar U13–3
taub (Gefühl) **U47**–3; U16–17
Taubheitsgefühl U13–6; U47–3
Tauchlöten U31–16
technisch durchführbar U21–4
teflonbeschichtet U26–10
Teilchenstrahlung U46–10
Teildosen U19–7
teiljustierbar U31–1
teilnahmslos **U4**–10,12
Teilnahmslosigkeit **U4**–13
Teilprothese U32–10; U42–2
Teilreaktion U18–11
Teilungskerbe U5–7
Teilverrenkung **U17**–4
Telekanthus U45–5
Teleskopbrücke U42–9
Teleskopkrone U40–18; U42–9
Teleskopschraube U42–9
Tempern **U31**–15
Tenalgie U16–21
Tendodynie U16–21
teratogen **U20**–33
Teratogenese U20–33
Termin U6–10
Terminabsage **U6**–12
Test, parameterfreier U14–34
–, toxikologischer U19–13
–, verteilungsunabhängiger U14–12
–, Wilcoxon U14–34
Testgruppe U15–10
Testmedikament **U15**–23,2; U5–3
Testperson **U14**–2
Teststärke, statistische U14–1
Tetanus U38–6
Textilpflaster U28–21
Therapeut U18–4
therapeutisch U18–4; U19–13
Therapie **U18**–1,4
–, physikalische U18–4

Therapieabbrecher U14–4; U15–14
Therapiearm **U15**–12
Therapieblock **U15**–11
Therapieergebnis **U15**–27
Therapiekontrolle U15–7
Therapieplan **U6**–13
therapierefraktär U16–9
Therapiereserve U18–4
therapieresistent **U18**–13
Therapieschema U19–1
Therapietreue U15–20; U18–15
Therapieversagen U18–1; U19–11
Therapieversager U15–21
Therapiewechsel **U15**–14
Therapiezugang, erweiterter
  U15–22
thermisch bedingt U40–21
Thoraxröntgen U21–1; U46–3
Thrombolytika U20–16
Tic(k) U16–12
Tiefbiss U36–12 f
Tiefenanschlag U43–10
Tiefenmarkierung **U43**–10
Tiefenschmerz U16–10
Tiefschlaf, künstlicher U4–14
Tiertransplantat **U50**–5
Timbre U11–8
Tinktur **U5**–10
Titan(ium) **U30**–10
Titanimplantatat U30–10
Titan-Keramikverbund U30–10
Titanoxid U30–10
Titanpfeiler U30–22
Titanschraube U29–16
titrieren U48–10
TMD-Gerät U37–13
Tod U15–27
tödlich U50–20
Toleranzentwicklung U19–12;
  U47–5
Toleranzstadium U47–20
Toleranztest U19–12
tolerierbar, klinisch U35–11
Toluidinblau U33–15
Tomographie **U46**–19
Ton U11–10; U30–5
Tonfall **U11**–10,13
Tonhöhe **U11**–10
Tonsilla lingualis U8–11
– pharygealis U8–12
Tönung U39–15
topisch **U19**–5
Torque **U36**–27
Torque-Zange U32–16
Torsion U3–16
Torsionsfraktur U17–1
Tortendiagramm U14–27
Torus **U44**–16
Totalprolaps U13–22

Totalprothese **U42**–3,2
Tourniquet U47–18
toxisch U19–13
Toxizität U19–13
Tracer U46–1,21 f
Tracheostoma U22–3
tragend U40–5
Träger U31–3
Trägheit U4–12
Tragkraft U43–14
Trainingszustand U3–17
Traktion (Fraktur) **U29**–3
Trance **U4**–15
Tränen U11–3
Tränensäcke U8–3
Tränenträufeln U3–18
Tranquilizer U20–23; U47–10
Transferkappe **U31**–11; **U40**–17
transfixieren U29–4
Transformator U33–1
Transillumination **U46**–17
transkutan U19–3
Translation **U36**–22; U38–5
Transluzenz U39–16
transmukosal (Anbindung) U43–5
transparent U39–16
Transplantat **U49**–14,9, **U50**–1;
  U22–20
–, allogenes **U50**–3
–, autogenes U38–17
–, autologes **U50**–2
–, mehrzeitiges U44–9
–, syngenes **U50**–4,1
–, xenogenes **U50**–5
Transplantatabstoßung U50–21
Transplantatannahme U50–1,21
Transplantatbeschaffung U44–9
Transplantatbett U50–1
Transplantatempfänger U14–24;
  U49–14; U50–3
Transplantatentnahme U49–12
Transplantat-gegen-Wirt
  Reaktion **U50**–20
Transplantatlebensdauer U14–25
Transplantatversagen U49–14
Transplantatzerstörung U50–1
transplantieren **U49**–14, **U50**–1
transponieren U49–11
Transposition U36–22
– (Lippenrot) U44–7
Transpositionslappen U49–13;
  U50–14
Transsudat U28–13
transversal (Kreuzbiss) U36–15
Trapezlappen U50–17
Traubenzucker **U12**–7
Trauma **U3**–2,4
–, okklusales **U35**–19
Traumapatient U3–4

traumatisiert U50–7
Tray U7–11; U24–1
Treacher-Collins-Syndrom U45–6
trennen U21–14
Trennmembran U35–28
Trennscheibe U32–5,8
Trepanation **U45**–20
Trepanbohrer U32–6; U41–22
Trepanfräser U43–10
Trichterbildung, apikale U41–13
trichterförmig U41–10; U49–4
Trifurkation U35–23
Trigeminusneuralgie U16–21
Triggerpunkt U48–5
Trinkwasserfluoridierung U34–13
Trismus **U38**–6
Trituration U31–14
Trokar **U24**–7
Trokardorn U24–7
Trokarhülse U24–7
Trommelfell U8–15
Trommelfellruptur U3–18
Tropfen **U5**–11
Tropfflasche U5–5
trüb (Sekret) U3–3
Trübungsstadium U39–16
Trümmerfraktur **U17**–7,3; U38–19
T-Scan **U33**–8
t-Test U14–34
Tuberculum mentale U8–6
Tubocurare **U48**–17
Tubus U47–17
Tuchklemme U24–13; U26–13
Tumeszenz U3–15
Tumor **U3**–5; U13–3,16
tunneliert (Furkation) U35–23
Tunnelmethode, subperiostale **U44**–13
Tüpfelung (Zahnfleisch) U9–12; U35–6
Tupfer **U24**–18; **U28**–23,11
–, chirurgischer U23–8,19
Tupferträger U24–18
Tupferzange U24–14,18
Tupfpräparat U24–18
Turmschädel U45–4
Turnusarzt U23–5

U

Übelkeit U20–12
übelriechend U34–20
Überanstrengung U3–17
Überbelastung **U3**–17; U42–16; U43–16
Überbiss **U36**–13
Überbissreduktion U37–24
überdecken U39–2

überdehnen **U3**–16f
überdenken U21–2
überdimensioniert U36–16
Überdosierung U19–13
Überdosis U19–7
Übereinstimmung U33–8
Überempfindlichkeit U13–10; U47–4
Überernährung U12–1
überessen, sich U1–1
Überfüllung U41–21
Übergang U43–13
Übergangsgebiss U10–1
Überhang U14–8
Überkappung (Pulpa) U40–6,18
überkonturiert U39–2,8
Überkronung U40–18
Überlagerung U36–16
Überlastung U42–16
Überlebensrate U14–25
Überlebensstatistik U14–1
Überlebensvorteil U14–25
Überlebenswahrscheinlichkeit, kumulative U14–31
Überlebenszeit **U14**–25
– (Transplantat) **U50**–21
Überlebenszeitanalyse **U14**–26,25; U15–28
überprüfen U15–17; U23–6; U32–25
Überprüfung U41–2
Überreizung U13–10
überschüssig U40–12
übertragen (Gewebe) **U49**–13; U45–23
Übertragung (Gewebe) U49–13
Übertragungsinfektion U27–9
Übertragungskappe **U31**–11,2
überwachen U23–6; U25–8
Überwachung **U25**–8; U18–7,14
–, anästhesiologische U47–2
–, intraoperative U21–2
Überwachungsgerät U25–8
Überweisung **U6**–11; U21–5
Überweisungsschein U6–11
überziehen U49–9
Überzug U5–6
Uhrzeigersinn U36–27
UK-Kollumfraktur U45–1
Ulcus **U13**–17
–, granulierendes U28–7
Ulkusabheilung U28–4
Ulkuskrater U13–17
ultrakurz (Strahlung) U46–20
Ultraschalldiagnostik **U33**–11
ulzerierend U13–17
Umbau (Knochen) U33–16
umformen U49–4
umhergehen **U25**–13

Umklappeffekt U46–13
Umlagerung U23–11
Umriss U33–12; U39–2; U46–12
umrühren U5–9
Umschlag **U28**–25,20,13; U29–8
–, feuchtwarmer U20–30
Umschlagfalte (Schleimhaut) U8–10
umschneiden (Präparation) U21–9
umschrieben (Läsion) U13–3
umspritzen (Nerv) U48–6
Umstechungsligatur U21–14; U26–3
umwandeln U1–6; U20–4
unangenehm U16–1,3
unansehnlich U3–11
unauffällig (Befund) U25–9; U46–3
unbeaufsichtigt U23–18
unbequem U16–1
unbeweglich U29–5
unbewusst U4–1
undeutlich (Sprache) U11–15
undicht U26–11; U47–15
Undurchlässigkeit (Strahlen) U46–11
unempfindlich **U47**–3; **U48**–4; U30–24
unerträglich U3–2; U16–2,9
unerwünscht U13–9; U18–12; U19–14
Unfalltod U3–4
Ungenauigkeit U31–6
ungenießbar **U1**–5
ungetrübt U4–1
ungezahnt U24–4
ungiftig U19–13
Unguentum **U5**–8
unheilbar U18–2
univariat U14–5; U14–33
Universalspender U49–15
unkorreliert U14–32
unlöslich U12–11
Unpässlichkeit **U16**–1
Unruhe U25–4
–, psychomotorische U4–12; U47–9f
unschön (Narbe) U28–10; U35–22
unter sich gehend U42–6
Unterarm U27–6
unterbelichtet (Film) U33–2
Unterbewertung U33–19
Unterbewusstsein U4–1
unterbinden **U26**–3
Unterernährung U1–3; U12–1
Unterfüllung **U40**–4,3; U41–21
unterfüttern U42–17
Unterfütterung, direkte **U42**–25
Unterfütterungsgerät U42–25
Unterfütterungslappen **U50**–18

Unterkiefer U8–6f; U38–7
Unterkieferast U38–10; U45–12
Unterkieferasymmetrie U3–16
Unterkieferdeviation **U38**–10
Unterkieferfraktur U45–1
Unterkiefermitte U38–8
Unterkieferosteotomie **U45**–12
Unterkieferrand U8–7
Unterkieferverrenkung **U38**–8
Unterkieferwulst **U44**–16
Unterlagen U15–15
Unterscheidungsparameter U14–5
unterschiedlich U14–14
Unterschnitt **U40**–13,4
unterspülbar U42–5
unterstützen U18–8,14
Untersucher U15–2
Untersuchung, diagnostische **U21**–11; U25–1
–, wissenschaftliche **U15**–1f; U14–16; U33–9
Untersuchungsobjekt **U14**–2
Unterton U11–10
unversehrt U3–3
unverständlich (Sprache) U11–17
Unverträglichkeit U19–12; U50–20
unverzerrt U14–18
unwahrscheinlich U14–31
unwirksam U15–8,26
unwohl fühlen, sich U16–1
unzerkaut (schlucken) U5–7; U19–3
unzugänglich (OP) U21–6
unzusammenhängend (Sprache) U11–1,17
unzuverlässig U14–30
Ursache (Krankheit) U13–8
Urteilsvermögen U4–12
usuriert U10–21
U-Test, Mann und Whitney U14–34
Uvula U9–10

V

Vakuumlöten U31–16
Validität U14–30
vaporisieren **U22**–15,5
Variabilität U14–14
Variable **U14**–5
Variante U14–14
Varianz **U14**–14
–, Inter-Beobachter- U14–14
–, Intra-Beobachter- U14–14
Varianzanalyse U14–14
Variation U14–14
Variationskoeffizient U14–14
Vaselin U20–30
Vasodilatanzien **U20**–17

Vasodilatation U20–17
Vasokonstriktion U20–17
Vasokonstringenzien U20–17
Vasopressin U20–21
vegetarisch **U1**–16
velopharyngeal U11–22; U45–3
Velum palatinum U9–10
Vena cava-Ligatur U26–3
Venae Sectio U3–6
Veneer **U39**–22
Venenkatheter, zentraler U22–19; U24–6
Venenpunktion U22–18
Venenschnitt **U22**–18; U3–6
verabreichen U19–3; U23–3
–, intranasal U48–5
Verabreichung **U19**–3,1; U5–1; U8–8; U18–6
Verabreichung (Testmedikament) **U15**–23
veränderlich U14–5
verankern, enossal U42–20; U45–23
Verankerung (Implantat) U45–21f
– (Prothese) **U42**–20,4,10; U40–14,17; U43–1
Verätzung U3–11
verbacken U31–18
Verband **U28**–17,3,20; U3–1
Verbandmull **U28**–18,23; U5–8; U24–18
Verbandraum U28–17
verbinden (Wunde) **U28**–17,1,20; U49–5
Verbinder **U42**–24
Verbindung U48–5; U14–32; U40–8; U49–6
–, chemische U39–20
–, künstliche U22–3
Verbindungselement **U42**–24,6
Verbindungssteg U43–5
Verbindungsstück U42–8
verblassen U13–27
verbleibend U41–23
Verblendkrone U40–18
Verblendmaterial U39–22
Verblendschale **U39**–22; U40–19
Verblendtechnik U39–22
Verblendung U39–2,22
verblinden U15–9
verblockt (Einheit) U42–22
verblüfft U4–8
Verbreitung (Keime) U27–8
verbrennen (Kalorien) U12–4
Verbrennung (Wunde) **U3**–11; U28–9; U50–5
Verbrennungsschorf U28–9
Verbrühung U3–11
Verbund **U39**–20

Verbundfestigkeit U39–20
verdampfen (Gewebe) **U22**–15,5
Verdauung U1–1
Verdauungstrakt U12–3
verdichten U32–17; U41–15
Verdichtung **U13**–14
Verdichtungsareale U13–14
verdickt U35–6
verdrahten U29–14
verdrehen U3–16
Verdünnungsmittel U5–9
Verdunstung U22–15
Vereinbarung, nur nach U6–10
vereisen U48–3
verengt U24–17
Verengung **U13**–19f
Vererbung U13–7
–, autosomal U13–7
Verfahren **U21**–4; U15–1; U45–18
Verfallsdatum U5–19
verfälschen (Ergebnis) U15–9
Verfärbung **U43**–18; U9–12; U34–11; U39–19
Verfestigung **U13**–14
verformbar U29–14
Verformung, elastische U37–10
Verfügbarkeit, biologische **U19**–10
Vergiftung U1–1
Vergiftungsnotfall U5–15
vergoldet U30–8
– (Metalldraht) U29–14
Vergoldungsbad U30–8
Vergrößerung **U13**–15; **U49**–19,2; U22–6
Vergrößerungsspiegel U32–4
Vergüten **U31**–15
Vergütungsofen U31–15
Verhalten, destruktives U3–18
Verhältnis U14–8
Verhärtung **U13**–13
verheilen **U28**–4; U18–2
verhungern **U1**–14
Verifizierung U15–17
Verjüngung U30–20
Verkalkung U10–22
verkeilen **U32**–22
Verklebung **U25**–10; U29–11
Verkleinerung U49–19
verknoten **U26**–6,4,16
verknüpfen **U26**–6
verkümmern U13–29
Verlagerung U23–13; U36–21; U38–5; U40–7
–, seitliche U36–21
Verlangen (Nahrung) U1–11
Verlängerung U29–3
Verlauf U13–5; U25–7
–, bogenförmiger **U39**–14
–, komplikationsfreier U25–7

Verlauf, postoperativer **U25**–7; U21–2
–, wellenförmiger **U39**–14
Verlaufskontrolle **U25**–15; U15–28; U18–14
Verlaufsuntersuchung U15–1
verlegen (Station) U23–17
Verlegung **U13**–18
verletzen **U3**–1,3
Verletzung **U3**–1 ff; U13–3; U16–1
–, stumpfe U17–3
verlieren (Zähne) **U10**–5
vermindern U20–18
vermischen U19–1
vernachlässigen U34–5
vernähen U24–5; U50–15
vernarben **U28**–10
vernebeln U47–1
Vernebler U47–14
Vernichtungsstrahlung U46–2
Verödung U13–18
verordnen **U19**–1; U18–15
verpacken **U5**–16
Verpackung U5–13,16
verpflanzen **U49**–13; **U50**–1
verreiben U31–14
Verrenkung **U3**–20, **U17**–4
Verriegelungsnagel U29–16
Verschattung, radiologische U13–14; U39–15; U46–11
Verschiebelappen **U50**–14; U44–5
verschieben U36–22
Verschiebung U3–20; U14–13; U17–4; U36–16; U38–5
verschlechtert U3–17
Verschlechterung U6–10; U13–2 U14–26
Verschleiß U3–18
Verschleißfestigkeit U30–3; U40–7
verschließen **U26**–11; U5–13
verschlingen U1–4
verschlucken (Fremdkörper) U1–1; U32–1
Verschluss **U26**–11; U13–18
–, luftdichter U34–16
–, undichter apikaler **U41**–16
Verschlussmechanismus U42–11
Verschmelzung U45–2; U30–4
verschmolzen (Wurzel) U9–8
Verschmutzung U27–9
verschnaufen U34–20
verschorfen **U28**–9; U22–9
verschrauben U29–16; U42–7
verschreiben **U19**–1
verschweißt U30–8
verschwollen U3–15
versehentlich U3–6
Versenkbohrer U32–6
versenken U43–11; U44–3

Verseuchung, radioaktive U27–9
Versicherung U3–1
Versiegelung **U26**–11; U30–6; U34–16; U40–3
Versiegelungslack **U34**–16
Versiegler **U34**–16; U26–11
Versorgung U18–1; U49–2
verspannt U8–13
verspritzen U39–21
Verstand, bei klarem U4–3
verständigen, sich U11–8
verständlich U11–1
verstärken U20–24; U26–15; U35–19; U48–11; U50–19
Verstärker U45–23
Verstärkungsnaht U49–8
Verstimmung U13–2
verstopfen U13–18; U11–6
Verstopfung U1–1; U20–13
Versuch U14–16
Versuchsserie U15–6
Versuchsteilnehmer U15–4
Vertebra U29–13
verteilen (Salbe) U5–8
Verteilung U14–13; U20–1
Verteilungskoeffizient U14–12
Vertikaldimension U36–3
vertragen (Medikament) **U19**–12
Verträglichkeit U19–12
Vertrauensbereich **U14**–17
Vertreter, gesetzlicher U25–3
verunreinigt U27–1 f; U28–12
Verunreinigung **U27**–9; U12–17; U31–15
verursachen (Verletzung) U28–16
verursacht, durch Arzt **U13**–9
Verwachsung **U25**–10; U38–12,15
Verwandtentransplantat U50–3
Verwirrtheit U4–8 f; U47–9; U48–4
Verwischung (Röntgenbild) U33–5
verwunden **U3**–1,3
Verwundung **U3**–3
Verzahnung **U36**–7
verzerrt (Gesicht) U3–16
– (Röntgen) U46–13
Verzerrung **U14**–18; U3–16; U15–9
Verzichterklärung U25–3
–, aufgeklärte U25–3
Verzögerer **U30**–23
verzögern U5–6; U20–7; U39–9; U48–4
Verzögerung U15–21
vestibulär U8–10
Vestibulum oris **U8**–10
Vestibulumplastik **U44**–7; U8–10
Vial **U5**–13
Videosubtraktion U33–16

Vierkrallen-Fasspinzette U24–14
Vigilanz **U4**–1 f
Virostatikum U20–9
virulent U27–11
Visier U27–18
Visier-Osteotomie **U45**–11,7
viskös U48–5
Vitalamputation U41–19
Vitalexstirpation **U41**–19
Vitalfunktionen U25–8
Vitalindikation U18–10
Vitalitätsprüfung U9–18; U32–20
Vitamin **U12**–13
Vitamin C **U12**–15
Vitaminanreicherung U12–13
Vitaminmangel U12–13; U20–25
Vogelgesicht U8–2
Vogelschnabelzange U32–16
Vokal U11–9,12
Vokalisation U11–8
volatil U48–4
Vollhautlappen U50–6
volljustierbar U31–1
Vollkeramikkrone U40–18
Vollnarkose **U48**–1
Vollprothese U9–9; U42–2
Vollwertprodukte U1–12
Volumen U40–4
voluminös U12–16
Vorbehandlung U18–5,1
Vorbelastung U43–14
Vorbereitungsraum U23–3
vorbeugend **U18**–6; U5–18; U34–2
Vorbohrer **U43**–8
Vorderzähne **U9**–2
voreingenommen U14–18
Vorfall **U13**–22; U14–19
vorgefertigt U30–7; U40–17
vorgeformt U49–4
Vorhersage **U14**–29
Vorhersagewert U14–29
vorhersehen U14–29
Vorhof (Mund) **U8**–10
Vorkehrungen U24–5
Vorkippung **U36**–23
Vorkontakte U36–9
Vormerksystem U6–15
voroperiert U21–1
Vorrichtung U24–1; U31–1; U32–1
vorschlagen U11–8
vorschriftsmäßig U19–1
Vorschub U46–19
Vorschubbewegung U38–5
Vorschubfeder U37–11
Vorsicht U5–18
Vorsichtsmaßnahme **U5**–18; U26–8; U23–9
Vorsorgeuntersuchung **U6**–15

vorspringen U8-6; U39-3
Vorsprung U40-7; U41-14
vorstülpen (Lippen) U8-6
Vorverlagerung U45-7
vorzeitig U37-12; U45-4

W

wach **U4**-2
Wachheit U4-1f
Wachheitsgrad U4-2
Wachkoma **U4**-17
Wachsaufstellung **U42**-13; U30-17
Wachsbiss U30-17
Wachseinprobe U30-17; U42-14f
wächsern U47-3
Wachsformling U30-17
wachsmodelliert U30-17
Wachsplatten U30-17
Wachsrückstand U30-17
Wachstum U20-9
-, progenes U37-20
-, rotierendes U36-27
Wachstumsschmerzen U16-5
Wachstumssteuerung U37-13
Wahleingriff U21-3,5
wahrnehmen, bewusst U48-4; U23-3
Wahrnehmung U4-1; U16-6
Wahrnehmungsvermögen U47-3
Wahrscheinlichkeit **U14**-31,1
Wahrscheinlichkeitsverteilung U14-12,31
Wanderlappen **U50**-16
wandern (Zahn) U36-21
Wange **U8**-5
Wangenabhalter **U32**-2; U24-16
Wangenbeißen U8-5
Wangenfettlappen U44-5; U35-16
Wangenschleimhaut U8-5
Warenzeichen U19-2
Wärmeausdehnung U31-6
wärmeerzeugend U12-4
warnen **U4**-2; U5-18
Wartezimmer **U6**-7
wasserabweisend U28-21
wasserdicht U26-11
wassergekühlt (Bohrer) U32-6
wasserlöslich U20-10
Wasserspritze **U7**-5
Wasserstoffionen U33-12
wässrig (Sekret) U28-13
Wattebausch **U28**-23
Wattepfropf U8-15
Watteträger U24-14
Wechselklinge U24-3
Wechselwirkung **U19**-11; U15-21
wecken U4-2

wegschneiden U3-6
wegspülen U7-8; U34-6
wegwerfen U27-4
wegwischen U5-10
weh **U16**-4
Wehwehchen **U16**-4f
Weiberknoten U26-6
Weichgewebemodell U31-2
Weichgewebeverlagerung U44-9
Weichlot **U31**-16
Weichteilauflösung U46-14
Weichteile **U33**-12
Weichteiltaschenbildung U35-11
Weichteilverletzung U3-2
Weichteilzerreißung U17-5
weinen U11-3
Weisheitszahn **U9**-8
weitmaschig U28-18
wellenförmig **U39**-14
Wendelappen U50-19
Werkzeug U24-1
Wert (stat.) **U15**-15; U14-6,16
-, kalorischer U12-4
Wertepaar U14-32
Wickel, feuchter **U28**-24,20
Wiederanheftung (Zahnfleisch) **U35**-27; U34-14
Wiederaufnahme, tägl. Aktivitäten **U25**-14
Wiederauftreten U45-9
wiederbeleben **U47**-25
Wiederbestellung U6-15
Wiederherstellung **U49**-1f; U35-26
-, Achsenausrichtung U29-2
-, kraniofaziale U45-21
Wiederherstellungschirurgie **U49**-3
Wiedervereinigung **U28**-2; **U49**-5
wiederverwendbar U27-4
Wilcoxon (Rangsummen)test U14-34
wildes Fleisch U28-7
wimmern U11-3
Wimpern U8-3
Winkelstück U32-5
winzig U22-5
Wirbelknochen U29-13
Wirkort U19-4; U20-3
Wirkprofil, pharmakodynamisches U19-8
Wirksamkeit **U15**-26; **U19**-9,8
Wirkstoff **U20**-2; U5-3
Wirkstofffreisetzung U19-4
Wirkung **U19**-8; U5-19; U15-26
-, biologische **U20**-3
-, koronardilatatorische U20-17
-, toxische U19-13
Wirkungsbereich, toxischer **U19**-13
Wirkungseintritt U19-8; U47-2

Wirkungsmaximum U19-7
Wirkungsmechanismus U19-8
Wirkungsspektrum U19-8
Wirkungsstärke **U19**-9,4
Wirkungsverlängerung U20-3
Wirkungsverzögerung **U15**-21
Wirkungsweise U5-17
Wissenschafter U15-2
wissenschaftlich U47-3
wohlschmeckend U1-5
Wölbung U39-8; U42-19
Wolframkarbid **U30**-11
Wort **U11**-11
wortkarg U11-12,18
Wucherung U20-31; U35-22; U44-16
Wulstnarbe U28-10
wund U13-17; U16-11
Wundabdeckung U49-9
Wundanfrischung U28-12
Wundauflage **U28**-17,3; U3-3; U24-14
Wundbehandlung **U28**-1
Wundbett U28-11; U50-8
Wunddehiszenz **U28**-16; U17-5
Wunde **U3**-3f; **U28**-11
-, klaffende U3-3; U28-16
-, offene U17-3
-, tiefe U28-1
Wundexzision U28-12
Wundhaken **U24**-16
Wundheilung **U28**-5
Wundhöhle U28-3
Wundkontrolle U18-7
Wundliegen U28-19
Wundnaht **U28**-3
Wundrand U28-2; U8-9; U26-17
Wundrandausschneidung **U28**-12
Wundränder U3-3; U24-16; U26-5; U28-17
Wundrandexzision **U28**-12
wundreiben U3-8
Wundsekret U3-3; U28-11,23
Wundspreizer **U24**-16
Wundspülung **U28**-11
Wundtoilette U28-12
Wundverband, antiseptischer U27-1
Wundverschluss **U28**-3; U26-1,4
Wundversorgung **U28**-1,5; U3-3
-, chirurgische U28-1
Würg(e)reflex U10-16; U32-3; U47-17
würgen **U10**-16
Wurzel(ab)deckung **U35**-12
Wurzel(kanal)behandlung **U41**-9,1,18f
Wurzel(kanal)füllung **U41**-15, 6,9,21; U9-19

Wurzel(kanal)füllung, orthograde U41 – 20
Wurzel, freiliegende U35 – 12
Wurzelamputation U41 – 23
Wurzeldentin U9 – 16
Wurzeldenudation U35 – 12
Wurzelfraktur U41 – 18
Wurzelfreilegung U35 – 12
Wurzelfüllung, retrograde U41 – 20; U44 – 4
Wurzelglättung U34 – 14; U24 – 10; U35 – 23
Wurzelhaut U9 – 13
Wurzelheber U32 – 15
Wurzelkanal U41 – 4
Wurzelkanalaufbereitung U41 – 11,9
Wurzelkanalerweiterer U32 – 11
Wurzelkanalfeile U32 – 12
Wurzelkanalinstrument U41 – 1
Wurzelkanalspülung U41 – 9
Wurzelkanalstift U30 – 12
Wurzelkanalstopfer U32 – 17; U41 – 15
Wurzelkanalzugang U41 – 10
Wurzelkronenabstand U39 – 12
Wurzelperforation, apikale U41 – 17
Wurzelresorption U10 – 20
Wurzelspitze U41 – 6,1; U9 – 19; U33 – 7
Wurzelspitzenfensterung U44 – 14
Wurzelspitzenresektion U41 – 20
Wurzelstift U29 – 15; U40 – 14 f
Wurzelzement U9 – 17
Wurzel-zu-Krone Quotient U43 – 16
würzen U2 – 18

X

x² Test U14 – 34
Xenotransplantat U50 – 5
Xeroradiographie U33 – 17

Z

Zahn U9 – 1
–, devitaler U41 – 3
–, gelockerter U37 – 16
–, impaktierter U44 – 3
–, luxierter U17 – 5
–, marktoter U41 – 3
–, mehrwurzeliger U9 – 19; U41 – 3
–, retinierter U44 – 3
–, unversehrter U30 – 1
–, vitaler U41 – 3
Zahnachsenneigung U36 – 23
Zahnäquator, anatomischer U39 – 8; U40 – 13

Zahnarzt U6 – 1; U44 – 1
Zahnarztassistentin U6 – 4
Zahnarztelement U7 – 2
Zahnarztpraxis U6 – 2; U31 – 14
Zahnaufhellung U39 – 19
Zahnband U34 – 5
Zahnbein U9 – 16
Zahnbelag U34 – 8
Zahnbeweglichkeit U9 – 1
Zahnbewegung, kfo. U36 – 22,1
Zahnbogen U9 – 9; U37 – 13
Zahnbogenbreite U9 – 9; U10 – 3
Zahnbogenform U36 – 4; U39 – 15
Zahnbogenkorrektur, kfo. U36 – 1
Zahnbogenlänge U36 – 4; U37 – 22
Zahnbogenverkürzung U36 – 4
Zahnbohrer U32 – 6
Zahnbreitendiskrepanz U36 – 18
Zahnbürste U34 – 4
Zahnbürstentrauma U34 – 4
Zahndurchbruch U10 – 1ff
Zähne (Wundhaken) U24 – 16
–, bleibende U10 – 6; U36 – 6
Zähneknirschen U10 – 18; U38 – 3
Zahnen U10 – 4
Zahnengstand U36 – 16,6
Zahnentfernung U10 – 7
Zähnepressen U8 – 7
Zahnerhaltung U6 – 1; U40 – 1
Zahnersatz U42 – 2; U10 – 1; U32 – 7
–, ästhetischer U39 – 1
–, implantatgestützter U6 – 13
Zahnextraktion U44 – 2
Zahnfach U9 – 13; U32 – 14
Zahnfarbe U39 – 15
zahnfarben U40 – 1
Zahnfäule U34 – 18
Zahnfehlstellung U9 – 1; U36 – 8
Zahnfleisch U9 – 12; U34 – 14
–, künstliches U42 – 19
–, Wiederanheftung U35 – 27
Zahnfleischabtragung U35 – 25
Zahnfleischbeweglichkeit U35 – 6
Zahnfleischbluten U35 – 3
Zahnfleischentzündung U35 – 13
Zahnfleischerkrankung U41 – 8
Zahnfleischfestigkeit U35 – 6
Zahnfleischfurche U35 – 4
Zahnfleischhyperplasie U35 – 3
Zahnfleischklammer U42 – 6
Zahnfleischlächeln U39 – 6
Zahnfleischlappen U44 – 5
Zahnfleischmaske U35 – 3
Zahnfleischmesser U24 – 3
Zahnfleischpapille U35 – 5
Zahnfleischplastik U35 – 26
Zahnfleischrand U35 – 3; U39 – 7; U9 – 12
Zahnfleischrückbildung U35 – 10

Zahnfleischsattel U35 – 18
Zahnfleischschwund U35 – 10
Zahnfleischtasche U35 – 11,24
Zahnfleischtaschenreduktion U34 – 14; U35 – 24
Zahnfleischtüpfelung U35 – 6; U39 – 7
Zahnfleischuntersuchung U35 – 6
Zahnfleischverlauf U39 – 7
Zahnfraktur U17 – 1
zahngestützt U42 – 12
Zahnhals U9 – 19; U42 – 19
Zahnhalskaries U34 – 17
Zahnhalsline U39 – 9
Zahnhalteapparat U35 – 1,5
Zahnhartsubstanz U34 – 18
Zahnheilkunde U6 – 1
–, ästhetische U39 – 1
–, konservierende U40 – 1
Zahnhöcker U9 – 4
Zahnhöhle U9 – 18
Zahnimplantat U43 – 2
Zahnintrusion U44 – 2
Zahnkaries U34 – 17f
Zahnkeimzyste U44 – 15
Zahnkrone U9 – 14
Zahnlockerung U44 – 2
zahnlos U10 – 7; U8 – 7; U42 – 5; U44 – 6
Zahnlosigkeit (Zahnentfernung) U10 – 7
Zahnlückenstand U36 – 16
Zahnluxation U44 – 2
Zahnoberhäutchen, erworbenes U34 – 10
Zahnpflege U34 – 1
Zahnpflegemittel U34 – 3
Zahnpressen U10 – 17; U38 – 3
Zahnprothese U10 – 8; U42 – 2; U49 – 18
Zahnpulpa U9 – 18
Zahnpulver U34 – 3
Zahnputztechnik U34 – 4
Zahnregulierung U36 – 1
Zahnreihe U9 – 9
Zahnreihen schließen U10 – 13
Zahnreinigungsband U34 – 5
Zahnschiene U42 – 22
Zahnschmelz U9 – 15; U24 – 11
Zahnschmerzen U16 – 4
Zahnschutz U8 – 8; U37 – 25; U42 – 22
Zahnseide U34 – 5
Zahnseidenspender U34 – 5
Zahnsonde U32 – 9
Zahnspange U37 – 1
Zahnspiegel U32 – 4
Zahnstein U34 – 9; U13 – 21; U32 – 13

zahnsteinanfällig U34–9
Zahnsteinentferner **U32**–13; U32–13; U34–9
Zahnsteinentfernung U34–9,14
Zahnsteinhaftung U34–9
zahnsteinhemmend U34–9
Zahnsteinlöser U34–9
Zahnstellung, lückige **U36**–17
Zahnstocher U34–4
Zahntaschentiefe **U35**–7
Zahntechniker **U6**–5
Zahnüberzahl **U36**–19
Zahnunterzahl **U36**–19
Zahnverbindungsschiene **U42**–22
Zahnverfärbung **U34**–11; U39–23
Zahnverlust U10–7
Zahnwanderung **U36**–21
Zahnwechsel U10–5
Zahnwurzel **U9**–19
Zahnzange U32–15
Zange **U24**–14; **U32**–16; U37–5
Zäpfchen **U5**–12; U9–10; U20–12
Zapfenzahn U9–1
Zeichen U18–10
Zeichensprache U11–8
Zeitpunkt der Wahl **U21**–5
Zellgift U20–32
zellschädigend **U20**–32
Zelltod **U13**–30
Zelltoxizität U20–32
Zelltrümmer U13–12; U28–12
Zellwachstum U15–18
Zement **U30**–6; U9–17
Zementfuge U30–6
Zementhaftung U30–6
Zementieren U30–6
Zementstopfer U30–6
Zementverbindung U30–6
Zentralwert U14–10
zentrisch U10–13; U36–2,13
zerbrechen U17–1
Zerfall U5–6
–, radioaktiver U46–22
zerfetzt (Gewebe) U3–7
zergehen lassen (im Mund) U5–7
zerkauen **U10**–15
Zerlegung (Quadratsummen) U14–34
zermahlen **U10**–18
zerreißen (Gewebe) U3–18; U17–5
Zerreißung **U3**–7,18; U17–3
zerren (Muskel) U3–17
Zerrung **U3**–16f
zersplittern (Knochen) U17–2,7
zerstören U3–18; U22–14
Zertrümmerung U17–7
Zeruminalpfropf U5–2; U17–6
zervikal U8–13
Zervix **U8**–13; U26–18

ziehen (Zahn) U44–2
Zielgewebe U19–4; U46–4
Zielgröße **U14**–20
Zielsetzung **U47**–3,2
Ziffer U14–6
Zink U12–17
Zinken U24–16
Zinkoxid-Eugenol-Zement U30–16
Zinkpaste U5–8
Zinn U30–1; U34–13
Zinn-Fluorverbindung **U34**–13
zischen U11–21
Zischlaute U11–21
zittern U4–16; U11–10
Zone, sterile U27–8
Z-Plastik U49–3; U50–14
zubeißen U10–11
zubereiten (Arznei) **U5**–5
zubereitet U1–1
Zubereitung U19–1
Zubereitungsform U5–6
zucken U16–12; U8–3
Zucker **U2**–16; **U12**–6
Zuckerverbindung U12–5
Zufall U14–1
zufällig U15–5
Zufallsgenerator U15–5
Zufallsprinzip U15–12
Zufallsstichprobe U14–4
Zufallszahl U15–5
Zufallszuteilung U15–5
Zufuhr (Nahrungsmittel) U1–1
zuführen U12–15; U19–4
Zug (Fraktur) **U29**–3
– (kfo.) **U36**–28
– (trinken) U1–4
Zugang U22–18; U44–13; U45–20
– erlangen U41–10
–, operativer **U21**–6,2; U41–17
zugänglich U32–2
Zugangsart U21–6
Zugangskavität **U41**–10; U40–2
Zugangsöffnung U30–12
Zugangsweg U21–6; U45–12
Zugbelastung U43–14
Zügel U29–8
zugelassen U20–2
zugeteilt U15–5
Zugfestigkeit U26–7
Zuggurtung U29–14
Zugkraft U36–28
zuheilen U28–4
Zunge **U8**–11
Zungenbändchen U9–11
Zungenbändchenexcision U44–7
Zungenbändchenplastik U44–7
Zungenbeweglichkeit U44–7
Zungenbrennen U9–1
Zungenentzündung U8–11

Zungengitter U37–15
Zungengrund U8–11
Zungenhalter U8–11
Zungenlappen U44–5
Zungenmandel U8–11
Zungenpapille U8–11
Zungenpressen **U36**–20; U37–15
Zungenreinigung U34–4
zungenseitig U8–11
Zungenspatel U8–11; U32–3
Zungenverwachsung U8–11
zurechtschneiden **U49**–4; U32–5
zurückbilden, sich U35–10
zurückführen auf U3–7; U12–17
Zurücklegen (Stichprobenerhebung) U14–4
zurückschneiden U26–13
zurückziehen, sich U4–12; U32–2
zusammenbeißen **U10**–17
Zusammenhang U14–32; U15–2
zusammenhängend reden U11–8
zusammenpressen **U10**–17
Zusammensetzung U5–17; U39–17
zusammenzucken (Schmerz) **U16**–12
Zusatzstift (Guttapercha) U41–15
Zusatztherapie U18–8,4
zuschreiben U20–20
Zustand (Pulpa) **U41**–2; U10–1
–, tranceähnlicher U4–13,15
zustopfen U28–24
Zuteilung U15–4
–, blockweise U15–11
Zuverlässigkeit **U14**–30,23
Zwangsernährung U1–3; U12–3
Zweck **U47**–3
zweiteilen U21–14
Zweiteingriff U21–1
Zweiterkrankung U14–9
zweizeitig (OP) **U50**–7; U21–4
Z-Wert **U14**–6
Zwillingsblock **U37**–14
Zwillingsbrackets U37–4
Zwischenglied **U42**–5
Zwischenmahlzeit **U1**–10; U12–2
Zwischenpfeiler U42–10
Zwischenraumbürstchen U34–4
Zwischenräume U50–9
Zyklus U5–1
Zylinderimplantat U43–6
Zyste **U13**–24
–, follikuläre U44–15
–, radikuläre U44–15
Zystotomie U22–2
Zystozele U13–23
Zytopathologie U13–1
Zytostatika **U20**–31f
Zytotoxin U20–32
Zytotoxizität **U20**–32

Grundsätzliches zur Aussprache

Obwohl in der medizinischen Fachsprache eine Vielzahl von Fachtermini aus dem Lateinischen oder Griechischen hergeleitet sind, ist deren richtige Aussprache selbst für amerikanische Ärzte immer wieder eine Quelle der Unsicherheit. Dies gilt umso mehr für den deutschsprachigen Arzt, denn viele Fachwörter sind zwar vom Schriftbild her vertraute Internationalismen, deren Aussprache im Englischen deckt aber sich nur selten mit jener im Deutschen. Deshalb ist die Aussprache eine wesentliche Voraussetzung für die Verständigung.

Der Benutzer findet die Aussprachehinweise in der weithin bekannten internationalen Lautschrift der International Phonetic Association (IPA). Die verwendeten Symbole, die auf der neuesten IPA-Version beruhen, sind auf der Innenseite der Umschlagklappe übersichtlich mit Beispielwörtern dargestellt. Grundsätzlich wird immer die Aussprache im *Standard American English (AE)* angegeben und durch Hinweise auf Varianten im *British English (BE)* überall dort ergänzt, wo Besonderheiten vorliegen. Als Grundlage für die Aussprache im AE diente vor allem das *Medical Audio Dictionary* (Merriam-Webster, 1997), ergänzt durch Recherchen unserer Mitarbeiter in den USA.

Hinweise zur Aussprache medizinischer Fachwörter		
-itis	[aɪtɪs]	gingiv**itis**, pulp**itis**, gastr**itis**, mening**itis**, sinus**itis**, arthr**itis**, periodont**itis**
h(a)ema-	[hiːmə]	**hema**toma, **hema**temesis, **hema**tocrit, **hema**turia
hemi-	[hemɪ]	**hemi**facial, **hemi**plegia, **hemi**block, **hemi**sphere, **hemi**anopsia, **hemi**zygous
syn-, sym-	[sɪn], [sɪm]	**syn**drome, **syn**desmosis, **syn**chronous, **syn**thetic, **sym**ptom, **sym**physis, **sym**pathetic
dys-	[dɪs]	**dys**function, **dys**plasia, **dys**trophic, **dys**phagia, **dys**crasia, **dys**ostosis
pn-, ps-, pt-	silent [p]	**pn**eumonia, **pn**eumatic, **ps**ychologic, **ps**oas, **pt**osis, **pt**yalin
ch	[k]	a**ch**e, tra**ch**ea, ta**ch**ycardia, splan**ch**nic, te**ch**nique, me**ch**anism, paren**ch**yma
sch	[sk]	i**sch**ial, i**sch**emia, **sch**edule, e**sch**ar, **sch**eme, **sch**ool
-myo-	[maɪoʊ]	**myo**cardial, **myo**metrium, **myo**neural, **myo**tomy, electro**myo**graphy, fibro**myo**ma
-cyto-	[saɪtoʊ]	**cyto**logic, **cyto**metry, **cyto**plasm, **cyto**toxic, **cyto**kine, leuko**cyto**sis, thrombo**cyto**penia
pyo-	[paɪoʊ]	**pyo**genic, **pyo**derma, **pyo**thorax, **pyo**cyst, **pyo**rrhea
micro-	[maɪkroʊ]	**micro**scope, **micro**surgery, **micro**bial, **micro**organism, **micro**flora
bio-	[baɪoʊ]	**bio**logic, **bio**psy, **bio**chemical, **bio**availability, **bio**assay, **bio**materials, **bio**compatible
eu-	[ju]	**eu**phoria, **eu**thyroid, **eu**thanasia, **eu**genic
-i *(lat. pl)*	[aɪ]	alveol**i**, vill**i**, bronch**i**, stimul**i**, calcul**i**, embol**i**, nucle**i**, ram**i**
-ae *(lat. pl)*	[ɪ]	sequel**ae**, vertebr**ae** [ɪ‖eɪ], papill**ae**, fistul**ae**, trabecul**ae**, fasci**ae**, conjunctiv**ae**
-(s)tomy -graphy -scopy*	main stress on vowel before the suffix!	an**a**tomy, lapar**o**tomy; ile**o**stomy; radi**o**graphy, arthr**o**graphy, son**o**graphy; end**o**scopy, bronch**o**scopy, colon**o**scopy

* Neben diesen hier aufgezählten Nachsilben gibt es noch eine Liste von weniger geläufigen, die durchwegs mit dem gleichen Betonungsmuster verbunden sind: **-lysis** (an**a**lysis, di**a**lysis, hem**o**lysis), **-metry/-ter** (cephal**o**metry, therm**o**meter), **-logy/-logist** (radi**o**logy/-gist), **-pathy** (neur**o**pathy), **-schisis** (cheil**o**schisis), **-rrhaphy** (herni**o**rrhaphy).

Unterschiede zwischen AE und BE in der Schreibweise

Standard American English			British English (RP)
f**e**tus, diarrh**e**a, **e**dema, man**e**uver, **e**sophagus, **e**strogen	e	oe	f**oe**tus, diarrh**oe**a, **oe**dema, man**oe**uvre, **oe**sophagus, **oe**strogen,
p**e**diatric, an**e**mia, h**e**morrhage, **e**tiology, c**e**cum, f**e**ces, an**e**sthesia	e	ae	p**ae**diatric, an**ae**mia, h**ae**morrhage, **ae**tiology, c**ae**cum, f**ae**ces, an**ae**sthesia
lit**er**, tit**er**, cent**er**, fib**er**, maneuv**er**, calib**er**, goit**er**	-er	-re	lit**re**, tit**re**, cent**re**, fib**re**, manoeuv**re**, calib**re**, goit**re**
catheter**ize**, paral**yze**, cauter**ize**, anal**yze**	-ize	-ise	catheter**ise**, paral**yse**, cauter**ise**, anal**yse**
hospital**iz**ation, mobil**iz**ation, local**iz**ation	-zation	-sation	hospital**is**ation, mobil**is**ation, local**is**ation
col**or**, lab**or**, behavi**or**, tum**or**, flav**or**, hum**or**	-or	-our	col**our**, lab**our**, behavi**our**, tum**our**, favo**ur**ite, flav**our**, hum**our**
homol**og**, catal**og**, dial**og**, anal**og**	-og	-ogue	homol**ogue**, catal**ogue**, dial**ogue**, anal**ogue**
diagr**am**, radiogr**am**, cystogr**am**, milligr**am**, sonogr**am**, cardiogr**am**	-am	-amme	diagr**amme**, radiogr**amme**, cystogr**amme**, milligr**amme**, sonogr**amme**, cardiogr**amme**
leu**ko**plakia, leu**ko**penia, leu**ko**cyte	leuko-	leuco-	leu**co**plakia, leu**co**penia, leu**co**cyte
*i**m**bed, i**n**quiry, i**n**close	in-/im-	en-/em-	e**m**bed, *e**n**quiry, e**n**close
offen**se**, licen**se**, defen**se**	-se	-ce	offen**ce**, licen**ce**, defen**ce**
counse**l**or, *insta**l**, tranqui**l**izer	-l	-ll	counse**ll**or, insta**ll**, tranqui**ll**iser

* Neben dieser Schreibweise existiert auch die *AE* bzw. *BE* Variante.